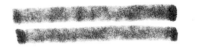

The Physics of Diagnostic Imaging

The Physics of Diagnostic Imaging

Second edition

David J. Dowsett MSc PhD
Consultant Medical Physicist, Dublin, Ireland

Patrick A. Kenny MA MSc PhD
Chief Medical Physicist, Mater Misericordiae University Hospital, Dublin, Ireland
Lecturer, Faculty of Radiology, Trinity College and University College, Dublin, Ireland

and

R. Eugene Johnston MA PhD
Professor Emeritus, University of North Carolina, USA

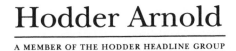
A MEMBER OF THE HODDER HEADLINE GROUP

First published in Great Britain in 1998 by International Thomson Publishing
This second edition published in 2006 by
Hodder Arnold, an imprint of Hodder Education and
a member of the Hodder Headline Group,
338 Euston Road, London NW1 3BH

http://www.hoddereducation.com

Distributed in the United States of America by
Oxford University Press Inc.,
198 Madison Avenue, New York, NY10016
Oxford is a registered trademark of Oxford University Press

© 2006 David J. Dowsett, Patrick A. Kenny and R. Eugene Johnston

All rights reserved. Apart from any use permitted under UK copyright law, this publication may
only be reproduced, stored or transmitted, in any form, or by any means with prior permission
in writing of the publishers or in the case of reprographic production in accordance with
the terms of licences issued by the Copyright Licensing Agency. In the United Kingdom
such licences are issued by the Copyright Licensing Agency: Saffron House, 6-10 Kirby
Street, London EC1N 8TS.

Whilst the advice and information in this book are believed to be true and accurate at the date
of going to press, neither the author[s] nor the publisher can accept any legal responsibility or
liability for any errors or omissions that may be made. In particular (but without limiting the
generality of the preceding disclaimer) every effort has been made to check drug dosages; however
it is still possible that errors have been missed. Furthermore, dosage schedules are constantly
being revised and new side-effects recognized. For these reasons the reader is strongly urged
to consult the drug companies' printed instructions before administering any of the drugs
recommended in this book.

British Library Cataloguing in Publication Data
A catalogue record for this book is available from the British Library

Library of Congress Cataloging-in-Publication Data
A catalog record for this book is available from the Library of Congress

ISBN-10   0 340 80891 8
ISBN-13   978 0 340 80891 7

2 3 4 5 6 7 8 9 10

Commissioning Editor: Joanna Koster
Development Editor: Sarah Burrows
Project Editor: Naomi Wilkinson
Production Controller: Joanna Walker
Cover Designer: Georgina Hewitt

Typeset in 10/12 pts, Minion by Charon Tec Ltd, Chennai, India
www.charontec.com
Printed and bound in the UK by CPI Bath

What do you think about this book? Or any other Hodder Arnold
title? Please visit our website at www.hoddereducation.com

To: 'mole, the bear and miles so far'

CONTENTS

Perhaps the major problem associated with teaching the physics of diagnostic imaging is its changeability. Over the last thirty years radiology has seen dramatic improvements in non-invasive imaging using X-rays, gamma rays, high frequency sound, and high frequency radio waves. Over the last fifteen years the quality of these images has enabled visualization of early pathological changes both in anatomy and function. The last ten years has seen the emphasis change to low radiation dose techniques which demand more efficient imaging methods. To some extent these have been supplied by digital image capture using either position sensitive phosphors (computer radiography) or purely electronic detector techniques enabling direct visualization (direct radiography). With digital systems a truly film-less environment can exist providing easy and rapid transmission of images, patient information and quality control data across countries, continents, and oceans. This complex scenario provides difficulties when trying to understand modern developments, teach students or set examinations. This book introduces current methods, fundamental principles, and applications. The reader is encouraged to explore specialist publications armed with this basic information.

DJD
PAK
REJ
2005

ACKNOWLEDGEMENTS

The authors wish to acknowledge the valuable constructive criticism given by Kwan-Hoong Ng, John Winder, Kimia Khalatbari, Tom O'Flaherty, and Greg Foley. We would also like to thank Penny Gore, Jonathan Swain, Andrew McGregor, Rob Cowan, and Michael Berkeley for their support and continuous presence.

We owe a very special thanks to Ruth Callan for her infinite patience and precision in correcting the manuscript and offering editorial advice. Any remaining errors that may have crept in are the responsibility of the authors.

ABC	automatic brightness control
AC	alternating current
ACE	automatic computing engine
ADC	analog to digital converter (*computing*); apparent diffusion coefficient (*MRI*)
ADSL	asymmetric digital subscriber line
AEC	automatic exposure control
AGC	automatic gain control
AIUM	American Institute of Ultrasound in Medicine
ALARA	as low as reasonably achievable
ALARP	as low as reasonably practical
ALI	annual limit on intake
ANOVA	analysis of variance
AOM	acoustic optical modulation
ARSAC	Administration of Radioactive Substances Advisory Committee (*in UK*)
BGO	bismuth germanate
BSF	back scatter fraction
CAD	coronary artery disease
CAT	computer aided tomography
CBF	cerebral blood flow
CBV	cerebral blood volume
CCD	charge-coupled device
CDD	contrast detail diagram
CF	conversion factor
CFOV	central field of view
c.g.s.	centimeter-gram-second
CIF	conversion improvement factor
CISC	complex instruction set computing
CLL	chronic lymphocytic leukemia
CLV	constant linear velocity
CNR	contrast to noise ratio
COR	center of rotation
CPU	central processing unit (*computing*)
CR	computed radiography
CREW	compression with reversible embedded wavelet
CRT	cathode ray tube
CT	computed tomography
CTDI	computed tomography dose index
CW	continuous wave Doppler
DAC	digital to analog converter
DAP	dose–area product

DC	direct current
DDREF	dose and dose rate effectiveness factor
DF	digital fluorography
DICOM	digital imaging and communication in medicine
DLP	dose–length product
DNA	deoxyribose nucleic acid
DOPA	(*see* L-DOPA)
dps	disintegrations per second
DQE	detective quantum efficiency
DR	direct radiography
DRAM	dynamic random access memory
DREF	dose rate effectiveness factor
DRL	dose reference level; diagnostic reference level (*given by ICRP 73*)
DSA	digital subtraction angiography
DSL	digital subscriber line (*see also, ADSL*)
DTPA	diethylenetriaminepentaacetic acid
DVD	digital versatile disc
EHIDA	diethyl variant of HIDA
EPI	echo planar imaging
ESD	entrance surface dose
FDA	Food and Drug Administration (*in the USA*)
FDDI	fiber optic distributed data interfaces
FFD	focus to film distance
FFT	fast Fourier transform
FID	focus to image distance (*in X-ray techniques*); free induction decay (*in MRI*)
FLASH	fast low angle shot
FOV	field of view
FPF	false positive fraction
FS	focal spot size
FWHM	full width at half maximum
FWTM	full width at tenth maximum
HVL	half-value layer
GFR	glomerular filtration rate
GRE	gradient recalled echo
GSD	genetically significant dose
GSO	gadolinium oxyorthosilicate
GUS	graphical user interface
HIDA	hepatic iminodiacetic acid
HIMSS	Hospital Information and Management Systems Society

HIS	hospital information system		**PACS**	picture archiving and communications system
HMPAO	hexamethylenepropylene amine oxime		**PD**	potential difference (*electricity*); pulse duration (*ultrasound*)
IAEA	International Atomic Energy Agency (*Vienna, Austria*)		**PE**	potential energy
ICMP	internet control message protocol		**PET**	positron emission tomography
ICRP	International Commission on Radiological Protection (*Didcot, UK*)		**PMMA**	polymethylmethacrylate
			PMT	photomultiplier tube
ICRU	International Commission on Radiation Units and Measurements (*Bethesda, USA*)		**PRF**	pulse repetition frequency
			PRP	pulse repetition period
ICU	intensive care unit		**PSL**	photostimulated luminescence
IDE	integrated drive electronics		**QC**	quality control
IHE	integrating the health care enterprise		**RAM**	random access memory
ISD	interscan delay		**RARE**	rapid acquisition relaxation enhancement
ISP	internet service provider		**RBC**	red blood cell
LAN	local area network		**RBE**	relative biological effectiveness
L-DOPA	3-hydroxy-L-tyrosine; a drug used for the treatment of Parkinson's disease		**RF**	radio frequency
			RISC	reduced instruction set computing
LEAP	low energy all purpose (collimator)		**RIS**	radiology information system
LET	linear energy transfer		**RL**	run length encoding
LFD	low frequency drop		**RMS**	root mean square
LOR	line of response		**RNA**	ribose nucleic acid
LSO	lutetium oxyorthosilicate		**ROC**	receiver operating characteristic
LVEF	left ventricular ejection fraction		**ROI**	region of interest
MAA	macro-aggregated albumin		**ROM**	read-only memory
MAG$_3$	mercaptoacetyltriglycine		**RSNA**	Radiological Society of North America
MDP	methylene diphosphonate		**RTS**	real-time sorter
mfp	mean free path		**SA**	spatial average
MGDS	mean glandular dose (*for a standard breast model*)		**SAR**	specific absorption rate
			SCSI	small computer system interface
MGD	mean glandular dose		**SDM**	selective dominant measurement
MIBG	*meta*-iodobenzylguanidine		**SDP**	slice dose profile
MIBI	sestamibi; hexakis-2-methoxy-isobutylisoni-trile		**SDSL**	symmetric digital subscriber line
			SID	source-to-image distance
MIRD	medical internal radiation dose		**SLL**	scan line length
m.k.s.	meter-kilogram-second		**SNR**	signal to noise ratio
MO	magneto-optical		**SP**	spatial peak
MPR	multi-plane reconstruction		**SPECT**	single photon emission computed tomography
MRA	magnetic resonance angiography			
MRI	magnetic resonance imaging		**SPL**	spatial pulse length
MRS	magnetic resonance spectroscopy		**SPR**	specific absorption rate
MSAD	multiple scan average dose		**SQL**	structured query language
MTF	modulation transfer function		**SRAM**	static RAM
MUGA	multiple gated acquisition		**SSP**	slice sensitivity profile
NMR	nuclear magnetic resonance		**STP**	standard temperature and pressure
NRPB	National Radiological Protection Board (*in the UK*)		**SUV**	standardized uptake value
			TA	temporal average
NTP	normal temperature and pressure		**TAP**	time average power
OD	optical density		**TE**	time-to-echo
OFD	object to film distance		**TEDE**	total effective dose equivalent
OID	object to image distance			

TFT	thin film transistor	**UFOV**	useful field of view
TGC	time gain compensation	**UHF**	ultra-high frequency
TIA	transient ischemic attack	**USB**	universal serial bus
TOF	time of flight	**UV**	ultraviolet
TPF	true positive fraction	**VDU**	video display unit
TR	time-to-repeat	**VHF**	very high frequency
UDP	user datagram protocol	**WAN**	wide area network

Basic mathematics for radiology

1.1 EXPRESSIONS

Mathematics plays a very important role in radiology and some knowledge of basic mathematics and formulas is necessary in order to fully appreciate certain applications. As radiology becomes more complex (e.g. radionuclide activity, digital imaging, magnetic resonance, axial tomography) quite simple mathematical procedures often explain complex details more effectively than words or diagrams.

Simple formulas can often be employed which reveal hidden difficulties, such as accuracy of counting radioactive samples or radiation dose measurements or X-ray exposure levels which can suggest corrective measures.

This chapter serves only for reference and identifies those areas of radiology where a knowledge of mathematics can reveal greater understanding.

1.1.1 The Système International d'Unités

The Système International d'Unités (SI units), the international system for units of measurement, is now the generally accepted international form of the metric system. Basic physical constants have standard

Table 1.1 *Basic physical constants (SI and c.g.s.).*

Quantity	SI unit: meter, kilogram, second	c.g.s unit: centimeter, gram, second
Mass	kilogram (kg)	gram (g) (gm)*
Length	meter (m)	centimeter (cm)
Time	second (s)	second (s)
(derived)	minute (min)	
	hour (h)	
	day (d)	
	year (a) (yr)*	

*Non-standard abbreviation.

SI abbreviations which are used throughout this book; these are given in Table 1.1. The year and gram sometimes have non-standard abbreviations and these are also included. The complete set of basic SI units along with their derived units, which are formed by combining base units for measuring physical quantities (e.g. pressure, radiation dose) are given in Chapter 2. Other systems of units are still in common use. The centimeter–gram–second (c.g.s. units) was used prior to the SI units and other units such as the micron (10^{-6} m), angstrom (10^{-10} m) and curie (3.7×10^{10} disintegrations per second) are frequently encountered in radiology. None of them is a recognized SI unit.

Table 1.2 *Common arithmetic symbols.*

Symbol	Function
+	Addition
−	Subtraction
× or *	Multiplication
÷ or /	Division
$\sqrt{x}$ or sqrt (x)	Square root
x^2	Square
$\log_{10} x$ or $\ln x$	Logarithm base 10 or e
$\tan x$	Trigonometry functions
$\sin x$	
$\cos x$	
=	Equals
≠	Does not equal
≈	Approximately equals
≡	Exactly equal to (identical to)
∝	Proportional to
>	Greater than
<	Less than
±	Range of + and − values
Δx	Small change in x
Σ	Sum of samples

Table 1.3 *Prefixes used for constants.*

Prefix	Symbol	Example	Factor
giga-	G	GBq	10^9
mega-	M	MJ, MBq	10^6
kilo-	k	kg, kW	10^3
centi-	c	cm, cGy	10^{-2}
milli-	m	mm, mGy	10^{-3}
micro-	μ	μs, μCi	10^{-6}
nano-	n	nm, ns	10^{-9}

1.2 NOTATION

The common symbols most frequently used in radiology are listed in Table 1.2. The order of priority when calculating a mixed equation is:

1 Bracketed functions, e.g. $(x + y)$
2 Squares and square roots, x^2, $\sqrt{x}$
3 Multiply and divide, × *, ÷ /
4 Addition and subtraction, +, −

Common prefixes which are used to express multiples or fractions of standard quantities are given in Table 1.3. Examples of prefix use would be kilogram (kg), microsecond (μs), millimeter (mm). Less common would be nanometer (nm), used for measuring wavelength and mega-becquerel (MBq), used for radionuclide activity levels.

1.2.1 Conventional notation

INTEGERS

A single whole digit, for example 1, 2, 3, 24, 135, 1 000 000 are all integers. Integers are used when only whole numbers make sense, such as sample numbers, radioactive counts or object numbers (e.g. patients, films).

FRACTIONS

Figures that are not whole numbers, e.g. 3.1416, are fractions. If the value has a fixed number of decimal places. e.g. 2.5, it is a **rational number**. If the fraction represents values such as π, e, $\sqrt{2}$ or ⅓ then the decimal places are infinite and it is an **irrational number**; for example, π is 3.14159…, e is 2.71828….

PRECISION

The precision or accuracy of a fraction is dependent on the number of **significant figures**. A value 1.23456 of six significant figures is accurate to five **decimal places**. Alternatively, a value such as π can be rounded off to four decimal places, so 3.14159 becomes 3.1416. The **least significant** figure is 9.

ROUNDING OFF

Rounding off is applied to calculations when extreme accuracy is not important. The value for π at 3.14159 is correct to six significant figures but in certain circumstances four significant figures are sufficient. Greater precision is required when measuring values with small differences in order to show a distinction, i.e. linear attenuation coefficients at high kilovoltages.

1.2.2 Scientific notation

This is used for describing very large and very small numbers in mathematical operations without introducing large quantities of zeros. The format is $a \times 10^n$ where the **mantissa** is a having values of 1 to 9 and the index is n which can be a positive or negative integer. Typical examples would be:

$$123.4 = 1.234 \times 10^2$$
$$0.0001234 = 1.234 \times 10^{-4}$$
$$12\,340\,000.0 = 1.234 \times 10^7$$

Box 1.1 Addition of mixed indices

Example 1: activities measured in curies

Adding 1.575 mCi to 43 μCi:

$$1.575 \text{ mCi is } 1.5750 \times 10^{-3} \text{Ci or}$$
$$1575.0 \times 10^{-6} \text{Ci}$$

$$43.0 \text{ μCi is } 43.0 \times 10^{-6} \text{Ci}$$

Add mantissas to give 1618×10^{-6}Ci (or 1.618 mCi).

Example 2: use of different units

Combine 1.75×10^{-6}m + 5.43×10^{-6}cm and give the answer in meters:

$$5.43 \times 10^{-6} \text{cm is } 0.0543 \times 10^{-6} \text{m}$$

Add mantissas to give 1.0843×10^{-6}m (or ≈1.08 μm).

Note. The integers could be subtracted using the same principle.

Box 1.2 Multiplication and division of values

Example 1: addition of indices

The speed of light is 3.0×10^8 m s^{-1}. How far will it travel in 2 ns (2×10^{-9}s)? Since distance traveled is speed × time, then the distance is

$$= (3.0 \times 10^8) \times (2 \times 10^{-9}) \text{ m}$$
$$= 6.0 \times 10^{-1} \text{m} = 0.6 \text{ m}$$

Example 2: addition and subtraction

A light year is the distance traveled by light in 1 year. There are $365 \times 24 \times 60 \times 60$ s in 1 year = 3.15×10^7s. So, the distance traveled in meters is

$$= 3 \times 10^8 \text{m} \times 3.15 \times 10^7 \text{s}$$
$$= 9.45 \times 10^{15} \text{m}$$

The distance in miles (1.6×10^3m = 1 mile) is

$$= (9.45 \times 10^{15}) \div (1.6 \times 10^3)$$
$$= 5.81 \times 10^{12} \text{ miles}$$

Practical examples of scientific notation used in radiology would be the old (non-SI) units of activity, the curie (Ci) where 1 μCi is 0.000001 Ci (or 1.0×10^{-6}Ci) and its equivalent SI unit, expressed in disintegrations per second, as the becquerel (Bq) where 1 μCi = 37×10^3Bq or 37 kBq.

The index 10^{-6} is shorthand for 'move the decimal point six places to the left' and the index 10^3 means 'move the decimal point three places to the right'. Similarly a mega-becquerel (MBq) is 1×10^6 disintegrations per second. When dealing with very large numbers it is convenient to use indices. For example, light travels at a speed of 30 000 000 000 cm s^{-1} through a vacuum. Such a large number is more conveniently written as 3.0×10^{10}cm s^{-1} or 3.0×10^8m s^{-1}.

Rules for addition and subtraction require that the units (e.g. gram, kilogram or meter, centimeter) and the exponents agree. An example of manipulating mixed indices and quantities is shown in Box 1.1. Only the integer numbers are added or subtracted: the exponents remain unchanged.

MULTIPLICATION AND DIVISION

In this case the integers are multiplied or divided; the exponents are added or subtracted. The units can be multiples of the same base (e.g. seconds, microseconds). Box 1.2 gives examples of multiplying and dividing dissimilar quantities.

FLOATING POINT

This notation is used to represent a very wide range of numerical values in a similar fashion to scientific notation but is found commonly associated with computer format. The notation as before is $a \times 10^n$ but the mantissa is restricted to be greater than 0.1 but less than 1.0 so:

123.4 is 0.1234×10^3
567.8 is 0.5678×10^3
0.0000789 is 0.789×10^{-4}

The index or **exponent** governs movement of the decimal point as before, to the right for positive values and to the left (adding zeros) for negative values.

The exponent is further simplified so the above numbers are represented with their relevant exponents as 0.1234E3, 0.5678E3 and 0.789E−4. This format is commonly accepted by calculators and computer programs (i.e. spreadsheets).

1.2.3 Negative numbers

Negative numbers simplify the handling of decreasing quantities. The answer to several subtraction calculations can give negative quantities, e.g. $7 - 9 = -2$. An **absolute** value to this sum, where the sign is removed, is 2 and can be obtained by squaring and then taking roots: $(\sqrt{7 - 9})^2 = 2$. This procedure is frequently used to remove negative quantities in statistics. An absolute number in an equation is bounded by vertical lines: $|7 - 9| = 2$.

BINARY NUMBERS

These use base 2 instead of the decimal base 10. Since only one of two conditions can exist (1 or 0 representing 'on' or 'off') this format is used by computers: each figure is called a **bit**. This format is more fully discussed in Chapter 11.

1.2.4 Complex numbers

If the equation $x^2 + 2x + 2 = 0$ is solved then it yields $(x + 1)^2 + 1 = 0$ which then simplifies to $x + 1 = \pm\sqrt{-1}$ where $x = -1 \pm \sqrt{-1}$. The quantity $\sqrt{-1}$ does not exist as an entity and is not a real number but the equations are not impossible so $\sqrt{-1}$ exists as an imaginary number and is denoted by i or j in an equation. A complex number has the form $a + ib$ where a and b are the real numbers.

Although complex numbers are rather artificial they are extremely useful for solving practical problems and play a very important role in waveform analysis involving frequency and phase that will be met when dealing with Fourier analysis and frequency–phase relationships in magnetic resonance imaging (MRI).

1.3 FRACTIONS AND RATIOS

Quantities are commonly compared with reference values either as fractions (e.g. one half, two thirds, three quarters) or as percentages (e.g. 33%, 50%, 33%).

1.3.1 Percentages

PERCENTAGE CHANGE

The term 'percentage' literally means 'for each hundred values'; abbreviated to %. Although this strict

---

Box 1.3 Application of percentages

Using eqn 1.1, the original value V_0 of 80 undergoes a reduction to a new value of $72V_n$. The new value as a percentage of the original is

$$\frac{V_n}{V_0} \times 100 = 90$$

The percentage change is

$$\frac{V_n - V_0}{V_0} \times 100 = 10$$

The ratio of signal to noise (SNR)

When a particular signal is measured in the presence of noise the pure signal is 12 units and the noise is 2 units. The SNR is 1:12/2, i.e. 1:6. If the noise content increases to 6 units the SNR is 1:12/6, i.e. 1:2.

Note. A decrease in the ratio signifies degradation of the perceived signal.

---

definition is commonly misused and expressions using '150%' and 'over 400%' are seen in some literature, this is not correct and should not be used in scientific work; $\times 1.5$ and $\times 4$ should be substituted. The symbol '%' (parts per hundred, or percent) has been modified as '‰' for parts per thousand.

FRACTIONAL ERROR

When measurements are carried out there is always inaccuracy associated with the measurement, whether it is a length, weight, activity or radiation exposure for example. If the original value V_0 is known, along with the nominal value V_n then the fractional error f is

$$f = \frac{V_n - V_0}{V_0} \tag{1.1}$$

Common examples of percentage calculations are given in Box 1.3.

RATIOS

Comparisons can also be made by comparing a reference with an unknown; the reference value is normalized to 1 so if the calculation yields 2.5 to 10 the ratio is 1:4. Box 1.3 also gives a worked example where ratios are commonly employed in radiology to give a 'signal-to-noise' ratio where a recorded signal is measured in the presence of noise.

1.4 RECIPROCAL VALUES

A reciprocal value describes quantities that are inversely related: as x increases then y decreases, i.e.

$$y = \frac{1}{x} \qquad (1.2)$$

Alternatively, eqn 1.2 can be expressed as

$$y = x^{-1} \qquad (1.3)$$

An inverse relationship plays an important role in radiology between distance d and radiation intensity I so that

$$I = \frac{1}{d^2} \qquad (1.4)$$

This forms the basis of the inverse square law which plays an important role in radiology.

Reciprocal values are frequently used for describing measurements. For example, kilometers per second or grams per cubic centimeter can be given as kg/s or g/cm^3 although, preferably, these should be expressed as kg s^{-1} and g cm^{-3}. An example demonstrating the derivation of this format is as follows. If an object moves a fixed distance (in meters) in a given time (in seconds) then the speed (in meters per second) at which the object moves is given by:

$$\frac{\text{distance (m)}}{\text{time (s)}} = \text{speed (m/s)} \qquad (1.5)$$

This can be rearranged as

$$\text{distance} \times \frac{1}{\text{time}} = \text{speed}$$

Since the reciprocal of time can be expressed as time^{-1} then from eqn 1.3:

$$\frac{1}{\text{time}} = \frac{1}{\text{second}} = s^{-1} \qquad (1.6)$$

So an object moving a distance (measured in meters) in a certain time (measured in seconds) has a velocity measured as meters per second or m s^{-1}. Similarly, thermal conductivity, measured as joules per second is J s^{-1} and acceleration, measured as meters per second per second is m s^{-1} s^{-1} or m s^{-2}. Volume measurements use the cube power so density is represented as kg m^{-3}.

1.5 LOGARITHMS

The logarithm of a decimal number is the exponent or power to which the base must be raised to produce the number. There are two common logarithmic bases:

- Base 10 (10^x), used for $\log_{10}$, the common logarithms.
- Base e (e^x) used for $\log_e$ (or ln), natural logarithms, where $e = 2.71828$ to six significant figures. It describes many common phenomena found in radiology, particularly the absorption of radiation (X-radiation, sound or radio frequencies) and decay of radioactive material.

For logarithms of both base 10 and base e the exponents have indices that are not whole numbers, i.e. $10^{2.6078}$ and $e^{0.693}$: the log values are 2.6078 and 0.693, respectively. Logarithmic quantities using base 10 and base e have the following inverse relationships:

$$\log_e 2 = 0.693, \quad e^{0.693} = 2, \quad e^{-0.693} = 0.5$$
$$\log_{10} 2 = 0.301, \quad 10^{0.301} = 2, \quad 10^{-0.301} = 0.5$$

1.5.1 Logarithm to base 10 ($\log_{10}$)

There is a difference between tables of logarithms and calculator/computer logarithms. Tables are designed to give convenient similar log values for numbers having the same digits, e.g. 2.0 and 0.2, which are both given a value 3010 so different tables for integers and fractions are not needed. Logarithms given by calculators and computers use the true log values where log 2.0 is 0.3010 as before but log 0.2 is -0.6989. Logarithms to base 10 were originally used for simplifying complex calculations but the introduction of scientific calculators has superseded their use for this purpose.

The manipulation of decimal numbers is simplified when using logarithms since complex calculations can be reduced to addition, subtraction, multiplication and division as shown in Table 1.4.

Table 1.4 *Logarithms simplify calculations.*

Decimal	Logarithm
Multiply ($a \times b$)	Add ($\log a + \log b$)
Divide (a/b)	Subtract ($\log a - \log b$)
Square (a^2)	Multiply by index ($\log a \times 2$)
Roots ($\sqrt[3]{a}$)	Divide by root ($\log a/3$)

Table 1.5 *Log values give decibel intensities.*

Intensity (W cm^{-2})	$\log_{10}$ value	Decibels (dB)
1	1.0000	0
2	0.3010	3
3	0.4771	5
4	0.6020	6
5	0.6989	7

Box 1.4 Film density as $\log_{10}$ values

The optical density of film (OD) is defined in eqn 1.7 as

$$\log_{10} \frac{I_i}{I_t}$$

If $I_i = 2000$ and $I_t = 200$ then

$$\log_{10} \frac{2000}{200} = 3.3010 - 2.3010$$

so the OD = 1 (i.e. 10% transmission).
   Similarly, if $I_i = 2000$ and $I_t = 20$ then the OD = 2 (i.e. 1% transmission).
   If $I_i = 2000$ and $I_t = 1000$ then the OD = 0.3 (i.e. 50% transmission).
Note. An OD value change of 0.3 doubles or halves the transmission. Compare this with the dB change of 3.0 in sound intensity.

EXAMPLES OF THE USE OF LOG$_{10}$ IN RADIOLOGY

Logarithms to base 10 are commonly used in radiology to calculate optical density and decibel ratings. Photographic optical density, OD, is measured as a $\log_{10}$ value of incident I_i and transmitted I_t light, where

$$OD = \log_{10} \frac{I_i}{I_t} \qquad (1.7)$$

A worked example of eqn 1.7 for film density, represented as light intensity transmitted by a light box through the film is given in Box 1.4.
   The $\log_{10}$ scale is also found in ultrasound imaging, where it is used for measuring sound intensity (W cm^{-2}) as the **decibel** (dB) which is represented as a rounded log value. Table 1.5 gives approximate decibel

levels showing that a change of 3 dB (a change from log 1.0 to log 2.0) doubles sound intensity.

1.5.2 Natural logarithms

Natural logarithms are logs to the base e, and they are indicated by the notation $\log_e x$ or $\ln x$. In biological and physical processes the exponential function e is common to many growth and decay processes and can be used to describe, for instance, absorption of radiation and decay of radioactivity.

GROWTH AND THE ORIGIN OF e

The process of growth can be expressed as

$$G = G_0 \left(1 + \frac{1}{t}\right)^t \qquad (1.8)$$

where G is the final value and G_0 the original value. The factor $1/t$ is the increment added at time t. For $t = 2$ the equation $e = (1 + 1/t)^t$ becomes $(1 + 1/2)^2 = 2.25$. For large values of t in eqn 1.8 the value e becomes 2.71828…. This irrational figure is adopted as the base of **Napierian** or **natural logarithms**.

The exponential law The common formula used in radiology which uses the exponential function e is

$$N = N_0 \times e^{-y} \qquad (1.9)$$

where N_0 is the original activity and N is the value representing new activity influenced by y. The parameter y is a mixed value whose components depend on the particular application. The general formula for **exponential decay** is eqn 1.9 above. It can also be applied to the absorption of radiation: the two components for the product y are:

- μ, which describes the absorption efficiency of the material
- x, the thickness of the material

So eqn 1.9 becomes

$$N = N_0 e^{-\mu x} \qquad (1.10)$$

As the two values N and N_0 now represent **radiation intensities** they now become I_0 (incident intensity) and I_x (intensity after adding absorber with thickness x). Eqn 1.10 becomes perhaps the most familiar equation in radiology:

$$I_x = I_0 \times e^{-\mu x} \qquad (1.11)$$

This formula was originally used by J. Lambert (1728–77; German physicist) to describe light absorption (Lambert's law). It is an important basic formula used in radiology where exponential change is seen such as the absorption of electromagnetic radiation (X- or gamma radiation) by various materials (e.g. tissue, aluminum, lead). It can also describe the decay of radioactive isotopes, e.g. ^{131}Iodine or $^{99\,m}$Technetium when I_x and I_0 become the activity levels.

If the radiation intensities are measured using eqn 1.11, then the separate indices can be found:

$$\frac{I}{I_0} = e^{-\mu x} \qquad (1.12)$$

Inverting eqn 1.12 removes the negative value so

$$\ln \frac{I_0}{I} = \mu x \qquad (1.13)$$

An example of the use of eqn 1.13 is in calculating absorber thickness necessary to reduce X-ray beam intensity as indicated in Box 1.5.

The thickness of absorber that reduces the beam intensity by ½ is the half-value layer and with this measurement the basic formula can be used to derive the attenuation coefficient of materials. This is shown in Box 1.5 and will receive added importance in Chapter 3.

APPLICATIONS

Applying the formula shown in eqn 1.11 to problems concerning radioactive decay the two exponent values (μ and x) now change to:

- Time t when activity is measured
- The **half-life** of the nuclide, $T_{\frac{1}{2}}$

so the formula now becomes

$$A_t = A_0 \times e^{-\lambda t} \qquad (1.14)$$

Box 1.5 Attenuation of radiation

What thickness x of lead is required to reduce radiation by 90% if the attenuation coefficient (μ) of lead is 27.72 cm^{-1} at the given kilovoltage?

Let $I_0 = 100$ and $I_x = 10$ then using eqn 1.13

$$\ln \frac{100}{10} = 2.3025$$

so $x = 0.08$ cm (0.8 mm).

where A_0 is the original activity and A_t is the activity at time t. The arguments are derived in Box 1.6, where μ can be obtained from the half-value layer (HVL). Instead of HVL a half-life is introduced so when the measurement time t equals $T_{\frac{1}{2}}$ a similar expression can be derived for λ:

$$\lambda = \frac{0.693}{T_{\frac{1}{2}}} \qquad (1.15)$$

Similarly, $e^{-\lambda T_{\frac{1}{2}}} = 0.5$ and $\ln 2 = \lambda T_{\frac{1}{2}}$. Since the fraction λ does not vary this is the **decay constant** for the isotope. Box 1.7 calculates the activity for a short half-life isotope ^{99m}Technetium using this constant.

EXPONENTIAL GROWTH

The exponential law also describes growth processes. An example from nuclear medicine would describe an increased growth of radioactivity in an isotope generator (^{99}Mo/^{99m}Tc), or in MRI for describing the rate at which the proton axis regains equilibrium during the T1 time in MRI.

1.6 PROPORTIONAL QUANTITIES

Although two quantities x and y may be directly **proportional** to each other they are not necessarily equal so: $y \propto x$ could signify $y \propto kx$ where k is a constant. In radiology X-ray intensity is proportional to tube current (in milliamps). Parameters are **inversely proportional** when $y \propto 1/x$, which restates eqn 1.2 and describes a function where if x is doubled y is

Box 1.6 Reducing intensity by half: the half-value layer (HVL)

Derivation of the attenuation coefficient

By definition adding a half-value layer (HVL) will reduce I_0 to $I_0/2$, so from eqn 1.11,

$$\frac{I_0}{2} = I_0 \times e^{-(\mu \times \text{HVL})}$$

and

$$e^{-(\mu \times \text{HVL})} = 0.5$$

or

$$e^{\mu \times \text{HVL}} = 2$$

Simplifying: $\ln 2 = \mu \times \text{HVL}$. Since $\ln 2 = 0.693$ then

$$\mu = \frac{0.693}{\text{HVL}}$$

Example

Find the attenuation coefficient μ if 4 mm (0.004 m) of aluminum reduces the beam intensity by half.

$$\mu = \frac{0.693}{0.004} \approx 173 \text{m}^{-1} (\text{i.e. } 1.73 \text{cm}^{-1})$$

Box 1.7 Isotope decay

Example 1

The half-life $(T_{\frac{1}{2}})$ for ^{99m}Tc is 6 h. If the original activity was 800 MBq how much remains after 1 day?

From eqn 1.14 $A_t = A_0 \times e^{-\mu \times t}$.

The original activity, A_0, is 800 MBq, the time, t, is 24 h, and the decay constant, λ, for ^{99m}Tc is 0.1155 h:

$$\begin{aligned} A_t &= A_0 \times e^{-0.1155 \times 24} \\ &= 800 \times 0.06253 \\ &= 50 \text{ MBq} \end{aligned}$$

This formula is also valid for mCi.

Example 2

The original activity of ^{131}I ($T_{\frac{1}{2}}$ 8 days) on day 0 was 400 MBq in 2 cm^3 saline. On day 5 130 MBq is required. What volume must be drawn up?

Total activity on day 5 is

$$\begin{aligned} A_t &= 400 \times e^{-(0.693 \times 5)/8} \\ &= 400 \times 0.65 \\ &= 260 \text{ MBq in 2 cm}^3 \end{aligned}$$

So 1 cm^3 will give the required 130 MBq.

---

halved. The radiation dose from a point source measured at a surface varies as the **inverse square** of the distance d already seen in eqn 1.4 restated now as $y \propto 1/d^2$, where y is the dose. The quantities dose and distance are not defined so an equals sign cannot be used. This important relationship will be discussed further in a later section.

1.7 GRAPHS

A graph illustrates the relationship between sets of numbers or quantities (usually two) plotted as a series of points or lines with reference to the set of axes. The most common type of graph is the Cartesian graph with uniform scales, shown in Fig. 1.1. This shows:

- The horizontal axis (the x-axis) or **abscissa** which usually contains the **independent variable** (e.g. time, distance, kilovoltage)
- The vertical axis (the y-axis) or **ordinate** contains the measured or **dependent variable** (e.g. size, exposure, attenuation)

1.7.1 Linear graphs

The straight-line relationships shown in Fig. 1.1 are given when:

$$y \propto x \quad \text{or} \quad y = c + mx \quad \text{or} \quad y = c - mx$$

(1.16)

where c is the intersect with the y-axis (the off-set) where the line does not intersect zero and m is the slope or angle of the line.

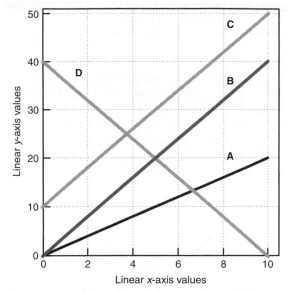

Figure 1.1 *Examples of three linear graphs described in the text. A and B have different slopes but the same origin (zero). C is offset by 10 and D shows a negative relationship with* y.

The examples in Fig. 1.1 show graphs A and B having different slopes but no offset. Graph C shows an offset from zero and graph D shows a negative relationship where $y = -mx$. If data are missing on a graph then it is valid to **interpolate** the missing values and fill in the unknowns by reference to neighboring points.

EXTRAPOLATION

Extrapolation infers the extreme values of a given range, either the highest or the lowest, but this can produce questionable results and must be used with care. A common radiology example where extrapolation is used is the relationship between radiation dose and the incidence of leukemia. Here the lower values are extrapolated since there are insufficient real measurements from observed results; this is investigated in Chapter 21 when exploring low radiation dose effects. In certain cases a series of experimental results are plotted and then a formula derived describing the relationship between x and y; this is an **empirical** approach. A series of measurements can also conform to a set formula; for example, a straight line or exponential and the measured values then fit a set formula (i.e. inverse or exponential function).

1.7.2 Nonlinear graphs

Nonlinear relationships are found when value x does not have a uniform relationship with value y. Common functions found in radiology are squared values, $y = x^2$, and inverse relationships, $y = 1/x$. Squared values, x^2 are plotted in Fig. 1.2a. Practical examples would be the intensity of X-ray output increasing as the square of the kilovoltage ($I \propto V^2$). **Inverse** values,

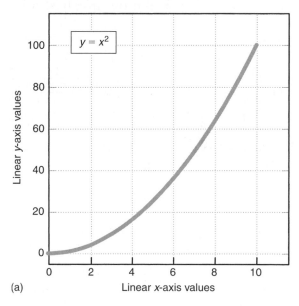

(a)

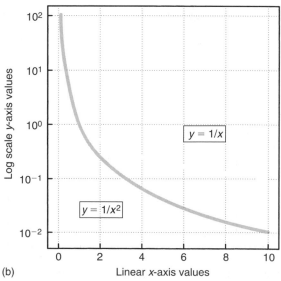

(b)

Figure 1.2 *(a) A nonlinear relationship plotted where* $y = x^2$. *(b) The inverse function showing* $y = 1/x$ *and* $y = 1/x^2$.

where $y = 1/x$, are plotted in Fig. 1.2b. Common examples in radiology would be $1/d^2$ (the inverse square law) and the probability of a photoelectric reaction with energy, E, varying as $1/E^2$.

1.7.3 Logarithmic functions

The common **exponential functions** of the type e^x and e^{-x} are plotted in Fig. 1.3a where the curve for e^x shows a rapidly increasing curve typically seen in X-ray tube rating charts plotting tube current versus filament current at high kilovoltage settings.

The negative curve for e^{-x} is a very common function in radiology because it describes both radioactive decay and photon (electromagnetic) attenuation. When dealing with a simple exponential function a **semi-log** plot, where the x-axis is linear but the y-axis is logarithmic, will yield a straight line. This is shown in Fig. 1.3b where the same functions e^x and e^{-x} are straight lines. This is most useful since it only requires the two or three points of a known exponential

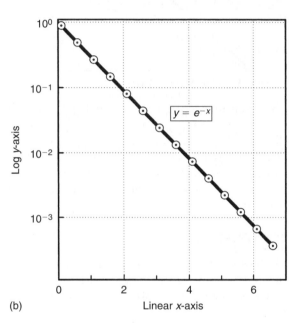

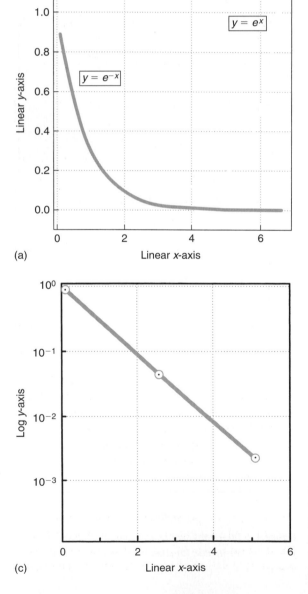

Figure 1.3 (*a*) The two exponential functions $y = e^x$ and $y = e^{-x}$ plotted on linear x- and y-axes. (*b*) The same functions e^{-x} plotted on a linear x-axis and a log y-axis (semi-log scale) yield straight lines. (*c*) An exponential curve only needs two to three readings for its completion (e.g. plot for the half-value layer).

function in order to plot the entire relationship. Figure 1.3c shows an example where radiation absorption is being measured and only two to three points are needed to give the complete function. A linear plot would require many points in order to give the same accuracy as a curve shown in Fig. 1.3a.

A multiple exponential function (two or more exponential functions combined) can also be separated on a semi-log plot. Figure 1.4a shows the fast and slow phases of a tissue clearance curve. These can be approximately separated by drawing a line along the flat section of the graph, representing the slow phase meeting the y-axis. These extrapolated values are then subtracted from the original graph revealing the fast slope.

OTHER LOGARITHMIC FUNCTIONS

The exponential function $1 - e^{-x}$ plotted in Fig. 1.4b is commonly seen in radiology since it describes conditions which are reaching saturation, e.g. growth of activity in isotope production (^{99m}Tc growth in a ^{99}Mo/^{99m}Tc generator) or returning to an equilibrium state such as a proton magnetic moment in nuclear magnetic resonance.

THE POWER LAW

The function $y = A + xn$ where A and n are constants may be rewritten as $\log y = \log A + \log x \times n$. As A is a constant then $\log A$ is also a constant so $\log y = \log x \times n$. This plots a straight line on log/log axes and obeys the **power law**. Examples of functions obeying the power law commonly found in radiology are:

$$y = x^2$$
$$y = x^{-2} \ (\text{or } 1/x^2)$$
$$y = x^{1/2} \ (\text{or } \sqrt{x})$$
$$y = x^{-1/2} \ (\text{or } 1/\sqrt{x})$$

In radiology they are seen for functions describing kV^2, Z^3, $1/d^2$ and $1/E^2$; each of these gives a straight line obeying the power law. An example for $1/d^2$ is shown in Fig. 1.5.

SPLINE FIT

If the number of data points are insufficient to produce a smooth curve (where one is expected) the data can be subjected to a smoothly joined polynomial. It resembles the position that a draftsman's spline (a thin flexible ruler) would occupy if it were constrained to

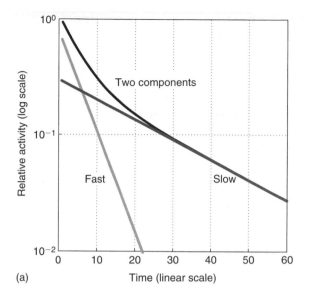

(a)

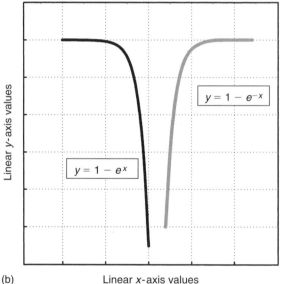

(b)

Figure 1.4 (**a**) A fast and slow phase tissue clearance which can be separated from the two-part composite exponential curve. The slow phase is first extrapolated back to time zero and these extrapolated figures subtracted from the composite curve to give the fast phase.
(**b**) Exponential growth using the function $y = 1 - e^{-x}$. The function $1 - e^x$ is rarely met in radiology but is included here for completion.

pass through the points. Cubic spline interpolation is a useful method for fitting the data points and smoothing discontinuities. It is an improvement on polynomial interpolation when the number of data points

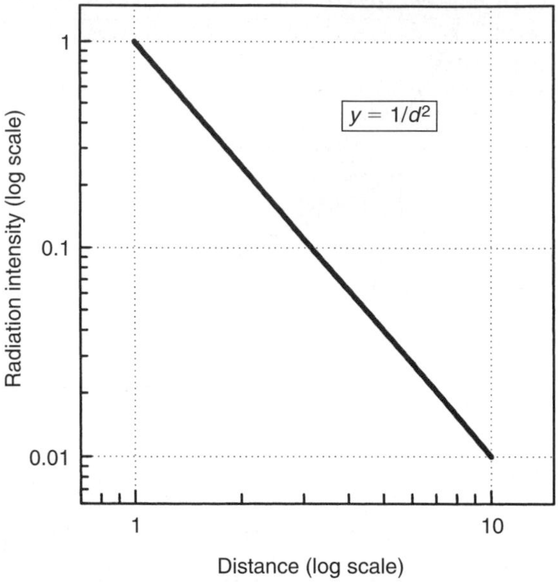

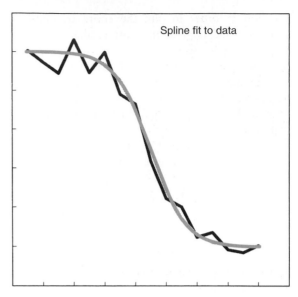

Figure 1.5 *A log–log plot obeying the power law. The general formula would be* y = xⁿ *where* n *is a fixed index: i.e. ½, −½, 2, 3. The example shows the inverse square law relationship (*y = 1/d²*).*

Figure 1.6 *Spline fit to sparse data points.*

increases. Figure 1.6 gives an example of a splice fit applied to a rough curve.

1.8 VECTORS AND SCALARS

SCALAR AND VECTOR QUANTITIES

Most quantities measured in science are classed as either scalar or vector quantities. A scalar quantity is one which has only magnitude (or size). Mass, volume, speed and temperature are scalar quantities.

A vector quantity has both magnitude and direction. However, force has a direction in which it acts so is therefore a vector quantity. Velocity and acceleration are examples of vector quantities. It can be represented by a line whose length is proportional to the magnitude and whose direction is that of the vector, or by three components in a rectangular coordinate system.

A **true vector**, or **polar vector**, involves a displacement or virtual displacement. Polar vectors include velocity, acceleration, force, electric and magnetic field strengths. The signs of their components are reversed on reversing the coordinate axes.

A **pseudovector**, or **axial vector**, involves the orientation of an axis in space. Pseudovectors include angular velocity, vector area, and magnetic flux density. The signs of their components are unchanged on reversing the coordinate axes.

Vector quantities are treated by **vector algebra**, for example, the resultant of two vectors may be found by a parallelogram of vectors.

A phasor is a rotating vector that represents a sinusoidally varying quantity. It is a valuable method of analyzing sine waveforms, common in radiology. Its vector length represents the amplitude of the quantity and it is imagined to rotate with angular velocity equal to the angular frequency of the quantity (sine wave frequency), so that the instantaneous value of the quantity is represented by its projection upon a fixed axis. The concept is convenient for representing the phase angle between two quantities; it is shown on a diagram as the angle between their phasors. This is further explored with sine wave functions in Chapter 2. It is applied again in MRI (Chapter 19).

1.9 CALCULUS

Problems often occur with graphed quantities where a rate of change of one measurement with another is required, such as the change of heat loss from an X-ray tube with time or the change of intensity with distance. The rate of change can be calculated by using **differential calculus**. The complete or part area under a

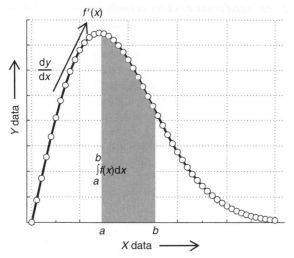

Figure 1.7 *The use of differential and integral calculus for analyzing a curve.*

Box 1.8 The exponential decay of an isotope

Using the basic form:

$$\frac{dy}{dx} = ky$$

where k = constant, and

$$\int \frac{dy}{ky} = \frac{1}{k}\ln y + C$$

which simplifies to $y = Ae^{-kx}$, where A is a constant.

Note. This is the basic formula for radioactive decay, attenuation of radiation through matter and heat loss.

---

curve is also a common requirement (the intensity of radiation given by a particular X-ray spectrum for instance) and this is calculated using **integral calculus**. The differential and integral calculus forms the foundation for many techniques used in radiology and a revision of its basic properties is relevant. This section is a springboard to further reading; a detailed description is not necessary at this point. The hypothetical function $f(x)$ where $y = f(x)$, describing the y value being some operation on x, is plotted in Fig. 1.7 which illustrates the fundamental points.

1.9.1 Differential calculus

This describes the **derivative** of a function or the gradient of a curve marked as the slope in Fig. 1.7. It is concerned essentially with the rate of change of one quantity with respect to another. If $f(x)$ denotes any function of x and $y = f(x)$ then the derived function is

$$\frac{dy}{dx} \tag{1.17}$$

Simple examples where differential calculus is used in radiology would be the rate of heat loss from an X-ray tube and the decay rate of a radioactive isotope together with the attenuation of radiation by an absorber. Film contrast is often expressed as a derivative curve superimposed on the characteristic curve.

EXPONENTIAL DECAY

Eqns 1.10 and 1.14 describing radioactive decay can be derived from first principles. Let the amount of undecayed nuclei at time t be $N = f(t)$, then $-dN/dt$ represents rate of decrease at that time so

$$\frac{dN}{dt} = -kN \tag{1.18}$$

where k is a positive constant. Eqn 1.18 is really the same as the basic equation in Box 1.8 expressed as a negative quantity so

$$\frac{dt}{dN} = -\frac{1}{kN} \tag{1.19}$$

and in a similar fashion to the second equation in Box 1.8:

$$t = \frac{1}{k}\ln N + C \tag{1.20}$$

This is usually expressed as $N = Ae^{-kt}$ where A is a constant. If at $t = 0$, N equals N_0 then A is replaced by N_0 and the formula becomes

$$N = N_0 e^{-kt} \tag{1.21}$$

This is the fundamental equation describing exponential decay or absorption. For radioactive decay the constant k is replaced by the decay constant λ.

HIGHER ORDER DIFFERENTIAL

If $f'(x)$ is the first derivative then $f''(x)$ is the second derivative taking the form

$$\frac{d^2 y}{dx^2} \qquad (1.22)$$

Second derivatives describe how the rate of change is itself changing; examples would be accelerations. This is sometimes applied to cardiology when studying the rate of change of wall motion. So the first derivative would be rate, s^{-1}, and the second derivative would be acceleration describing second per second or s^{-2}.

1.9.2 Integral calculus

Integration is the inverse of differentiation. The integral of a function $f'(x)$ with respect to x is written as $\int f'(x) \cdot dx$. The symbol $\int$ is the old English for S which is used here to represent 'sum'. The **definite integral** $f(x)$ as defined by an interval a to b in Fig. 1.7 takes the form

$$\int_a^b f(x) \cdot dx \qquad (1.23)$$

where a and b are the lower and upper limits of an area for the variable x.

Numerous approximations are available for calculating integrals. The trapezoidal rule places strips under the curve having trapezium shapes whose individual areas are summed to give the required curve area. Simpson's rule improves accuracy by using strips bounded by a parabolic shape which more closely approximates the shape of the curve.

IMPROPER OR INFINITE INTEGRAL

This is the case if one or both of the limits tends to infinity (a or $b = \infty$) such as the area under a continuous X-ray spectrum. Eqn 1.23 now takes the form

$$\iint f(x, y) \cdot dx \cdot dy \qquad (1.24)$$

This is an example of double integration for a two-dimensional array (x, y matrix), often seen in image analysis and manipulation.

1.10 VOLUMES AND SURFACES

The emission of radiation from a point source occurs equally in all directions creating a sphere of radiation. This is **isotropic** emission and applies commonly to a radioactive source. The X-ray tube focal spot does not emit isotropically due to forward absorption by the anode.

When measuring isotropic radiation sources with a flat detector it is important to realize that the detector surface, being flat, can only capture a very small proportion of the total activity emanating from the source. A basic knowledge of planar and volume geometry is therefore useful in radiology for understanding detector efficiency.

1.10.1 Volumes

SOLID GEOMETRY

The geometry of a three-dimensional (3-D) body is applicable to irradiation of volumes and surfaces from a point source (X-ray or gamma ray). The relevant formulas are:

- Surface area $4\pi r^2$
- Spherical volume $4\pi r^3/3$

THE INVERSE SQUARE LAW

This can be derived by reference to spherical geometry shown in Fig. 1.8a. It is a very important concept in radiation exposure. The intensity of radiation from an isotropic source is measured at r_1 and r_2: this is the photon density per unit area. The energy emitted is E so the intensity at the surface of the small sphere Ir_1 is

$$Ir_1 = \frac{E}{4\pi r_1^2} \qquad (1.25)$$

and for the intensity Ir_2 is

$$Ir_2 = \frac{E}{4\pi r_2^2} \qquad (1.26)$$

The intensity of radiation varies as $1/r^2$, the inverse square of the distance – if the intensity at 2 m is 100 then at 4 m it will be 25.

and can only be achieved by a detector which completely surrounds the source.

DETECTOR EFFICIENCY, *e*

This is given by the equation

$$e = \frac{\Omega}{4\pi} \times 100\% \qquad (1.27)$$

where Ω is the solid angle subtended by the detector surface. The efficiency of a spherical detector having 4π geometry is approached by a nuclear medicine 'dose calibrator' where a radioactive source is placed inside a gas detector. There is a slight loss of efficiency due to the sample aperture which is the detector entrance. This is described in Chapter 16.

1.10.2 Surface detectors

Flat or surface detectors are manufactured in a variety of sizes, rectangular as well as round. If a circular detector shown in Fig. 1.8b is taken (radius *r* or diameter *d*) and the hypotenuse is *L* then the geometry of a cone can be employed:

- Detector area πr^2
- Detector circumference $2\pi r$ or πd
- Conic angle $\Omega = \pi r^2/L^2$

Using these formulas the efficiency of a planar detector can be calculated as shown in Fig. 1.8b (examples would be a gamma camera or an image intensifier face). For surface detectors with a detector area $A = \pi r^2$ then the conic angle subtended by the detector is

$$\Omega = \frac{A}{r^2} \qquad (1.28)$$

The value of 6.28 steradians is the central angle of a hemisphere representing a surface detector; this is called **2π geometry**. Geometrical detector efficiency for 2π geometry (surfaces) is determined by two factors:

- Area of detector
- Source to detector distance

These factors define the solid angle 'subtended' by the detector relative to the source and eqn 1.28 is used for calculating the efficiency. Calculated examples are given in Box 1.9.

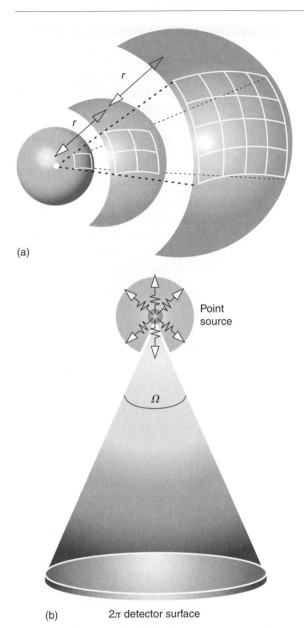

(a)

(b) 2π detector surface

Figure 1.8 *(a) Isotropic emission from a source. Intensity measured at the surface of two spheres having radius* r$_1$ *and* r$_2$ *(in text). (b) Planar detector efficiency showing the detector surface subtending the solid angle Ω with the point source.*

STERADIAN

This is the solid angle used in spherical geometry so $4\pi = 12.56$ steradians, to four significant figures, which is the complete central angle of a sphere; the 100% collection efficiency is known as **4π geometry**

Box 1.9 Detector efficiency

Use eqn 1.28 for the angle $\Omega = A/r^2$, to find the efficiency for a $10\,mm^2$ detector at (a) 25 mm and (b) 50 mm.
(a) At 25 mm:

$$\frac{10}{25^2} = 1.6 \times 10^{-2}\,\Omega$$

$$e = \frac{1.6 \times 10^{-2}}{4\pi} \times 100\%$$

At 25 mm = 0.127% which would be 1.27% for a $100\,mm^2$ detector surface.
(b) At 50 mm

$$\frac{10}{50^2} = 4.0 \times 10^{-3}\,\Omega$$

$$e = \frac{4.0 \times 10^{-3}}{4\pi} \times 100\%$$

$$\text{At 50 mm} = 0.032\%$$

Note. The geometrical efficiency of a 2Ω detector is extremely small.

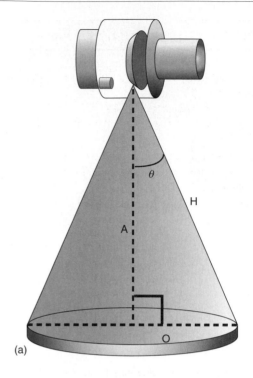

(a)

RADIAN

This is the basic unit for a plane angle Ω shown in Fig. 1.8b, which is $360/2\pi$ or 57.2958°, to six significant figures. The radian is based on the constant proportionality between the radius and the circumference of a circle. The definition of a radian is the angle subtended (at the center) by an arc equal in length to the radius of the circle. The circumference equals $2\pi r$ so a circle contains 2π radians. A complete 360° rotation is 2π radians or 6.283... so 1 radian $\approx 57.3°$. The radian and steradian are supplementary SI units.

1.11 TRIGONOMETRY

TANGENT

The geometric definition is a straight line which touches the circumference of a circle at only one point. However, it is also a trigonometric value relating the angle of a triangle to side dimensions. If a right-angled triangle represented in Fig. 1.9a has sides adjacent A,

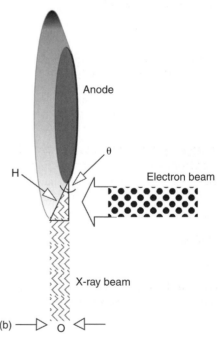

Figure 1.9 *(a) The useful field of view given by an X-ray tube can be calculated using* tan θ *as shown in the text. A = adjacent side, O = opposite side, H = hypotenuse. (b) The effective focal spot size of an X-ray tube target can be calculated from the anode angle and length of the target area.*

Box 1.10 Trigonometry examples

Tangent example from Fig. 1.9a and using eqn 1.29: angle $\theta = 20°$.

  Adjacent side $A = 100 \, cm$
  Field of view $= 2 \times (0.364 \times 100) = 36 \times 2$
  $= 72 \, cm$

Sine example from Fig. 1.9b and using eqn 1.30.
  If the hypotenuse H (real focal length) is 3 mm and the anode angle $\theta = 20°$ then the effective focal spot:

$$H \times \sin \theta = 3 \times 0.342 = 1 \, mm$$

opposite O and the hypotenuse H, relative to angle θ then

$$\tan \theta = \frac{O}{A} \qquad (1.29)$$

The useful field of view can be calculated with the dimensions given in Fig. 1.9a.

SINE

A sine of an angle in a right-angled triangle is given by the ratio of the opposite to the hypotenuse:

$$\sin \theta = \frac{O}{H} \qquad (1.30)$$

The effective focal-spot size of an X-ray tube can be calculated from knowledge of the anode angle and its sine value: Fig. 1.9b shows the dimensions involved and a worked example is given in Box 1.10. The important geometry of **sine waves** will be covered in later chapters.

COSINE

This is the third member of the family of trigonometry functions having the relationship

$$\cos \theta = \frac{A}{H} \qquad (1.31)$$

It is included for completeness and its value in radiology is discussed in Chapter 2 where sine/cosine values play an important role in waveform analysis and alternating current power supplies.

1.12 OSCILLATIONS AND WAVES

Signals used in radiology for image formation are commonly either continuous (video) or undergo a decay process after a finite length of time (radio waves). Continuous signals are **periodic** and decaying signals are **transient**. A continuous sound wave, an electromagnetic emission or the AC mains supply would demonstrate a periodic signal whilst a magnetic resonance signal or an ultrasound pulse would be transient.

1.12.1 The sine wave

The simplest type of periodic signal is the sine wave, shown in Fig. 1.10a where the signal varies as

$$y = A \times \sin(\omega + \theta) \qquad (1.32)$$

where A is a constant representing amplitude and ω is the angular frequency, $2\pi f_o$ where f_o is the number of repetitions per unit time or the wave **frequency** measured in hertz (Hz). The variable θ is the initial **phase angle** with respect to the time origin, in radians. The distance between zero crossing points is the wavelength λ so that if n oscillations pass a given point in unit time the velocity, V, of the wave is $\lambda \times n$.

Angular velocity The waveform repeats itself every 360° so the phase relationships between waveforms, where one leads or lags the other, can be simply described by using a circular **phase diagram** shown in the top right of Fig. 1.10a, b and c. For two waveforms having different phase relationships in Fig. 1.10b, the angular velocity is $\theta_2 - \theta_1 = \Delta\theta$ expressed in **radians**. Figure 1.10b shows two sine waves with the same frequency but different amplitudes, A_1 and A_2, and phase. The phase diagram indicates the amplitude difference and 90° phase shift.

A 3-phase sine wave with equal amplitude and 120° phase shift is shown in Fig. 1.10c. Its phase diagram shows the same 120° phase shift between each waveform. This is the common waveform in 3-phase AC power supplies.

1.12.2 Waveform analysis

The signals most commonly encountered in radiology (e.g. ultrasound, MRI, image data) consist of mixed waveforms, each having a different frequency, amplitude, and phase. These signals can be separated

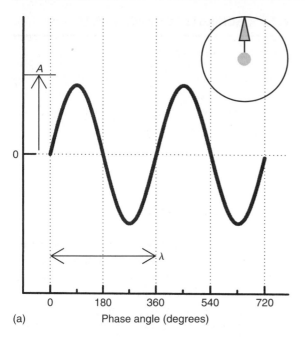

(a)

Phase angle (degrees)

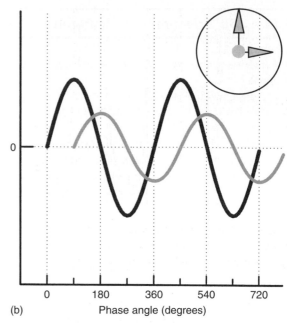

(b)

Phase angle (degrees)

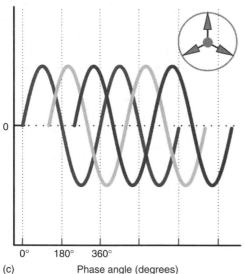

(c)

Phase angle (degrees)

Figure 1.10 (*a*) *The geometry of a sine wave showing wavelength and amplitude. The two waveforms in (**b**) have a different amplitude and phase which is identified by the arrow position and size in the phase diagram (90° phase difference). The 3-phase waveform in (**c**) (AC power supply) shows a 120° phase difference.*

and their individual characteristics measured by using Fourier analysis (J.B. Fourier, 1768–1830; French mathematician). Fourier's theorem states that a composite waveform or function $x(t)$ comprising different frequencies, phase and amplitude can be treated as a series of the form

$$x(t) = A_0 + A_1 \times \sin(\omega_t + \theta_1) + A_2 \times \sin(2\omega_t + \theta_2)$$
$$+ A_3 \times \sin(3\omega_t + \theta_3) + A_4 \times \sin(4\omega_t + \theta_4)$$
$$+ \cdots A_n \times \sin(n\omega_t + \theta_n) \qquad (1.33)$$

$A_1, \ldots, A_n$ represent the peak amplitude of the fundamental and harmonic component of the series; $\theta_1, \ldots, \theta_n$ represent the phase relationships between the fundamental and harmonics at time t. So a complex waveform seen in image data (computed tomography) or ultrasound, for instance, can be decomposed into the sum of its individual sine waves where the fundamental frequency is

$$f_0 = \frac{\omega}{2\pi} \qquad (1.34)$$

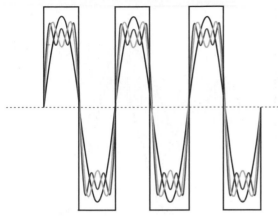

Figure 1.11 *An example of Fourier analysis of a rectangular waveform (square wave) showing the results of using increasing numbers of terms in eqn 1.35.*

In order to simplify the principle of Fourier analysis without introducing complex variables a demonstration of its analytical ability is given in Fig. 1.11 for a rectangular waveform combining eqns 1.33 and 1.34 to give

$$x(t) = \frac{A}{2} + \frac{2A}{\pi} \times \sin(\omega_t) \times \frac{2A}{3\pi} = \sin(3\omega_t)$$
$$+ \frac{2A}{5\pi} \times \sin(5\omega_t) + \cdots + \frac{2A}{n\pi} \times \sin(n\omega_t)$$

$$(1.35)$$

The first two terms then the next three in eqn 1.35 are plotted in Fig. 1.11 showing that increasing the number of terms more closely approaches the original rectangular waveform.

When a waveform analysis is attempted the more terms that are included the greater the accuracy but a large number of terms is obviously impractical so a truncated Fourier series is employed.

1.13 BASIC STATISTICS IN RADIOLOGY

Statistical analysis allows accurate predictions and sensible decisions to be made, sometimes on incomplete measurements or data sets. Each **data set** or sample may come from the same **population** (e.g. population heights or weights) or may come from two different populations (e.g. population heights in country A versus country B).

In radiology the data sets are commonly count or density measurements taken from different organs or tissues in an image or sample activity counts (e.g. counts when determining glomerular filtration rate) or a group of physiological measurements (e.g. heart rate, body temperature) from a group of patients undergoing a particular investigation (new contrast agent or drug). These quantities taken from a population are **variables**. It is rarely possible to measure an entire population so a population sample must be taken. The size of the sample depends on the variation within the population.

1.13.1 Sample distribution

The degree of variability of a series of measurements such as photon flux on a detector surface, is subject to random variations. For comparative measurements it is not necessary to count the total number of events (usually impossible anyway) providing the equipment is stable. A sample series of count rates or densities is only required. However, even under the most careful experimental conditions a series of repeat observations with a constant level of activity will give variable results. The distribution of this variability can be analyzed to give useful information about counting characteristics, for example.

Three basic distributions are used for describing different data characteristics. These are, in order of complexity: binomial, Poisson and Gaussian (normal) distributions.

BINOMIAL DISTRIBUTION

This describes the probability of an event occurring p or not occurring q. If a certain population has a disease content of 10% then the probability of a certain selected person having the disease is $p = 0.1$ or not having the disease is $q = 0.9$, then $p + q = 1$. The probability that two people selected from this population will have the disease or be normal is obtained by expanding $(p + q)^2$ which is p^2 for both having the disease, $2pq$ for one being normal and one having the disease and q^2 for both being normal. The simple algebraic relationship leads to the expansion

$$p^2 + 2pq + q^2 = (p + q)^2 \qquad (1.36)$$

Similarly the probabilities from a population of n individuals can be derived by expanding $(p + q)^n$. This forms the binomial distribution which plays an important role in population sampling and having

Box 1.11 Example of binomial distribution

A certain radiology department has a 20% rejection rate for its film radiographs (processor spoilage, technical error etc.). This is particularly high so a study was designed where a group of five films ($n = 5$) was selected at the end of each clinical session. There were 12 sessions per day so at the end of the year 4380 groups of five films had been analyzed. For a 20% rejection rate $p = 0.2$ and $q = 0.8$. Since $(p + q)^n = (0.2 + 0.8)^5$ this expands to give

$$p^5 + 5p^4q + 10p^3q^2 + 10p^2q^3 + 5pq^4 + q^5$$

Inserting the figures gives the individual values:

$$(0.2)^5 + 5(0.2)^4(0.8) + 10(0.2)^3(0.8)^2 \ldots \text{etc.}$$

This expansion is the binomial distribution for the different outcomes as the relative expected frequencies.

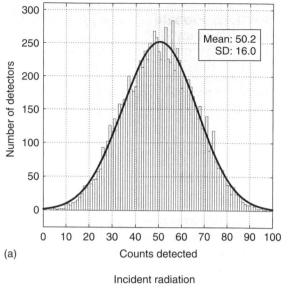

(a)

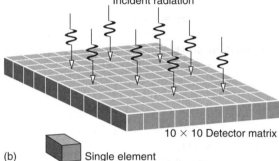

(b)

Figure 1.12 *(a)* A Poisson and normal distribution superimposed. *(b)* A detector surface and a single detector exposed to a uniform X-ray fluence.

confidence that a sample from this population accurately represents the population distribution.

During sampling we do not know the value of p but are trying to infer its value. In application a sample of a definite size is taken and a note is made of the number of times a certain event is observed. The binomial distribution can be a useful tool for quality control procedures in radiology where equipment performance is being documented. An example of this application for estimating the film rejection rate in a department and judging whether the rejection rate has gone up or down is calculated in Box 1.11.

From the above distribution we may calculate the mean μ and standard deviation σ values of the number of reject films per sample. These are $\mu = np$ and $\sigma = \sqrt{npq}$. Substituting the values from this exercise gives $\mu = 1.0$ and $\sigma = 0.894$.

POISSON DISTRIBUTION

In most practical applications the binomial distribution is not appropriate since we do not know the value of n in the expression $(p + q)^n$. This is true, for example, when studying the number of counts registered by a detector or intercepted by an imaging surface.

A Poisson distribution (S.D. Poisson, 1781–1840; French mathematician) is shown as a histogram

portion in Fig. 1.12a representing the random distribution of counts collected over a uniformly exposed detector surface, represented in Fig. 1.12b, constructed from 10×10 detectors having individual areas of 1 cm^2.

The Poisson distribution can be used to answer the question 'How many X-rays m are intercepted by a detector in an array of detectors?' (or a certain fixed area of an imaging surface). If the number N of individual detectors (or areas shown in Fig. 1.12b) is large and the probability P of an X-ray photon falling on a single detector is small then the variable x is the number of X-rays detected. The Poisson probability $P(x)$ which would describe this is

$$P(x) = \frac{m^x}{x!} \cdot e^{-m} \tag{1.37}$$

where e is the exponential constant.

Box 1.12 Probability of registering a certain count

From a detector counting background activity, what is the probability of registering a count of 7 when the average count is 5 using eqn 1.33?

$$P(x) = \frac{(5)^7}{7!} \times e^{-5}$$
$$= 0.10$$

Box 1.13 Expected probability

For a middle-aged population of 2000 the bone mineral concentration was measured as $1.0\,g\,cm^2$ with a standard deviation of $0.01\,g\,cm^2$. What would be the expected number of people having a bone mineral concentration of $0.98\,g\,cm^2$ from this population?

$$t = \frac{0.98 - 1.0}{0.01} = -2.0$$

Consulting a table of t values gives a probability value of 0.023 for $t = 2.0$ and $2000 \times 0.023 = 46$, which would be the expected number of normals having this low value in our population of 2000.

The probability of recording a certain count value is calculated in Box 1.12. Since factorials are used this example uses low count values. The variance of this distribution is

$$\sigma^2 = (x - m)^2 = m \qquad (1.38)$$

The standard deviation of a Poisson distribution is $\sqrt{m}$. This is very useful in radiology when the distribution or noise of a particular measurement is required. If a particular count is 100 the expected noise or signal variation would be 10 or 10% whereas if the count is increased to 10 000 the expected noise is 100, reducing its effect to 1%.

The Poisson distribution may only be applied in cases where the expectation of m is constant from reading to reading as would be the case when collecting counts for a fixed period of time.

NORMAL OR GAUSSIAN DISTRIBUTION

The frequency of occurrence of a certain random event can be assigned to the mathematical families described by the binomial or Poisson distributions. While these distributions enable the study of discrete events (i.e. probability of occurrence or counts seen per unit time) it does not allow the study of continuous random variable distributions where the investigation does not involve individual counts or events but estimations or measurements of the entire population are made.

Continuous variables seen in radiology would be:

• Weight of individuals in a population
• Attenuation coefficient of separate tissue samples (e.g. bone) in a population
• Uptake of radioactive tracer in normal tissue of a population group

• Bone mineral concentration in a population
• T1 and T2 times of various discrete tissue types

If a large number of events described by these examples are recorded then the Poisson distribution approaches a continuous distribution shown by the curve envelope in Fig. 1.12a. This is a bell-shaped curve commonly referred to in statistics which describes a continuous, normal or Gaussian distribution (K.F. Gauss, 1777–1855; German mathematician). The bell shape is described by the general formula

$$y = \frac{1}{\sigma\sqrt{2\pi}} \cdot \exp(t^2/2) \qquad (1.39)$$

where $t = x - \bar{x}/\sigma$. The normal curve extends to infinity in either direction (asymptotic) and the area under the curve represents probability and the constant $1/\sqrt{2}$ ensures that the total area is unity. The parameter σ in eqn 1.39 is the standard deviation of the mean value x.

Probability tables can be used for estimating the number of items in a certain population which would fall into a specified standard deviation band and Box 1.13 gives an example of their use in a calculation concerning numbers of individuals in a population having a certain bone density. The standard deviation will be described later.

1.13.2 Measures for data spread

The crudest measure of overall spread is the distance between highest and lowest data values; this is the

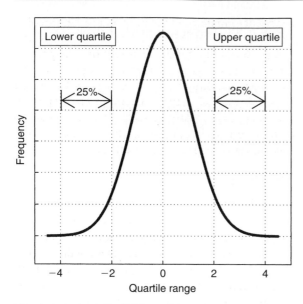

Figure 1.13 *Quartile divisions of the normal curve.*

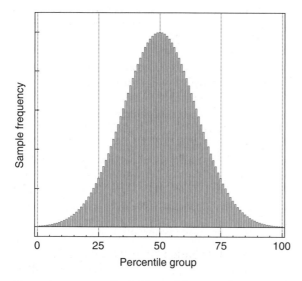

Figure 1.14 *Percentile divisions of the normal curve.*

range but this is strongly influenced by **outlier** presence or abnormally high or low values.

The population can be simply divided into four groups (Fig. 1.13) giving **quartiles**. The lower quartile being the lowest 25% and the upper quartile being the highest 25%, the inter-quartile range occupies the middle 50% and is a good measure of dispersion, being immune from outlier interference. The median and quartiles are special cases of a general scheme for dividing a distribution by **quantiles**. The normal distribution can be divided into 100 equal portions to give a

Table 1.6 *Data for exposure dose during chest radiography plotted in Fig. 1.15a.*

Dose, x (mSv)	Frequency, f	The product fx
0.1	98	9.8
0.2	160	32.0
0.3	120	36.0
0.4	65	26.0
0.5	45	22.5
0.6	15	9.0
0.7	7	4.9
0.8	3	2.4
0.9	1	0.9
Totals	$\Sigma f = 514$	$\Sigma fx = 143.5$

percentile distribution. Figure 1.14 shows this division. This is useful for representing radiology patient dose levels since dose reference levels (DRLs) take the 75th percentile as the acceptable dose limit.

The data in Table 1.6 show a frequency range stretching from an exposure dose of 0.1 to 0.9 mSv but from 0.6 onwards only small numbers are involved and this range of figures gives a false impression. Other measures of dispersion are therefore required. The data given in this table are plotted in Fig. 1.15a. These measurements represent the surface doses reported by various hospitals for chest radiography. The itemized dose values x, their frequency of occurrence f and the product of fx listed in the table are used in calculations. These data show a skewed distribution and separate mean, median and mode values of the distribution can be identified in the figure.

THE MEAN

The arithmetic mean $\bar{x}$ is the most common average value quoted for a set of data and is commonly found by adding together the individual values and dividing by the number of items. The data set featured as a grouped frequency distribution in Table 1.6 does not lend itself to this method of calculation so the mean is calculated from the frequency distribution in the table as

$$\bar{x} = \frac{\sum fx}{\sum f} \tag{1.40}$$

where Σf and Σfx values are the sum values. The arithmetic mean value for this data set is 0.28 and is marked on Fig. 1.15a.

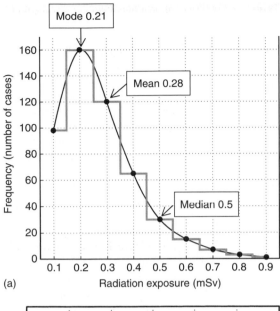

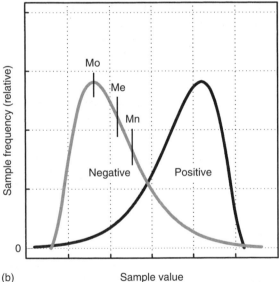

Figure 1.15 *(a) Data example of chest exposure during plain film radiography representing the spread of entrance dose from a selection of hospitals. These data are used to calculate the mode, mean and median of this negative skewed distribution. (b) Continuous distributions showing negative and positive skewness. The mean Mn, mode Mo and median Me points are marked.*

THE MEDIAN

This is the value of the item x which lies in the center of the distribution with half the data on one side and half on the other. It is calculated as $(n + 1)/2$ where n is

the number of items in the distribution. The median of the data plotted in Fig. 1.15a is 0.5. If the position of the central point in the distribution is important then the median can be a useful average. This is the case where the data set contains extreme values which distort the overall picture. The median is immune to these and gives a more correct picture of frequency distribution. The disadvantage, however, is that the median value is unsuitable for calculation.

THE MODE

In some instances neither the mean nor median gives the best description of a data set (this is the case for the skewed distribution in Fig. 1.15a). The mean value is influenced by all the values and does not draw attention to extreme values which may be of significance. The median is the central value, dividing the data set in half but this value may be unrepresentative; so it is in this case. The mode, however, is that value in a data set which occurs most frequently. The mode can be obtained by inspection (roughly) or by calculation (exactly) using the formula

$$\text{mode} = L + \frac{f_m - f_L}{(f_m - f_L) + (f_M - f_H)} \times C \quad (1.41)$$

where L is the lower limit of the modal group (0.15) as the class intervals are 0.5–1.5, 1.5–2.5, etc.; f_M is the frequency of the modal group (160); f_L the frequency of the neighboring lower group (98) and f_H the frequency of the higher neighboring group (120). The class or item interval distance C is 0.1. Using this equation the exact modal value is found to be 0.21.

The mean, mode and median values are identical in a normal distribution but if the distribution is not normal, containing extreme values (larger or smaller) then the distribution is skewed and the mean, mode and median do not coincide; negative and positive skewed distributions are demonstrated in Fig. 1.15b. These are commonly found in image distribution maps where localized high count regions (organ uptake) will skew the data.

1.13.3 Standard deviation

A more stable value of data spread in a distribution comes from calculating how each variable differs from the mean value. This is the derivation of **variance** and the square root of the variance is the standard

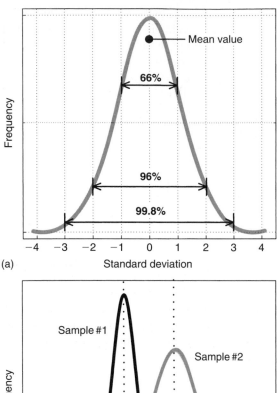

(a)

(b)

Figure 1.16 *(a) The standard deviation plotted on the x-axis and the areas under the normal curve that they cover. (b) Sample spread showing sample #1 with a narrow standard deviation and sample #2 with a larger standard deviation. These samples could be from different populations (e.g. diseased and normal).*

deviation, σ. Standard deviations have been calculated already for binomial and Poisson distributions. A continuous distribution of n items requires a more complex calculation, however:

$$\sigma = \sqrt{\frac{\sum (x - \bar{x})^2}{n - 1}} \qquad (1.42)$$

The normal distribution shown in Fig. 1.16a plots the standard deviation as the x-axis, the various areas

Table 1.7 *Coefficient of variation (CV).*

Observed count	σ	CV (%)
10	± 3.2	31.6
100	± 10.0	10.0
1000	± 31.6	3.16
10 000	± 100.0	1.0

of the normal curve and shows that the area covered from $\sigma = -1$ to $+1$ is 66% and from σ -2 to $+2$ covers 96% and $\sigma = -3$ to $+3$ covers 99.8%.

The two sample populations shown in Fig. 1.16b are of different sizes and give different standard deviations. They could be superimposed so giving the same mean value but their standard deviation value would distinguish them.

STANDARD ERROR

When samples are taken from a large population there is always an uncertainty between the sample mean and the parent population mean (the mean value for the entire count distribution). This is simply measured as

$$\text{standard error} = \frac{\sigma}{\sqrt{n}} \qquad (1.43)$$

The standard error becomes smaller as the number of items increases. The standard error is most useful when calculating confidence limits which a selected quality control measurement should keep within.

COEFFICIENT OF VARIATION

A measure of spread within the sample uses the standard deviation expressed as a percentage of the mean:

$$\text{CV} = \frac{\sigma}{\bar{x}} \times 100 \qquad (1.44)$$

where CV is the coefficient of variation, in percent. From Table 1.7 it can be seen that larger sample sizes give smaller variations.

1.13.4 Statistics of counting

There will always some degree of error when collecting count data for imaging or sample quantification. The sample accuracy or image quality depends on the number of counts taken or stored, as seen in

Table 1.7. If the total counts collected are 100, 1000, 10 000 then the standard deviations are roughly 10, 32 and 100 showing that it requires about 1000 counts to achieve a coefficient of variation of 3%. To express the deviation in terms of counting rate the total time taken is used as a divisor. For 1000 counts in 10 s the deviation is

$$\sqrt{\frac{1000}{10}} = 10 \text{ counts s}^{-1} \qquad (1.45)$$

The counting rate would be expressed as 100 ± 10 counts s^{-1} which indicates that there is a 68.3% probability (1σ) that the counting error is >10 counts s^{-1} or 10%. If 10 000 counts are collected over 100 s the uncertainty remains the same (10 counts s^{-1}) but the accuracy is now 1%. The greater the number of counts collected (which could be met either as a count rate sample or in an image pixel) the smaller the error due to statistical fluctuations.

BACKGROUND COUNTS

There is always a background count due to either natural radiation or interfering radiation sources. These can be caused by:

- Other radioactive sources in the vicinity, for example patients, natural radiation or other active samples, in the case of sample counting
- Scattered radiation from other parts of the body in the case of radiography

When the sample count is large compared with the background the standard error can be estimated with little error. When the background and sample counts are not greatly different then the background must be considered. It should be noted that percentages and ratios are comparative measurements and so should not be used as data in any form of statistical analysis.

SAMPLING INTERVAL

This plays an important role when measuring dynamic events. Figure 1.17 illustrates two sampling intervals A and B. The under-sampling in A misses detail of the fast changes in the initial stages of a tissue or organ uptake which is shown in B having many more samples. Over-sampling does not add to the information but requires more storage space and takes longer to analyze.

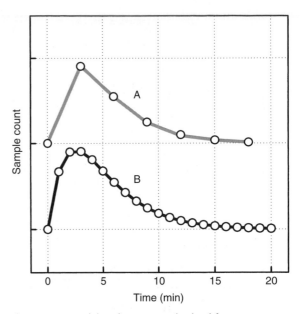

Figure 1.17 *Activity–time curves obtained from a glomerular filtration rate study. Under-sampling (**A**) misses the fast vascular changes revealed in (**B**), which has more samples.*

1.13.5 Sample data analysis

Problems which require the use of statistics can usually be reduced to one of three basic tests:

- A **significant difference** between two data sets from different populations
- Finding a trend in a sample: the **regression**
- Testing for the similarity between samples: the **correlation**

DIFFERENCE BETWEEN SAMPLES

This is broadly divided into:

- **Parametric** tests where population quantities are used, i.e. means, variances or standard deviations
- **Non-parametric** tests that do not use population parameters and present the data often in the form of scores or ranks

If we wish to test the hypothesis that two data sets plotted in Fig. 1.16b are significantly different and do not form part of the same larger population, then a simple Student's t-test will indicate if the sample mean value could have come from a population with a known mean and estimated standard deviation value.

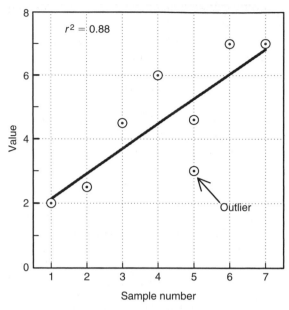

Figure 1.18 *A set of data which shows some positive correlation characteristics (r = 0.88). A regression analysis shows a rough linear relationship using a least squares calculation.*

Most books on statistics will give the basic Student's 't' formula for this computation giving also the corrections that must be made for small sample numbers. More rigorous methods of analysis are available, as for example the analysis of variance (ANOVA) tests for the variance within each sample.

Non-parametric tests that have a lower overall power than their parametric equivalent utilize scores or ranking marks in their data set. These, of course, would be distribution free, not having means, variances or standard deviations. Examples would be a ranking of (say) 1 to 5 to describe the confidence of visualizing a lesion in a particular radiograph, which has been processed in two different ways (gray scale or color for instance).

The Tukey quick test decides whether two independent ranked samples could have been drawn from the same population. A Mann–Whitney test is equivalent to the t-test which scores the difference between the medians of two distributions. The Kruskal–Wallis test is the non-parametric version of an ANOVA.

REGRESSION AND CORRELATION

These tests determine how variables x and y are related linearly. The graph in Fig. 1.18 is a scatter diagram which gives a rough idea how the variables x and y are related (if at all). A number that is a measure of how linear the relationship is between x and y is needed, however: this is the **sample correlation coefficient**, r, ranging from -1 to $+1$. A value of $+1$ indicates a perfect linear relationship, where y increases with x; a value of -1 indicates a perfect negative relationship, where y decreases with x. Zero indicates a total random distribution between x and y.

The correlation coefficient is a measure of the linear relationship between x and y but it does not indicate what the relationship is. It is often necessary to know the trend of the relationship for certain values of x, so that a prediction can be made: if a value for x is given then the probable value of y can be calculated. The slope of the **regression line** will give this.

Both x and y for the correlation coefficient are random variables; the distribution or relationship is not known beforehand. The regression analysis, however, can select certain values of x (fixed population characteristics) so they are not random. The y values retain their random nature since these are not controlled.

KEYWORDS

2π surface: relating to a flat radiation detector
4π surface: relating to a volume radiation detector
abscissa: the horizontal x-axis of a graph. Usually holds the independent variable
coefficient of variation: a measure of dispersion as the standard deviation expressed as a percentage of the mean
correlation coefficient: a measure of association between two random variables. If one variable changes with the other then they are said to be correlated
data set (or set): a collection of numbers that usually have one common property
decimal place: the figures to the right of the decimal point giving a specified degree of accuracy
deterministic: a model where all events are inevitable consequences of antecedent causes. An effect seen at a predefined point (e.g. count rate, dose)
dispersion: the spread of a distribution (see standard deviation and quartile)
e: symbol for the transcendental number 2.718 282. . . used as the base for the natural logarithm (also see exponential)
extrapolation: estimation of a value of a variable beyond known values

exponent: indicator for decimal point shift (left or right) in scientific notation, or in an exponential function x^n then n is the exponent

exponential: most commonly used when the exponent is the power of e. The exponential of x is e^x

floating point: a method of writing real numbers as $a \times 10^n$ or $a\mathrm{E}n$ where $a < 1$ but $\geqslant 0.1$ and n is the integer exponent directing decimal point position '$-$' left, '$+$' right. For example $0.564\mathrm{E}{-}1 = 0.0564$. A format also used in computing

Fourier analysis: a method of waveform analysis

histogram: a chart which displays grouped data

integer: a whole number

interpolation: estimation of a value of a variable between two known values

isotropic: emitting in all directions (spherical emission)

least squares: a way of estimating the best fit straight line for a plotted set of values

logarithm: the power to which a fixed number, the base, must be raised to obtain a given number. Abbreviated to log for base 10 and ln for base e

normal distribution: a continuous distribution of a random variable with its mean, median, and mode equal

null hypothesis: usually based upon the assumption that nothing special is different between two samples. A statistical test challenges this assumption. If the significance of the difference (probability) is sufficiently large then the null hypothesis is rejected

ordinate: the y-axis of a graph

outlier: observation which is far removed from the others in a set

parametric (non-parametric): pertaining to exact measurement (e.g. count density, weights, temperature). Non-parametric measurements are scores or ranks

power law: a function giving a straight line when plotted on log–log axes

quantile: general name for the values of a variable which divide its distribution into equal groups

quartile: the value of a variable below which three quarters (first or upper quartile) or one quarter (third or lower quartile) of a distribution lie

radian (rad): the SI unit of plane angle where 1 rad is $57.2958°$

rational (irrational) number: having a fixed number of decimal places. An irrational number would be π or e

regression: a test which calculates the best fit for a straight line through a set of points on a graph when y is the dependent variable and x the independent (see least squares)

scientific notation: a numerical form similar to floating point: $a \times 10^n$ or $a\mathrm{E}n$ where a is a number 1 to 10 and n is a whole number as before, i.e. $5.64\mathrm{E}{-}2 = 0.0564$

significance: a probability of rejecting the null hypothesis. $p = 0.05$ borderline significance, $p = 0.01$ significant, $p = 0.001$ highly significant

sine wave: a wave function where $y = \sin x$

skew: a distribution where mean, mode, and median do not coincide

standard deviation: a measure of sample dispersion. Square root of the variance

standard error: standard error of the sample mean. A comparison of the sample mean with the parent mean $\sigma/\sqrt{n}$

steradian: the solid angle in spherical geometry

stochastic: an entirely random process

variable, continuous: a variable that may take any value

variable, dependent: a variable dependent on another. Usually placed on the y-axis

variable, discrete: the opposite to continuous. A variable that may only take certain values

variable, independent: a variable not dependent on another. Usually placed on the x-axis

variance: a measure of dispersion

Basic physics for radiology

2.1 INTERNATIONAL SYSTEM OF MEASUREMENT

The early system of measurement used centimeter–gram–second (c.g.s) as the standard but this has been replaced by the meter–kilogram–second–ampere (MKSA) system or the Système International d'Unités (SI units) which is now the standard measurement system in physics. Confusion exists when these two systems are quoted together since the two systems not only differ in their nomenclature but also in defining fundamental quantities.

2.1.1 Basic units

A few SI units have already been given in Chapter 1, a complete set of basic units is given in Table 2.1.

Table 2.1 *SI base units.*

Quantity	Name	Symbol
Length	meter	m
Mass	kilogram	kg
Time	second	s
Temperature	kelvin	K
Electric current	ampere	A
Luminous intensity	candela	cd
Amount of substance	mole	mol

If all the quantities in a calculation are expressed in SI units then the answer will hold the SI unit format.

2.1.2 Derived units

A table of derived SI units is given at the end of this chapter, along with two supplementary units: the **radian** and the **steradian**, which are units for plane and solid angles respectively. Non-metric measurements, e.g. mile, pound, inch and gallon are not used, although certain metric non-SI units are still retained and the equivalent SI units are given in Table 2.2 for these.

Table 2.2 *Frequently encountered non-SI units and their equivalents.*

Non-SI	SI unit	Application
angstrom 10^{-10} m	nanometer 10^{-9} m	Wavelength
micron 10^{-6} m	nanometer 10^{-9} m	Wavelength
erg	joule ($1\,J = 10^7\,erg$)	Energy
curie (Ci)	becquerel ($37\,GBq = 1\,Ci$)	Activity
gm cm^3	kg m^3	Density
mmHg	Pascal ($1.33 \times 10^2\,Pa = 1\,mmHg$)	Pressure

2.2 VELOCITY AND ACCELERATION

2.2.1 Linear velocity (v)

The velocity of a moving point or of a body is the rate of its displacement or the rate at which it changes its position, in a given direction. The rate of displacement of the body is the distance it moves during each unit of time. If it moves through s meters in t seconds then $v = s/t \, \mathrm{N\,m\,s^{-1}}$. Velocity is a vector quantity having both magnitude and direction, but when the direction is constant (a straight line) and the body covers equal distances in equal times, the velocity is uniform and is measured by the displacement per unit time, as above.

Box 2.1 shows the distance traveled by electromagnetic radiation in one nanosecond is 30 cm or approximately 1 foot. Velocity is different from **speed**; speed is the rate of displacement regardless of direction. Velocity and speed are equal only when the body is moving in a straight line, speed can then be changed by a change in magnitude alone, while the velocity of a body can be changed by either a change in its speed or a change in its direction of motion.

2.2.2 Linear acceleration (a)

If the velocity of a moving mass is changing the mass is accelerating. The rate at which the velocity of a mass is increasing is its acceleration, measured as the change of velocity (x/t) per unit time t expressed as 'per second, per second':

$$\text{acceleration} = \frac{x}{t} \, \mathrm{cm\,s^{-1}\,s^{-1}} \qquad (2.1)$$

When the rate of change of velocity is increasing in eqn 2.1, acceleration is $+a$, although the + sign is

Box 2.1 Photon time of flight

The distance traveled by a 0.511 MeV gamma photon after 1 nanosecond (10^{-9} s) can be calculated utilizing the fact that all electromagnetic radiation has a velocity of approximately $3.0 \times 10^{8} \, \mathrm{s^{-1}}$. Therefore,

distance traveled = $(3.0 \times 10^{8}) \times 10^{-9} = 0.3 \, \mathrm{m}$

not usually shown. If the rate of change of velocity is decreasing, the body is retarding (or decelerating), and this is negative acceleration $-a$. Acceleration due to **gravity** differs according to position on the globe. The measured values vary from $9.780 \, \mathrm{m\,s^{-2}}$ on the equator to $9.832 \, \mathrm{m\,s^{-2}}$ at the North Pole. These values of g are influenced by both gravity and rotation of the Earth; the approximate value of $9.8 \, \mathrm{m\,s^{-2}}$ is taken as the general value.

SUMMARY: UNITS OF LINEAR VELOCITY

SI	$\mathrm{m\,s^{-1}}$	
c.g.s	$\mathrm{cm\,s^{-1}}$	$1 \, \mathrm{cm\,s^{-1}} = 1 \times 10^{-2} \mathrm{m\,s^{-1}}$
Other	miles $\mathrm{hr^{-1}}$	$1 \, \mathrm{m.p.h.} = 0.44 \, \mathrm{m\,s^{-1}}$

2.3 FORCE AND MOMENTUM

These fundamental concepts play an important role in X-ray tube design since a heavy rotating metal anode gives considerable problems concerning force and **momentum**.

2.3.1 Force (F)

Richard Feynman (1918–1988; US physicist) remarked that to seek a precise definition of force is futile. The question is complex because as well as **gravitational** force, there are three other distinct fundamental forces: **electromagnetic** (or Coulomb), **strong** and **weak** forces. Gravitational and electromagnetic forces are long range 'macro' forces; strong and weak forces are very short range nuclear forces.

The gravitational force with which the Earth attracts a body is the weight of a body; its mass is the amount of substance in the body. Weight differs according to the object's position on Earth. The **newton** (N) is the gravitational force F which gives a mass of 1 kg an acceleration of $1 \, \mathrm{m\,s^{-2}}$, so

$$F = ma \qquad (2.2)$$

All objects fall with the same acceleration due to the Earth's gravity which is about $9.8 \, \mathrm{m\,s^{-2}}$ (neglecting air resistance). The force on a mass of 1 kg due to gravity, from eqn 2.2, is $1 \times 9.8 = 9.8$ N; mass and weight are proportional (mass $\propto$ weight). A common balance compares masses but a spring balance will indicate weights since it will be influenced by gravity.

Box 2.2 Mammography compression paddle

Assume that the stated maximum range (F) is 150–200 N. Since mass $m = F/a$ and acceleration due to gravity $a = 9.8\,\mathrm{m\,s^{-2}}$ the actual pressure felt by the patient under maximum compression is equivalent to 15 to 20 kg.

Box 2.3 Radiation dosimetry: nuclear recoil

We will use the ^{238}U nuclear recoil due to alpha particle emission as an example. The nuclear mass m_n due to 92 protons and 146 neutrons is $3.97 \times 10^{-25}\,\mathrm{kg}$. The mass of an alpha particle (m_α) (two protons and two neutrons) is $6.68 \times 10^{-27}\,\mathrm{kg}$. The velocity of the alpha particle (v_α) is measured as $6.25 \times 10^7\,\mathrm{m\,s^{-1}}$. The original nucleus, before emission of the alpha particle, is at rest so linear momentum is zero (v_n and $v_\alpha = 0$). Conservation of momentum requires that $m_n v_n + m_\alpha v_\alpha = 0$. The nuclear recoil velocity (v_n), which is a minus value, is therefore

$$-\left(\frac{m_\alpha}{m_n}\right) \times v_\alpha = 1.05 \times 10^6\,\mathrm{m\,s^{-1}}$$

Box 2.2 shows how the pressure delivered by a mammography compression paddle is calculated in newtons.

To resolve the ambiguity in the meaning of the word 'weight' it is important to differentiate between whether mass or force is meant. This can be achieved by using SI units properly, i.e. using kilograms when mass is intended and newtons where force is intended. A gravitational force can also be defined as an agency which tends to change the momentum of a body, and can be measured as the rate of change of **momentum** it produces; being proportional to the rate of increase of momentum mv. Force is therefore given as

$$F = \frac{\mathrm{d}(mv)}{\mathrm{d}t} = \frac{m\,\mathrm{d}v}{\mathrm{d}t} = ma \qquad (2.3)$$

Objects have a reluctance to move when they are at rest. They also have a reluctance to stop when they are moving; this is the object's inertia. An applied force must overcome this inertia before the body can be set in motion, or before the direction of its motion, or the rate at which it is moving, can be changed. The braking force required to bring an object to rest depends on time to rest. Rotating parts in radiology (X-ray tube anode, fan beam assembly in computed tomography) produce problems during acceleration and braking; in practice their momentum change is reduced by decreasing the object mass.

To illustrate the conservation of momentum consider the worked example in Box 2.3 which calculates the recoil velocity of a uranium nucleus undergoing alpha emission. Radiation dosimetry, to some extent, considers the recoil velocity of the nucleus. The range of the alpha particle and recoiling nucleus in matter (tissue) is very short and the energy is deposited very close to the location of the decay. However, for an ingested radionuclide this may be near a radiosensitive area (e.g. DNA).

2.3.2 Linear momentum (p)

When a force has set a body in motion, the body is stopped only by the application of other forces (such as friction, braking, magnetic force). The moving body possesses linear momentum; the product of the mass (m) and the velocity (v) of the body, so $p = mv$. Since force is momentum change per second (mass × velocity change) and velocity change per second is acceleration a then momentum change (ΔI) is also described by $F = ma$. The **conservation of momentum** is a fundamental law of physics which is central when considering elastic and inelastic collisions between objects (radiation and orbital electrons). Although there may be a change in energy the total momentum is conserved. The recoil of a nucleus after emission of a particle is an example of the conservation of momentum as described in Box 2.3.

FRICTION

Friction causes energy losses which are commonly seen as an increase in system heat. Since friction always opposes motion a moving body experiences a frictional force. This is not confined to solids, it is also experienced by fluids and gases, and is caused by viscous drag between layers of molecules.

SUMMARY

Units of mass

SI	kilogram, kg	Kilogram
c.g.s.	gram, g	$1\,g = 1 \times 10^{-3}\,kg$
Other	pound, lb	$1\,lb \approx 0.45359\,kg$

Units of force

SI	newton, N	$1\,N = 1\,m\,kg\,s^{-2}$
c.g.s.	dyne, dyn	$1\,dyn = 1\,cm\,g\,s^{-2} = 10^{-5}\,N$

2.4 ROTATIONAL MOTION

Rotational motion (angular velocity, momentum and acceleration) is concerned with particle motion (e.g. nucleus, electrons) in an angular or circular orbit and will become more familiar when nuclear magnetic resonance is discussed.

If a force is being applied to a disk or wheel so as to produce rotary motion, variation of the force will usually cause a proportional variation in the speed of rotation and therefore of the kinetic energy of the rotating part. Any mass when in motion tends to resist being retarded. In the case of a rotating anode it can be shown that its tendency to preserve its state of motion (its **inertia**) is determined by its mass and its radius. The inertia I of a disk of uniform density having mass M and radius R is given by

$$I = \tfrac{1}{2} MR^2 \qquad (2.4)$$

from which it is seen that the inertia can be increased by increasing either the mass or the diameter of the disk. The mass of the object is a measure of the amount of matter and its inertia and is expressed in kilograms. A fixed point on a uniformly rotating disk or wheel

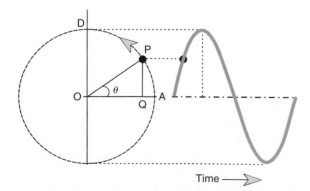

Figure 2.1 *Rotating frame where radius + angular velocity traces a simple sine wave.*

will show a constant speed but since the direction of motion is continuously changing the velocity is not constant. In Fig. 2.1 a point P describes a circular path round the axis O, OA being the radius. Some of these relationships play an important role when describing oscillating functions (particularly electromagnetic waveforms and sound) in terms of frequency, wavelength and phase.

2.4.1 Centripetal acceleration and force

When a mass m moves with a circular motion of radius r with uniform velocity v there is an acceleration toward the center called the **centripetal acceleration** (a) acting radially inward, where $a = v^2/r$. Although the circular motion has uniform velocity its direction is continuously changing, so the body experiences acceleration toward the center; the velocity changes only in direction, not in magnitude. The inward force that must be applied to keep the body moving in a circle is the **centripetal force** (F) where $F = m(v^2/r)$. It is sometimes convenient to picture a counteracting force acting radially outward termed the **centrifugal force**. Box 2.4 calculates the forces involved in a rotating arm of a computed tomography (CT) system having a section time of 0.5 s, a radius of 0.6 m and a mass of 100 kg. The considerable force of almost $10\,000\,N$ must be carefully balanced and places very high demands on mechanical precision and robust construction.

2.4.2 Angular velocity (ω)

This is the rate at which the angle (θ) between OP and OA changes; the angular velocity of point P about O

Box 2.4 CT fan beam support and X-ray tube

Calculate the centripetal/centrifugal forces on a CT X-ray tube and support of mass 100 kg and 0.6 m radius revolving at 0.5 s or 2 revolutions per second.

Force $= ma = m(v^2/r)$
Velocity $= 2\pi r \times 2\,m\,s^{-1} = 7.54\,m\,s^{-1}$

Therefore, the centripetal or centrifugal force is

$$\left(\frac{100 \times 7.54^2}{0.6} \right) = 9466\,N$$

(Fig. 2.1). It is the angle θ in radians that would be swept by the radius in 1 s. As P rotates uniformly, angle θ will increase uniformly with time, and the angular velocity will be a constant value. As P rotates anticlockwise from A toward D the length of the perpendicular PQ increases as the angle θ increases, and for any given position of P, $\sin\theta = \text{PQ/OP}$ but since OP is fixed as the radius, then $\sin\theta \propto \text{PQ}$ and its magnitude traces a **sine wave**. Angular velocity is related to linear velocity v by $\omega = v/r$. For a constant speed the angular velocity (or **frequency**) ω is the number of complete revolutions per second. One revolution is $2\pi r$ so angular velocity can be expressed as $\omega = 2\pi/t$ or $2\pi v$ rad s^{-1}; the time t to complete one revolution. Box 2.5 describes an anode of length 100 mm rotating at constant angular velocity ω (or angular frequency).

ANGULAR DISPLACEMENT (θ)

Angular displacement (θ) is the angular change in angular motion defined as $\theta = x/r$ where x is the linear displacement and r the radius of angular motion. Since r (the radius) is fixed then $\theta \propto x$. Angular displacement is in radians (rad) where $360° = 2\pi$ rad and 1 rad $= 57.3° = 180°/\pi$ rad.

ANGULAR ACCELERATION (α)

Angular acceleration (α) is the rate of change in angular velocity; related to linear acceleration (a) by $\alpha = a/r$ or v^2/r.

Box 2.5 The rotating anode of an X-ray tube

For an anode radius (r) of 100 mm (i.e. 0.1 m), mass (m) of 2.0 kg, rotating at 9000 revolutions per minute, the angular velocity, moment of inertia, angular momentum, and linear velocity are:

Angular velocity:
$\omega = 9000 \times 2\pi \times 1/60 = 942.5$ rad s^{-1}

Alternatively, $\omega = v/r = 942.5$ rad s^{-1}.

Moment of inertia: $I = \frac{1}{2}mr^2 = 0.01$ kg m^2
Angular momentum: $L = I\omega = 9.425$ kg m^2 s^{-1}
Linear velocity: $2\pi r \times (\text{rpm}/60) = 94.25$ m s^{-1}

Alternatively, $v = \omega r = 942.5 \times 0.1$ m $= 94.25$ m s^{-1}, or just over 200 mph.

ANGULAR MOMENTUM

If a body of mass m is in circular or rotational motion, its linear velocity, in the direction of the tangent to the circle at any given moment, is v. Its linear momentum is mv. Its linear velocity is equal to the product of its angular velocity ω and the radius r of its circle of motion, so that $v = \omega r$. Linear momentum is mv or $m\omega r$. Rotational motion is described by its angular momentum, a vector quantity $m\omega r^2$. Angular momentum may be changed by applying a **torque** to the rotating body. An applied torque may increase or decrease the rotation motion, or it may change the direction of the rotation axis. Angular momentum is a quantity that is used to describe rotation motion of an object with mass. Angular momentum is also a vector quantity. Electrons and protons possess an intrinsic magnetic moment that is distinct from any 'orbital' motion, associated with and proportional to the 'spin' angular momentum of the particle. Box 2.6 calculates the angular momentum of the electron orbit in a hydrogen atom.

TORQUE (τ)

Torque (τ) is the effective force on a rotating body turning the body about its center or pivot point. The torque exerted by a force is also known as the moment of the force. It will be further described in the chapter on magnetic resonance imaging. Angular momentum may be changed by applying a torque to the rotating body. An applied torque may increase or decrease the rotation motion, or it may change the direction of the rotation axis. For rotating objects, torque (t) is equal to the time rate of change of angular momentum. When an object possesses angular momentum and a **magnetic dipole moment** is placed in a uniform external magnetic field, the resulting motion can be complex. A torque will be produced which will cause a rotation motion at a constant angular frequency. This is referred to as the 'precession frequency'. Table 2.3 compares the linear and angular quantities.

The value of the angular momentum is a very important physical constant, designated $\hbar$ (h-bar), from which Planck's constant (h) can be derived since $h = 2\pi\hbar$. From the value calculated in Box 2.6 this is 6.62×10^{-34} to three significant figures or $6.6260755 \times 10^{-34}$ to eight significant figures. Planck's constant is discussed in more detail later in this chapter.

Box 2.6 The electron orbit of a hydrogen atom and angular momentum of an electron

Electron orbit

An electron moves in a circular orbit at constant velocity. Given that the radius r of the orbit $= 0.5 \times 10^{-10}$ m, then:

Linear velocity of the electron $= 2.2 \times 10^6$ m s^{-1}

Since $\omega = v/r = (2.2 \times 10^6)/(0.5 \times 10^{-10})$ then

Angular velocity $\omega = 4.4 \times 10^{16}$ s^{-1}
Angular acceleration $\alpha = v^2/r = 9.7 \times 10^{22}$ m s^{-2}
(where s^{-2} is s^{-1} s^{-1})

Angular momentum

To calculate the angular momentum (L) of an orbiting electron in a hydrogen atom take the radius r as 5.29×10^{-11} m, the rest mass, m, of an electron as 9.11×10^{-31} kg, and the linear velocity v as 2.2×10^6 m s^{-1}.

Angular momentum is

$$L = mr^2\omega,$$

where ω is the **angular velocity**

$$= v^2/r = 4.4 \times 10^{16} \text{ rad s}^{-1}$$

$$= 1.054 \times 10^{-34} \text{ kg m}^2 \text{ s}^{-1}$$

2.5 DENSITY AND PRESSURE

2.5.1 Density

The physical **density** of a body ρ is its mass (kg) divided by its volume (m^3). The density will be the same for any object made of the identical material; it will vary if the material's composition is changed. The density of a substance ρ is its weight relative to volume, so:

$$\rho = \frac{\text{mass}}{\text{volume}} \tag{2.5}$$

The SI unit is kg m^3 although non-SI g cm^3 is often used. A conversion factor of 10^3 converts g cm^3 to kg m^3. So if 50 g of aluminum displaces 18.5 cm^{-3} of water its density is

$$\rho = \frac{50}{18.5} = 2.70 \text{ g cm}^{-3} \text{ or } 2700 \text{ kg m}^{-3}$$

The densities of elements (e.g. aluminum, tungsten, uranium) usually follow their atomic number (Z) but there are exceptions, as shown in Table 2.4. Water has a density of 1000 kg m^{-3} (1 g cm^{-3}) and this liquid is used as a reference for density measurements. The relative density for aluminum is therefore just 2700. The density of a substance divided by the density of water is the specific gravity or relative density; for a gas the relative substance is usually air.

THE MOLE

The mole is the amount of substance which contains as many elementary entities as there are atoms in

Table 2.4 *Density of some materials.*

Z	Material	Density (kg m^{-3})
	Air	1.225
	Water	1 000
	Muscle	1 000
	Fat	900
	Bone	1 650 to 1 800
13	Aluminum	2 700
26	Iron	7 870
29	Copper	8 900
42	Molybdenum	10 200
73	Tantalum	16 600
74	Tungsten	19 320
76	Osmium	22 480
79	Gold	19 300
82	Lead	11 340

Table 2.3 *Linear and angular parameters compared.*

Linear parameter	Angular parameter
distance l (m)	angle θ (rad)
velocity v (m s^{-1})	angular velocity ω (rad s^{-1})
acceleration a (m s^{-2})	angular acceleration α (rad s^{-2})
mass m	moment of inertia, I
force $F = ma$	torque $\tau = I\alpha$
momentum $p = mv$	angular momentum $L = I\omega$
work $W = Fs$	work $W = \tau\theta$
power $P = Fv$	power, $P = \tau\omega$
kinetic energy $\frac{1}{2}mv^2$	kinetic energy $\frac{1}{2}I\omega^2$

Box 2.7 Molar quantities

As an example calculate how much solid sodium chloride is needed to make 1 L of a 1 molar solution (saline).

Sodium chloride has a molecular weight of $23 + 35 = 58$ and so 58 g are required to make 1 L of a 1 M solution. Similarly, 5.8 g are required to make 1 L of a decimolar solution (0.1 M).

Table 2.5 *Electron density in common elements relevant to radiology.*

Element	Z	A	e ($\times 10^{23}$)
H	1	1	6.02
O	8	16	3.01
N	7	14	3.01
C	6	12	3.01
I	53	127	2.50
Ba	56	138	2.44
Pb	82	207	2.38

0.012 kg of carbon (^{12}C). The elementary entities may be atoms, molecules, ions, electrons or other particles, or groups of particles, as shown in Box 2.7. The number of elementary particles is a constant known as **Avogadro's constant** and is 6.022×10^{23} mol^{-1} atoms per mole. The atoms per unit mass $= N/A$, where A is atomic mass. Since Z (atomic number) also represents the number of electrons then electron density $e = N \times (Z/A)$. From Table 2.5 it can be seen that lighter elements have greater electron density. This plays an important part in X-ray interactions.

2.5.2 Pressure

Pressure is caused by the weight of material pressing on its surface or by collisions of atoms or molecules of gas within a container (e.g gas radiation detectors), where it acts in all directions. The SI unit is the **pascal** (B. Pascal, 1623–62; French mathematician) and one pascal (1 Pa) equals $1 \, N \, m^{-2}$. Atmospheric pressure is about 1.01×10^5 Pa or approximately $10^5 \, N \, m^{-2}$. The non-SI unit, mmHg, is used extensively in medicine and is retained by agreement. It is related to the pascal: 1 mmHg $= 1.33 \times 10^2$ Pa.

Standard atmospheric pressure previously given as 760 mmHg is now taken as 10^5 Pa. Pressure p is defined as the force per unit area ($N \, m^{-2}$):

$$p = \frac{F}{A} \qquad (2.6)$$

where F is the total force on the surface and A is the surface area. Hence pressure is not the same as force and the result of eqn 2.6 is measured in newtons per square meter ($N \, m^{-2}$). This is true for incompressible substances: solids and liquids.

Box 2.2 has already demonstrated how the compression force of a mammography compression paddle can be represented in newtons.

GAS LAWS

The effects of varying the pressure, volume, and temperature of a gas are described by Boyle's law (Robert Boyle, 1627–91; Irish physicist) and Charles' law (J.A. Charles, 1746–1823; French physicist). Together these laws form basic relationships in physics and also feature in the propagation of sound through air. Boyle's law states that pressure is inversely proportional to volume at constant temperature and Charles' law states that volume and temperature are proportional at constant pressure. Summarizing these two statements gives

$$\frac{PV}{T} = \text{constant} \qquad (2.7)$$

The gas laws play an important academic role in the derivation of the SI scale for temperature. The increase in volume per unit volume of gas at 0°C per °C rise in temperature, keeping pressure constant, forms a volume coefficient a:

$$\frac{\text{increase in volume from 0°C}}{\text{original volume at 0°C} \times \text{temperature rise}} \qquad (2.8)$$

This is a constant whose accurate measurements indicate a value of 3.6609×10^{-3} or 1/273.15°C^{-1} for all gases. Charles' law states that a given mass of gas increases by 1/273.15 of its volume at 0°C for every degree rise in temperature at constant pressure. Lord Kelvin (1824–1907; British physicist) originated his kelvin temperature scale where 0°C is 273.15 K and 0 K (zero K or absolute zero) is −273.15°C; the magnitude of each division is identical: 1°C is the same size as 1 K. The **kelvin** (K) is the SI unit of temperature.

STANDARD TEMPERATURE AND PRESSURE (STP)

In order to make comparisons (e.g. relative density) many measurements are made at standard temperature and pressure (STP). The standard temperature is 298.15 K (25°C) and the pressure is 10^5 Pa (about 760 mmHg).

SUMMARY

Force, mass, momentum and radiology density, pressure and radiology.

Units of density

SI	$kg\,m^{-3}$	
c.g.s.	$g\,cm^{-3}$	$1\,g\,cm^{-3} = 1 \times 10^{-3}\,kg\,m^{-3}$
Other	$lb\,ft^{-3}$	$1\,lb\,ft^{-3} = 16.0\,kg\,m^{-3}$

Units of pressure

SI	pascal, Pa	$1\,Pa = 1\,N\,m^{-2}$
		$= 1\,m^{-1}kg\,s^{-1}$
c.g.s.	$dyn\,cm^{-2}$	$1\,dyn\,cm^{-2}$ (μbar)
		$= 10^{-1}\,Pa$
Other	mmHg;	$1\,mmHg \approx 133.322\,Pa$
	atmosphere	$1\,atm \approx 101\,325\,Pa$

2.6 WORK, ENERGY, AND POWER

Units of work, energy, and amount of heat are physical quantities of the same dimension and should therefore be measured in a common unit.

2.6.1 Work

When a force F moves a body a certain distance d the work done is $F \times d$ and is measured in **joules** (J). Work W is the force F multiplied by the distance d moved by the force:

$$W = F \times d \qquad (2.9)$$

One joule of work is done by a force of 1 N moving through a distance of 1 m or $1\,J = 1\,N\,m$. The capacity to do work involves either kinetic energy or potential energy.

Work done by constant pressure, as seen in pumps such as the heart, is $W = PV$ where P is force per unit area and V the volume. The example shown in Box 2.8 describes the work done by the human heart, at rest and exercise.

Box 2.8 The cardiac stress test

Use the formula $W = PV$. Cardiac output, at rest, is approximately 5 L of blood per minute. Since $1\,L = 10^{-3}\,m^3$ then the volume of blood pumped per second is $8.3 \times 10^{-5}\,m^3$. Taking the average systolic/diastolic pressure in the left ventricle as 100 mmHg or $1.33 \times 10^4\,Pa$ (where $1\,mmHg = 1.33 \times 10^2\,Pa$) and the average right ventricle pressure as 20 mmHg or $2.66 \times 10^3\,Pa$, then the work done by left ventricle is 1.1 J and that done by the right ventricle is 0.22 J, giving a total **work** at rest as 1.32 J per contraction or a **power** rating of 1.32 W. Under strenuous exercise conditions cardiac output can rise to 30 L with average pressures at 120 mmHg and 25 mmHg. This would increase the work done by the rapidly beating heart to approximately 10 J or a power rating of 20 W (120 beats per min).

2.6.2 Energy

Energy is the ability to do work. Work, energy and the amount of heat are physical quantities having the same dimensions and measured in a common unit, the joule – a unification made possible by the SI system, and so the units of energy are also measured in joules. Energy may take the form of **mechanical energy** which can be either **potential energy** or **kinetic energy**. Other forms of energy are **electrical**, **chemical** and **heat**. Potential energy is the energy of a body due to its condition or state. Examples would be given by batteries (power supplies) or gravitation. The amount of potential energy is measured by the work the system performs until the energy source reaches its ground state. Kinetic energy (E_k) increases with mass m and velocity v. If an object is brought to rest in time t the final velocity is zero as $F = ma$ or momentum change per second $= mv/t$. If over distance d, moved by the object in time t, the velocity diminishes uniformly from v to zero, then d = average velocity $\times$ time $= vt/2$.

Work done (kinetic energy) is $E_k = F \times s = (mv/t) \times (vt/2)$, canceling t to give

$$E_k = \frac{1}{2}mv^2 \qquad (2.10)$$

Box 2.9 Energy/mass conversion

As an example we will calculate the fuel consumption (m), per day, in a nuclear power station for a commercial 600 MW advanced light water reactor (LWR). The energy E (in joules) is $(600 \times 10^4) \times (8.64 \times 10^4) = 5.184 \times 10^{13}$ J (where 8.64×10^4 is the number of seconds in 1 day). Since $m = E/c^2$ then, by substituting the appropriate values,

$$m = \frac{5.184 \times 10^{13}}{\left(3 \times 10^8\right)^2} = 5.76 \times 10^{-4} \text{ kg}$$

or just over 0.5 g of fuel per day! Compare this to the many thousands of kilograms of coal or oil consumed by conventional power stations.

Box 2.10 Electron energy

Computer display screen

Calculate the velocity of an electron beam with kinetic energy of 30 kV (a typical applied display tube voltage).

As 1 eV = 1.602×10^{-19} J so 30 keV = 4.906×10^{-15} J. The electron mass is 9.109×10^{-31} kg. Since $E = \frac{1}{2}mv^2$ then $v = \sqrt{2E/m} = 1.02 \times 10^8$ m s^{-1}. The electron is traveling at half the speed of light.

X-ray tube

The applied voltage is 100 keV. Electron beam velocity is 1.87×10^8 m s^{-1} or almost two thirds the speed of light.

This equation defines **kinetic energy**. The forms of kinetic energy include:

- **Translational**, where the entire object moves.
- **Vibrational**, where small masses move back and forth. Simple gas molecules composed of one element (e.g. hydrogen, helium, oxygen) only have translational kinetic energy. More complex gas molecules (e.g. H_2O, NH_3) may have rotational and vibrational kinetic energy.
- **Rotational**, which is given by object spin. The total kinetic energy of a rotating mass is the sum of its rotational kinetic energy about its axis and through its center of mass and its translational kinetic energy of the object's center of mass.

The **conversion of energy** obeys a basic physical law that states: in a given system, the total amount of energy is always constant although the energy may change from one form to another (e.g. electrical energy into light and heat energy). The total amount of energy is obtained by adding the kinetic and potential energies. From the equation $E = mc^2$ a **mass/energy relationship** can be calculated so a 1 kg mass is equivalent to 9×10^{16} J; 1 g is equivalent to 9×10^{13} J. The mass energy transformed in a nuclear power station is calculated in Box 2.9. The resting mass of an electron is 9.1×10^{-31} kg which is equivalent to 8.1985×10^{-14} J or 0.511 MeV. This will be further explored in the section on nuclear medicine.

The electron velocity can be calculated from its kinetic energy. The examples in Box 2.10 show that the kinetic energy of the electron depends on the applied kilovoltage.

2.6.3 Power

Power is the rate of doing work; that is

$$\text{power} = \frac{\text{work done}}{\text{time taken}} \qquad (2.11)$$

In the SI the rate of doing work or the time taken to do an amount of work is given by the **watt** (W), and 1 J = 1 W s. This is defined as the rate of doing work (spending energy) per second. This quantity is frequently too small so the multiple unit watt-hour (Wh) and kilowatt-hour (kWh) are used. Since 1 J is 1 W s, 1 Wh = 3600 J and 1 kWh = 3.6×10^6 J.

Electrical energy is measured in joules and electrical power in watts.

SUMMARY

Work, energy, power, and radiology.

- Mass (units: km) is a measure of inertia. Force (units: N) is mass $\times$ acceleration.
- Momentum is mass $\times$ velocity.
- Work (units: J) is force $\times$ distance.

- Energy (units: J) is the capacity for doing work.
- Power (units: $J s^{-1}$ or W) is the rate of doing work.
- The efficiency of a system is power obtained divided by power supplied. This is never 100% due to heat production and loss.

Units of work and energy

SI	joule, J	$1 J = 1 W s = 1 N m = 1 m^2 kg s^{-2}$
eV		$1.60218 \times 10^{-19} J$
keV		$1.60218 \times 10^{-16} J$
MeV		$1.60218 \times 10^{-13} J$
c.g.s.	erg	$1 erg = 1 cm^2 g s^{-2} = 10^{-7} J$

Units of power

SI	watt, W	$1 W = 1 J s^{-1} = 1 N m s^{-1}$
		$= 1 m^2 kg s^{-3}$
	kW hour	$10^3 W \times (3.6 \times 10^3 s)$
		$= 3.6 \times 10^6 J$
c.g.s.	$erg s^{-1}$	$1 W = 1 \times 10^7 erg s^{-1}$

2.7 HEAT

Heat is a form of energy that gives atoms and molecules increased movement or kinetic energy. Thermodynamics is the study of heat transfer. Since heat is a form of energy it can be measured in joules and watts.

Heat is transmitted from one place to another by **conduction, convection,** and **radiation**. All of these play a very important part in radiology equipment (e.g. X-ray tubes, generators).

2.7.1 Temperature

Two temperature scales are used for measuring change in heat output:

- Celsius or centigrade: On this scale the temperature of melting ice is 0°C and of boiling water is 100°C both at normal pressure $10^5 N m^{-2}$.
- Kelvin: Zero kelvin (0 K) is absolute zero, equivalent to -273.15°C. The melting point of ice is therefore 273.15 K.

(Note that the Fahrenheit scale has now been discontinued in Europe.)

Temperature scales are compared in Table 2.6. The Celsius and Kelvin scales have the same magnitude so a 1° change in either scale is the same. The kelvin is the SI unit and its derivation has been given from the gas laws stated above.

Temperature conversion from Fahrenheit to Celsius uses a polynomial function where:

$$T_f = \frac{9}{5}(T_c + 32) \quad \text{and} \quad T_c = \frac{5}{9}(T_f - 32)$$

$$(2.12)$$

where T_f and T_c are the Celsius or Fahrenheit scales. Since the Celsius and Kelvin scales have the same magnitude conversion is simply $T_c = T_k - 273.15$.

2.7.2 Heat units

The heat capacity of an anode is sometimes expressed in heat units HU for 3-phase and single-phase supply. This is slightly larger than the joules value since it does not consider voltage ripple in these generators: HU = V × mAs. Converting to joules takes account of the voltage ripple in these generators so HU × 0.7 = J. Heat units were common when single-phase and 3-phase electrical generators supplied X-ray sets, since the high voltage electrical supply had a ripple component which produced a cyclic variation in X-ray (and hence heat) production. Contemporary X-ray equipment now uses high frequency supplies for their generators and are virtually constant current; the ripple component is negligible. The heat unit, consequently, has been superseded by measuring heat capacity in joules (J) and heat dissipation in joules per second or watts (W). Table 2.7 compares measures of heat energy. About 4.2 J is required to raise 1 g of water by 1 K, measured as its thermal capacity. When

Table 2.6 *Units of temperature: Fahrenheit, Celsius and kelvin.*

Physical state	°F	°C	K
Absolute zero	−460	−273.15	0
Freezing point water	32	0	273.15
Boiling point water	212	100	373.15

Table 2.7 *Units of heat measure.*

Units	Joule equivalent
Heat unit (HU)	1.4 J (1 J = HU × 0.7)
1 W	$1 J s^{-1}$
1 cal	4.186 J
1 Btu	1055 J
1 kWh	$3.6 \times 10^6 J$

electrons bombard the anode of an X-ray tube their energy is converted into X-rays and heat. Less than 1% of this energy is converted into X-radiation; the rest is heat produced in the target.

For constant-current generators (voltage ripple = zero) the heat loading of an X-ray tube is the product of applied kV, tube current and exposure time. For an X-ray tube operating at 100 kV with a constant tube current of 400 mA the energy delivered is 40 kW. If the exposure time is 0.05 s then 2000 joules (2 kJ) of heat needs to be dissipated; enough energy to boil 5 cm^3 water in 0.05 s.

2.7.3 Heat capacity (C)

This is measured in $J\,K^{-1}$ (or $°C^{-1}$) and is the characteristic of the material independent of its size or shape and is the heat required to raise its temperature by 1 K or 1°C. Heat capacities of common materials are listed in Table 2.8. The thermal capacity of 1 L of water ($4200\,J\,K^{-1}$) is larger than 1 cm^3 of water. It is the characteristic of the material independent of its size or shape. The heat capacity of a body, such as a piece of metal (e.g. an X-ray tube anode), is the heat required to raise a particular mass by 1 degree. It is expressed in joule per kelvin ($J\,K^{-1}$), so heat capacity C = mass × specific heat capacity. The heat capacity of a 2 kg rotating anode if manufactured from copper would be 2×386 or 772 J. However, copper has a low melting point so tungsten, molybdenum or an alloy of titanium, zirconium, and molybdenum (TZM) is used. The relevant heat capacities for a 2 kg anode manufactured from various materials are shown in Table 2.8.

2.7.4 Specific heat or specific heat capacity (c)

This is the heat capacity per kg of the substance. Specific heat capacities are expressed in $J\,kg^{-1}K^{-1}$.

Table 2.8 Heat capacity of anode materials.

Anode material (2 kg)	Heat capacity J K^{-1}
Tungsten	272
Titanium	1046
Zirconium	560
Molybdenum	492
TZM	692

Table 2.9 Specific heats and thermal conductivities of common materials.

Substance	Specific heat (J kg^{-1} K^{-1})	Melting point (°C)	Thermal conductivity (W m^{-1}K^{-1})
Water	4200		0.59
Oil	2130		0.15
Aluminum	910	660	237
Graphite	711	~3550	~130
Titanium	523	1660	23
Copper	386	1083	401
Zirconium	280	1852	22
Molybdenum	246	2607	140
Rhenium	138	3180	48
Tungsten	136	3377	178
Glass	67	1127	0.9–1.3

The **specific heat** of a substance is the heat required to increase the temperature of 1 kg by 1 K (or $°C^{-1}$). So 42 J of heat raises:

2 g water	by 5°C
2 g aluminum	by 20°C
2 g copper	by 50°C

Table 2.9 lists values of specific heat for common substances. The reason for choosing water and oil for heating and cooling liquids is obvious from their capacity to both store and transport heat. Water is a good reservoir for excess heat or a good cooling medium whereas aluminum and copper take up heat rapidly and, since they are also good heat conductors, are able to conduct it away rapidly. The specific heat of gases varies according to pressure.

2.7.5 Heat loss

The speed of heat transfer is measured in watts per meter per kelvin (or Celsius) W m^{-1} K^{-1} ($°C^{-1}$) as **thermal conductivity**. It is the characteristic of the material independent of size or shape. Table 2.9 includes thermal conductivities of some important substances to radiology. For comparison silver has the highest value ($427\,J\,kg^{-1}\,K^{-1}$) and air has one of the lowest: $0.02\,J\,kg^{-1}\,K^{-1}$.

Generally the heat Q gained (or lost) by an object is given by $Q = mc\Delta T$, where m is the mass of the object, c its specific heat capacity and ΔT its temperature change. Since $\Delta T = Q/mc$, a given loss of heat

Table 2.10 *Heat loss from two X-ray tube designs.*

	Conventional	Fluoroscopy
Anode heat storage capacity	426 kJ	1.8 MJ
Anode heat loss	88.75 kJ min^{-1}	672 kJ min^{-1}
Anode heat loss		
Radiation	1.5 kW	9.2 kW
Conduction	negligible	2 kW

Q to the surroundings, the temperature fall ΔT of a small mass of material is greater than a large mass of material at the same temperature. The rate at which a hot solid or liquid cools also depends on the nature and area of its surface, in addition to its temperature, mass and specific heat capacity. Table 2.10 compares heat loss from two X-ray tube designs, one using ball races and the other using sleeve bearings. The latter, owing to its greater surface contact, allows significant heat loss through conduction.

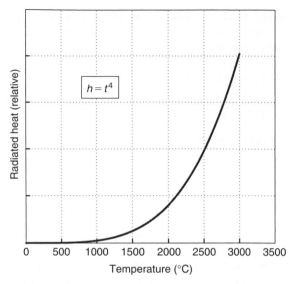

Figure 2.2 *Heat radiated from a surface proportional to the fourth power of its temperature.*

CONDUCTION

The heat transfer can be large for materials with high values of thermal conductivity; these are good heat conductors such as silver and copper. Copper is used for conducting heat in the X-ray tube. Tungsten is a fair conductor of heat but has a high melting point so is ideal for the X-ray tube target. Molybdenum is a poor heat conductor so is used as the anode stem protecting the bearings from conducted heat. Substances with small values would be poor heat conductors but good insulators (air and oil) transfer heat by convection. The **conduction** of heat is by molecular vibration along the material and sets up vibrations which are communicated to other molecules. Heat is transferred along the substance without any alteration in the position of the molecule.

CONVECTION

In liquids heat causes a fluid to expand making it less dense so it rises. The cold, denser fluid takes its place. The heat in this case is carried by moving molecules. This can be achieved by natural **convection** or by pumping (forced convection). In gases the convection of heat occurs more readily since gases expand considerably more when heated. Convection currents in air remove heat from an X-ray tube housing to the atmosphere. Oil and then water circulation (forced convection) remove heat from large X-ray installations (e.g. CT systems).

RADIATION

The transfer of heat by conduction and convection requires a material medium either solid, liquid or gas for its transport, but heat can be transmitted through a vacuum by radiation (infrared).

The radiation from an X-ray tube anode depends on the nature of its surface, temperature t, and surface area A so that the **intensity** I of radiation emitted by a body is proportional to t^4. So a doubling of temperature increases the heat intensity by 2^4 or $\times16$. Conversely, a reduction of surface temperature from 1000°C to 500°C reduces the heat radiated to 6% of the original. The relationship $I \, \alpha t^4$ for a fixed anode size is plotted in Figure 2.2 showing the rate of heat loss increasing rapidly with the temperature of the surface. This is a most important factor when operating an X-ray tube near its maximum rating since heat loss radiated from the anode is highest at this point.

EMISSION AND ABSORPTION

For a given temperature a body radiates most heat when its surface is matt black and least when it is highly polished; graphite is an ideal radiator so it is most useful in the construction of X-ray tube anodes.

A blackened surface is both a good emitter and absorber. A polished surface is a poor absorber and emitter but is a good reflector of heat.

RELEVANCE TO RADIOLOGY

From the simplified sketch of an X-ray tube housing in Fig. 2.3 it is evident that conduction, radiation, and convection play a vital role in removing excess heat from an X-ray tube during operation. The choice of materials and the dimensions influence heat transfer. The tungsten target reaches extremely high temperatures (about 3000°C) and although it has a high melting point it also has a low specific heat so excess heat must be removed quickly. This is achieved by radiation from the anode surface ($\propto t^4$). Surface area is best increased by adding graphite which increases the surface area without adding undue weight. Molybdenum is chosen as a support stem since its low thermal conductivity protects the bearings of the rotating anode (see Table 2.9).

Radiated heat is absorbed by the X-ray tube envelope (glass or ceramic/metal) which is then conducted to an oil bath which loses heat by convection to the atmosphere. Oil is chosen as a heat conducting medium mainly for its insulating properties and high boiling point. Its thermal conductivity is poor but since it has a relatively high specific heat (Table 2.9) it acts as a good heat reservoir.

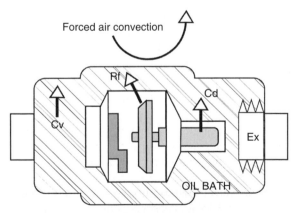

Figure 2.3 *Heat loss from an X-ray tube housing. Heat radiated from the anode (Rf) is conducted away from the glass/ceramic tube case by conduction through the bearing (Cd) and convection currents through the oil (Cv) then by the surrounding atmospheric air. Expansion of the oil is taken up by the bellows (Ex).*

2.7.6 Latent heat

LATENT HEAT (J KG^{-1})

Latent heat ($J\,kg^{-1}$) is the amount of heat per unit mass that is added to or removed from a substance undergoing a change of state, i.e. from solid to liquid or liquid to gas. If heat is applied to ice the temperature of the ice remains at 0°C until all the ice has changed to water. The heat required to change the ice to water is the 'hidden' or 'latent' heat. The **latent heat of fusion** is the quantity of heat required to change 1 g of a solid, at its melting point, to a liquid at the same temperature. Ice has a latent heat of fusion of 336 J. The **latent heat of vaporization** is the quantity of heat required to change 1 g of a substance from a liquid state to a vapor state at its boiling point. This is 2260 J for steam, so a great deal of energy is removed from the system when water changes from liquid to steam.

EVAPORATION

This is the change of liquid to vapor at a temperature below the boiling point. Liquids vary in the ease with which they change. Those which evaporate easily have a low boiling point: they are known as volatile liquids. Latent heat is needed to change from liquid to vapor and this heat is absorbed (taken) from the surface. Liquids with large latent heats (e.g. water) remove heat more effectively. Table 2.11 lists the latent heats for two liquids, water and alcohol, in $MJ\,kg^{-1}$ showing the much larger latent heat for water.

2.7.7 Expansion

Most materials expand when their temperature increases. Gases show the greatest expansion of all on heating. Expansion in metals is measured as a coefficient of linear expansion which is defined as the increase in length, per unit length, for a temperature change of 1 K. An example is given in Box 2.11.

The coefficients of expansion for materials used in radiology are listed in Table 2.12. Expansion causes

Table 2.11 *Latent heats ($MJ\,kg^{-1}$) of two liquids.*

Substance	Latent heat (vaporization)
Water	2.260
Alcohol	0.850

Box 2.11 Expansion of metal

One meter of steel increases its length to 1.10 m when the temperature rises by 90°C.
The linear coefficient of expansion is

$$\frac{1.10}{1000 \times 90} = 1.22 \times 10^{-5} \text{ K}^{-1}$$

Note. As the coefficient is a percentage value no units of measurement are included.

Table 2.12 *Expansion of some common materials.*

Solid	Expansion (10^{-6} K^{-1})
Lead	29.0
Aluminum	25.0
Steel	12.0
Copper	17.0
Molybdenum	5.0
Tungsten	4.0
Glass	9.0–12.0
Glass (Pyrex)	3.0
Invar	0.9

problems in the construction of X-ray tubes where conducting metal contacts are brought out through the insulating glass envelope. The excessive heat produced during X-ray production would cause failure at these joints unless glass and metal are closely matched for their expansion properties. Low expansion glass (Pyrex) and metal alloys are used to achieve this.

The relatively small expansion shown by molybdenum and tungsten makes these ideal metals for X-ray tube construction where considerable heat is experienced, but heavy duty anodes are protected from non-uniform expansion by placing stress cuts along their circumference (Fig. 2.4).

The volumetric expansion of liquids and gases under pressure and the derivation of various gas laws has been discussed in Section 2.5.

HEATING EFFECT BY COMPRESSION

This is the converse of expansion by heating and can only be observed in gases, since solids and liquids are incompressible. Compression increases the gas density so more molecules collide with the surface and therefore more kinetic energy is converted into heat.

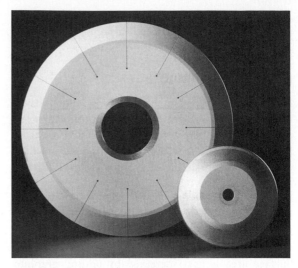

Figure 2.4 *Two anodes of 100 mm and 200 mm diameter. The larger anode showing radial cuts. (Courtesy Philips Medical Inc.)*

2.7.8 X-ray tube rating

The energy rating for X-ray anodes ranges from 250 kJ to 3.5 MJ. Heat dissipation is given in watts or joules per second. Table 2.13 shows some heat ratings for typical X-ray tubes. The anode heat capacity and anode heat dissipation are shown in heat units, joules per minute, and watts.

LOADABILITY

The principal factors affecting the choice of an X-ray tube for a particular application (e.g. conventional X-ray examination, CT, fluoroscopy, mammography) are:

- The maximum tube voltage
- The thermal loadability for short, medium and long exposure times
- The focus size

The thermal loadability of an X-ray tube for short, medium, and long exposures is determined by the anode's heat capacity and heat loss (cooling rate).

An X-ray tube with high loadability, such as used in CT and fluoroscopy, would have a large diameter anode with high heat capacity and an efficient loss of heat through radiation and conductivity through a sleeve rather than ball bearings. Forced cooling (by air,

Table 2.13 *X-ray tube specifications.*

Use	Anode heat capacity	Anode heat dissipation	Anode diameter
Conventional	300 kHU 210 kJ	60 kHU min^{-1} 44.4 kJ min^{-1} 740 W	80 mm
CT	6.3 MHU 4.7 MJ	840 kHU min^{-1} 621.6 kJ min^{-1} 10.3 kW	120 mm
Fluoroscopy	300 kHU 210 kJ	908 kHU min^{-1} 672 kJ min^{-1} 11.2 kW	200 mm

Table 2.14 *Comparison between a modern sleeve bearing X-ray tube (Philips MRC 200) and an earlier tube design using a ball race to support the anode.*

	Conventional ball race	High rating spiral-groove	Increase
Anode heat capacity (AHC)	1688 KJ	1688 KJ	
Anode diameter	113 mm	200 mm	
Focal track diameter	113 mm	180 mm	
Max. cooling rate at max. capacity	5.2 kW	11.2 kW	×2
Cooling rate at 50% capacity	0.6 kW	2.5 kW	×4

oil or water) increases tube loadability. An ideal high-output tube has two distinguishing characteristics:

- An anode disk with a large diameter, providing greater heat radiation and greater heat storage
- Higher conduction through larger surface area sleeve bearings

The anode disk cools by heat radiation. The hotter the disk, the greater the loss of heat radiation. A large disk diameter means increased heat radiation. A smaller disk diameter with the same disk volume means less heat radiation with the same heat capacity. Heat conduction through sleeve bearings provides direct cooling and is more effective than heat radiation at lower temperatures and remains relatively high when little heat storage capacity is used. Table 2.14 shows the significant improvement in loadability for two X-ray tubes: one using a ball race for rotor support and another using sleeve bearings.

The **short-term loadability** is a measure for very short exposure time (0.1 s or less) and is determined by the size of the region which is directly bombarded by the electrons. The focal track of a rotating-anode tube is exposed to direct bombardment by electrons, and therefore represents the region with the highest thermal load. It is this region that determines the short-term loadability.

In a rotating-anode tube, short-term loadability depends on the speed of rotation, the length of the focal track, and on its width. In order to achieve a relatively wide focal track, while keeping the virtual focus size to the minimum, the focal track is traced out on an angled section of the anode. In general, the smaller this angle is, the wider the focal track can be and the short-term loadability will be correspondingly greater. However, the size of the angle is also determined by geometrical considerations, as a given field size at a given source-image distance requires a certain anode angle. At the end of a short exposure, the heat from the focus or focal track is distributed by conduction over the anode disk. If this is not followed by immediate and effective dissipation of the heat from the anode disk, the next exposure can only take place if it is still possible for the heat to be distributed over the anode. As soon as the whole of the anode disk is hot, additional exposures must be postponed until the heat has been dissipated from the anode by radiation or conduction. The heat storage capacity for series of images is determined by the mass of the anode.

Another possibility for X-ray tube design is that of rapidly restoring the heat capacity by providing suitable cooling (heat loss) for the anode. The anode cooling rate determines the **long-term loadability**.

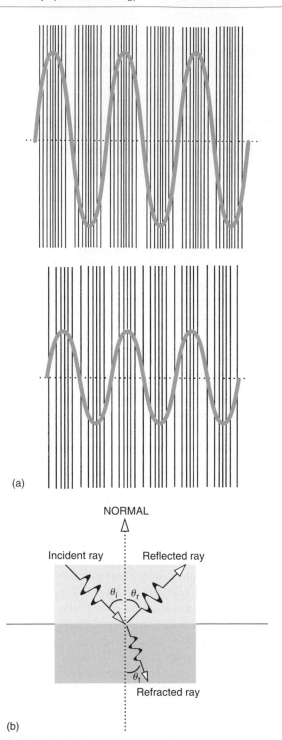

(a)

NORMAL

Incident ray   Reflected ray

θ_i θ_r

θ_t

Refracted ray

(b)

Figure 2.5 *(a) Sound energy transmitted by compression and rarefaction giving a pressure equivalent sine waveform. (b) Reflection and refraction of the incident sound wave. The incident angle θ_i and angles of reflection θ_r and refraction θ_t are marked.*

2.8 SOUND

Sound is a longitudinal wave made up of areas in a material (e.g. air, tissue, water) where the density and pressure are higher (compression) or lower (rarefaction) than normal. Figure 2.5 illustrates the compression and rarefaction events. The amplitude of the wave corresponds to denser compression events. High frequency is represented by denser packing of the compression and rarefaction events.

Velocity of sound in medium depends on density ρ and elasticity K: the velocity of sound v in a gas obeys

$$v = \sqrt{\frac{K}{\rho}} \qquad (2.13)$$

Boyle's law states that gas volume is inversely proportional to pressure:

$$V \propto \frac{1}{P} \qquad (2.14)$$

and as gas density is proportional to pressure then sound velocity is independent of pressure changes. From Charles' law at constant pressure $V \propto T$; since $V \propto 1/\rho$ then $1/\rho \propto T$. Therefore at constant pressure:

$$\text{velocity} \propto \sqrt{T} \qquad (2.15)$$

A list of sound velocities is given in Table 2.15 where the velocity of sound in air is approximately $330\,\text{m s}^{-1}$ being independent of pressure but proportional to $\sqrt{T}$ as stated above.

REFLECTION AND REFRACTION

Sound is reflected from a smooth surface. Smooth is defined as any unevenness in the surface is much less than the wavelength; this gives **specular reflection**. A rough surface will give **non-specular** reflection. For specular reflection, shown in Fig. 2.5b, the angle of

Table 2.15 *Sound velocity in $m\,s^{-1}$.*

Material	Velocity
Air	330
Helium	1000
Water	1540
Soft tissue	1500–1540
Bone	4080
Aluminum	6400

incidence is equal to the angle of reflection. The angle of incidence θ_i between the direction of motion of the incident wave and the normal (perpendicular from the surface) is equal to the angle of reflection θ_r. The sound wave may be partially reflected and the remaining wave front traveling through the new medium. The *transmitted* wave will change direction depending on material composition. The beam is *refracted* and is due to the fact that the speed of sound is different in the two materials. The frequency of the sound will not change but the wavelength will. This will be less in the material in which the wave travels more slowly. The angle between the refracted wave and the normal is the angle of **refraction**.

SNELL'S LAW

(W. Snell, 1591–1626; Dutch physicist) The sine of the incident angle divided by the sine of the angle of refraction is a constant. This constant is the **refractive index**.

$$\text{refractive index} = \frac{\sin \theta_i}{\sin \theta_t} \qquad (2.16)$$

INTENSITY

Intensity is the sound power per unit area and proportional to pressure squared: $I \propto P^2$. Sound intensity is measured in $J\,s^{-1}\,m^{-2}$ or $W\,m^{-2}$. As an example normal conversation has an intensity of 10^{-7} to $10^{-4}\,W\,m^{-2}$ and the threshold of hearing is $10^{-12}\,W\,m^{-2}$. The ultrasound unit is $10^{-3}\,W\,m^{-2}$ ($mW\,cm^{-2}$). A sound pressure wave P passing through two spheres of radius r_1 and r_2 (see Section 1.10) gives an intensity

$$I = \frac{P}{4\pi r^2} \qquad (2.17)$$

The total energy passing through sphere 1 must equal sphere 2. Since $4\pi r^2$ is the surface area of a sphere then the average intensity falls off as the **inverse square** from the point source. So the intensity of a spherical wave decreases as $1/r^2$.

The **amplitude** A decreases with distance as $1/r$ since:

$$A_2 = A_1 \left(\frac{r_1}{r_2} \right) \qquad (2.18)$$

Further properties of sound as related to medical imaging are discussed in Chapter 17.

THE DECIBEL

(Alexander Graham Bell, 1847–1922; British inventor). The decibel is a ratio measure of relative powers or intensities. It uses a logarithmic scale. Relative **intensities** are measured as

$$dB = 10 \log_{10} \frac{I}{I_0} \qquad (2.19)$$

where I_0 is the reference sound level, commonly $10^{-12}\,W\,m^{-2}$ at 1 kHz at audible levels. A sound level of 20 dB is ×10 is more intense than a 10 dB sound level. A 3 dB change halves or doubles the sound intensity. When comparing the pressure or amplitude differences a factor of 20 is used:

$$dB = 20 \log_{10} \frac{A}{A_0} \qquad (2.20)$$

Whereas the half-power value is 3 dB in eqn 2.19, the half amplitude is 6 dB in eqn 2.20. The attenuation given by a material is quoted as dB mm^{-1}; this is the attenuation coefficient α. The speed of sound is frequency independent but α is influenced strongly by frequency. For soft tissue $\alpha = 0.1$ dB mm^{-1} so 3 cm of tissue will reduce the intensity by 50%; bone will give $\alpha = 1.3$ dB mm^{-1} attenuation. The attenuation coefficient is the sum of the individual coefficients for scatter and absorption.

2.9 WAVES AND OSCILLATIONS

Oscillations in the form of sound or radio-frequency waveforms play a most important part in radiology. The interactions of sound waves and radio waves show the same general behavior:

- Harmonic motion
- Signal decay
- Signal resonance
- Interference between signals having different frequency and phase

The waveform characteristics of oscillating signals can be analyzed using a Fourier transform as described in Chapter 1.

2.9.1 Simple harmonic motion

When the force acting on a system is directly proportional to its displacement x from a fixed point then the variation of x with time follows a sine relationship (see Section 2.4):

$$x = a \sin \omega t \qquad (2.21)$$

where a is the amplitude of the waveform or the greatest displacement from the equilibrium position. The constant ω equals $2\pi f$ where f is the frequency of oscillation measured in cycles per second or hertz (Hz). The period T of the waveform which is a measure of the time to undergo one complete cycle is $1/f$ so $\omega = 2\pi/T$. Each time the waveform completes a cycle it moves forward a distance λ, the wavelength. Eqn 2.21 is used to plot the sine wave in Fig. 2.6a. In 1 s when f vibrations occur the wave moves forward a distance $f\lambda$. Hence the velocity c of the waves, which is the distance a peak moves in 1 s is

$$c = f\lambda \qquad (2.22)$$

2.9.2 Damping and resonance

The amplitude of vibration of a simple harmonic motion shown in Figure 2.6a does not remain constant but becomes progressively smaller (the exception here is an electromagnetic wave). A vibration undergoing loss of energy shows damping (Fig. 2.6b).

The amplitude of a mechanical vibration (pendulum swing) undergoes damping due to the air's viscosity, an electrical waveform undergoes damping due to energy loss within the circuit. As damping is increased the oscillations die away more quickly. So a waveform is influenced by energy input. If this oscillating energy is influenced by a retarding force, electronic or mechanical (friction), then the oscillation amplitude decreases exponentially which is shown by the decay envelope of Fig. 2.6b.

RESONANCE

In order to keep a damped system, which is losing energy, in continuous oscillatory motion some outside periodic force must be introduced. The frequency of this force is called the forcing or driving frequency. The frequency of the undamped waveform is the system's natural frequency.

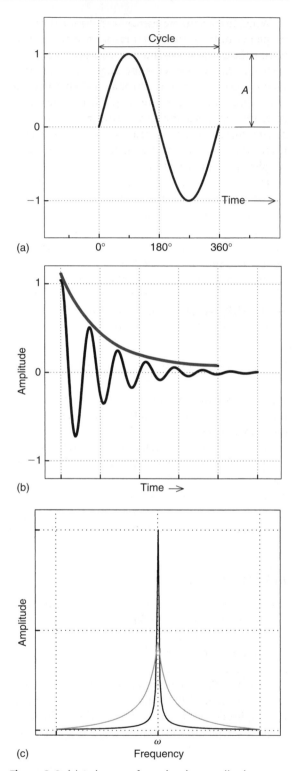

Figure 2.6 *(a) A sine waveform showing amplitude, wavelength, measured as a complete cycle. (b) A damped sine wave showing exponential loss of amplitude. (c) A frequency ω at resonance giving a strong peak intensity.*

When the forcing frequency is equal to the natural frequency of the system then **resonance** occurs producing the greatest power output; the peak frequency ω in Fig. 2.6c is the resonant frequency. This is of practical use in radiology where an oscillating system (e.g. ultrasound transducer crystal or tuned MRI inductive circuit) is the same as the frequency of the driving force (electrical pulse). Considerable energy is absorbed at resonant frequency from the system supplying the external force.

The two resonant signals shown in Fig. 2.6c are a strong resonant signal and a slightly damped signal. The amplitude of the oscillations at resonance will be less if the system is strongly damped and the curve will also be broader. The resonance coupling is enhanced when the frequencies are equal; resonance causes a dramatic increase in signal amplitude at the resonant frequency. This is the principle behind radio frequency (RF) reception: an RF receiver is tuned to be in resonance with the RF transmitter.

2.9.3 Interference

When waveforms having the same frequency but slightly different phase combine they interfere with each other as shown in Fig. 2.7a. Waveforms **in phase** (coherent) show **constructive interference** and produce a resultant of greater amplitude (*Cn*). Waveforms **out of phase** (incoherent) show **destructive interference** (*Ds*). Increasing phase differences give greater degrees of destructive interference until a 180° phase difference causes the signal to disappear giving a zero resultant.

BEAT FREQUENCY

If two waveforms have slightly different frequencies (Fig. 2.7b) then phase differences will change with time and wave interference alternate between constructive and destructive. These alterations of intensity cause an overlaying beat frequency. The beat frequency is the difference between the two original wave frequencies. The frequency variation modulates the amplitude of the resultant wave which will have a frequency equal to the average frequency of the two waves.

TRANSVERSE WAVES

Transverse waves are propagated by vibrations perpendicular to the direction of the wave travel.

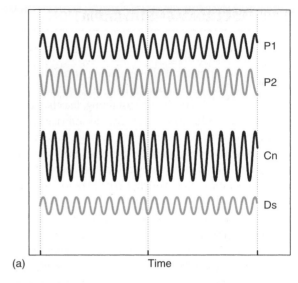

(a)

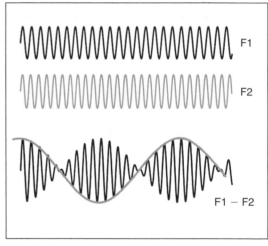

(b)

Figure 2.7 (*a*) Constructive (Cn) and destructive (Ds) interference of two waveforms with the same frequency but different phases P1 and P2. (*b*) A beat frequency caused by slightly different frequency waveforms F1 and F2.

Examples of these are seen on water and **electromagnetic waves** (light waves).

LONGITUDINAL WAVES

Longitudinal waves have vibrations that occur in the same direction as the direction of travel. The most common example is a **sound wave** where compressions and rarefactions move along with the speed of the waveform, each particle vibrating about a mean position transferring energy to the next particle.

2.10 ELECTROMAGNETIC RADIATION

Electromagnetic energy is transmitted by both an electric and magnetic field oscillating together and opposed 90° to each other; this is diagrammatically shown in Fig. 2.8. This is self-sustaining, the changing electric field producing a magnetic field and vice versa. All electromagnetic waves travel through a vacuum with the same speed c which is $3.0 \times 10^8 \, \mathrm{m \, s^{-1}}$; this is a constant. There is no known limit on wavelength, which can range from several kilometers to 10^{-14} m. The energy content of an electromagnetic wave is a multiple of the basic quantum: the **photon**.

The electromagnetic spectrum encompasses extremely low frequencies and wavelengths from radio waves and visible light to ultraviolet, X-rays and gamma radiation. Each frequency band has unique properties but the wave character is identical having an electrical and magnetic component.

2.10.1 Dual characteristic of electromagnetic radiation

Electromagnetic radiation behaves both as particles (photons) and waves. Discrete packets of energy are called **quanta** or **photons** and have energy which is related as

$$E = hf \qquad (2.23)$$

where f is the frequency, in hertz (Hz ≡ cycles s^{-1}), and h is Planck's constant (Max Planck, 1858–1947; German physicist). This is a conversion factor used in eqn 2.23 to enable the answer to be expressed as joule seconds where $h = 6.62 \times 10^{-34} \, \mathrm{J \, s}$.

Wave energy increases with frequency. The frequencies f of some electromagnetic radiations are:

Red light	3.7×10^{14} Hz
Blue light	7.5×10^{14} Hz
Ultraviolet	4×10^{15} Hz
X-rays	5×10^{17} Hz
Gamma radiation	5×10^{19} Hz

In comparison, radio and television waves (frequency modulation (FM) and ultrahigh frequency (UHF)) are much lower down the scale having frequencies between 80 MHz and 1 GHz (80×10^6 to 1×10^9 Hz).

2.10.2 Radiation energy

This is a function of wavelength λ and frequency f since

$$c = \lambda f \qquad (2.24)$$

and consequently

$$f = \frac{c}{\lambda} \qquad (2.25)$$

where c is the speed of light ($3.0 \times 10^8 \, \mathrm{m \, s^{-1}}$). Albert Einstein (1879–1955; German physicist) introduced the idea of photon energy E being a function of frequency and **Planck's constant** broadened Planck's equation (eqn 2.23) so:

$$E = hf = mc^2 \qquad (2.26)$$

The mass–energy relationship demonstrated by this equation enables electron mass to be expressed as either 9.1×10^{-31} kg or 0.511 MeV (mega-electron volts).

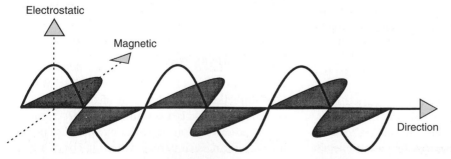

Figure 2.8 *Electromagnetic energy is transmitted with a 90° opposed dual electrical and magnetic component.*

The **electron volt** is a measure of radiation energy since the joule is too large a quantity being 6.24×10^{18} eV or conversely 1 eV equal to 1.6×10^{-19} J. Wavelength and energy can be converted by utilizing eqn 2.24: since it then follows from eqn 2.25 that this function can be substituted for f in eqn 2.26 to give

$$E = \frac{hc}{\lambda} \tag{2.27}$$

Using the constants stated above: $hc = (6.62 \times 10^{-34}) \times (3.0 \times 10^8) = 1.98 \times 10^{-25}$ J m.

Since 1 keV $= 1.6 \times 10^{-16}$ J the answer can be expressed in kiloelectron volts (keV) providing the wavelength is given in nanometers (nm) so:

$$E = \frac{1.24}{\lambda} \tag{2.28}$$

where E is in kV and λ is in nm. Alternatively the answer can be given in electron volts if the wavelength is in meters:

$$E = \frac{1.24 \times 10^{-6}}{\lambda} \tag{2.29}$$

The interrelationship between frequency, wavelength, and energy is explored in Box 2.12 for visible light, ultraviolet and X-rays.

ELECTROMAGNETIC SPECTRUM PROPERTIES

A summary of the formulas and values that are commonly used in radiology is given in Table 2.16. Electromagnetic radiation exhibits the following:

- Electric and magnetic vectors are 90° opposed
- Wave/particle–photon duality.
- Very broad range of frequency and wavelength.
- Polarization of the wave (orientation in a single plane commonly seen in radio and visible wavelengths).
- Speed in vacuum 3.0×10^8 m s^{-1} (is a constant).
- Unaffected by external electrical or magnetic fields.
- Absorption by material follows an **exponential** law.

2.10.3 Optics

The production of light from an intensifying screen, video screen or laser is an essential process in radiology for producing images. The behavior and distortion of light when passing through different materials

---

Box 2.12 Radiation energy as electron volt

Red light

The wavelength is 700 nm (7×10^{-7} m).

$$f = c/\lambda = 4.28 \times 10^{14} \text{ Hz}$$

$$E = \frac{1.24 \times 10^{-6}}{7} \times 10^{-7} = 1.77 \text{ eV}$$

Blue light

The frequency f is 7.5×10^{14} Hz.

$$\lambda = \frac{c}{f} = \frac{3.0 \times 10^8}{7.5} \times 10^{14} = 4 \times 10^{-7} \text{ m}$$

$$E = \frac{1.24 \times 10^{-6}}{4} \times 10^{-7} = 3.1 \text{ eV}$$

Alternatively $E = hf$ (where $h \equiv 4.13 \times 10^{-15}$ eV), then $(4.13 \times 10^{-15}) \times (7.5 \times 10^{14}) = 3.1$ eV.

Ultraviolet

Frequency $= 4 \times 10^{15}$ Hz

$$\lambda = \frac{3.0 \times 10^8}{4} \times 10^{15} = 75 \text{ nm}$$

$$E = 16 \text{ eV}$$

X-rays

A continuous spectrum from 60 to 120 keV has a wavelength range from 0.02 to 0.0099 nm and a frequency range from 1.5 to 3.0×10^{19} Hz.

Table 2.16 *Summary: electromagnetic units.*

Measure	Formulas	Values
Velocity c	$c = f\lambda$	$c = 3.0 \times 10^8$ m s^{-1}
Wavelength λ	$\lambda = c/f$	λ in m or nm
Frequency f	$f = c/\lambda$	f in Hz
Planck's constant h		6.62×10^{-34} J s
		4.13×10^{-15} eVs
Electron mass e		$e = 9.1 \times 10^{-31}$ kg
		$= 0.511$ MeV
		$= 1.6 \times 10^{-19}$ C
Energy E	$E = hc/\lambda$	$hc = 1.24 \times 10^{-6}$ eV

determine the quality of the final image whether on film or video screen.

Light undergoes reflection, refraction, and interference in a similar fashion to sound waves. Constructive interference occurs when two waves, in phase, combine to give a wave of larger amplitude. Destructive interference occurs when the waves are out of phase. Coherent sources have the same frequency and are in phase. This short description of light behavior will be covered in more detail in the relevant chapters.

UMBRA AND PENUMBRA

A point source of light projects a sharp shadow onto a screen. Figure 2.9a demonstrates that when this ceases to be a point source then image unsharpness causes shadowing. The degree of shadowing depends on the size of the focal spot f and its position relative to the object and image plane. The parameters i and o in Fig. 2.9b determine the penumbra dimension p (unsharpness) so that

$$p = \frac{i \times f}{o} \qquad (2.30)$$

Umbra and penumbra effects are shown by X-rays since they are produced by fine and broad focal spots and mimic the light effects described here. The geometry of an X-ray beam also obeys eqn 2.30.

COLOR RGB

Video color displays use the primary colors of red, green, and blue to form their images. These can be mixed to give any particular color scale. The thermal scale has become popular as a logical continuous scale using a 'temperature gradient' of red, orange, white to represent increasing count densities or activities.

THE LASER

(Light amplification by stimulated emission of radiation) A strong monochromatic coherent light source can be produced by causing many atoms to make transitions from one excited state to another so that all the light waves are in phase (coherent). Many materials can be made to lase: ruby, carbon dioxide, helium/neon. These are high power devices commonly found in laser film formatters.

Semiconductor lasers are low power devices producing red/infrared light used for optical transmission and reading laser disks and CD-ROMs.

FIBER OPTIC EFFECTS

Light travels at a constant $3 \times 10^5 \mathrm{km\,s^{-1}}$ in a vacuum. However, when it enters a transparent medium (e.g. glass) the speed of light is reduced by a factor of about 1.5 ($2 \times 10^5 \mathrm{km\,s^{-1}}$). This factor is the refractive index of the material. When light passes from one medium to another this change in speed causes the light to bend. Under certain conditions the light ray will be reflected back into the more dense medium: this is **total internal reflection**. Light rays in glass are totally internally reflected if their angle of incidence is increased beyond a critical angle (42°). Figure 2.10a

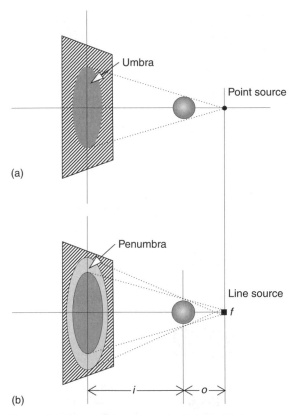

Figure 2.9 (a) A point source projecting an object as a pure shadow (umbra). A broader light beam from a line source (b) causes a secondary shadow (penumbra) whose dimensions are determined by parameters f, i and o identified in the text.

shows light rays within glass being refracted at the interface with a less dense medium (air).

Images can be transferred along a bundle of **coherent** fibers where the position of the fibers is identical at the start and the end of the bundle length. Figure 2.10b shows an optical fiber plate (short length of coherent fibers) applied to a phosphor screen; this light pipe prevents light scatter so reducing image data loss that would occur by viewing the phosphor screen directly. Tapering the fiber bundle can either minify or magnify the image.

The light beam can be piped along a glass rod or fiber. An optical fiber for this purpose is typically 0.125 and 0.5 mm in diameter and signal losses are about 0.5 dB km^{-1} resulting in a small signal loss of about 10% per km. Signals can be transmitted over about 50 km without amplification. A simplified transmission scheme is shown in Fig. 2.10c.

Fiber optics play an important part in image intensifier signal collection in fluoroscopy, explained in Chapter 10. It is also playing an increasing role in computer data transmission over local area networks (LANs) (see Chapter 11).

RADIO WAVES AND TRANSMISSION

Radio waves are a form of electromagnetic radiation produced by oscillating electrons in an inductor

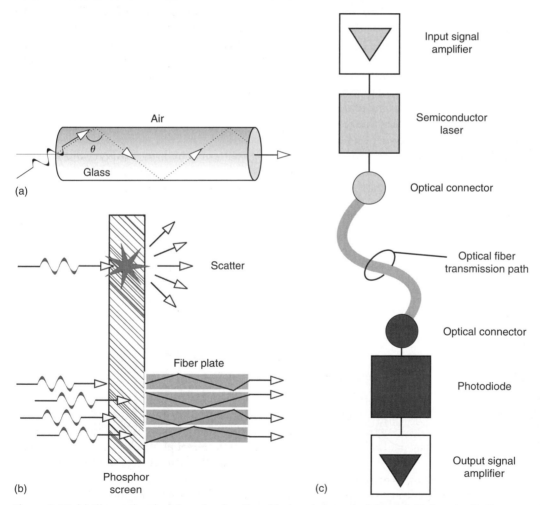

Figure 2.10 (*a*) *Fiber optic principle, only when the critical angle is reached does total internal reflection occur.* (*b*) *A fiber optic plate on a phosphor screen (image intensifier) prevents light diffusion.* (*c*) *Fiber optic fiber used for digital signal transmission between two computer workstations.*

(coil). The waves are transferred to an aerial which at low frequencies can be a short length of wire but at higher frequencies a system of conductors is necessary to shape the transmitted beam or increase the ability to detect radio waves of a certain frequency band.

Very high frequency (VHF) radio waves (20 to 80 MHz) are the signal in magnetic resonance imaging. At these frequencies it is essential to maintain impedance matching otherwise the signal strength will be reduced.

Interference from other radio transmissions is reduced by using efficient narrow-band transmission and receiving circuits (high Q). These resonate at narrow precise frequencies (see resonance in Fig. 2.6c).

2.11 MAGNETISM

Ferro-magnetic materials are crystalline and small regions within these crystals have strong resultant magnetism but this is randomly distributed so the bulk material shows no magnetism. These tiny regions are called **domains**. It is the realignment of these domains which achieves the magnetic property. Total realignment gives saturation and magnetization of the material is at a maximum when all domains point in the same direction.

The domains can be disturbed by heat and vibration so the magnetic property is gradually lost. Audio or video magnetic recordings gradually become noisier as the magnetic signal on the tape is lost over time. MRI permanent magnets very slowly lose magnetic strength for the same reason.

2.11.1 Magnetic units (intensity, flux)

A magnetic field B is the force equivalent in magnetism to an electrostatic charge producing an electrostatic field which sets up lines of charge around an object. The SI unit for the magnetic field is the **tesla** (T) (N. Tesla, 1856–1943; Croatian physicist). A **magnetic flux** is set up by the magnetic field. The unit for the magnetic flux per unit area at right angles to the direction of the magnetic field B (magnetic line density) is the **weber** (Wb) where $1\,\text{Wb} = 1\,\text{T m}^{-2}$. The motion of an electric charge (a flowing current) is always accompanied by a magnetic flux. The insertion of ferro-magnetic material (iron, cobalt, nickel) within a magnetic flux causes the atoms within the material to align themselves and a permanent magnet is formed. Permanent magnets have a north and south pole (compared to positive and negative charges in electrostatics). Lines of force connect these poles which form the magnetic flux lines shown in Fig. 2.11a.

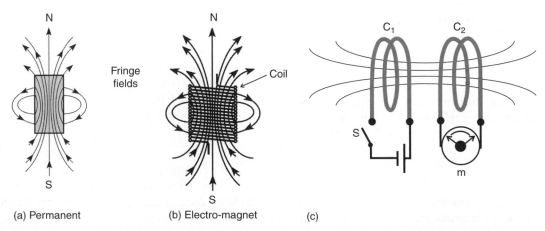

Figure 2.11 *(a) Magnetic flux field lines surrounding a permanent magnet. (b) Magnetic induction seen in a coil carrying an electric current. (c) Current induction in a second solenoid.*

2.11.2 Magnetic induction

A current carrying wire shows the following points:

- A magnetic field surrounds it.
- The magnetic field is perpendicular to the current.

The magnetic effect shown by a current carrying wire can be increased by winding the wire into a coil (a solenoid), so concentrating the lines of magnetic force. A solenoid is constructed from a multi-turn coil, shown in Fig. 2.11b; an iron core will concentrate the magnetic flux still more, this is the basis of an electromagnet which loses its magnetization when the current is switched off.

ELECTROMAGNETIC INDUCTION

If a magnet is moved within a coil a current is induced in the coil. The coil can be moved producing the same effect. This is the principle behind the dynamo and alternator, producing electric energy from mechanical energy.

INDUCTION BY CURRENT

If two coils (C_1 and C_2 in Fig. 2.11c) are placed closely together and C_1 energized by switching a battery in circuit, causing a growth of a magnetic field, then this induces a current in C_2. The current in C_1 must be changing to induce a current in C_2. This is the principle behind the transformer to be discussed later.

2.11.3 Magnetic strength

This is dependent on the pole strength m_1 and m_2 at a distance d. These attract or repel each other with a force F so that

$$F = K \times \frac{m_1 \times m_2}{d^2} \qquad (2.31)$$

where K is a constant; the force obeys the inverse square law. Intensity of the magnetic field is measured as

$$F = \frac{m_1 \times m_2}{p \times d^2} \qquad (2.32)$$

where p is the permeability of the medium which is large for ferro-magnetic materials (p for air = 1). In coils C_1 and C_2 (described above) the magnetic flux would be p times as great if the coils are wound over

a magnetic core material (soft iron); this is exploited in transformer design.

FIELD CHANGE

A small field produces strong magnetization in soft iron so this is an ideal ferro-magnetic material but steel requires a stronger electric field so is not an ideal magnetic material. Ferrite (a ceramic iron material) gives a large field change for a large electric field; it quickly saturates and retains this saturated condition when the electric field is removed. This property makes ferrite a valuable magnetic material for recording analog and digital information on tape or disk.

EDDY CURRENT LOSSES

A changing magnetic flux in the coil produces a flux change in the core material (soft iron) which causes eddy current losses seen as heat. Eddy currents can be reduced if the core is laminated. At higher frequencies (radio frequencies) soft iron is not suitable so sintered iron particles are used (ferrite). Eddy current losses cause serious problems in MRI.

SHIELDING

It has already been seen that ferro-magnetic materials serve to concentrate the magnetic flux. Soft iron (mu-metal) is a common material used for shielding against magnetic interference and can be placed around sensitive equipment (e.g. image intensifiers, photomultiplier tubes), since it can concentrate quite weak magnetic fields reducing the external magnetic flux and so protecting devices which are surrounded by the material.

2.12 ELECTRICITY

Electricity and the properties of electricity are obviously of prime importance to radiology. The high voltages associated with **static electricity** and their electrostatic effects are essential for electron beam control in X-ray tubes, image intensifiers and video display tubes. As the name electrostatics implies the properties do not depend on organized electron flow but rather distribution of positive and negative charges on a body. **Current electricity** is concerned with the flow of electrical energy by charge carriers (electrons) between two points having a potential difference between them. This difference is the **electromotive force** (emf) measured in volts and can be treated as a form of potential energy in both static and current electricity.

2.12.1 Electrostatics

This is the branch of physics that deals with static or very high voltages (relevant to X-ray generators and X-ray tubes). The static **electric charge** arises when electrons are transferred from one object to another. An object with excess electrons has a negative charge and, conversely, an object having lost electrons has a positive charge. The basic measurement of charge is the **coulomb** (C) (Charles Coulomb, 1736–1806; French physicist): 1 coulomb = 6.24×10^{18} electrons.

Each electron has a charge Q of 1.6×10^{-19} C per electron. This is a fundamental constant usually called the elementary charge. The rest mass of the electron is also a fundamental constant being 9.1×10^{-31} kg. The charge and energy of an electron beam are calculated in Box 2.13.

The **laws of electrostatics** state that similar charges ($-$, $-$ or $+$, $+$) on separate bodies repel; unlike charges ($+$ and $-$) attract. The force of two charged bodies is proportional to their charge $F \propto q$. The attractive or repulsive force F of a charge q over a distance d has the relationship

$$F \propto \frac{1}{d^2} \qquad (2.33)$$

This has already been expressed as the inverse square law in Chapter 1.

Also

$$F = \frac{q_1 \times q_2}{d^2} \qquad (2.34)$$

which is analogous to the magnetic force in eqn 2.31. Here F is the force exerted on two objects with charges q_1 and q_2 at a distance d. The inverse square law also applies to charged bodies. This equation describes Coulomb's law which plays an important part in X-ray tube design for defining electron beam dimensions.

The force is proportional to the charge ($F \propto q$) and every charge produces an **electric field** in the space around it:

$$\text{electric field} = \frac{F}{q} \qquad (2.35)$$

Box 2.13 The charge of an electron beam

If Q coulombs flows during t seconds then

$$I = \frac{Q}{t} \text{ amps}$$

$$Q = I \times t$$

Example 1

If $I = 4\,\mathrm{C\,s^{-1}}$ and $t = 10\,\mathrm{s}$ then

$$Q = 40 \text{ coulombs}$$

Example 2

For an X-ray exposure for 100 mA at $t = 0.5\,\mathrm{s}$ (50 mAs), $I = 0.1\,\mathrm{C\,s^{-1}}$ and $Q = 0.05\,\mathrm{C}$ or 50 mC (millicoulombs). So X-ray exposure in mAs is equivalent to mC.

Energy gained by an electron beam in an X-ray tube

If 3×10^{17} electrons representing 50 mA (1.6×10^{-19} C each electron) move along an X-ray tube at 120 keV, then energy gained is

$$E = QV \text{ joules}$$

$$= (3 \times 10^{17}) \times (1.6 \times 10^{-19}) \times (120 \times 10^3)$$

$$= 5760 \text{ J}$$

The charges will be closer giving a stronger electric field where the conductor is most curved. A sharp edge will have a very high electric field; this property has valuable applications to the design of focusing cups in X-ray tubes. Figure 2.12a shows how sharp edges can be used for controlling the dimensions of an electron beam produced by an electrically heated filament. Before an electric current can flow there must be a pressure difference or driving force between the electrodes. This is called a potential difference (PD) which is measured as the **volt** (V) (A.G. Volta, 1745–1827; Italian physicist) and applies to both static and current electricity. It is the work done in moving 1 C, so $1\,\mathrm{V} = 1\,\mathrm{J\,C^{-1}}$. The volt as a unit exists as multiples listed in Table 2.17. The **electron volt** has been previously mentioned in Section 2.10.2 and is a measure of energy necessary since traditional units of

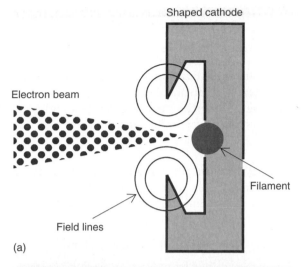

Shaped cathode

Electron beam

Field lines

Filament

(a)

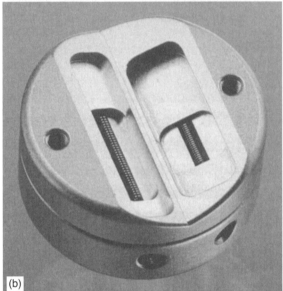

(b)

Figure 2.12 (**a**) Static field set up around shaped points in an X-ray tube filament cup assembly. (**b**) The cathode of a dual filament X-ray tube showing each filament in shaped cup with sharp edges.

Table 2.17 Multiples of the volt.

Unit	Occurrence or use
megavolts (MV: 10^6)	Static electricity (millions of volts)
kilovolts (kV: 10^3)	X-ray high voltage (20–150 kV)
volts	Domestic supply and batteries (1.5–240 V)
millivolts (mV: 10^{-3})	Physiological signal level (ECG) (10–100 mV)
microvolts (μV: 10^{-6})	Radio signal strength e.g. MRI (1–10 μV)

Box 2.14 The energy equivalence of an electron volt

The electron velocity v at 1 V is $6 \times 10^5\,\mathrm{m\,s^{-1}}$. The rest mass m is $9.1 \times 10^{-31}\,\mathrm{kg}$ so

$$\tfrac{1}{2}mv^2 = 0.5 \times (9.1 \times 10^{-31}) \times (6 \times 10^5)^2$$

$$\text{or} \quad 1.6 \times 10^{-19}\,\mathrm{J}$$

This is the **energy equivalent** of 1 eV.

Similarly, the electron velocity at 100 kV is

$$1.6 \times 10^{-19} \times (1 \times 10^5) = 1 \times 10^{-14}\,\mathrm{J}$$

so

$$\tfrac{1}{2}mv^2 = 1.6 \times 10^{-14}$$

Velocity v is $1.88 \times 10^8\,\mathrm{m\,s^{-1}}$ at 100 kV, which is about two thirds the speed of light.

Note. Relativistic effects (mass–velocity) play a small part in electron velocity.

---

energy (joule) are much too large to describe electrostatic attractive forces. The electron volt (eV) is the energy acquired by an electron when it moves between a potential difference of 1 V. The electron volt has multiples keV and MeV. Equivalent values of the electron volt are:

$$1\,\mathrm{eV} = 1.6 \times 10^{-19}\,\mathrm{J}$$
$$h = 4.13 \times 10^{-15}\,\mathrm{eVs}$$

There is a clear distinction between electrical potential difference (voltage: 50 kV, 100 kV etc.) and energy (electron volt: 50 keV, 100 keV etc.). Energy equivalence and velocity of an electron beam are calculated in Box 2.14.

Electrostatic forces are responsible for accelerating electrons in an X-ray tube. Electrostatics are also employed to control the dimensions of an electron beam. Figure 2.12b shows a filament cup whose sharp edges carry a strong electric field and this negative potential can repel the electron beam, controlling its dimensions and also switching off the beam, if the charge is high enough.

2.12.2 Direct-current electricity

Direct current (DC) is given by batteries, dynamos and rectified power supplies and is used as the final power supply for radiology equipment whether driving high voltage X-ray tubes or low voltage semiconductor circuits. Electrical current is caused by the transport of electrons and is measured in **amperes** (A) (A.M. Ampère, 1775–1836; French physicist):

1 ampere = 1 coulomb per second (C s^{-1})

Box 2.15 Electrical energy

Energy gain

If the energy is W then, since $Q = I \times t$,

$$W = IVt \text{ joules}$$

For a voltage of 50 000 V (50 kV) at 50 mAs (i.e. 50 mA for 1 s), the energy consumed is

$$0.1 \times 50\,kV \times 0.5\,J = 2500\,J$$

Note. $1\,V = 1\,J\,C^{-1}$

Electric power

A 100 W electric light bulb at 220 V consumes $W/V = 0.45$ A, and 110 V consumes 0.9 A. Commercial electric power is measured in kilowatts (kW). Electrical energy consumed is expressed as kW × time, which is the kW hour (kWh).

So four 100 W lamps burning for 8 h consume: $100 \times 4 \times 8 = 3.2\,kWh$ regardless of the supply voltage.

Note. $1\,kWh = 3.6 \times 10^6\,J$

As 1 C represents the charge on 6×10^{18} electrons 1 A would be this number of electrons per second passing in a conductor. Smaller currents are measured in milliamps (mA; 10^{-3} A) and microamps (mA; 10^{-6} A). The volt can be described in terms of current flow since it is the difference of electrical potential between two points on a wire carrying a constant current of 1 A when the power dissipation is 1 W, so:

$$1\,V = 1\,W\,A^{-1}$$

X-ray tube current is measured in mA and X-ray exposure is measured in mA per unit time, i.e. mA seconds (mAs) and from the above definition of a coulomb:

$$1\,mAs = 1 \times 10^{-3} \text{ coulomb } (1\,mC)$$

The energy gained by an electron when it is accelerated from one electrode to another (video/television tube, X-ray tube) can be calculated as shown in Box 2.15. A summary of electrical measurements is given in Table 2.18 along with constants useful for radiation calculations.

POWER AND RESISTANCE

(George Simon Ohm, 1787– 1854; German physicist) Ohm's law states that current I and voltage V are proportional providing temperature and resistance R of the conductor are constant. So $I \propto V$ and V/I is a constant.

The unit of resistance is the **ohm** (Ω). One ohm maintains a current of one amp at one volt so that

$$R = \frac{V}{I} \tag{2.36}$$

Variations of this basic formula of eqn 2.36 are

$$I = \frac{V}{R} \quad \text{and} \quad V = IR \tag{2.37}$$

Table 2.18 *Summary: electrical units.*

Measure	Parameter	Relationships
Electric charge (Q)	coulomb (C)	$1\,C = 6.24 \times 10^{18}\,e$
	charge/electron	$1.6 \times 10^{-19}\,C$
Potential difference (PD)	volt (V)	$1\,V = 1\,J\,C^{-1}$
Energy (E)	joule (J)	$J = QV$
	electron volt (eV)	$1\,J = 6.24 \times 10^{18}\,eV$
		$1\,eV = 1.6 \times 10^{-19}\,J$
Current (I)	ampere (A)	$Q = I \times t\ 1\,A = 1\,C\,s^{-1}$
		$(6.24 \times 10^{18}\,e\,s^{-1})$

If a is the cross-sectional area of a conductor then providing the length L is constant its resistance is proportional to cross-sectional area. So that

$$R \propto \frac{L}{a^2} \qquad (2.38)$$

If the diameter of the wire is doubled (increasing the area a) then resistance decreases by ¼.

The heating effect of electric current depends on:

- The electric current being passed I
- The resistance of the circuit R
- The time spent t

The following relationships can be established: (1) for a constant current I and fixed resistance the heat produced $\propto$ time spent and (2) for a constant resistance and fixed time the heat produced $\propto I^2$. Joules' laws of electrical heating summarize these findings. The heat developed in a wire is proportional to:

- The time spent
- The current squared I^2
- Resistance of the conductor (wire) $P = I^2Rt$ joules

Electrical power P relationships are derived as

$$\frac{\text{energy delivered}}{\text{time taken}} \quad \text{so} \quad P = \frac{IVt}{t} = IV \quad (2.39)$$

where P is in $J\,s^{-1}$. Since $1\,W = 1\,J\,s^{-1}$ and $P = IV$ then: $W = IV$ watts.

Examples of electrical power calculation are given in Box 2.15 and a summary of units in Table 2.19. **Power loss** is calculated by deriving electrical power P as

$$P = IV \qquad (2.40)$$

and restating Ohm's law as $V = IR$. Then

$$P = I \times (IR) \quad \text{or} \quad P = I^2R \qquad (2.41)$$

Similarly, since $I = V/R$ then

$$P = V \times \left(\frac{V}{R}\right) \quad \text{or} \quad P = \frac{V^2}{R} \qquad (2.42)$$

which gives three standard formulas (eqns 2.40, 2.41, and 2.42) relating power with voltage, current and resistance. Since all conductors have some electrical resistance, no matter how small, power is always lost when transporting electricity. Box 2.16 illustrates this for 500 V, 10 kV, and 100 kV power lines.

2.12.3 Alternating current and voltage

Alternating current (AC) is produced by generators/alternators and electrically oscillating circuits. It is used for transmitting electrical power over long distances, eventually appearing as the domestic mains supply; it is more easily controlled than DC.

Alternating current is produced at the power station by a generator capable of delivering many thousands of volts at a very high current. This is stepped up prior to transmission along the high voltage power lines; the voltages sometimes exceed 500 000 volts. High voltage transmission reduces power lost in the cables as demonstrated in Box 2.16. Power loss can be reduced by either:

- Increasing the supply voltage
- Reducing cable resistance

The transmitted high voltage is successively stepped down in order to supply cities, towns, streets, and eventually individual consumers. A single and 3-phase AC waveform is shown in Fig. 2.13. Each phase of the 3-phase supply is separated by 120° and transmits electrical energy with much greater efficiency than a single-phase supply.

Table 2.19 *Summary: resistance and power.*

Measure	Parameter	Relationships	
Resistance (R)	ohm (Ω)	$I = V/R$	
		$R = V/I$	
		$V = IR$	
Power (P)	Watt (W)	$P = IV$	$1\,W = 1\,J\,s^{-1}$
		$P = I^2R$	$1\,J = 1\,W\,s$
		$P = V^2/R$	$1\,kWh = 3.6 \times 10^6\,J$
		$E = W/Q$	$W = EQ$
			$W = I^2Rt = V^2\,t/R = VIt$

Box 2.16 Power loss and power transmission

Power loss

Consider a cable of resistance $2\,\Omega$ supplying a 100 W lamp.

At 110 V, approximately 1 A is flowing so the power lost in the cable is

$$I^2R = 1 \times 2 = 2\,W$$

Hence 2% of the lamp power is lost in the cable. At 220 V, approximately 0.5 A is flowing and the power lost in the cable is

$$0.25 \times 2 = 0.5\,W$$

Hence 0.5% of the available power is lost.

Power transmission

Consider the supply of 1 MW to a small town over a cable with a resistance of $10\,\Omega$. This can use

500 V at 2000 A or

10 000 V at 100 A or

500 000 V at 2 A

These all deliver the required 1 MW. The power loss is I^2R so

at 500 V there is *total* power lost in the cable
at 10 000 V, 10% of the power is lost
at 100 000 V, 0.1% of the power is lost

(*Note.* Power transmission uses the highest practical voltage to minimize power loss.)

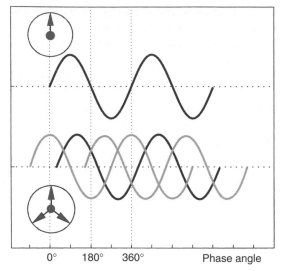

Figure 2.13 *A single-phase and a 3-phase supply. The polar diagram indicates that the three phases are 120° out of phase with each other.*

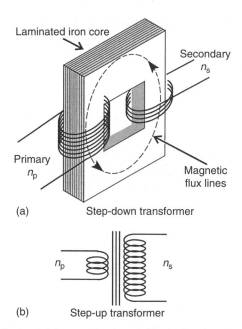

Figure 2.14 *(a) A step-down transformer showing the primary and secondary windings on an iron core and (b) an electrical schematic for a step-up transformer.*

The valuable property of alternating current is that it can be easily changed from high to low values and vice versa with very little loss; this is achieved with a **transformer**. A transformer (Fig. 2.14a) consists of two coils, primary n_p and secondary n_s, wound on a soft iron core in the case of low frequency power supplies (50 or 60 Hz) and shown diagrammatically for sintered ferrite cores which are used for high frequency transformers >1000 Hz.

The following relationship applies to transformers, where E_p and E_s are the voltages at the primary (n_p) and secondary (n_s) windings:

$$\frac{E_s}{E_p} = \frac{n_s}{n_p} \tag{2.43}$$

The parameters n_p and n_s are the number of turns so the ratio n_s/n_p is the turns ratio in eqn 2.43. A step-up transformer has a turns ratio >1 and a step-down transformer <1.

The current in a transformer changes inversely with the voltage; the energy in the transformer obeys the conservation of energy, thus the energy in the secondary at any instant equals the power supplied to the primary. If I_s and I_p are the secondary and primary currents then:

$$I_s \times E_s = I_p \times E_p \qquad (2.44)$$

and

$$\frac{I_s}{I_p} = \frac{E_p}{E_s} = \frac{n_p}{n_s} \qquad (2.45)$$

thus for a step-up transformer (shown schematically in Fig. 2.14b) with a turns ratio 60:1 (voltage increases) the currents are stepped down in the ratio 1:60. A step-down transformer will increase current in the secondary winding but at a reduced voltage. In practice there is a loss of energy in the transformer due to eddy currents which are induced in the iron core by the changing magnetic flux in the windings; these losses can be reduced if the core is laminated.

The current needed for an X-ray machine is calculated in Box 2.17 and shows that very high mains supply currents are necessary for the high voltages required.

The voltages induced in the secondary winding of a transformer depend on the size of the primary and secondary windings. For 50/60 Hz supplies the average X-ray generator transformer is particularly large and occupies a great deal of space in the X-ray room (approximately a 0.5 m cube).

Extremely compact high voltage transformers can be designed by increasing the AC supply frequency since the induced secondary voltage E_s is influenced by the cross section area of the transformer core A and the number of turns n and the frequency:

$$E_s = (A \times n) \times f \qquad (2.46)$$

The **high frequency transformer** size can be reduced substantially by increasing the supply frequency and maintaining E_s constant in eqn 2.46. This is accomplished by first converting the 50/60 Hz supply to DC and then electronically converting this to a much higher frequency using a high frequency converter. High voltage transformers can be small enough to fit with the X-ray tube itself in CT machines. Box 2.18 illustrates the reduction in transformer size with increasing frequency of supply.

The X-ray system contains various transformer designs. A step-up transformer supplies the very high voltage necessary to generate the X-rays. A step-down transformer supplies the low voltage for the filament of the X-ray tube. These are commonly combined in the

---

Box 2.17 X-ray generator supply

What is the mains current I_p required to supply an X-ray generator capable of giving $125\,\mathrm{kV_p}$ at 100 mA? The mains voltage is 220 V.

$$I_p = \frac{E_s \times I_s}{E_p}$$

$$= \frac{\left(125 \times 10^3\right) \times \left(100 \times 10^{-3}\right)}{220}$$

$$= 56\,\mathrm{A}$$

A 110 V supply would require 112 A.
Note. X-ray equipment requiring high currents commonly employs high voltage 3-phase supplies.

Box 2.18 High frequency transformer

Transformer size decreases with increased frequency. The basic formula is $E_s = (A \times n) \times f$.

For an X-ray tube supply of 100 keV and a relative overall size $(A \times n)$, for 50 Hz transformer being 2000.

$$2000 \times 50\,\mathrm{Hz} = 100\,\mathrm{keV}$$
$$1666 \times 60\,\mathrm{Hz} = 100\,\mathrm{keV}$$
$$1000 \times 100\,\mathrm{Hz} = 100\,\mathrm{keV}$$
$$20 \times 5\,\mathrm{kHz} = 100\,\mathrm{keV}$$
$$10 \times 10\,\mathrm{kHz} = 100\,\mathrm{keV}$$

So operating a generator frequency of 10 kHz, instead of 50 Hz, reduces the transformer size by 200 times.

same transformer tank complete with oil coolant. An isolation transformer with equal turns ratio is used in order to separate the mains supply from the machine power supply; this reduces electrical shock hazards to personnel using the equipment. A single winding auto-transformer is sometimes employed in order to compensate for power loss in the high voltage cables.

The AC parameter analogous to resistance in a DC circuit is the **impedance**. For AC supplies it is a complex function of resistance, inductance, and capacitance of the circuit as well as the frequency of supply. The unit of impedance is the same as the DC unit (the ohm Ω; see Ohm's law) and similarly we can write $V = IZ$ or $I = V/Z$. In certain AC circuits it is important to match the impedances when the supply is connected in order to prevent undue power loss. This is most important when dealing with radio-frequency (high frequency AC) circuits that are used in magnetic resonance imaging.

AC POWER

The electrical power in a DC circuit is the product of current and voltage. **AC power** in alternating current circuits is measured similarly but this is only valid when the current and voltage waveforms are in phase, which is the case with purely resistive circuits, e.g. heaters and light bulbs. With electrical loads that include inductors, e.g. motors, transformers, the voltage and current are not in phase as shown by Fig. 2.15. The degree of phase shift is expressed by the power factor (cos ϕ) or phase angle. So the relationship between true power P measured in kW and apparent power S measured in kVA is

$$P = S \times \sin \varphi \qquad (2.47)$$

Box 2.19 gives an example of real and apparent power measurements when the voltage and current waveforms are out of phase.

Comparing the electrical energy W produced by a direct current I flowing through a resistance R for a time t with an alternating current flowing through the same resistance requires a measure of the **root mean square** for the alternating current. This is defined as that value of steady current which would dissipate heat at the same rate in a given resistance which for direct current is given by

$$W = I^2 \times R \times t \qquad (2.48)$$

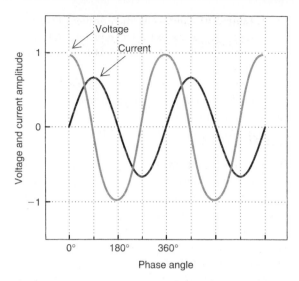

Figure 2.15 *AC power voltage and current waveform for an inductive load where voltage and current show a 90° phase difference.*

Box 2.19 Real and apparent power

The applied AC voltage and current to a system including an inductor (inductive load) is 440 V at 50 A. The **apparent power** is $440 \times 50 = 22\,kVA$. A 12° phase shift gives a power factor of 0.84, so the **true power** is $22 \times 0.84 = 18.5\,kW$.

If a current is continuously varying (AC) the electrical energy is not converted into heat energy at a constant rate. The sine wave for a mains supply shows maximum energy when the current is maximum and zero when the current is zero. For this reason a mean value is derived called the root mean square (RMS) value. The RMS value of an AC power source, restating the above definition, is simply that value of DC which produces the same heating effect. For any sinusoidal waveform the RMS value is

$$\frac{\text{peak value}}{\sqrt{2}} \qquad (2.49)$$

The quoted mains supply is always given as its RMS value, the peak voltages are obtained by multiplying by $\sqrt{2}$ (or 1.414) which gives the results listed in Table 2.20. It is planned to 'harmonize' UK with other European voltages to a common 230 V.

Table 2.20 *Mains supply voltages.*

RMS value	Peak value
115	162 (USA)
220	311 (Europe)
240	339 (UK)

RECTIFICATION

The convenience of an AC supply for transmitting electric current and its ease of voltage change by transformers are offset by the problems associated with converting the alternating waveform to a DC supply by rectification, since the AC supply cannot be used for driving X-ray generator units or electronic equipment. Rectification is achieved by using one-way current devices (diodes) which in early machines used thermionic emission but in present day equipment use semiconductors. Figure 2.16a shows rectified waveforms derived from an AC waveform undergoing half- and full-wave rectification. The configuration of half- and full-wave rectifiers is shown in Fig. 2.16b.

These rectifiers only allow passage of current in one direction so their output has a single polarity. A half-wave rectifier uses a single diode and is 50% efficient since it does not utilize the negative half of the AC waveform. A full-wave rectifier uses four diodes and is 100% effective in utilizing all the AC power.

2.13 ELECTRONICS

The control of electrical circuits by thermionic or semiconductor devices is central to the equipment used in diagnostic imaging. The control of high voltages associated with X-ray production was, in the past, performed by mechanical switching but is now almost universally performed by electronic devices. Electronics is divided into analog and digital circuits. Analog devices are amplifiers which deal with varying signal voltages representing the X-ray spectrum, sound or radio waves. Digital devices act as very fast switches and feature mostly in logic circuits of control systems and computers.

2.13.1 High voltage electronics

When heat is applied to a wire filament, electrons close to the surface gain energy and leave the metal due to

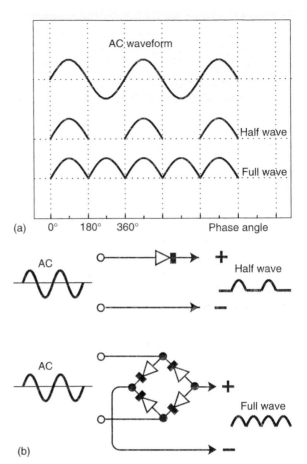

Figure 2.16 *(a) The rectified AC waveform undergoing half-wave rectification (only positive cycles used) and full-wave rectification where both positive and negative cycles are used for the rectified DC supply. (b) The half-wave and full-wave circuits using diode rectifiers.*

thermionic emission, forming a cloud. The concentration of electrons causes a negative space charge which repels further electron emission. Placing a positive charged electrode (anode) above the filament will draw electrons so a current will flow. Electrons only flow from the negative cathode (filament) to the positive anode. Figure 2.17a shows this effect and the direction of current flow between cathode and anode. As the filament temperature is increased from T_1 to T_3 in the simple device shown in Fig. 2.17b the curves show that the current increases nonlinearly reaching a saturation point or plateau. The saturation current level depends on the applied voltage between anode and cathode (x-axis).

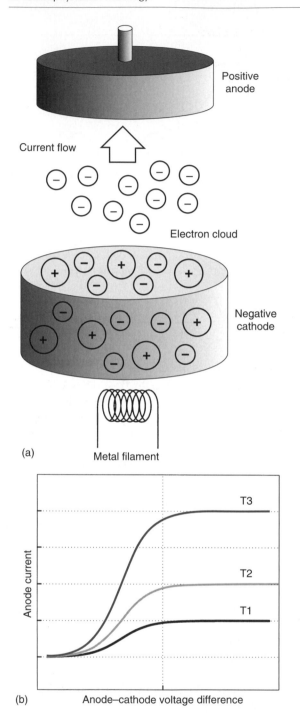

(a)

Metal filament

(b)

Anode–cathode voltage difference

Figure 2.17 *(a) Thermionic emission from a heated metal filament creating an electron cloud. There is a high potential difference between anode and cathode causing a current flow. (b) The thermionic emission efficiency depends on the temperature of the filament. The current flow (anode current) increases with increased filament temperature (T1 to T3).*

As well as being nonlinear this device is also unidirectional (a diode), allowing current to pass from cathode to anode (not vice versa) which removes the negative half of the alternating current; this is the rectification action.

2.13.2 Low voltage electronics

Vacuum tube devices (valves) have all but been replaced by **semiconductors**. The X-ray tube is perhaps the remnant vacuum tube device that has not been replaced. Semiconducting materials include silicon, germanium, and gallium arsenide: the former predominates. These materials are doped with impurities to produce n-type and p-type semiconductors. Electrons are the main conductors or majority carriers in n-type semiconductors. The p-type semiconductors have 'holes' or orbital gaps as majority carriers.

The n-type and p-type semiconductors are combined to form the **p–n junction diode**. The junction diode exhibits different properties when connected to different polarity (+, −). Before current supply is connected a small **depletion layer** exists between the p- and n-boundary. Electrons migrate from the n-type a small way into the p-type layer. Holes from the p-type also migrate into the n-type material. If the positive pole of a battery is connected to the p-type and the negative pole to the n-type then a current flows (Fig. 2.18a); the diode is then **forward biased**. Reversing the polarity causes a wide depletion layer to be formed (Fig. 2.18b) and no current is able to flow; the diode is **reverse biased**. When a p–n junction is part of a circuit and the voltage varied from negative to positive as plotted in Fig. 2.18c current only flows when the diode is forward biased. Current flow does not obey Ohm's law since current flow shows an exponential relationship. The junction diode acts as a rectifier for AC waveforms. They have replaced all thermionic diodes in X-ray equipment giving a large reduction in size and cooler operation.

Three layer semiconductor devices are used for **signal amplification**. These are transistors which include two p–n junctions in a sandwich (Fig. 2.18d). A transistor can be either p–n–p or n–p–n. The three regions are **collector**, **base**, and **emitter** with the load commonly in the collector circuit (common emitter circuit). In the absence of a current (I_b) in the circuit (base-emitter) there is only a very small current through the load resistor (I_c). When a voltage V_b is

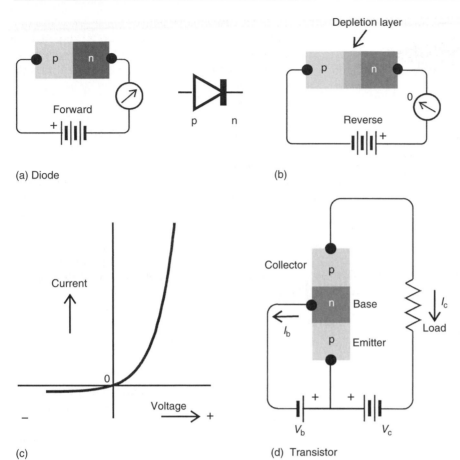

Figure 2.18 *(a) Forward biased diode conducting current. (b) Reverse biased diode where a depletion layer has formed preventing current flow. (c) The response of a diode to a negative and positive voltage showing its nonlinear response in the forward direction. (d) A 3-layer device, a transistor, which amplifies a small base signal.*

applied charge carriers called 'holes' (electron vacancies) are introduced which cause a current to flow in the base-collector circuit. The current I_c through the load is much higher than the current I_b and so amplification has taken place; a small base current controls a much larger collector current. Basic semiconductor devices are shown as schematics in Fig. 2.19a: a diode, pnp and npn transistors, a thyristor which is used as a fast switching device in high power circuits (X-ray generators) and a general symbol which represents an amplifier circuit.

The basic transistor circuit can be modified to form a **switching device** where a small signal can switch large collector loads on and off. Millions of micro-transistors can form fast switching devices which are incorporated into integrated logic devices for computers.

A reversed bias junction diode is sensitive to penetrating **radiation** (X-rays, gamma rays). Ionization causes carriers to be formed and a current flows proportional to radiation intensity. This is represented in Fig. 2.19b. Efficiency is low for X- and gamma radiation since the depletion zone is small. The depletion layer width is determined by the applied voltage and is typically 10–30 μm. Since Z for germanium (32) is higher than silicon (14) then germanium makes a more efficient detector. Small pn diodes are used for small scale X-ray detectors, useful for surface dose measurements and automatic exposure controls.

2.14 ATOMIC AND NUCLEAR STRUCTURE

The atom is the fundamental unit from which all matter is made. The essential features are shown in Fig. 2.20. All atoms consist of:

- Electron shells forming orbits
- A nucleus which is the central mass consisting of protons and neutrons

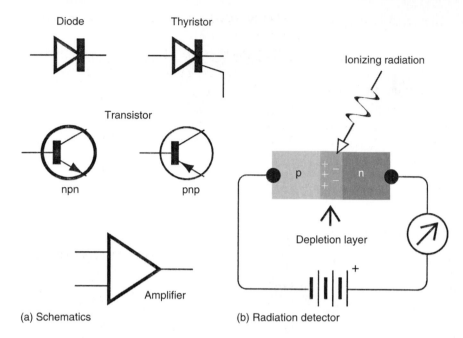

Figure 2.19
(*a*) *Semiconductor circuit symbols commonly used in radiology equipment.* (*b*) *A semiconductor radiation detector.*

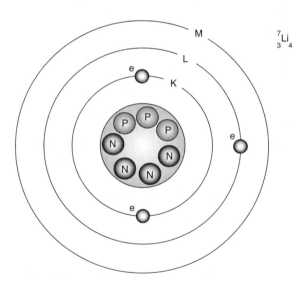

Figure 2.20 *Representation of the atom showing a nucleus with three protons and four neutrons together with the K, L and M electron orbits; the three proton charges being balanced by three electrons. This would represent a lithium atom.*

The atom is neutral, having an **electron charge** equal to the nuclear charge. Atoms of the separate elements have different numbers of protons forming the nuclear charge (+) balanced by different numbers of electrons (−).

Table 2.21 *Fundamental atomic particles.*

Particle	Charge	Mass
Electron	−1	~0
Positron	+1	~0
Proton	+1	1
Neutron	0	1
Neutrino	0	0
Photon	0	0

2.14.1 The nucleus

This is a small positively charged mass at the center of the atom; its size is approximately $\times 10^4$ to 10^5 smaller than the atom itself but contains almost all the mass of the atom since an electron is about $\times 2000$ less massive than a proton. The important components of an atom are listed in Table 2.21 giving their electrical charge and mass. The neutrino, which takes part in beta decay, and the photon, which forms the electromagnetic radiation (gamma radiation), have neither charge nor mass. The positron can be treated as a positively charged electron and will be further discussed in Chapter 15, which deals with nuclear medicine. The neutron is a neutral particle that only increases the nuclear mass without altering the nuclear charge.

The nucleus of an atom is characterized by its charge:

- The atomic number, Z, representing the number of protons in the nucleus
- Atomic mass or mass number, A; the total number of protons and neutrons in a nucleus.

The atomic number Z is the number of protons, while N represents the number of neutrons. The atomic mass A is the sum of protons and neutrons. The full description of the element X is given symbolically as

$$^A_Z X_N$$

Examples for hydrogen, carbon, and lead would be:

$$^1_1H_0, \quad ^{12}_6C_6, \quad ^{208}_{82}Pb_{126}$$

More simply they can be represented as:

$$^1H \quad ^{12}C \quad ^{208}Pb$$

The proton adds mass and charge to the nucleus; the neutron, being neutral, adds mass without charge. Isotopes are defined as a change in atomic mass without change in atomic number (loss or gain of neutrons). An unstable nucleus produces alpha, beta or gamma radiation in order to achieve stability; this is fully discussed in Chapter 15.

EFFECTIVE ATOMIC NUMBER

This has been estimated for a variety of compounds since it is an important factor in dosimetry. Care should be taken when applying these calculated values since they will alter with photon energy. Photoelectric effect depends on Z^3 and will vary with keV: Compton scatter will not be so affected. PMMA thermoplastic polymers of the type polymethyl methacrylate ester including Plexiglas, Lucite, Perspex are used as tissue equivalent materials. Table 2.22 lists the effective atomic numbers accepted for a range of radiologically important tissues and compounds.

2.14.2 The electron

This is a negatively charged particle discovered by J.J. Thomson (1856–1940; British physicist). **Electron orbits** form shells around the nucleus; the closest orbit to the nucleus is designated K followed by L, M, N etc., drawn in Fig. 2.20. The nucleus and its surrounding concentric shells of orbiting electrons make up the

Table 2.22 *Effective atomic numbers for radiologically important compounds.*

Material	Effective atomic number ($\bar{Z}$)	Density (kg m^{-3} × 10^3) (ρ)
Air	7.78	1.205
Muscle	7.64	1.04
Water	7.5	1.0
Bone	12.3–14.0	1.65
Fat	6.46	0.916
PMMA	6.56	1.18
Polystyrene	5.74	1.044
LiF	8.31	2.675

Table 2.23 *K-shell binding energies.*

Element	Z	K-shell energy (eV)
Carbon	6	0.28
Nitrogen	7	0.4
Oxygen	8	0.5
Phosphorus	15	2.1
Sulfur	16	2.5
Calcium	20	4.0
Molybdenum	42	20.0
Barium	56	37.4
Iodine	53	33.2
Tungsten	74	69.5
Lead	82	88.0
Uranium	92	115.6

complete atom. There are maximum numbers of electrons that can occupy each orbit (quantum number):

K	2 electrons
L	8 electrons
M	18 electrons
N	32 electrons
O	50 electrons

Electrons and some other fundamental particles (protons) have **spin** or **angular momentum**. This is always the same for a certain particle type and is a whole number. Angular momentum for protons is important in radiology when describing nuclear magnetic resonance.

The electrons are held in their orbits by electrostatic forces called **binding energies**; these are greater for the K-shell electrons and get successively weaker for the outer orbits. Binding energies for any particular K-shell will be greater for nuclei with large positive charges (large atomic number, Z). Examples of some of the binding energies are given in Table 2.23.

The removal of an electron from an orbit can only be achieved if the binding force is overcome. Most energy is needed for the K-shell electrons; these are more closely bound. The outer shell electrons are more easily removed and take part in chemical reactions; these are the **valency** electrons.

The electron orbit energy levels in an atom and the energies necessary to eject the electron from its orbital during the **ionization process** play an important role in the interaction of radiation with matter (Fig. 2.21a). The electron undergoes a transition when moving from one orbital to another either absorbing energy when going to a higher orbital from its ground state or emitting energy (usually in the form of a photon) when descending into a lower orbital.

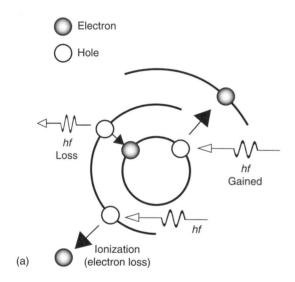

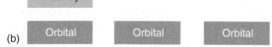

Figure 2.21 (a) Electron orbits showing transition from one energy level to another. A transition is accompanied by energy equal to the energy difference between the two levels taken in (photon absorbed) or given out (photon emitted). (b) Bands of conduction and valency separated by a varying width band gap in solid insulators, semiconductors and conductors.

If an atom gains or loses an electron it acquires an electrical charge and becomes an **ion**. Metals commonly lose electrons and become positive ions; nonmetals gain electrons becoming negative ions. This is commonly seen in ionizing salt solutions which dissociate, so NaCl in solution $\rightarrow$ Na$^+$ + Cl$^-$, also sodium and chlorine in their elemental state: Na $-$ e$^-$ $\rightarrow$ Na$^+$ and Cl + e$^-$ $\rightarrow$ Cl$^-$. In both cases Na$^+$ and Cl$^-$ are ions. If energy is delivered to a system (e.g. a gas) in the form of X- or gamma radiation then it will ionize giving a positive ion and a free electron: Xe + hf $\rightarrow$ Xe$^+$ + e$^-$.

When the xenon is irradiated it is ionized and the ionized events (Xe$^+$ + e$^-$) can form an electrical signal, which is the basis of a gas detector for ionizing radiation. Ionization events can occur with any element and are a most important reaction in radiology.

IONIZATION

Since the positive charge on the nucleus is balanced by the negative charges of the electrons, removal of any electrons gives the remaining structure a positive charge. The positive ion is unstable until the vacant orbit is filled by a free electron. If the K-electron is removed then the vacancy can be filled by an electron from the L-shell leaving a vacancy which then attracts its neighboring electron and so on, producing a cascade.

Figure 2.21a illustrates electron movement between orbits. The L-electron jumping into the K-orbit loses energy in the form of electromagnetic radiation. Other electron jumps involve less energy for their transition and give lower energy radiation (ultraviolet). A transition from a higher orbit to a lower one (the ground state) emits electromagnetic radiation. The K- and L-shell transitions emit X-ray photons which are **characteristic** for the atom.

Electrons in the outer shells can receive enough energy to be moved into an upper orbit, placing the atom into a state of **excitation** (Fig. 2.21a). They stay there for a short time before returning to their original orbit emitting electromagnetic radiation: visible or ultraviolet. These events play an important role in luminescence, which is found in some radiation detectors and screen materials (Chapter 6). Excited atoms are also more active chemically and are considered in tissue radiation dosimetry (Chapter 21).

2.14.3 Elements and compounds

At the atomic level electrons are attracted to the positively charged nucleus and are bound to the nucleus in stationary states known as orbitals. Groups of orbitals that differ only in the **angular momentum** of the electrons are combined together in **electron shells**. Electrons in the outermost shell are valency electrons and take part in the chemical properties of the atom.

The periodic table places the elements in order of their atomic number. Each row of the periodic table signifies the start of a new electron shell so elements which have similar chemical properties appear in the same part of the table. Metals tend to be on the left (e.g. Na, Ca) and nonmetals (e.g. I, Xe) tend to be on the right of the table. When atoms form **solid** compounds or crystals the energies of the orbitals change slightly so single energy levels become ranges of energy called energy bands shown in Fig. 2.21b, these are:

- The **valence band** where the valence electrons are found.
- The **conduction band** where there are both electrons and spaces for more electrons. The electrons are mobile and materials which have a conduction band are the only ones which can conduct electricity at room temperature.
- The **forbidden band** is the range of energies between two energy bands which is not occupied by electrons. The electron must cross this band gap to occupy a higher electron band. The band gap is large in insulator materials, very narrow in semiconductors and does not exist at all in conductors.

These bands are most important in radiology since they play a significant role in semiconductor electronics and radiation detector operation.

2.14.4 Solids

Solid materials (elements or compounds) can be classified as **insulators**, **metals** or **semiconductors** depending on electronic configuration; these have crystalline (structured) or amorphous (unstructured) form. Every solid material, or compound, is bound by their outer orbital electrons in an 'electronic cloud' differing according to the solid configuration. The electron cloud within the solid occupies either the valency or the **conduction bands**. Electrons in conduction bands are freely mobile over quite large distances but valency electrons are not mobile taking part in chemical reactions, so can be considered as tightly bound electrons in an atom.

Metals have a quantity of freely mobile electrons in the conduction band, as their unpaired electrons in the outermost shell become localized in this region. The degree of conductivity depends on the availability of electrons in this conduction band. Silver and copper have high electrical conductivity due to large numbers of electrons in their conduction band. Semiconductors and insulators have no electrons in their conduction band and their valence bands are completely filled. They do not conduct electrical current except at high temperatures.

The **energy difference** between an electron in a valency band and an electron in the conduction band is high in insulators (several eV). In a semiconductor it is so low (around 1 eV) that electrons can be elevated from valency to conduction bands.

An insulator has very few electrons in the conduction band.

2.14.5 Semiconductors

In an intrinsic semiconductor the valency and conduction bands are so close in energy that an appreciable number of electrons will have enough thermal energy to be found in the conduction band. These electrons and the corresponding 'holes' in the conduction band, which have a positive charge, are freely mobile. This means that an intrinsic semiconductor such as silicon or germanium can conduct current under certain conditions (see Section 2.13).

In order to achieve appreciable conductivity even at room temperature or with very small activation energy, semiconductors are carefully **doped** with impurities so that the crystalline structures contain defects. The impurities function as localized electron donors just below the conduction band and the energy required to lift an electron into the conduction band is much smaller. Such doping creates semiconductors that are called **n-type** where the n depicts conduction due to negative charges (electrons). If doping introduces electron acceptor states close to the valence band, these states can accept electrons from a valence band when only a small amount of energy (electrical) is put into the system. This doping leaves positively charged electron holes in the valence bands which are highly mobile and can conduct an electrical current. Such semiconductors are **p-type** since the current is supported by positive electronic charges.

In semiconductors the forbidden band is relatively small and only a small amount of energy is necessary to move valence electrons into the conduction band. In a **photoconductor**, this energy can be supplied by incident electromagnetic radiation (e.g. light, heat X-rays) when electrons are elevated to the conduction band and the semiconductor can conduct an electric current under the influence of an applied voltage.

The property of **luminescence** is discussed in Chapter 6.

KEYWORDS

2π surface: relating to a flat radiation detector
4π surface: relating to a volume radiation detector
abscissa: the horizontal x-axis of a graph usually holding the independent variable
ampere, A: is a measure of electrical current; $1\,C\,s^{-1}$ represents 6.24×10^{18} electrons per second
Avogadro's constant: number of particles in 1 mole; 6.022×10^{23}
coefficient of variation: a measure of dispersion as the standard deviation expressed as a percentage of the mean
correlation coefficient: a measure of association between two random variables. If one variable changes with the other then they are said to be correlated
coulomb, C: the SI unit of charge $1\,A = 1\,C^{-1}$
data set (or set): a collection of numbers that usually have one common property
decimal place: the figures to the right of the decimal point giving a specified degree of accuracy
density, ρ: mass per unit volume; $kg\,m^{-3}$ or a non-SI unit of $g\,cm^{-3}$
deterministic: a model where all events are inevitable consequences of antecedent causes. An effect seen at a predefined point (e.g. count rate, dose)
dispersion: the spread of a distribution (see standard deviation and quartile)
e: symbol for the transcendental number, 2.718 282, used as the base for the natural logarithm (also see exponential)
elastic collision: in which the kinetic energy of the colliding bodies is the same after collision as before. No energy change

electron charge, e: the charge on the electron; $1.602 \times 10^{-19}\,C$ and $1\,C = 6.24 \times 10^{18}$ electrons
electron volt, eV: a measure of electromagnetic radiation energy, particularly photons $1\,eV = 1.59 \times 10^{-19}\,J$
energy: ability to do work (potential and kinetic energy)
exponent: indicator for decimal point shift (left or right) in scientific notation, or in an exponential function x^n then n is the exponent
exponential: most commonly used when the exponent is the power of e. The exponential of x is e^x
extrapolation: estimation of a value of a variable beyond known values
floating point: a method of writing real numbers as $a \times 10^n$ or aEn where $a < 1$ but $\geqslant 0.1$ and n is the integer exponent directing decimal point position '−' left, '+' right. For example $0.564E - 1 = 0.0564$. A format also used in computing
Fourier analysis: a method of waveform analysis
gravity, g: gravitational constant $9.78\,m\,s^{-2}$ at the equator, $9.832\,m\,s^{-2}$ at the North Pole
histogram: a chart which displays grouped data
integer: a whole number
intensity: the power carried by a wave or oscillation divided by the area over which it arrives ($W\,m^{-2}$)
internal reflection: this occurs when the reflection angle is $>90°$
interpolation: estimation of a value of a variable between two known values
isotropic: emitting in all directions (spherical emission)
joule, J: the SI unit of work; $1\,J = 1\,N\,m^{-2}$
kelvin, K: the SI unit of temperature; $0\,K = -273.15°C$
kinetic energy: the energy due to motion; $E = \frac{1}{2}mv^2$
least squares: a way of estimating the best fit straight line for a plotted set of values
logarithm: the power to which a fixed number, the base, must be raised to obtain a given number. Abbreviated to log for base 10 and ln for base e
momentum: mass $\times$ velocity, measured as $kg\,m\,s^{-1}$
newton, N: the SI unit of force; $F = ma\ kg\,m\,s^{-1}$
normal distribution: a continuous distribution of a random variable with its mean, median, and mode equal
null hypothesis: usually based upon the assumption that nothing special is different between two samples. A statistical test challenges this assumption. If the significance of the difference (probability) is sufficiently large then the null hypothesis is rejected
ohm, Ω: the measure of electrical resistance when $1\,A$ flows at a potential difference of $1\,V$

ordinate: the y-axis of a graph

outlier: observation which is far removed from the others in a set

parametric (non-parametric): pertaining to exact measurement (e.g. count density, weights, temperature). Non-parametric measurements are scores or ranks

pascal, Pa: the SI unit for pressure in $N m^{-2}$ and $1 mmHg = 1.33 \times 10^2 Pa$

potential energy: chemical, gravitational, electrical, and elastic are all examples

power: the rate of work done per unit time, as $J s^{-1}$

power law: a function giving a straight line when plotted on log–log axes

quantile: general name for the values of a variable which divide its distribution into equal groups

quartile: the value of a variable below which three-quarters (first or upper quartile) or one-quarter (3rd or lower quartile) of a distribution lie

radian, rad: the SI unit of plane angle, where 1 rad is $57.2958°$

rational (irrational) number: having a fixed number of decimal places. An irrational number would be π or e where the number cannot be represented as a ratio

refraction: the change in the direction of a wave front when passing from one medium to another

refractive index: the product of the sine of angle of incidence to the sine of the angle of refraction

regression: a test which calculates the best fit for a straight line through a set of points on a graph when y is the dependent variable and x the independent (see least squares)

scientific notation: a numerical form similar to floating point: $a \times 10^n$ or aEn where a is a number 1 to 10 and n is a whole number as before, i.e. $5.64E-2 = 0.0564$

significance: a probability of rejecting the null hypothesis. $p = 0.05$ borderline significance, $p = 0.01$ significant, $p = 0.001$ highly significant

sine wave: a wave-function where $y = \sin x$

skew: a distribution where mean, mode, and median do not coincide

specular reflection: reflection at a smooth border where the surface unevenness is much less than the wavelength

standard deviation: a measure of sample dispersion. Square root of the variance

standard error: standard error of the sample mean. A comparison of the sample mean with the parent mean $\sigma/\sqrt{n}$

steradian: the solid angle in spherical geometry

stochastic: an entirely random process

tesla, T: the SI measure of magnetic field strength, where $1 T = 1 N m^{-1}$ at 90° to the field

variable, continuous: a variable that may take any value

variable, dependent: a variable dependent on another. Usually placed on the y-axis

variable, discrete: the opposite to continuous. A variable that may only take certain values

variable, independent: a variable not dependent on another. Usually placed on the x-axis

variance: a measure of dispersion

volt, V: a measure of electrical potential difference, where $1 V = 1 J C^{-1}$

watt, W: the SI unit of mechanical or electrical power, where $1 W = 1 J s^{-1}$

wavefront: a line that joins all points on a wave that have the same phase

weber, Wb: the unit of magnetic flux

3

X-ray production and properties: fundamentals

3.1 INTRODUCTION

On Friday 8 November 1895 Wilhelm Conrad Röntgen (1845–1923; German physicist) while experimenting with high voltages using a Crooke's tube (an evacuated tube with electrodes inserted) noticed that invisible radiation was being produced that penetrated the soft tissue of his hand revealing skeletal structure. He called the radiation 'X-rays': X denoting their unknown origin. Within a year of their discovery X-rays were being used for medical imaging. In 1901 Röntgen received the first Nobel Prize for physics. In 1913 W.D. Coolidge (1873–1975; USA engineer) produced the electrically heated cathode tube: the forerunner of all modern X-ray tubes.

3.1.1 X- and gamma radiation

The principle of X-ray generation is relatively simple. A beam of high energy electrons from a heated **filament** (situated in a cathode assembly) bombards a positively charged heavy metal target, the **anode**.

The electrons mostly react with the target's orbital electrons producing heat (99%): the remaining electrons interact with the target nuclei giving a **continuous** X-ray spectrum made up of many photon energies; a **poly-energetic** spectrum. X-ray photon energy from the tube can be controlled by varying the electrical supply high voltage. The diagnostic range has a **peak energy** (kV_p) from 40 to 140 kV_p; mammography utilizes a lower energy from 20 to 30 kV_p.

Figure 3.1a shows that an X-ray tube can be treated as a electronic diode since the electrons only travel in one direction, having a heated filament at one end which acts as the source of electrons and an anode at the other.

Electrons emitted by the filament are accelerated across a vacuum by applying a high voltage, colliding with the anode to produce X-radiation. X-rays are formed by electrons changing direction within the vicinity of a heavy nucleus (tungsten). Since there is a direction change the electrons lose energy in the form of electromagnetic radiation.

GAMMA RADIATION

In contrast to X-rays gamma radiation, although similar to X-radiation in many respects, is produced during nuclear decay and has discrete energies forming a line spectrum. It is mostly mono-energetic although some nuclides emit more than one gamma energy. Gamma radiation, having discrete energies, is measured in keV and MeV; the useful diagnostic imaging range being 100 keV to 0.511 MeV.

A non-nuclear source of gamma radiation is positron annihilation. X-rays are also produced from some types of nuclear decay: these processes are

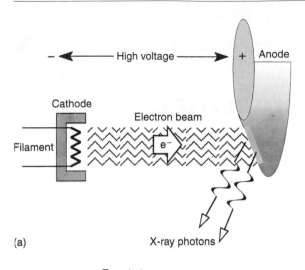

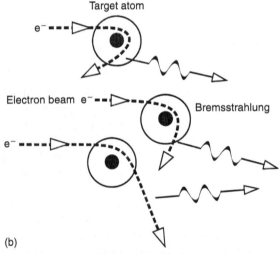

Figure 3.1 *(a) The basic components of an X-ray tube. A hot filament is the electron source embedded in a metal cathode (negative charge). The electron beam is attracted toward the target anode (positive charge) causing Bremsstrahlung events. (b) Bremsstrahlung production caused by electron deflection by heavy metal nuclei.*

covered more fully in Chapter 15 (which deals with nuclear medicine).

3.1.2 Bremsstrahlung

The potential energy of the electron is the product of the electrostatic charge between the cathode and anode seen in Fig. 3.1a. Potential energy is transformed into kinetic energy as they accelerate between cathode and anode.

The electrons penetrate the anode material passing close to its atomic nuclei. They are deflected from their initial path by the nuclear coulomb field of the heavy atoms (e.g. tungsten) causing changes in velocity (both acceleration and deceleration) simply illustrated in Fig. 3.1b. During their changes in velocity (deflection) they lose energy in the form of electromagnetic radiation which is called braking radiation or **Bremsstrahlung**. The deflection is dependent on the nuclear charge (atomic number Z) of the anode. Loss of kinetic energy through interactions with target electrons causes a great deal of heat energy which must be removed effectively in order to prevent anode melting. Heat and light production (99%) together with X-rays (1%) obey the basic equation from Chapter 2:

$$E = hf \qquad (3.1)$$

where h is Planck's constant and f the frequency of the electromagnetic radiation.

The X-ray tube has a high vacuum so that gas molecules do not impede the electron beam and since very high voltages are used (from 20 to 150 kV) the tube must be manufactured from robust insulating materials, e.g. glass or ceramic.

CONTINUOUS X-RAY SPECTRUM

Only a small proportion of the X-rays are created at the surface of the target, those formed deeper within the target material are absorbed. Energy transformations that yield X-radiation vary since the bombarding electrons approach the nuclei differently; there is, consequently, a spread of Bremsstrahlung energies from maximum (where the entire electron energy is transformed into X-radiation) to the lowest energy X-ray emission when the electron is only slightly deflected by the nuclear field. Electron velocity increases with the applied high voltage but very few electrons lose all their energy in a single event giving a photon of maximum energy; most of them undergo multiple events where energy loss results in a mixed energy X-ray photons. The peak high tension applied to the tube does not represent the maximum X-ray photon energy (kV peak or kV_p) owing to relativistic effects which reduce electron velocities. The resulting X-radiation takes the form of a continuous X-ray spectrum which is shown in Fig. 3.2.

The lowest energy photons are removed since the beam of X-rays leaving the tube is filtered by the glass envelope. If low energy X-rays are required (e.g.

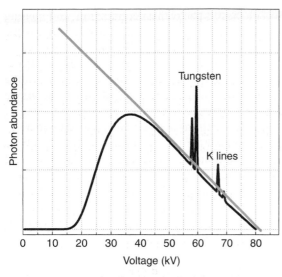

Figure 3.2 *Continuous spectrum (gray line) shows that the lowest photon energies (below about 20 keV) are removed by the X-ray tube glass wall giving an exit spectrum which is peaked. Characteristic line spectra are superimposed on this spectrum.*

mammography) then a thin metal beryllium window must be used with its much lower density (1800 kg m⁻³) than glass (4200 kg m⁻³) giving a greater transparency to lower energy X-radiation.

CHARACTERISTIC RADIATION

The collisions between the beam electrons and the inner orbital electrons (K and L shells) of the target create orbital vacancies. These are quickly filled accompanied by the emission of characteristic radiation in the form of line spectra which are seen superimposed on the continuous X-ray spectrum in Fig. 3.2. The line spectra for tungsten occur at roughly 59 and 69 keV.

3.1.3 X-ray beam intensity

X-ray production is a very inefficient process, most of the electrical energy is lost as heat. The approximate balance is:

Electron beam intensity	100%
Heat and light production	99%
X-radiation from anode surface	1%
Remaining after inherent filtration	0.5%
Remaining after added filtration (available X-rays for imaging)	0.1%

Table 3.1 *Efficiency of X-ray production.*

Element and kilovoltage	Efficiency (%)
Tungsten ($Z = 74$)	
20 kV	0.162
60 kV	0.48
100 kV	0.814
140 kV	1.14
Molybdenum ($Z = 42$)	
20 kV	0.092

The **probability** p for Bremsstrahlung events is low, about 1–5%, but increases with both atomic number Z of the anode material and the electron beam energy E, so that $p \propto ZE^2$. Substituting kV for E yields

$$p \propto Z * kV^2 \qquad (3.2)$$

This function follows a power law relationship. The **efficiency** η of Bremsstrahlung production depends on

$$\eta = k * E * Z \qquad (3.3)$$

where k is a constant, being 1.1×10^{-9} for tungsten. The efficiency of Bremsstrahlung production for tungsten and molybdenum, over a range of energies, is listed in Table 3.1. X-ray intensity increases with applied kilovoltage and density of anode material since both the probability and efficiency are influenced by these two factors.

Knowing the electron charge and the tube current together with the exposure time (mA s) the available photons which form a chest radiograph can be estimated as in Box 3.1. If allowances are made for X-ray production efficiency an approximate quantity can be derived that is useful for future calculations.

SUMMARY

- X-rays are produced by bombarding heavy metal targets with electrons: the probability of production increases as the kilovoltage squared.
- Efficiency increases with applied kilovoltage and with target Z.
- Bremsstrahlung radiation gives a continuous X-ray spectrum. The peak energy (kV_p) equals the applied kilovoltage.
- The lowest photon energies are absorbed by the tube wall. Lower energies can be retrieved by using a beryllium window.
- Characteristic X-rays are produced by dislodging K- and L-shell electrons from the target.

Box 3.1 Chest radiograph photon number

The number of X-ray photons produced during a standard radiograph of 60 kV at 5 mAs can be calculated approximately:

Electron charge is 1.6×10^{-19} C.

Since $1 \text{ A} = 1 \text{ C s}^{-1}$ then $\text{C s}^{-1} \times$ seconds represent coulombs.

$$5 \text{ mA s} = \frac{5 \times 10^{-3}}{1.6 \times 10^{-19}} = 3.13 \times 10^{16} \text{ electrons}$$

but owing to low production efficiency at 60 kV only 0.5% produce useful X-rays (Table 3.1). So 60 kV at 5 mAs would give:

$$3.13 \times 10^{16} \times 0.005 = 1.5 \times 10^{14}$$

available X-ray photons.

3.2 X-RAY TUBE DESIGN

Diagnostic X-ray tubes are high precision units which are engineered to very close tolerances and are largely hand finished; they are therefore costly items. The major problems of X-ray tube design are:

- Efficient production of X-radiation and efficient heat removal
- Constant X-ray beam quality with desired geometry (beam profile)
- Reliable performance under a wide variety of loading conditions such as short duration/high loading (pulsed computed tomography (CT) and digital subtraction angiography (DSA)) and long duration low loading (fluoroscopy)

The majority of X-ray tubes employ **rotating anodes** since stationary anode X-ray tubes are only suitable for low output applications experienced in dentistry and small mobile X-ray units. Consequently rotating anodes are the most common X-ray tube design.

The important components can be identified from the detailed diagram of Fig. 3.3.

METALS USED IN CONSTRUCTION

The various materials used in X-ray tube construction are listed in Table 3.2 along with their properties.

Specific heat capacity, heat conduction, and melting point are very important parameters owing to the excessive heat produced by X-ray tubes.

Molybdenum has a larger heat capacity than tungsten and is used as a backing for the target and in the manufacture of the supporting stem for the anode disk.

Carbon, in the form of graphite, is used for increasing the radiating surface of the anode. It is ideal since it is a good heat radiator (black), has a low mass and a high melting point.

Copper has a large heat capacity together with superior heat conduction but a lower melting point which restricts its use and is mainly found as electrical wires and as part of the anode rotor.

3.2.1 The cathode assembly

The basic design for the X-ray tube shown in Fig. 3.3a shows the cathode and filament assembly consisting of a **filament**, made from tungsten wire, which is heated electrically to a high temperature so that electrons are 'boiled-off' from its surface. These electrons form the **tube current**. The filament is located within a negatively charged nickel **cathode** which is shaped so that a precise beam geometry is obtained.

THE FILAMENT

This is manufactured from tungsten wire and is part of the cathode assembly. Together they provide a carefully shaped electron beam which bombards a precise target area on the anode. The cathode assembly is connected to the negative high voltage supply.

FILAMENT SUPPLY

The power supply, which heats the filament, is low voltage AC from a filament transformer supplying 8 to 12 V. Since this is AC there is a superimposed low frequency ripple on filament emission and the X-ray tube current. High frequency transformers do not have this problem.

THE CATHODE

This houses the filament and is manufactured from nickel. The filament is located within a depression or **cup** having sharp contoured edges which electrostatically focus the electron beam. Figure 3.4a shows the complete cathode assembly. Exact focusing is achieved

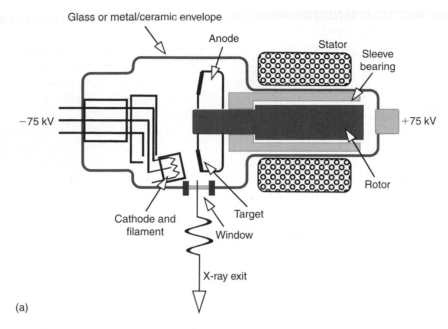

Glass or metal/ceramic envelope

Anode

Stator

Sleeve bearing

−75 kV

+75 kV

Rotor

Cathode and filament

Target

Window

X-ray exit

(a)

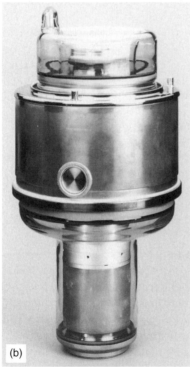

(b)

Figure 3.3 *(a) The details of a typical X-ray tube showing the position of the filament– cathode assembly with respect to the anode. A molybdenum axle supported by bearings (rotor) is driven by the external stator. High voltage negative and positive connections are shown. (b) Commercial X-ray tube (Siemens) showing glass/metal construction.*

by altering the depth of the filament in the cathode during manufacture. The cathode cup can also be independently supplied with a high negative voltage which can dynamically alter the focal size or, if the negative charge is big enough, switch off the electron beam entirely. This is the **grid controlled** X-ray tube and is used in cine-fluorography, DSA units and CT where rapid pulses of X-rays are required.

Table 3.2 *Melting point, specific heat and thermal conductivity of some important materials.*

Material	M. pt (°C)	Specific heat ($J\ kg^{-1}K^{-1}$)	Thermal conductivity ($W\ m^{-1}K^{-1}$)
W	3410	137	176
Mo	2617	253	138
Ni	1726	455	59
Cu	1356	385	385
C	3800	730	5
Glass	1400	670	1.5

Figure 3.4b shows three examples of beam control obtained by using an increasing negative voltage on the cathode cup. A broad focus beam (top diagram) is about 1 to 2 mm wide and a fine focus beam (middle) is typically about 0.4 to 0.1 mm wide. A high negative charge on the cathode edges (bottom diagram) switches off the electron beam entirely, and this control mechanism is used for giving precise X-ray pulses.

TUBE LIFETIME

The available electron density from the heated filament (emission current density) depends on the filament temperature. The relationship between filament temperature and emission current density is plotted in Fig. 3.5a and shows that for small changes in filament temperature there are large changes in emission current and hence X-ray tube current. Stable filament power supplies are therefore essential for consistent X-ray exposure.

The level of filament current significantly determines the lifetime of the X-ray tube. This is indicated by a typical life-time graph in Fig. 3.5b. For short exposures the filament temperature is 2500°C but would be lower for continuous use as in, say, fluoroscopy.

SPACE CHARGE EFFECT

As electrons leave or are 'boiled-off' from the filament it becomes increasingly more positive owing to the loss of negative charge. The electrons tend to be attracted back towards the filament surface. At higher filament temperatures a cloud of electrons develops containing a constant stream of electrons both leaving and returning from the filament surface shown in Fig. 3.6a. It has already been demonstrated

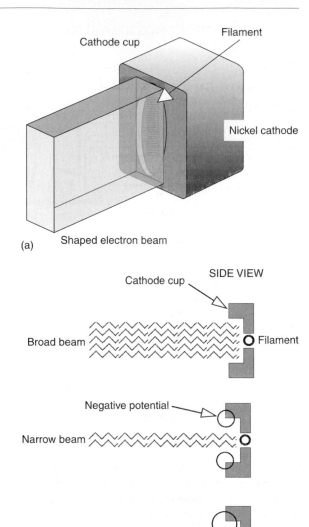

(a) Shaped electron beam

(b)

Figure 3.4 *(a) The filament encased in a nickel cathode. The sharp edges of the cup shape the electron beam. (b) The geometry of the electron beam is controlled by the applied negative voltage to the cathode. The bottom diagram shows how the beam can be switched off by applying a much higher negative voltage.*

in Chapter 2 that a positive charged body (anode) placed near the filament will attract some electrons from the cloud and therefore a current will pass between the filament and the anode. Electrons are injected into this dynamic system by the negative high voltage supply (-75 kV) connected to the filament circuit.

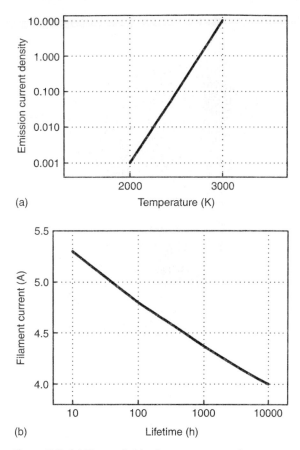

(a)

(b)

Figure 3.5 *(a) The available electrons measured as an emission current increases rapidly with relatively small increases in filament temperature. (b) Increasing the filament current shortens tube life.*

The tube current (current flow in the diagram) depends on the applied anode voltage. At lower voltages (between 20 and 40 kV) not all the available electrons are attracted from the filament. This limits the tube current and is the **space charge** effect. This effect is demonstrated by the shoulder region of the graph in Fig. 3.6b between a tube voltage of about 10 to 50 kV. Increasing the tube voltage overcomes this problem allowing higher tube currents shown by a large increase in tube current with applied tube kilovoltage in the graph.

3.2.2 Anode construction

Dental units and some small mobile X-ray units use stationary or fixed anode designs. The most efficient design however uses a rotating-disk anode which enables higher X-ray output owing to more effective cooling.

The basic design of a simple rotating anode consists of a tungsten disk, typically between 90 and 200 mm diameter, with an accurately beveled edge giving the **anode angle**; this has already been seen in Fig. 3.1a but is given in more detail in Fig. 3.7a. It is attached to a molybdenum stem which connects with a rotor forming, together with the stator windings, an induction motor which rotates the anode at speed.

Since useful X-rays are produced at the surface of the anode the target area itself is made from thin metal alloy (tungsten–rhenium), about 1 mm thick. This has the added advantage of easier heat removal and the rhenium content reduces surface pitting.

Graphite, being a very low mass material with a high melting point, is brazed onto the back of the anode which increases heat radiating efficiency in tubes that will experience high loading (DSA and CT).

ANODE SIZE

Rotating anode disks are manufactured in many designs, the anode diameter determines the heat rating of the X-ray tube and therefore its thermal loading. The disk mass and surface area also play an important part.

From Fig. 3.7b a larger anode diameter at the same rotational speed offers a longer track length of target and so the heat generated is spread over a greater area of metal. Larger disks therefore take higher loading (higher output). The 150 mm anode gives a target length × 1.5 more than the 100 mm anode and its target area is also larger. Anode disk diameters vary from 75 to 200 mm depending on loading required. Larger anode diameters are used for high power applications such as fluoroscopy and CT. A larger disk diameter increases the heat capacity and also the area radiating heat but there is potential mechanical damage in the larger anode due to localized expansion.

This is prevented by cutting radial slots into the anode (the 150 mm anode in Fig. 3.7b); these are **stress relieved** anodes. This technique is not usually applied to CT tubes since the slit surface would interfere with the high speed grid control producing the pulsed X-ray beam.

Exposure overload monitoring devices (such as Loadix, a thermal detector device) placed behind the anode to monitor heat output prevent X-ray tube ratings from being exceeded. Anode speed affects rating

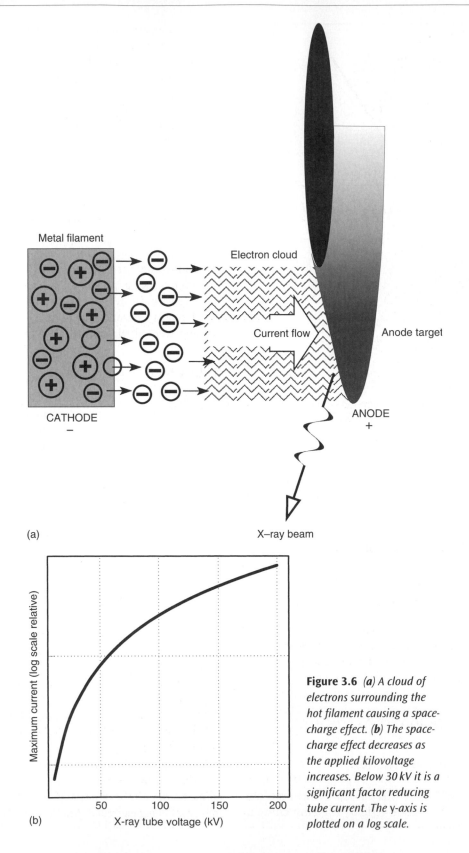

Metal filament

Electron cloud

Current flow

Anode target

CATHODE
−

ANODE
+

X–ray beam

(a)

Maximum current (log scale relative)

X-ray tube voltage (kV)

50   100   150   200

(b)

Figure 3.6 *(a) A cloud of electrons surrounding the hot filament causing a space-charge effect. (b) The space-charge effect decreases as the applied kilovoltage increases. Below 30 kV it is a significant factor reducing tube current. The y-axis is plotted on a log scale.*

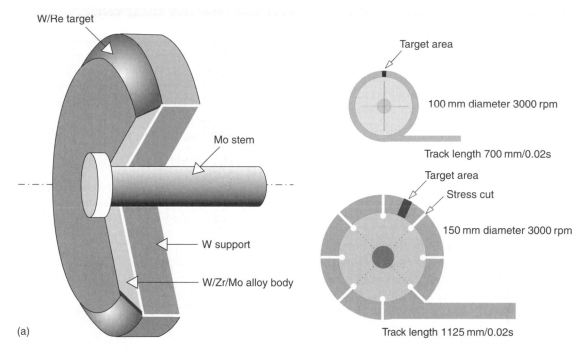

Figure 3.7 (*a*) *The rotating anode construction showing a solid tungsten/zirconium/molybdenum base supporting a pure tungsten layer on which the thin (1 mm thick) tungsten–rhenium alloy target is fused.* (*b*) *A 100 mm diameter anode (top) showing the track length available during a 0.02 s exposure time. Increased track length (150 mm) allows greater heat dissipation for the same exposure time.*

Box 3.2 Anode disk size and power rating

Anode diameter and power rating

With reference to Fig. 3.7b, for a 100 mm diameter anode and a 7 mm track width, the mean radius is $(100 - 7\,\mathrm{mm}) = 93\,\mathrm{mm}$ and the track length is $2\pi \times 93/2 = 292\,\mathrm{mm}$.

Anode rotation speed of 3000 rpm

The complete target area is exposed every $60/3000 = 0.02\,\mathrm{s}$. For 9000 rpm this would be $0.0066\,\mathrm{s}$ so the electron energy deposited in the anode is spread over a greater target area for faster rotational speeds (also see Fig. 3.7b).

and Box 3.2 gives some examples for anode size and speed.

3.2.3 Rotor and stator

The rotating anode forms part of an induction motor shown as the rotor and stator in Fig. 3.3. The rotor, made from copper, is attached to the anode by a molybdenum stem. This revolves about a central axle which forms the positive electrode $(+75\,\mathrm{kV})$. The axle bearing can consist of either ball races, lubricated by a silver paste, or sleeve bearings. The latter allow greater surface contact and therefore more rapid cooling by conduction. Excessive heat transfer along the anode stem is restricted since molybdenum has relatively poor heat conductivity and most of the heat loss is by radiation from the anode surface toward the X-ray tube envelope (glass or metal). In some tubes, employing sleeve bearings, an oil circulation path passes along the axle. The anode rotational speed is either 3000 or 3400 rpm at 50/60 Hz supply frequency or 850–10 000 rpm using high frequency waveforms. For these higher speeds either the overall tube loading can be increased or finer focal spot sizes can be selected. Larger disk diameters require better support and the anode stem in these tubes is carried forward and supported by its own bearing, giving support both in front and behind.

3.2.4 Focal spot

The X-rays do not originate from a single point on the anode surface, but from a rectangular area, the dimensions and angle of which are carefully calculated. This is shown as a target area in Fig. 3.8a and forms the **real focal spot** of the electron beam. The anode angle determines the projected or **effective focal spot** size of the X-ray beam (sometimes called the apparent focal spot). The focal spot size influences the sharpness of the image and the tube rating.

REAL AND EFFECTIVE FOCAL SPOTS

The size of the effective focal spot is determined by the **line focus principle** and a calculation is given in Box 3.3 using the geometry shown in this figure. This calculation shows that the formation of a symmetrical effective focal spot from an angled real focal spot on the anode surface is achieved by choosing an angle that projects the same length as the real focal spot width.

USEFUL FIELD OF VIEW

The smaller the angle θ the wider the track can be, as seen in Fig. 3.8b. In general the smaller the anode angle the wider the focal track which increases the power

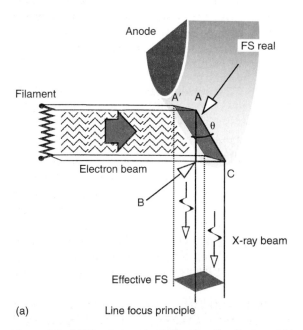

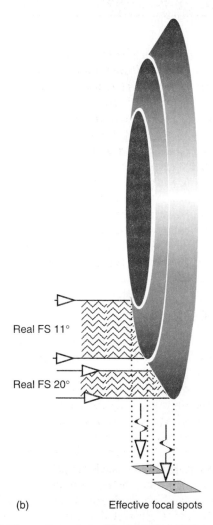

(a)   Line focus principle   (b)   Effective focal spots

Figure 3.8 *(a) The electron beam bombarding the target (shaded area). The anode angle θ of the triangle A,B,C is used for calculating the effective focal spot size. (b) Increasing the anode angle decreases the real focal spot area which reduces anode rating.*

Box 3.3 The line focus principle

From Fig. 3.8a the electron beam of width A–A' strikes the anode target area. The dimension f (which equals CB) is determined by

$$\sin\theta = \frac{\text{opposite}}{\text{hypotenuse}}$$

So the effective focal spot BC $= \sin\theta \times$ AC. If AC is 2 mm (real focal spot) the effective or apparent focal spot is then 0.2588×2 or 0.5 mm. Doubling the real focal spot size (4 mm) will give a 1 mm effective focal spot.

rating, however angle size also influences the field size of the X-ray beam at a given source-to-image distance (SID). Field size increases with anode angle, but so also does the effective focal spot size which will degrade image resolution, so a large area radiograph would be obtained at the expense of resolution.

Conversely, a smaller anode angle would give a smaller field size but a better resolution. The choice of anode angle depends on the application required and the SID. A smaller anode angle yields a larger focal spot and consequently higher heat rating or load. Stationary anode tubes have an energy dissipation of about 200 J mm^{-2}s^{-1} of the actual focal spot size. A rotating anode has an energy dissipation of 1500 J mm^{-2}s^{-1}.

DUAL FOCAL SPOTS

For many applications two focal spot sizes are necessary; a second smaller spot is used for higher resolution or magnified radiographs. Two methods are shown. In Fig. 3.9a a single filament refocuses the electron beam electrostatically varying the negative voltage on the cathode cup, so bombarding a smaller area on the anode track (see narrow beam in Fig. 3.4b). Alternatively Fig. 3.9b shows a double filament, each one directed to a different angled target, which requires a dual track anode to give two focal spot sizes.

Each method has its disadvantages. Figure 3.9(c) shows that the single track dual focus anode uses the central portion of the track for both fine and broad focus beams so greater wear will take place shortening tube life. Wear is reduced for a dual track dual focus

design (lower picture in (c)) but the track length for the fine focal spot is shorter which will reduce its loading capability.

EFFECT

Photon intensity across the X-ray beam is not uniform. The uniformity changes with anode angle and gives a **heel effect** to the beam intensity. Collimating the useful field of view reduces the heel effect but does not eliminate it; Fig. 3.10a. The diagram of the field intensity patterns in Fig. 3.10b shows that the heel effect decreases with increase in anode angle: 7°, 12°, and 20° but increasing the angle adversely effects image resolution and thermal rating (loadability). The heel effect only occurs in line with the cathode/anode axis and the plot of intensity across the beam in this axis, Fig. 3.10(c), indicates the substantial drop (up to 25%) in beam intensity at the anode end of the tube. This is improved with increased SID as shown by the two plots for 70 and 110 cm SID.

3.2.5 Tube enclosure

X-RAY TUBE ENVELOPE

Boro-silicate glass is the common material for tube construction since it conforms with manufacturing requirements. A high vacuum must be maintained in the X-ray tube for the electron beam so the surrounding envelope must be:

- Strong enough to withstand atmospheric pressure
- Heat resistant to withstand considerable heat production by the anode
- Transparent to the heat radiated from the anode

During the life of the tube metal atoms from the incandescent filament and those vaporized from the focal spot are deposited on the glass walls; this slowly reduces its insulator properties. The closer the electrodes are to the wall the more serious is this problem and gives design restrictions. Glass envelopes are particularly prone to breakdown but metal/ceramic enclosures repel ion deposits reducing the tungsten coating build-up.

More compact tube design can be obtained by using a metal envelope which will be unaffected by vaporized metal and be a more efficient heat exchanger, it is also stronger. The insulating regions in metal tubes are made from ceramic material.

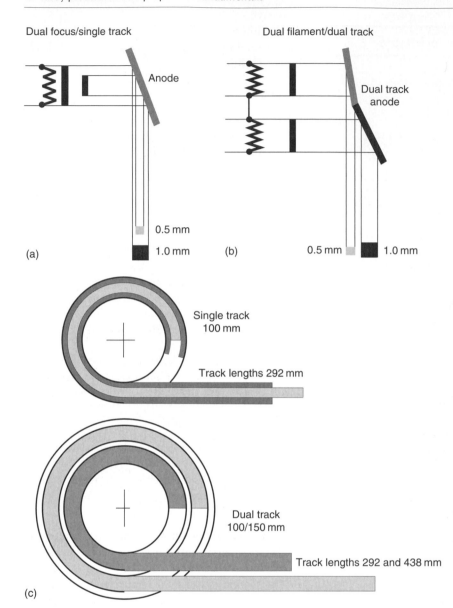

Dual focus/single track

Anode

0.5 mm

1.0 mm

(a)

Dual filament/dual track

Dual track anode

0.5 mm   1.0 mm

(b)

Single track
100 mm

Track lengths 292 mm

Dual track
100/150 mm

Track lengths 292 and 438 mm

(c)

Figure 3.9 *(a) Dual focal spot sizes can be obtained by altering the target size with different negative potentials on the filament cup or (b) employing two filaments focused on different target angles. (c) Anodes showing single and dual target areas.*

HOUSING

The X-ray tube itself is enclosed in a sealed housing which is shown in Fig. 3.11. Efficient removal of heat produced by X-ray production by the tube is essential. Circulating air is sufficient to cool mobile and mammography units (fan assisted cooling can halve tube cooling time), but circulating oil is necessary within the enclosure for cooling conventional and DSA equipment. The total heat capacity of the tube enclosure is largely dependent on the volume of oil it contains.

RADIATION SHIELDING

Radiation shielding X-rays are emitted from the tube in all directions and overall lead shielding must cover the complete housing assembly. Any leakage of radiation is measured with the collimator diaphragms closed and should be less than $1 \, mGy \, h^{-1}$ (100 mR) at 1 m and is usually less than $0.3 \, mGy \, h^{-1}$ (30 mR). An acceptable leakage figure for current X-ray equipment would be $\times \, 0.5 \, mSv \, h^{-1}$ at $150 \, kV_p$. Since the beam intensity varies across the beam width in the anode–cathode axis (heel effect) a fixed lead diaphragm

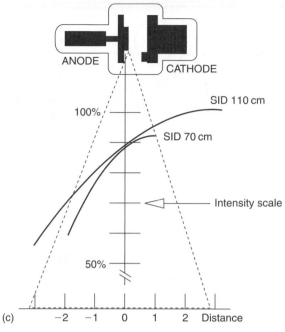

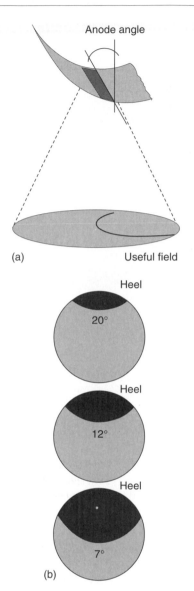

Figure 3.10 *(c) The plot of beam intensity shows the variation along the anode to cathode axis for two source-to-image distances (SIDs): 70 cm (shaded curve) and 110 cm (black curve).*

Figure 3.10 *(a) The useful X-ray field is contained by the central beam and the outside margins of the beam are blocked by collimating the beam. (b) This useful field is still non-uniform due to the heel effect, influenced by anode angle.*

restricts beam dimensions yielding the useful beam width. Other adjustable diaphragms/collimators are used for varying the overall beam size for different fields of view.

3.2.6 X-ray window

The glass window of the X-ray tube removes low-energy X-ray photons (from 0 to ≈ 20 keV) and so provides **inherent beam filtration** (seen in Fig. 3.2). Further filtration is still necessary, however, as photons from the low energy end of the spectrum play no part in image formation and are absorbed in the first few centimeters of soft tissue which contributes to the patient radiation dose.

Fixed or **added filtration** is added to the beam to remove lower energies. Inherent and fixed filtration together give the **total filtration**. The inherent filtration is equivalent to about 0.5 mm aluminum but as the tube ages this increases due to vaporized tungsten and the fixed filtration (about 1.5 to 2.0 mm aluminum) must be altered to compensate for this.

3.3 THE X-RAY SPECTRUM

The theoretical complete spectrum from an X-ray tube has already been shown as a straight gray line in Fig. 3.2 but in practice several factors remove the lower energy photons:

- The depth of interactions within the target
- X-ray tube wall thickness
- Additional beam filtration

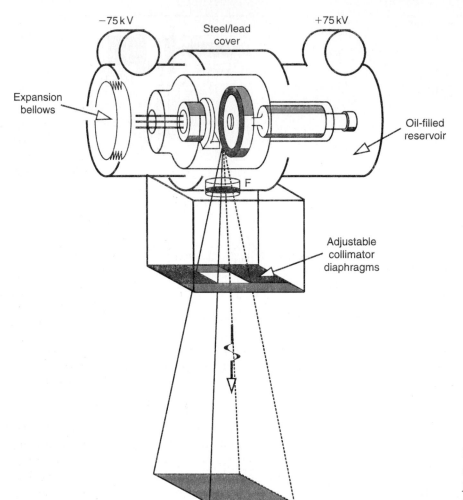

-75 kV

Steel/lead
cover

+75 kV

Expansion
bellows

Oil-filled
reservoir

F

Adjustable
collimator
diaphragms

Figure 3.11 *X-ray tube housing showing position of fixed filtration (F) and beam collimators.*

The **maximum** beam energy (kV_{peak} or kV_p) depends on the applied voltage which directly influences speed of the electron beam (kinetic energy). The X-ray **minimum** energy depends on the material through which the bremsstrahlung must pass.

3.3.1 Characteristic radiation

The common target materials tungsten, rhenium and molybdenum yield line spectra for their characteristic K energies:

Tungsten	69.5 and 59.3 keV
Rhenium	71.6 and 61.1 keV
Molybdenum	20.0 and 17.3 keV

Figure 3.12 shows an unfiltered (A) and filtered (B) continuous spectra from a tungsten anode showing the K-shell radiation as superimposed line spectra which result from interactions with the electron beam and the K-shell electrons. Smaller line spectra from the L shells would also be present.

3.3.2 Beam energy

Increasing the high voltage increases the overall intensity of the continuous spectrum. In Fig. 3.13a the kilovoltage has been increased in three steps from 75, 100, and 125 kV; the peak energy values (kV_p) follow this. The choice of kilovoltage determines object (patient) penetration and image quality. Low kilovoltages give high contrast images (distinguishing soft tissue differences in mammography) since low energy X-ray photons are easily absorbed. Higher kilovoltages, due to their increased penetration, reduce contrast differences

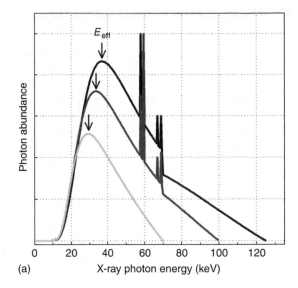

Figure 3.12 *Continuous X-ray spectra from tungsten targets, before (**A**) and after (**B**) filtering showing increase in effective energy (E_{eff}) and tungsten's characteristic K lines.*

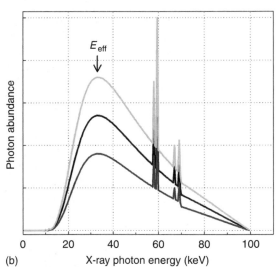

Figure 3.13 *(**a**) The change of the X-ray spectrum with applied kilovoltage. Peak kilovoltages of 50, 80, and 120 kV$_p$ show how the effective energy also changes. (**b**) Intensity of the X-ray beam increases with tube current (mA) but the effective energy remains the same.*

and since beam intensity increases as the kilvoltage squared (Equation 3.5) the overall radiation reaching the film also increases (higher penetration). It will be seen in later chapters that film-screen sensitivity also improves with kilovoltage.

EFFECTIVE ENERGY

This is the modal output identified on the curves in Fig. 3.13a as E_{eff}. The beam's effective energy can be influenced by changing kV$_p$ and filtration. The intensity Q of the beam is seen to increase as Q is proportional to the kilovoltage squared so a 30% increase in kilovoltage approximately doubles X-ray beam intensity along with an increase in effective energy. The effective energy of a moderately filtered X-ray spectrum is very roughly two thirds kV$_p$ so 100 kV$_p$ would translate as 70 kV$_{eff}$.

IMAGE DENSITY

In order to achieve the same film density when increasing the kilovoltage in the 50 to 70 kV range then the exposure should be altered according to

$$\left(\frac{kV_{p,old}}{kV_{p,new}} \right)^4 \text{ so } \left(\frac{50}{60} \right)^4 < 0.5 \qquad (3.4)$$

For each 10 kV the exposure doubles or halves. Either the tube current (in millamps) or the exposure time

(in seconds) can be altered to maintain the same image (film) density. This effect lessens at higher kilovoltages (85 to 120) for each 15 kV increase doubles or halves exposure.

The characteristic radiation energy does not change with voltage but its intensity increases, contributing about 10% for a tungsten anode in the diagnostic range.

3.3.3 Current

Increasing the tube current does not influence beam quality as its penetration is unaltered since only the intensity or **quantity** of X-ray photons increases as Q proportional to the tube current. Although the height of the curve changes, the overall shape remains the same so beam penetration is unaltered; beam quality remains the same (Fig. 3.13b). In summary, the overall quantity of X-ray photons produced by an X-ray tube depends on:

• Material atomic number (Z)
• Applied kilovoltage (V)
• Tube current (I)

The beam intensity is the product of

$$Z \times V^2 \times I \qquad (3.5)$$

where the voltage V is in kilovolts and the current I is in milliamps. This intensity value is influenced by the degree of beam filtration.

3.3.4 Beam filtration

The two spectra in Fig. 3.12, A and B, show the effect of adding filters which remove the lower X-ray energies. This changes the proportion of high to low energy photons in the spectrum so the effective energy increases. Aluminum is the common filter material for conventional radiography but at higher kV_p settings (CT at 125 or 140 kV_p) copper is used, together with aluminum. Both aluminum and copper have low K-edges (Al at 1.6 keV; Cu at 8.0 keV) so these do not interfere at diagnostic energies. Removing low energy radiation from the beam significantly reduces patient entrance dose shown in Fig. 3.14 where dose versus added beam filtration is plotted. Fixed filtration for a conventional X-ray tube is typically 1.2 to 1.5 mm aluminum. The effect of filtration on the X-ray spectrum in Fig. 3.12 shows the lower energies are preferentially removed and overall beam intensity is reduced but the effective energy E_{eff} is increased.

K-EDGE FILTRATION

Metals with higher K-edge values (20 to 30 keV) are useful filters in radiology since they preferentially remove higher energy photons. These filters are commonly found in mammography where they reduce patient radiation dose by removing energies above

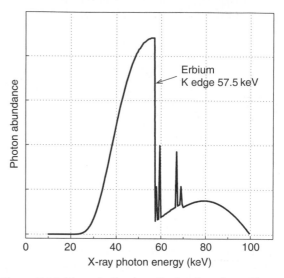

Figure 3.14 *The reduction in patient surface dose with increased tube filtration. The thickness of fixed filtration depends on kV_p.*

Table 3.3 *K-edge metals used as beam filters.*

Metal	K-edge (keV)
Molybdenum	20.0
Rhodium	23.2
Palladium	24.3
Tin	29.2
Samarium	46.8
Erbium	57.5

28 keV which only play a minor role in image formation for this examination. Common K-edge metals used for X-ray beam filtration are shown in Table 3.3.

Samarium is sometimes encountered as a K-edge filter in conventional radiography along with erbium whose effect on an X-ray spectrum in shown in Fig. 3.15. The K-edge for tin is useful since this allows this metal to be used as lightweight shielding in lightweight protective aprons (see Chapter 5).

3.3.5 X-ray beam quality

BEAM QUALITY

This is defined as the penetrating power of the X-ray beam and subjectively describes the shape of the continuous spectrum. Changing the kilovoltage changes beam quality since the penetrating power alters and the increased cut-off point (kV_p) changes the spectrum

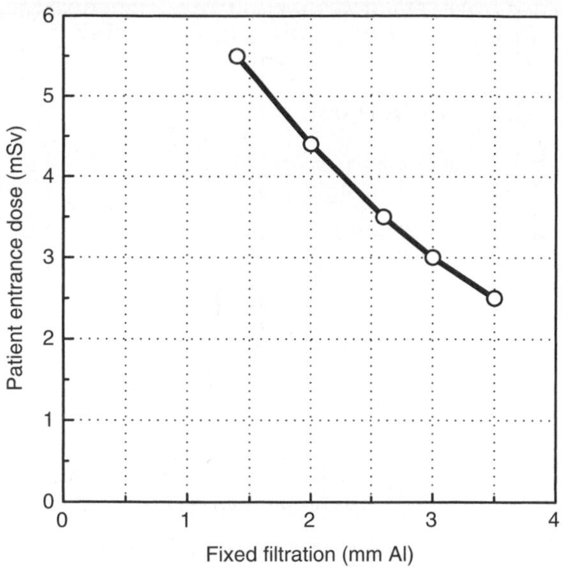

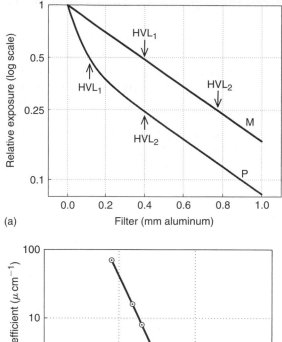

Figure 3.15 *Certain metals have K edges that appear in the diagnostic range. There is maximum absorption at their K edges. Erbium is shown here.*

shape; the effective energy also changes. Other factors such as filtration and high voltage supply characteristics (single and 3-phase supply etc.) also change beam quality.

Tube current, although it changes the quantity of radiation, as seen in Fig. 3.13b, has no effect on the spectrum's effective energy so has no influence on the quality of the beam.

THE HALF-VALUE LAYER

This is a practical measure of X-ray beam **quality**. Thin aluminum foil of known thickness (from 0.1 to 2 mm) is placed in a narrow beam of X-rays until the original intensity is reduced by half. The thickness of aluminum producing this is the half-value layer (HVL) for the beam and is normally between 2.5 and 3.0 mm for $80\,kV_p$ X-rays. The half-value layer will alter depending on spectrum shape. This is described further in Chapter 5.

BEAM HOMOGENEITY

A homogenous photon beam (gamma source) would be attenuated in a simple exponential fashion by increasing the aluminum thicknesses (Fig. 3.16a).

For a single energy photon beam the HVL reduces beam intensity to half. A second HVL will bring the

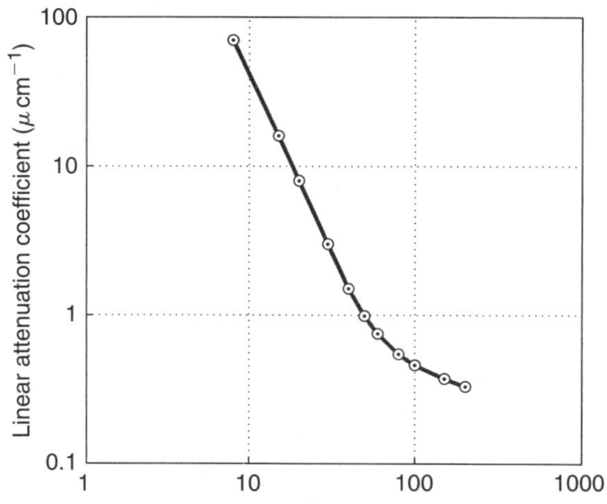

Figure 3.16 *(a) The reduction of beam intensity to half its original value is a measure of its half-value layer (HVL). (b) Attenuation coefficient versus kilovoltage for aluminum. This curve can be used for finding the equivalent energy of a poly-energetic beam.*

intensity to a ¼. For a homogeneous beam shown in Fig. 3.16a the first and second (primary and secondary) HVL are equal; slope M gives an HVL_1 of 0.375 mm and HVL_2 of 0.75 mm.

For a continuous spectrum (non-homogeneous beam) of X-rays (slope P) the primary and secondary HVL are not equal since lower energy photons are preferentially removed and the simple exponential law is not obeyed (HVL_1 is 0.125 mm but HVL_2 is 0.375). A predominance of low energy photons in the X-ray beam will cause more inhomogeneity since the majority of these will be removed in the primary HVL leaving fewer to be removed in the secondary HVL. The difference between mono-energetic and poly-energetic radiation is shown when this second half-value layer is measured. A low first HVL indicates the presence of low energy photons which play no part in image formation and only increase patient surface dose since the low energies are removed by the surface tissue. A high HVL indicates loss of useful medium energy X-ray photons which would have influenced image contrast. The HVL does *not* represent the fixed filtration of the beam but is influenced by it. The fixed filtration can be derived from the HVL value.

EQUIVALENT ENERGY

This is defined as the energy of the mono-energetic beam which gives the same HVL as the X-ray spectrum. In other words, the single energy whose photons would be attenuated to the same extent as those of the mixed energies of the X-ray beam continuous spectrum. As an example a $100\,kV_p$ X-ray spectrum having an HVL of 5 mm Al gives an attenuation coefficient of:

$$\mu = \frac{0.693}{\text{HVL}} = 1.38\mu \text{ cm}^{-1} \qquad (3.6)$$

From the graph in Fig. 3.16b this shows an equivalent energy of 40 keV. This should *not* be confused with the effective energy which is the X-ray spectrum modal point; a rough approximation for this would be $100 \times 2/3$ or $\approx 70\,kV_{eff}$. See Chapter 5 for more information on the half-value layer and equivalent energy.

3.3.6 X-ray beam quantity

A subjective assessment of spectrum shape is given by beam quality. The **quantity** of X-radiation incident on a surface (e.g. patient) depends on area, time and energy. Measurements of radiation quantity are important for estimating the sensitivity of imaging devices and calculations in radiation dosimetry. There are four important parameters that describe intensity and these are given in Box 3.4.

PHOTON FLUENCE

For N photons of energy E incident on a surface area A m^{-2} for time t then the **photon fluence** Φ

Box 3.4 X-ray beam quantification

The photon fluence

From the photon number 1.5×10^{14} calculated in Box 3.1 the X-ray fluence Φ for a chest radiograph of $60\,kV_{eff}$ 5 mA s over an area of 1500 cm^2 would be

$$\Phi = \frac{N}{A}$$

where N is the number of photons and A is the area in centimeters squared. So, Φ is

$$\frac{1.5 \times 10^{14}}{1.5 \times 10^3} = 1.0 \times 10^{11} \text{ photons cm}^{-2}.$$

The photon flux

For the same conditions the photon flux ϕ is

$$\phi = \frac{\Phi}{t} = \frac{1.0 \times 10^{11}}{0.05}$$
$$= 2.0 \times 10^{12} \text{ photons cm}^{-2}\text{s}^{-1}$$

The energy fluence

$$\phi = \frac{NE}{A} 1.0 \times 10^{11} \times 0.06$$
$$= 6.0 \times 10^{9} \text{ MeV cm}^{-2}$$

The energy flux

$$\psi = \frac{\Psi}{t} = \frac{6.0 \times 10^{9}}{0.05}$$
$$= 1.02 \times 10^{11} \text{MeV cm}^{-2}\text{s}^{-1}$$

(in photons m^{-2}) is a measure of photon intensity per unit area expressed as

$$\Phi = \frac{N}{A} \qquad (3.7)$$

PHOTON FLUX

The photon flux ϕ per unit time t is

$$\varphi = \frac{N}{At} \qquad (3.8)$$

The photon flux is given as photons m^{-2}s^{-1}.

ENERGY FLUENCE

The energy fluence Ψ is the photon energy E deposited per meter. For a mono-energetic beam this is simply expressed as $\Psi = \Phi E$ measured in either joules or MeV m^{-2}.

ENERGY FLUX

For a mono-energetic beam the energy flux ψ is simply ϕE but for a poly-energetic beam the proportion of each energy per unit time (E_i) gives the energy flux density (in J or MeV m^{-2}s^{-1}) which is the sum of all the different energy components:

$$\psi = \sum (\psi \times E_i) \qquad (3.9)$$

The complete family describing the quantity of X-ray photons is used in Box 3.4 for calculating the quantity of X-rays used in a chest radiograph, using the basic quantity already calculated in Box 3.1.

Energy flux density depends on the anode material, tube current and applied kilovoltage so that as already seen in Equation 3.5:

$$\psi \propto Z \times I \times E^2 \qquad (3.10)$$

where Z is the atomic number, I the tube current and E the applied kilovoltage. A change in tube kilovoltage has a much greater effect on intensity than a change in tube current. From the above formula, increasing the kilovoltage by 10 kV from 60 to 70 has the same effect on the energy flux density as increasing the tube current by roughly $\times 1.5$.

3.4 ELECTRICAL CHARACTERISTICS

Factors influencing an X-ray tube electrical performance are:

- Filament current
- Maximum kilovoltage
- Stationary anode: 70–90 kV$_{p}$
- Rotating anode: 100–150 kV$_{p}$
- Tube current
- Exposure time

3.4.1 Filament current

The filament must be large enough to give a practical electron density but not too large, since this will cause focusing problems. The controlling factors are maximum operating filament temperature and filament size. Filament current is increased for low kV$_{p}$ work (mammography) to maintain tube current and compensate for the space charge limitation shown in Fig. 3.6b for low kV values 20 and 40 kV. Increasing filament emission with temperature has already been demonstrated in Chapter 2, the space charge effect restricts tube current and its influence can be seen in Fig. 3.17a and b.

In practice the filament current is not switched on and off after each exposure but is kept in a standby mode (about 5 mA) and increased to operating currents (4.5 to 5.5 A) for exposures. When an exposure is made a preparation switch is first depressed which starts the anode rotating and increases the filament temperature from standby mode.

3.4.2 Tube voltage

The response of an X-ray tube to voltage is shown in Fig. 3.17a. When the filament is heated with electric current electrons are emitted from its surface as already described in Chapter 2 (space charge effect). When a high voltage is applied across the filament (part of the cathode) and the anode, some of the electrons from the space charge will travel across the tube providing the tube current; the higher the voltage the higher the current as the graph shows.

The rising part of the curve is 'space charge limited' but as all the available electrons are removed the curve shows a plateau region where increasing the voltage does not produce an increased tube current. At this point the tube is 'saturated'. The tube current, therefore, does not depend on the tube voltage but on the filament electron emission (i.e. filament temperature), the tube current is emission or temperature controlled; the height of the plateau region alters with filament temperature.

Figure 3.17a demonstrates this saturation effect by plotting tube current against filament current for separate high voltages. At low voltages (mammography) there is a tube current that cannot be exceeded in spite of filament current increase. Increasing the kilovoltage overcomes the space charge limitation and allows a higher tube current at 40 kV. The operating tube voltage is determined by use. Mammographic tubes are designed for low voltage work (20 to 30 kV$_{p}$), modern CT up to 140 kV$_{p}$ and some high voltage chest X-ray tubes can approach 180 kV$_{p}$. Much lower filament currents are required for high kV work since the space charge effect is much less (see Fig. 3.6b).

3.4.3 Tube current

Tube currents vary between 50 and 400 mA for conventional radiography and up to 1000 mA for fluorography, DSA, and CT. Mammography X-ray tubes operate at lower voltages (from 25 to 30 kV$_p$) placing their operating region below the saturation region seen in Fig. 3.17b. Increasing filament current, at fixed voltage, will not influence tube current under these conditions and so filament current is limited to

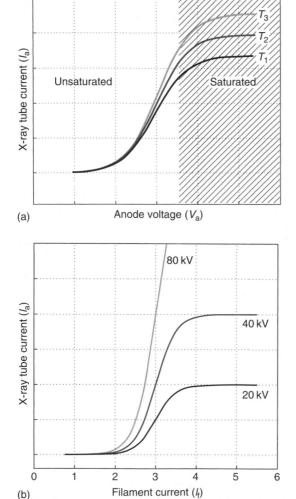

(a)

(b)

Figure 3.17 (a) *The variation of anode current with anode voltage showing space-charge limited region and saturated region for increasing filament temperatures (T_1 to T_3).* **(b)** *Tube kilovoltage and X-ray tube current for three kilovoltages showing saturation at 20 and 40 kV.*

prevent tube damage (see Fig. 3.5b). Emitted electron density can be increased by increasing the temperature or surface area of the filament. This is commonly achieved in mammography by operating dual (side-by-side) filaments focused on the same anode target area.

GRID CONTROL

If a sufficiently high negative voltage is applied to the sharp edges of the cathode cup (about 2 kV) then the electron beam issuing from the filament can be cut off entirely (Fig. 3.4b). A pulsed control voltage can be applied which can switch the beam on and off with very little inertia, so very sharp X-ray pulses, of the order of a few milliseconds duration can be obtained. This is the method chosen for switching the X-ray beam in fluoroscopy (digital and cine) and computed tomography (CT).

3.5 X-RAY TUBE RATING

This is the total workload that can be placed on a tube combining the effects of kilovoltage (kV$_p$), tube current (in milliamps) and exposure time (in seconds) for a certain focal spot size; this is the **electrical rating**. Anode **heat gain** and **heat loss** determine the **thermal rating** of the X-ray tube, commonly referred to as loadability. The workload (loading) or rating of an X-ray tube depends on factors which can be varied i.e.:

- Tube kV$_p$
- Tube current
- Filament current and temperature
- Focal spot size
- Exposure time

Other factors, which are not variable but significantly influence tube rating are anode diameter and anode rotation speed.

3.5.1 Electrical rating

MAXIMUM KILOVOLTAGE

This is usually limited by the insulation of the tube and its oil filled housing. The maximum tube kilovoltage is limited in practice by electrical overload detection.

MAXIMUM TUBE CURRENT

The curve in Fig. 3.18a shows the maximum tube current for an X-ray tube operating at 80 kV. Above the curve the X-ray tube will be overloaded and damaged by excess heat. In order to keep within the electrical rating the permissible maximum tube current decreases as the kilovoltage increases (Fig. 3.18b). The tube current is varied by the filament current (filament heating) and the maximum allowable tube current depends on the tube kilovoltage. Increasing the size of the anode increases the maximum allowable tube current (Fig. 3.18c).

MAXIMUM POWER

The product of the current I and maximum kilovoltage V is the tube power (in watts): $P = IV$. This is the maximum power or rating that can be used without damaging the anode; however the rating at fast exposure times must be modified. At 3000 rpm the target lengths shown in Fig. 3.7b are completely exposed

every 0.02 s so exposure times less than 20 ms only use a part of this target length; for these the anode rating is independent of the exposure time so the rating curves flatten at shorter exposure times.

KILOWATT RATING

This is usually measured from the rating curve for an exposure of 0.1 s. In order to find the tube rating locate the intersection of the curve at the 100 ms (0.1 s) point on the x-axis (dotted line marked on graph in Fig. 3.18b). This determines the tube current for the chosen kilovoltage on the rating curves. Since $P = IV$ watts then:

$$500 \text{ mA for } 60 \text{ kV} = 30 \text{ kW}$$
$$375 \text{ mA for } 80 \text{ kV} = 30 \text{ kW}$$
$$300 \text{ mA for } 100 \text{ kV} = 30 \text{ kW}$$

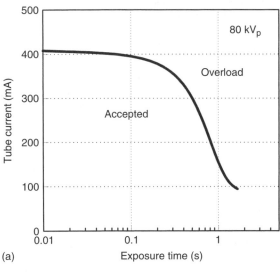

(a)

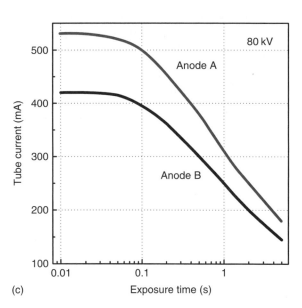

(c)

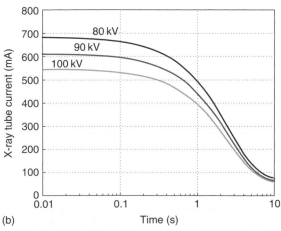

(b)

Figure 3.18 *(a) A simplified rating curve plotting time of exposure against maximum allowable tube current. Exposure rates below the curve are acceptable. The rating curve flattens for fast exposure times (<0.1 s). (b) Tube rating for three kilovoltage settings 60, 80, and 100 kV; allowable tube current decreases as the kV increases. (c) Rating increases with size of anode; size A has a larger diameter than B.*

Box 3.5 demonstrates that increasing the real focal spot size can yield higher electrical rating. The anode angle is adjusted to give the same effective focal spot (line focus principle).

For very short exposure times (0.1 s or less) **short-term loadability** is determined by the size of the anode target. This depends on:

- Speed of anode rotation
- Length of focal track
- Width of focal track

The smaller the anode angle the more the short-term loadability can be increased but the anode angle size also determines the field size and heel effect. Anode cooling determines the **long-term loadability** which is influenced by tube specification. If radiation is to be produced continuously, as in fluoroscopy, the

tube loading is determined by the rate at which the heat can be dissipated. High mAs exposures permitted at low mA and long exposure times (e.g. 200 mA at 1 s) may not be permitted at high mA and short exposure times (1000 mA at 0.2 s). If the tube rating is exceeded then:

- Use a larger focal spot.
- Use a higher speed rotation.
- Reduce mA and increase exposure time.
- Increase kV_p and reduce mA or time.
- Choose a sensitive film-screen combination which requires less exposure.

Radiographic techniques that use the maximum ratings of an X-ray tube produce target track roughening, so resolution slowly deteriorates and more tungsten becomes vaporized inside the tube enclosure, including the window area. This markedly reduces X-ray output since it acts as an effective filter. Operating at maximum ratings will considerably shorten the tube life so the tube should only be used at maximum rating if diagnostic quality demands it. Some specifications for three types of X-ray tube are given in Table 3.4.

A large focal spot gives increased loading and reduced heel effect (Fig. 3.10b), but the effective focal spot will be large giving poor resolution images. A finer focal spot improves this but the tube's rating is reduced.

Improved resolution (smaller focal spot) leads to:

- Lower rating, where a possible could be a larger anode diameter and/or faster rotation
- Increased heel effect and less film coverage. A possible solution is to increase FFD but therefore less intensity $1/d^2$ requiring increased tube output (kV, mA or time)

FALLING LOAD

If it can be arranged for the tube current to be high in the initial part of the exposure and then fall steadily

---

Box 3.5 Power rating for spot size and angle

Focal spot size and rating

For a focal spot size and anode angle:

$$11.6 \times 3 \text{ for an angle of } 15°$$
$$10.26 \times 3; \text{ angle of } 17°$$
$$8.7 \times 3; \text{ angle of } 20°$$

Each gives an effective focal spot size of 3×3 mm (see line focus principle). The power rating for a typical rotating anode is 1500 W mm^{-2}, so for an anode angle of:

$$15°: 3 \times 11.6 \times 1500 = 52 \text{ KW}$$
$$17°: 3 \times 10.26 \times 1500 = 46 \text{ KW}$$
$$20°: 3 \times 8.77 \times 1500 = 39 \text{ KW}$$

Note. Smaller anode angles have higher ratings but give a larger heel effect.

Table 3.4 *Commercially available X-ray tube specifications.*

Tube type	Anode size (mm)	Angle	Focal spot	Heat storage	Long term loadability
Ceramic/metal	200	9°	0.5/0.8	1.8 MJ	3.2 kW
CT metal	100	10°	1.0	1.1 MJ	1.5 kW
Glass/metal	90	9°	0.5/1.0	590 kJ	300 W

during the exposure the same mAs can be achieved in a shorter time than would be the case for a constant current.

The falling load principle enables rapid multiple exposures to be made by driving the X-ray tube at near its maximum rating over the entire exposure time. Heat loss from the anode is most efficient at high working temperatures and the falling load principle keeps the high heating level constant.

The falling load principle is not suitable for very short exposure times when there would not be sufficient time for the multiple steps. The rating curve in Fig. 3.19 shows the principle for the example in Box 3.6.

3.5.2 Thermal rating

The operating limits of an X-ray tube are influenced by three exposure factors:

1. Kilovoltage, chosen for particular investigation and penetration
2. Exposure timing, chosen to reduce movement unsharpness
3. Focal spot size, chosen for optimum resolution

The heat generated at the anode by a combination of these factors determines the choice of tube design

and its thermal rating. The overall heat loss from the X-ray tube and its housing is represented in Fig. 3.20.

HEAT GENERATED

Factors 1 and 2 in the above list are a measure of the energy dissipated in the tube anode. This energy is proportional to kV and mA and exposure time. Since the majority of this energy appears as heat this product is the measure of power as described above. For a constant potential generator operating at 100 kV and 300 mA (see graph in Fig. 3.18b) an electrical power of 30 kW is dissipated in the anode. Since 1 J = 1 W s then for an exposure time of 0.02 s the total heat energy is 30 kW × 0.02 = 600 J. This heat is deposited over a small area of the anode associated with the focal

> ### Box 3.6 Falling load calculation for Fig. 3.19
>
> From the example 60 kV at 150 mAs is required. The timing is proportioned as:
>
> $$500 \text{ mA at } 0.05 \text{ s} = 25 \text{ mAs}$$
> $$400 \text{ mA at } 0.1 \text{ s} = 40 \text{ mAs}$$
> $$300 \text{ mA at } 0.15 \text{ s} = 45 \text{ mAs}$$
> $$200 \text{ mA at } 0.2 \text{ s} = 40 \text{ mAs}$$
> $$\text{Total time } 0.5 \text{ s giving } 150 \text{ mAs}$$
>
> The falling load provides 150 mAs in 0.5 s (point A in Fig. 3.19). A constant load would require 1.0 s (point B).

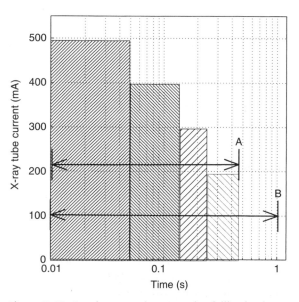

Figure 3.19 *A rating curve demonstrating falling load showing the proportional exposures giving the required mAs calculated in Box 3.6. The shaded area shows the equivalent time for a constant current mAs.*

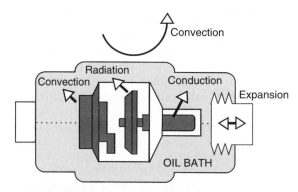

Figure 3.20 *General heat loss from an X-ray tube enclosure relies on radiation from the anode, conduction through the bearings and convection currents set up in the surrounding oil bath. All this heat is eventually lost from the tube housing to the surrounding air.*

spot dimensions. Excessive heat can melt the target surface causing pitting and unequal expansion of the anode itself. A moderate form of this damage affects all X-ray tubes over their working life. A gradually pitted surface increases the size of the focal spot so resolution deteriorates and scatter from the uneven surface reduces tube output. Exposure factors are increased to compensate which accelerates the damage.

TARGET COOLING

If there is no anode cooling then exposure (mAs) would depend only on focal spot size and the applied kilovoltage. Increased mAs or kilovoltage could only be used with large focal spots. This is not the case, however, since cooling by radiation, conduction and convection all remove heat from the anode during operation as Fig. 3.20 demonstrates. Forced air cooling accelerates heat loss further increasing possible tube loading.

EXPOSURE TIME

The optimum quality radiographs are achieved as a trade-off between tube current and time. The shortest time is usually chosen in order to minimize patient or organ movement (lung, heart). Since very short times would require damagingly large tube currents, exposure time is extended. This will, in turn, increase the total amount of heat generated and depend on its heat loss capabilities.

3.5.3 Anode heating and cooling

At the end of a short exposure the heat from the target is distributed by conduction throughout the anode mass. If this is not removed then the next exposure cannot take place without damaging the tube. Thus the heat capacity of the anode limits the number of exposures that can be made per unit time. Loadability can be seen in three separate applications:

- Series loadability, where the tube is switched on and off for short periods over a long study time (angiography)
- Single exposure, maximum rating demanded for a short time (high kV chest radiography)
- Continuous loadability, where the tube is kept switched on at a lower level but for a long time

HEAT STORAGE CAPACITY

The heat energy deposited in the target limits the workload and depends on:

- Exposure time
- Disk rotation
- Focal track length
- Focal spot size

The heat stored in an anode mass depends on its heat capacity expressed in heat units (HU) or joules. Maximum heat storage capacity is related to: anode mass $\times$ specific heat $\times$ temperature rise. Since the first two are constant in any one tube, temperature rise is dependent on the anode heat capacity. The early methods of measuring X-ray tube power used heat units which were the product of:

- Tube kV $\times$ tube mA $\times$ exposure time (single phase)
- Tube kV $\times$ tube mA $\times$ time $\times$ 1.35 (3-phase)

An increase of 35% is added for a 3-phase or constant potential (or high frequency) supply due to improved efficiency. For an exposure of $70\,kV_p$ at 10 mAs the heat deposited would be $70 \times 100 \times 0.1 = 700\,HU$ for a single phase supply or $700 \times 1.35 = 945\,HU$ for a 3-phase. Converting these values into joules uses the conversion figures: HU $\times$ 0.71 = joules or conversely: joules $\times$ 1.41 = HU. A conventional anode would have a typical heat storage capacity of 100 kHU. This would increase to a few MHU for heavily loaded tubes (fluoroscopy and CT). Current metal/ceramic tubes can have a heat storage approaching 5 MHU and a continuous load of 7 kW.

ANODE HEATING

Anode heating is a considerable quantity of heat produced by bombarding the anode with an electron beam. During operation it glows red and sometimes white hot. This heat is removed by radiation from the anode to the enclosure wall (glass or metal) and also by conduction along the bearing. Sleeve bearings are replacing ball bearings in X-ray tube construction since they allow a greater heat loss by conduction which allows a higher tube rating. Reflector plates behind the anode prevent excessive radiant heat from reaching the rotor-bearing mechanism.

Excessive heating of the anode will vaporize the target giving a rough surface which degrades the focal spot geometry, reducing X-ray output due to photon scatter from the rough target surface; it will also cause bearing damage. The vaporized anode material (tungsten) will increase the beam filtration (increased HVL), lowering image contrast.

ANODE COOLING

The cooling curve in Fig. 3.21 shows the number of heat units remaining per minute. The heat stored in an anode mass depends on its heat capacity. This is the heat storage capacity expressed in heat units or joules explained above.

If the maximum heat capacity of the anode is 100 000 HU, then at a rate of 850 HU s^{-1} this can be exceeded in 2.5 min continuous exposure. For long exposure times, as in fluoroscopy thermal equilibrium occurs when the heat generated by the electron beam is balanced by factors influencing heat loss (radiation, conduction, convection). The heating curves in Fig. 3.21 show that equilibrium would be achieved for this tube at about 500 HU s^{-1}, leveling out at the maximum heat rating of 100 kHU. The rate of radiant heat lost from the anode T_{loss} to the surrounding oil depends on the temperature difference between the anode T_a and the oil T_o so that:

$$T_{loss} = T_a^4 - T_o^4 \qquad (3.11)$$

The greatest heat loss occurs at high temperature differences. Doubling the values of T_a and T_o increases heat loss by ×16. Heat loss from the anode is most effective when the anode is operating near its maximum rating (falling load principle).

KEYWORDS

anode: the positive electrode of a thermion device. Commonly applied to the X-ray tube

beam filtration: the use of thin metal foil to remove low energy components from a poly-energetic beam

beam homogeneity: a measure of how a poly-energetic beam compares to a mono-energetic beam of the same effective energy (E_{eff})

beam intensity: the number of photons per unit area (photon fluence)

beam quality: the penetrating power of the X-ray beam. Dependent on range of beam energies

bearings: rotational support for X-ray tube anode. Either ball or sleeve bearings are used

Bremsstrahlung: generation of X-rays due to loss of electron energy (braking radiation)

cathode: a negatively charged nickel support for the filament

continuous spectrum: poly-energetic X-ray spectrum

energy (effective) E_{eff}: the modal energy of a poly-energetic beam

energy (equivalent): energy of a mono-energetic beam which would have the same HVL as the filtered X-ray beam

energy (fluence): Ψ, measured in MeV cm^{-2}

energy (flux): ψ, measured in MeV cm^{-2} s^{-1}

falling load: using the maximum electrical rating to give a shorter exposure time

filament: coiled tungsten wire which is heated electrically to produce an electron cloud

filament cup: part of the cathode assembly surrounding the filament which concentrates the negative charge so shaping the beam

filter (K-edge): a high atomic number metal foil having a K-absorption edge in the diagnostic energy range

filtration (fixed): additional filter material added in order to remove low energy X-rays

filtration (inherent): the filtration offered by the X-ray tube glass envelope

filtration (total): Inherent + fixed filtration which should be at least 1.5 mm aluminum for a 80 kV$_p$ beam energy

focal spot (effective): calculated from the line-focus principle

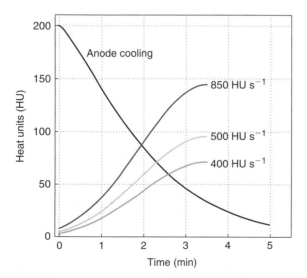

Figure 3.21 *Example of a cooling curve and HU curves for a specific X-ray tube.*

focal spot (real): the dimensions of the anode target area

half-value layer(HVL): the thickness of aluminum which reduces the X-ray beam intensity by half. This should be at least 2.5 mm aluminum at $80\,kV_p$

heat units (HU): a measure of heat storage for an X-ray tube

heel effect: the diminishing intensity across the X-ray beam toward the anode

keV: thousands of electron volts. Used as a precise measure of X-ray photon energy

kV_{eff}: see effective energy

kV_p: the peak photon energy of an X-ray beam

line-focus principle: a formula for calculating a symmetrical focal spot using the electron beam angle and the real focus dimensions

mAs: the product of tube current (in milliamps) and exposure time (in seconds)

photon (fluence): Φ, photons cm^{-2}

photon (flux): ϕ, photons cm^{-2}s^{-1}

rotor: an integral part of the anode stem making up the induction motor

space charge: accumulation of an electron cloud around a filament. More pronounced at low kilovoltages

stator: the external winding surrounding the rotor section which completes the induction motor (see rotor)

useful field: the extent of the collimated X-ray beam

window: the tube exit for the X-ray beam in the housing, which holds the fixed filtration

4

X-ray production and properties: specific machine design

4.1 THE SUPPLY GENERATOR

A classic examination question in radiology physics: 'If an X-ray unit requires a highly stable DC supply for consistent X-ray output why is an AC supply used?' This question requires some thought before an accurate answer can be given.

The ideal generator is a **constant potential** generator which does supply the X-ray tube with a non-fluctuating constant DC using DC regulators for altering the high voltage. A DC battery supply for this unit would be absurd since a bank of batteries supplying 100 kV for a reasonable length of time would occupy a very large space and would be excessively expensive.

The only practical solution is to use a **rectified** mains supply (single or 3-phase). All voltage fluctuations in the constant potential generator are equalized by regulating triode electronic tubes (valves) in the high voltage lines, giving a constant voltage with no ripple to the X-ray tube. The control circuits are in the high voltage side which provides very fast response times of <1 ms. A constant potential generator is very expensive and occupies a large space; they are rarely found in diagnostic departments.

BASIC GENERATOR DESIGN

A typical X-ray generator derives its power from a single or 3-phase mains supply. The AC voltage levels are increased or decreased by using power **transformers**. The AC is converted to a DC supply for the X-ray tube high voltage by using **rectifiers**. A general design for a **conventional** X-ray generator, that is a generator using mains frequency supplies, is shown in Fig. 4.1. The specific features of a conventional generator are:

- Input transformer which allows adjustment of input mains voltage (primary) and output (secondary)
- A timer (older equipment only)
- A high voltage transformer increasing voltage levels up to 150 000 V for the X-ray tube
- A rectifier system converting high voltage AC to DC
- A low voltage transformer reducing voltage levels to supply the tube filament 8–12 V

The main supply can be either single-phase (110 or 220 V) or 3-phase (220 to 440 V). An auto- or step-transformer (T1) allows adjustment to variations in the line supply (line compensation: M) manually or automatically. The reproducibility of the X-ray tube voltage is only ensured with stable line voltages. Response of automatic stabilizers is about 100 ms so rapid changes in the mains supply may still be transferred to the X-ray tube voltage.

The X-ray tube high voltage of about 150 kV maximum is obtained from a step-up transformer (T2).

The exposure timing and switching takes place in the primary low voltage circuit (kV selector and timer). Timers in conventional generators are mainly

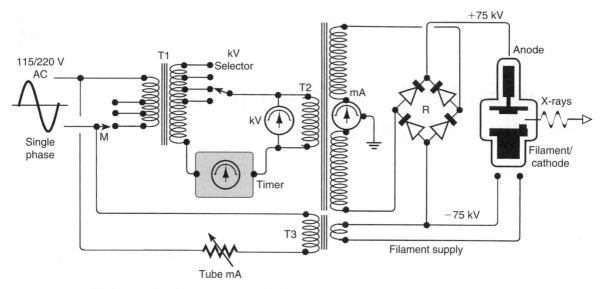

Figure 4.1 *Simplified conventional generator showing basic components and controls described in the text.*

electronic as mechanical timers are too slow and unreliable. Current equipment does not rely on a timer mechanism for halting the exposure. This is accomplished by feedback from an ionization chamber placed in the X-ray beam.

The high voltage generator itself consists of an oil filled tank which contains the high voltage transformer (T2) with its rectifiers (R). Also included in the bath is the filament transformer (T3) and high voltage switches. The high voltage is split as −75 kV and +75 kV with respect to earth so the insulation is only subjected to half the potential difference. The meter measuring the tube current (in mA) is placed halfway in the secondary winding of T2 which is at earth potential.

4.1.1 Supply frequency

The AC mains supply has a cyclic frequency of 50 Hz in Europe and 60 Hz in the US. This variation can be responsible for small differences in generator performance.

SINGLE PHASE SUPPLY

Single phase supply is the domestic mains supply at 115 V in the US and 220, 240 V in Europe. The waveform is shown in Fig. 4.2a and b. X-ray generators using this supply use two types of rectification. **Half-wave** or **single-pulse** generators produce the pulsatile

waveform shown in Fig. 4.2a where only the shaded area is useful for X-ray production. Their efficiency is low giving power levels of about 2 kW and these supplies are found in low power X-ray sets, such as dental and small mobile units. Single phase, **full-wave** rectified units produce the waveform in Fig. 4.2b; this is also known as a **two-pulse** generator for obvious reasons. This design makes better use of the supply power using both halves of the AC waveform and consequently higher X-ray outputs can be obtained; about 50 kW maximum.

The half-wave system is the simplest requiring only a single rectifier. The full-wave system requires a four rectifier-bridge. A capacitor (C) can be added to smooth the pulsatile DC and reduce ripple. Supply frequency is superimposed on the rectified DC as 'ripple'. This causes serious fluctuations in output and so broadens the X-ray spectrum. Typical ripple percentages are given in Table 4.1 for single and 3-phase supplies.

THREE-PHASE SUPPLY

This waveform is shown in Fig. 4.2c and has already been described in Chapter 2 as three sine waves with a 120° phase difference. The supply is obtained from a special 3-phase mains supply (228 V in the US, 440 V in Europe) using a star-delta transformer design. Half-wave rectification is produced from a **six-pulse** generator using twelve rectifiers in parallel as a double-star circuit shown in Fig. 4.2c. It gives a substantially higher

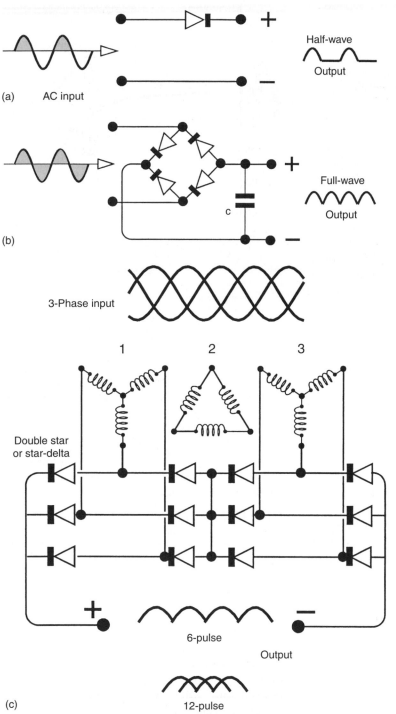

Figure 4.2 *(a) Single-phase waveform half wave rectified using a single diode and (b) full-wave rectified using four diodes. (c) A 3-phase supply showing star, delta, star transformer input and half-wave (6-pulse) or full-wave (12-pulse) rectified output.*

output than two-pulse (single-phase) generators. They are found in medium power units of about 50 kW or small generators used in older mammography equipment.

Full-wave rectification in 3-phase circuits uses a star-delta configuration as the input. This is a **twelve-pulse** generator and is used for high power supplies (≤150 kW) such as old model DSA or CT machines.

Table 4.1 *Ripple values for generators.*

Generator	Ripple
Single phase, half-wave	100%
Single phase, full-wave	100% (15–20% smoothed)
3-Phase, 6-pulse	13%
3-Phase, 12-pulse	3%

The outputs for a 6- and 12-pulse generator are shown in Fig. 4.2c. The higher the pulse number the higher the efficiency of the power unit, producing an X-ray spectrum with a higher effective photon energy as shown in Fig. 4.3a for the same kV_p. This will allow faster exposures (less patient movement artifact) and less low energy photons, reducing patient dose. Anode heating during exposure can be kept constant (constant load) or can be reduced by feedback control under falling load conditions as described in Chapter 3.

The mains supply to the generator, whether it be single- or 3-phase, can show variation particularly if it also supplies other equipment. This produces significant variation in supply voltage which is compensated manually or automatically by a separate transformer (an auto-transformer) which is shown in Fig. 4.1 as 'M'. Single- and 3-phase rectified power supplies now commonly feed high frequency generators since these offer superior control and stability.

4.1.2 High frequency generators

Medium and high frequency generators are now common for all X-ray equipment from mobiles, conventional, fluoroscopy, DSA and CT. They have many of the advantages of a constant potential generator giving very low ripple (<1%).

Figure 4.3b shows how the low frequency mains supply is first rectified to give a DC voltage which then supplies a high frequency generator (2 to 10 kHz) which is rectified and supplies the X-ray tube circuits. The high frequency is rectified to give a very constant DC high voltage. The generator design can utilize either single- or 3-phase main supplies. These are full wave rectified and smoothed to give a steady DC voltage which supplies a thyristor converter which switches the DC voltage producing a medium (up to 2000 Hz) or high (up to 20 kHz) square waveform. A high frequency transformer then converts this low voltage high frequency AC to kilovolt levels.

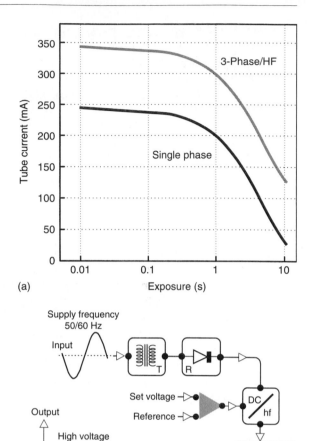

(a)

(b)

Figure 4.3 *(a) Increased rating given by a 3-phase or a high frequency generator over the single phase (2-pulse) generator. (b) A high frequency waveform showing the mains frequency which is rectified to supply the high frequency generator. When rectified this gives a stable DC supply.*

Rectification and smoothing gives the high voltage DC for the X-ray tube. The thyristor converter can be controlled by low voltage signals to regulate its high-voltage output. There is a significant decrease in transformer size with increasing frequency for the same power output. Extremely compact transformer design is possible since cross-section A and number of turns n are related to output voltage V and AC frequency f as

$$V = A \times n \times f \qquad (4.1)$$

This has obvious size advantages when designing compact generators for mobiles and CT units. There can be up to an 80% reduction in transformer size over conventional 50/60 Hz units for the same power output.

The tube kilovoltage can be electronically switched on and off at any point in time (no phase restrictions, unlike single- and 3-phase units). Tube voltage is preset according to reference input control value shown in Fig. 4.3b. Variation will influence output voltage and so can be regulated by slight frequency variation as plotted in Fig. 4.4a and is independent of tube current. For power rating up to 50 kW the generator is small enough to be built into a single housing with the X-ray tube. This is a 'single-tank' generator. For power ratings higher than 50 kW the tube and generator housing are usually separate. Converter frequencies vary between 5 and 10 kHz depending on manufacturer and after rectification yield a very low ripple DC voltage. Feed-back regulation of the high voltage can give a response time of 200 μs, so extremely stable output is possible giving <5% variation compared to between 10 and 20% for conventional single-phase and 3-phase generators. The high frequency generator can derive its power from either a single- or 3-phase line supply which is rectified and then supplies the converter with power DC.

4.1.3 Generator performance

The general symbols used for describing high frequency generators are shown in Fig. 4.4b. Three types of transformer are commonly found: isolation, step-up and step-down. A common rectifier symbol serves for both medium voltage (115–240 V) and high voltage (150 kV); this is typically a full-wave semiconductor device. A DC to high frequency converter provides the 5 to 10 kHz by switching the DC input; there is a third input for controlling the frequency level. A single input amplifier and a dual input comparator are common components; the comparator gives a signal output when input levels are different. An X-ray tube with stator windings completes the symbol family.

A general schematic for a high frequency generator unit is given in Fig. 4.5 where high frequency converters, of different kinds, supply the X-ray tube high voltage, the filament low voltage and also control the speed of the anode induction motor. Comparators are used as control devices accepting a reference input which can represent rotor speed, tube voltage or current and constantly comparing this with the measured value. A comparator circuit also monitors exposure

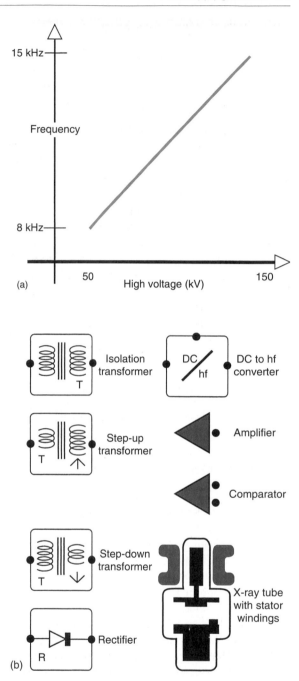

Figure 4.4 (*a*) *Variation of voltage output with small changes in generator frequency.* (***b***) *Block diagrams used in generator schematics showing three types of transformers and a full-wave semiconductor rectifier for both medium and high voltage rectification. The DC to high frequency converter has a frequency control input. There is a single input/output amplifier and a two input comparator which detects signal differences. An X-ray tube assembly is also represented.*

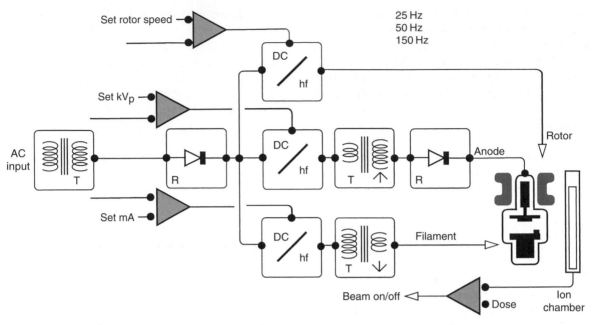

Figure 4.5 *Basic high frequency design showing the basic building blocks: DC/high frequency converters, transformers (T) step-up T↑ and step-down T↓ and the various feedback controls for controlling kilovoltage, anode rotation speed and tube current respectively.*

from the X-ray beam and switching this off when a certain level has been reached.

MAXIMUM RATING

The insulation of the X-ray tube and housing has a maximum voltage rating usually less than the generator output. Maximum tube-current is controlled by both the filament current and tube kilovoltage as already seen in Chapter 3. The maximum tube current is determined by the filament rating and reduces with increasing tube kilovoltage.

Since the 3-phase or high frequency generator is more efficient a higher **effective energy** can be obtained. In the electrical rating graphs of Chapter 3 the tube current plateau decreases as the kilovoltage is raised due to electrical power limitations which are the product of kilovoltage and current. This represents the maximum power that can be focused on the anode for the shortest time without damage. It is not a filament current limitation but a thermal limitation and is relevant when very short exposures are taken (<0.1 s). Heat produced can be calculated from the electrical consumption. If the tube is being operated at 10 kW for 0.05 s then the total heat produced will be 10 000 × 0.1 J or 1000 J. For shorter exposure times

and a constant mAs this amount of heat will be produced in a shorter time over a smaller target area.

OVERLOAD PROTECTION

The automatic overload monitors of the generator (excessive power) that prevent electrical overload cannot protect against thermal overload due to too short intervals between exposures. Thermal overload protection is provided by a small temperature detector (Loadix) placed in the X-ray tube housing behind the anode. This indicates when the anode radiant heat exceeds a safe value and can feed information to a high frequency generator so that power input can be reduced from say 100% to 80%, which enables uninterrupted operation.

CABLE RESISTANCE

High voltage generators are connected to the X-ray tube by means of two high voltage cables which deliver a split voltage i.e. −75 kV and +75 kV. This is for safety reasons since it gives symmetrical potential with regards to earth.

Supply cable resistance plays an important role in machine installation and these must be kept short if significant voltage drops at the generator are to be avoided during operation. A 10 kW generator will draw up to 50 A from the supply (depending on supply voltage) so even a small resistance of between 0.5 and 1 Ω will cause a substantial voltage drop of the order of 50 V. Any voltage drop is usually compensated by adjusting the auto-transformer setting.

RIPPLE

The cyclic variation, pulsation or ripple on the high voltage, described earlier, depends on the type of supply (single-phase, 3-phase or high frequency). This is measured as the percentage of the peak value:

$$R = \frac{V_{max} - V_{min}}{V_{max}} \times 100\% \qquad (4.2)$$

The peak value of the X-ray tube supply is critical to image quality, since the proportion of ripple influences the X-ray spectrum. A large ripple content will reduce the available maximum voltage. Reproducibility of the generator output (stable kilovoltage) also influences the consistency of image quality. Variation in power output should be very low; 5–10% for conventional work and between 1 and 2% for mammography and DSA. It is less than 1% for CT. Advantages of a high frequency supply are:

- Either a single- or 3-phase supply can be used to provide the DC for the converter
- Precise electronic control of the output with a response time of about 200 μs
- Fast switching of the tube voltage on and off during exposure
- The tube voltage is independent of tube current
- Extremely compact high voltage generator can be incorporated into tube assembly
- Higher radiation output than conventional 3 phase supplies
- Feedback controls vary or stabilize the X-ray tube voltage and current

4.2 CONTROL CIRCUITS

Controlling high frequency generator kilovoltage output (eqn 4.1) is achieved by altering the frequency by a feedback control signal. In this way the kilovoltage can be finely adjusted within very close tolerances (better than 1%).

4.2.1 High voltage control

The high voltage control is shown in Fig. 4.6. The sample signal is derived from a resistor divider circuit in the high voltage line and feeds one input of a comparator. When this difference is found between sampled voltage and the set reference, a DC control voltage alters the frequency of the converter which alters high voltage level. Tolerance levels better than 1% are essential for special applications such as subtraction angiography and CT. The X-ray beam is switched off rapidly after the required exposure by applying a low voltage logic signal to the converter; the speed of switching is compared in Table 4.2. Low inertia switching giving pulsed beams in CT and DSA uses grid-controlled X-ray tubes.

4.2.2 Filament control and tube current

Slight variations in filament current produce large variations in the tube current which has already been seen in Chapter 3. The filament receives its power from an individual low voltage 'step-down' transformer shown both in the conventional circuit in Fig. 4.1 and high frequency circuit in Fig. 4.5. The transformer supplies between 8 to 12 V at 6 A. Since the filament current is 50/60 Hz in the conventional AC supply, filament temperature alternates with the supply frequency giving a current ripple of about 10% which is super-imposed as ripple on the tube current.

The electron emission from the filament surface provides the tube current. Precise stabilization of the filament current by means of feedback controls is shown in Fig. 4.6. Both kilovoltage and tube current are monitored so that when either is changed the filament current is adjusted to provide consistent output. If this feedback stabilization fails then there will be abrupt unregulated changes in the tube current when the kilovoltage settings are changed. Rapid response feedback control is most easily carried out with high frequency units. There are three levels of filament current control during operation of the X-ray unit:

- A pre-heating current to maintain the filament winding in standby mode: about 2 to 3 A. There is no electron emission so the X-ray tube current is zero
- Filament operating at lowest rating gives a low tube current 0.1 to 4 mA for fluoroscopy

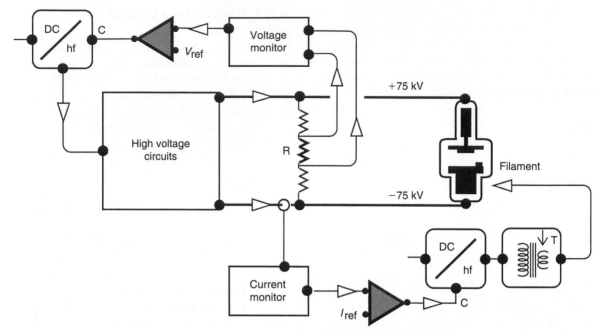

Figure 4.6 *Stabilizing tube voltage and current by means of feedback controls from the high voltage output via a resistor chain (R). Tube current is monitored by a separate comparator circuit and is stabilized by adjustments to the filament supply.*

Table 4.2 *Generator switching and rating.*

Generator	Speed	Rating
Two-pulse	20 ms	2–50 kW
Six-pulse	10 ms	50 kW (at 100 kV)
Twelve-pulse	3 ms	70 kW (at 100 kV)
Constant potential	20 μs	150 kW (at 100 kV)

- High filament current for routine work. Exact pre-set values are used since a very small deviation in filament current gives significant tube-current variations.

4.2.3 Starter

An asynchronous motor consisting of a rotor (connected to the anode) and an external stator at ground (zero volts) potential drives the rotating anode. The asynchronous motor design allows a large gap between the stator and rotor. X-ray tubes with ball bearings are accelerated before an exposure is made and then braked after exposure when the inertia of the anode plays an important part in braking. X-ray tubes with sleeve bearings are kept running throughout the working day since most wear occurs during braking, which is not necessary with this bearing.

The speed of starter rotation is the supply frequency $\times$ 60. Conventional starters use either the line frequency direct which would give speeds of 3000 rpm for 50 Hz and 3600 rpm for 60 Hz, or use the third harmonic from a 3-phase supply which would give 9000 or 10 800 rpm respectively.

Figure 4.5 shows a starter circuit as part of the high frequency generator. Slow rotation of the anode (15 to 20 Hz) is used for low output continuous screening (fluoroscopy) since there is reduced anode heating and slower speeds will reduce bearing wear. Medium frequency 50 to 180 Hz is used for conventional work while 200 to 300 Hz is reserved for special fast exposure times. Circuits monitor the anode rpm in order to indicate warning of worn bearings.

4.2.4 Exposure timing

TIMING CIRCUITS

Control of X-ray exposure in conventional, mains driven, X-ray units was obtained by using mechanical timers, either clockwork or electrical. These have been discontinued since they are unable to offer fast switching rates necessary for effective X-ray exposure (0.01 to 0.05 s) and have been replaced by either electronic, frequency controlled or exposure controlled timers.

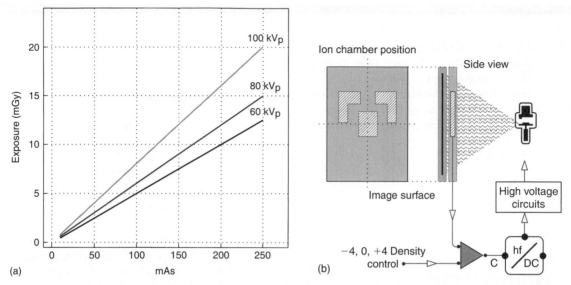

Figure 4.7 (a) There is a linear relationship between mAs and radiation output (mGy) for each kilovoltage setting. This is a good test for overall accuracy of generator regulation. (b) Automatic dose control from ion chambers placed in front of the film cassette. Regions can be selected which cover the anatomy of interest (shaded areas). When the ion chamber output records an exposure commensurate with the density setting the X-ray beam is switched off.

TIMER LINEARITY

The radiation output should increase linearly with time for a given kilovoltage and tube current (in mA). Tube current and exposure time both cause linear change in radiation output so their product, mAs, should also show a linear relationship. Figure 4.7a shows values of mAs plotted against exposure radiation dose (mGy) for 60, 80, and $100 \, kV_p$ showing the expected linear response which indicates that both exposure timing and the tube current regulation are working to specification. Exposure timing can be set manually or typically by feedback from an exposure meter. Dose rate is measured by the built-in ion chamber situated either in front or behind the film cassette and switches the X-ray beam off when the integrated dose reaches a predetermined value set in the machine (dependent on film type and intensifying screen speed). Figure 4.7b shows such an arrangement fitted into a film cassette holder.

Several parameters control the exposure timing from a built-in ionization chamber. The output (radiation dose) from a generator is related to kilovoltage V, tube current I and exposure time t as

$$D = k \times V^n \times I \times t \qquad (4.3)$$

where k is a constant depending on anode material, filtration etc. and the power n depends on tube

kilovoltage (for 50 kV it is about 5, reducing to 3 at 150 kV). The parameters in eqn 4.3 are used by the exposure control to give consistent film density over a range of settings.

ELECTRONIC TIMING

Electronic timing devices use an R/C circuit (see Chapter 2) for producing switched variable time fractions. These are placed in the primary of the high voltage circuit of conventional machines controlling either a mechanical (relay) or electronic (thyristor or thyratron) switch: this is shown as the timer in Fig. 4.1. Modern units use semiconductor timers. Frequency or pulse counting timers monitor the tube current for an appropriate number of cycles then switch off the high frequency generator.

FREQUENCY OR PULSE COUNTING TIMERS

The product Q of tube current I and time t describes the exposure as the product of milliamps and seconds (mAs):

$$Q = I \times t \qquad (4.4)$$

When an exposure is made the selected tube kilovoltage is applied and the tube current, as measured by the feedback controls in Fig. 4.6, is integrated over time t until the mAs product reaches its predefined value.

The tube voltage is then immediately switched off. Accurate reproducibility of the mAs value must be ensured since a small variation in mAs will cause a visible density change on the film image. The variation ΔQ in mAs value, given by the high frequency generator depends on the tube current and switching frequency f so that

$$\Delta Q = \frac{I}{2f} \qquad (4.5)$$

So for 1000 mA and a 5 kHz converter frequency the reproducibility would be ± 0.1 mAs.

4.3 EXPOSURE CONTROL

Ion chambers are commonly employed as automatic exposure control (AEC) devices for maintaining optimum film density for each kV and mA setting. Usually all that is required from the operator is a kV_p setting; mAs is then chosen by the AEC for the particular film type and examination. The position of some commonly used automatic exposure controls (AECs) is shown in Fig. 4.8.

4.3.1 Automatic dose control devices

AEC units control exposure time for a predetermined kilovoltage and current (in mA). They are mostly flat ionization chambers made from radiolucent plastic which are placed in front of the film cassette in a common array pattern shown in Fig. 4.7b. This arrangement allows choice of AEC position for any patient study. Film density variation is selected by means of a feedback control to the generator converter as shown in the diagram. The dominant region of an image containing diagnostic information should maintain a specific optical density and these selected areas are placed within one of the separate automatic exposure controls (shaded areas on the diagram). These are either ion-chamber detectors or semiconductor device(s) which monitor the X-ray intensity in the chosen dominant area. AEC systems are used in fluoroscopy, conventional radiography and DSA.

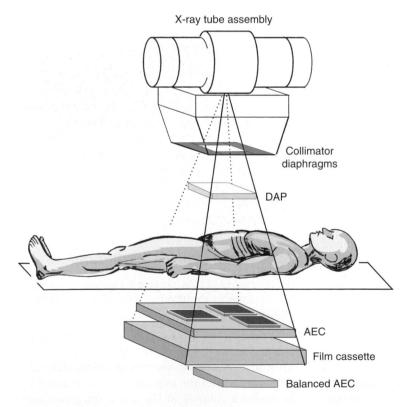

Figure 4.8 *A variety of exposure controls and measuring devices fitted to the X-ray unit. The typical AEC is fitted in front of the film cassette but for mammography it occupies a central area behind the cassette. A dose–area product (DAP) meter is fitted directly to the collimator housing.*

Mammography uses a special balanced detector system behind the cassette. The reference signal which controls each exposure contains information about patient absorption and film-screen sensitivity. Three types of AEC are currently in use:

- Flat plate **ionization chamber** placed in front of the cassette. This is almost transparent to X-rays so does not interfere with the film image.
- **Semiconductor detector(s)** placed behind the cassette prevent image shadowing and are found in low exposure techniques such as mammography.
- **Photomultiplier** (Chapter 2) measures light intensity from an image intensifier acting as a brightness control and indirectly measuring radiation dose.

All AEC systems have preset controls covering various radiographic procedures (extremities, chest, abdomen etc.). An over-ride film density correction control allows adjustment in detector sensitivity for variations in different film-screen sensitivities. This is shown as a −4, 0, +4 variable input in Fig. 4.7b. A mammography automatic exposure control is made behind the cassette and this is fully described in Chapter 6.

4.3.2 Dose–area product meters

A valuable requirement for any X-ray examination is to know the total dose received by the patient during a particular study. This information is provided by a dose–area product meter (DAP or diamentor).

The dose–area product is measured with a large area ion chamber placed directly below the tube collimator housing. Its position is shown in Figs 4.8 and 4.9a.

The dose–area product meter is not an exposure control. It allows the radiation exposure to patients to be recorded and is the area integral of the air kerma over the surface area of the useful beam. It is measured in $Gy\,m^{-2}$ (replacing $R\,cm^{-2}$). Conversion factors are $1\,R\,cm^{-2} \equiv 0.87\,cGy\,cm^{-2} = 0.87\,mGy\,m^{-2}$.

The DAP enables the total dose to be recorded for each patient examination, it can also display the total elapsed fluoroscopy time. With regular use the dose–area product meter can compare exposures for different patients and different techniques which is particularly useful for training. The detector consists of a large parallel-plate ionization chamber connected to a high input impedance amplifier. The charge collected by the chamber is proportional both to the chamber area and the X-ray dose. The chamber is

fixed close to the X-ray tube housing (usually the diaphragm housing) where the X-ray dose is high and backscattered radiation from the patient is minimal.

Figure 4.9a shows the independence of dose measurement with distance from the X-ray source. Since

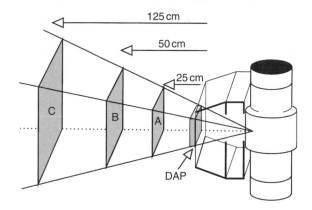

	A	B	C
Distance (d)	25	50	125 cm
Area (A)	10^2	20^2	50^2
Dose (D)	10	2.5	0.4 mGy
$A \times D$	1000	1000	1000 mGy cm^2

(a)

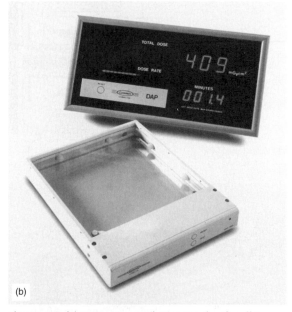

(b)

Figure 4.9 *(a) Dose–area product meter showing distance independence as it registers dose (mGy or Gy) per unit area (cm²). (b) A commercially available example (courtesy Gammex).*

the chamber is transparent it does not interfere with any light beam positioning device. Table 4.3 lists the factors that do alter the dose–area product. Under-couch X-ray fluoroscopy units are not ideal for dose–area product meters since the table acts as an additional filter in front of the patient.

This is not the case (obviously) with over-couch designs. A commercial DAP is shown in Fig. 4.9b with a large ion chamber and digital readout which can feed a paper printer for a permanent patient record.

Table 4.3 *Factors influencing dose–area product.*

Factor	Units
Tube kilovoltage	kV_p
Tube current	mA
Filtration	mm Al
Time	minutes
Area	cm^2

4.4 X-RAY TUBE DESIGN

4.4.1 Tube envelope

Glass has been the traditional material for X-ray tube construction but the modern metal/ceramic X-ray tube has several advantages over glass:

- Scattered electrons from the anode are collected by the metal envelope.
- Improved heat conduction for size and increased rating possible due to more effective heat removal.
- Vaporized metal from the anode condenses on the metal envelope rather than glass which slowly destroys its insulating properties, giving longer tube life.

The general features of a modern metal/ceramic X-ray tube are shown in Fig. 4.10a and the appearance of a modern metal cased X-ray tube is shown in the photograph of Fig. 4.10b. Additional improvements have increased tube performance by enlarging

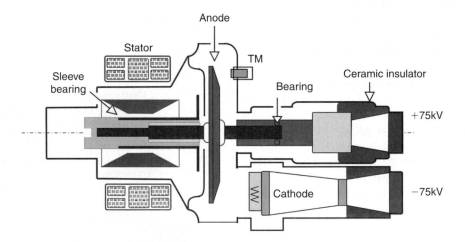

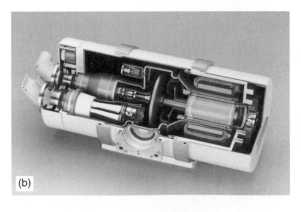

(b)

Figure 4.10 *(a) Metal/ceramic X-ray tube with a double bearing to carry the large anode. There is a thermal monitoring device (TM) for the anode. (b) Photograph of a modern metal/ceramic X-ray tube (Philips Rotalix).*

anode diameters and improving the bearings and their lubrication.

4.4.2 Anode design

The design of the anode disk plays a crucial part in the performance of the X-ray tube. The body of the anode disk is a refractory alloy of molybdenum, titanium and zirconium (Fig. 4.11a). The surface target is about 0.7 mm thick consisting of a tungsten–rhenium alloy on a similar thickness of pure tungsten.

Tungsten–rhenium alloy permits higher thermal loading since it is not subjected to pitting. Increasing the diameter of the anode from the conventional 90/100 mm to 200 mm also gives higher loading and shorter exposure times. Special precautions are necessary to prevent distortion of larger anode disks due to local thermal expansion and Fig. 4.11b shows stress slots are cut around the disk circumference which prevent this. Disk volume is increased by backing the anode disk with graphite which gives minimum increase in weight but doubling the heat storage shown in anodes (b) and (c). A CT anode is sometimes flat in order to provide maximum metal thickness behind the focal spot; the angulation is achieved by a 9–11° cathode offset. Direct cooling of the anode is achieved in some tubes by circulating oil through a channel in the anode shaft.

LUBRICATION OF ANODE BEARING

Air, water and oil are all obviously unsuitable for bearing lubrication at the high working temperatures of an X-ray tube. The lubricant commonly used is a metallic gallium alloy which is liquid at room temperatures. It has an extremely low vapor pressure, which is essential to maintain the vacuum conditions and provide good conduction of both heat and electric current. Some rotor bearings now use a sleeve design instead of a ball bearing; the rotating shaft fits tightly into a hollow sleeve. Spiral grooves cut into the shaft improve metal lubricant circulation. The wear of these bearings is small and occurs during anode braking when there is direct mechanical contact between bearing surfaces. It is therefore recommended that the anode for these tubes is kept continuously rotating.

4.5 EQUIPMENT

Conventional radiography uses short exposures having a small value for mAs and so X-ray tubes and generators can be of a moderate rating for certain investigations but are more demanding and operate tube and generator near the maximum limits.

4.5.1 Tube thermal workload

The principal criteria involved for X-ray tube selection are the maximum tube voltage, the focal spot size and the thermal loadability for short, medium, and long exposure times. The workload capacity of the X-ray tube is determined by the rapid rise in temperature of the focal spot.

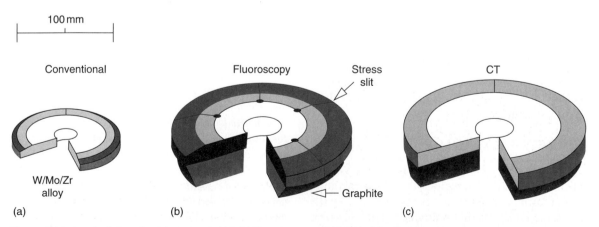

Figure 4.11 *Anode designs for (a) conventional, (b) fluoroscopy and (c) CT applications.*

A distinction is made between the rise in temperature for short load times (<0.1 s: short-term loadability) and the rise in temperature for longer load periods. Very short exposure times (0.01 s) affect the rating of an X-ray tube since if the tube rotates at 3000 rpm equivalent to one revolution in 0.02 s then the focal spot area occupies only half the target circumference and the heat produced must be dissipated from this reduced area.

Figure 4.12a shows that only partial use is made of the available target area of 3000 rpm anodes during fast exposure times; larger anodes rotating at increased speeds provide a solution to this problem. For short exposure times the current rating remains constant as shown by the electrical rating graphs of Chapter 3; the heat input rate remains constant even though the exposure time may vary from 0.1 to 0.02 s. The tube rating is therefore independent of exposure time at <0.1 s so for very short time exposures the rating can clearly be improved by increasing the anode rotation speed. For very long load periods (e.g. fluoroscopy: long term loadability) a further limit is imposed by the thermal capacity of the anode and thermal dissipation to the surrounding cooling medium (oil). If an X-ray tube has experienced high load conditions then either the exposure power must be reduced or a pause must be made before the next set of exposures.

LOAD MONITORING

The thermal state of the anode is monitored by a temperature sensor incorporated into the rear of the tube envelope behind the envelope (Loadix). The sensor is part of a feedback control circuit that considers the permitted load values for the tube, the intended number of exposures, and the duration of each exposure so that tube ratings are not exceeded. Figure 4.12b illustrates the magnitude of the temperature rise that an anode may experience for different clinical applications: a single exposure from a high voltage chest-unit, a series of exposures during cardiac angiography and low power continuous use experienced in fluoroscopy screening.

SHORT-TERM LOADABILITY

This applies to very short exposure times of 0.1 s or less which applies to the flat region of the electrical rating graph shown in Chapter 3. This is determined by the size of the target region bombarded by the electron beam, which depends on the speed of anode rotation,

length of the focal track and its width. The target angle is also critical since, in general, the smaller the angle the wider the focal track and therefore the greater the short-term loadability. Choice of anode angle is also determined by field size considerations.

MEDIUM-TERM LOADABILITY

This is considered when the heat storage capacity for series of images is determined by the mass of the

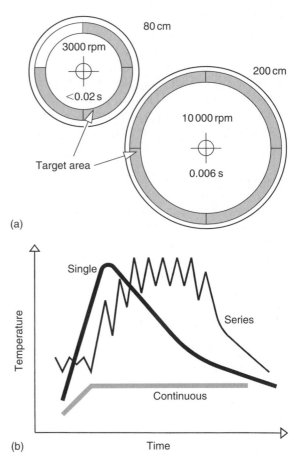

(a)

(b)

Figure 4.12 *(a) The area of anode used when making a very fast exposure, showing the difference between a small diameter anode and a rapidly rotating large area anode used in high load applications such as chest radiography, fluoroscopy, and CT. (b) The thermal load or loadability for various clinical examinations. The single exposure taken during a chest radiograph imposes a high thermal load which is then dissipated. A series of high exposures (angiography) places high demands on the tube whereas low tube current fluoroscopy imposes a continuous low thermal workload.*

anode. The large thermal build-up and dissipation during a single exposure (chest radiograph) and a series of exposures (cine-angiography) are compared with a low continuous exposure (screening during fluoroscopy) in Fig. 4.12b.

LONG-TERM LOADABILITY

This requires rapid restoration of heat capacity by providing efficient cooling of the anode.

SERIES LOADABILITY

This measure is defined as the load that the tube can withstand continuously for a period of say 20 s with a suggested cooling period of 120 s. It is proportional to the quantity of anode material or anode heat storage capacity. Series loadability is proportional to the diameter of the focal track. It is also determined by the length of the series of exposures but also the cooling period between.

BATCH LOADABILITY

Batch loadability is the term used for describing a set of exposure series as would be experienced in CT examinations. An example of an acceptable load would be a batch of 2 min with a cooling period of 15 to 20 min before repeating the batch series. Doubling heat storage only usually gives an increase of about 40% in the batch loadability since heat dissipation plays an important role.

4.5.2 Applications

The specific requirements for clinical applications place different demands on the X-ray tube and generator. **General radiography** for dentistry or small mobile applications uses only short-term loadability so simple stationary anode X-ray tubes can be used for these low power mobile X-ray sets. **Chest radiography** using high kilovoltage techniques also considers short-term loadability but since the source-to-image distances (SIDs) are large the focal spot size can be quite large. Unsharpness is a minimum for a 1.6 mm focal spot at 2 m SID and also a small anode angle can be used since field of view is not a critical factor at these distances. However, since X-ray intensity obeys the inverse square law large tube currents are necessary in order to give adequate beam intensity for the

very short exposure times (20 ms) and tube loading is close to maximum. **Skeletal and abdominal** examinations demand critical tube loadability and focal sizes. Kilovoltages commonly employed are between 60 and 85 kV to give sufficient contrast. The SID is usually small – between 40 and 100 cm – requiring a larger focal spot size to give the field of view at these distances. However, large focal spot sizes may be a limiting factor so dual focus tubes are employed giving a finer spot size for high definition work. A high tube load, upwards of 80 or 100 kW, is sometimes required in order to give short exposure times.

The requirements for combined **radiography and fluoroscopy** are for high tube loadability particularly when long SIDs are used, but where under-table work is carried out using short SIDs the anode angle is critical to enable a practical field of view. Continuous loadability is commonly found in fluoroscopic screening. During screening or fluoroscopy conditions continuous low tube currents are required. Directly controlled R/F systems (under-couch tube) require relatively small tube currents for fluoroscopy allowing simple heat loss from the tube. It is common practice to use a more slowly rotating anode (20 Hz).

In order to cover a useful image field at an FFD of <100 cm a large field of view is obtained if the anode angle is not too small (12° to 15°). Remote controlled R/F systems (over-couch tube) use larger SIDs (≈100 cm) demanding greater output (doubling loadability up to 100 kW) so a high output tube is necessary in order to freeze intestinal motion for spot filming by using fast exposure times of the order of 0.01 to 0.02 s. Basic specifications for high, medium, and low rated X-ray tubes are given in Table 4.4; recent CT machines have demanded even higher rated tubes.

Table 4.4 *Specifications of three X-ray tubes of different rating.*

	High load	Medium load	Low load
Anode diameter	200 mm	100 mm	60 mm
Focal spots	0.5 and 0.8 mm	0.2–1.0 mm	0.4–0.6 mm
Anode heat storage	1.8 MJ	250–500 kJ	70–100 kJ
Application	CT, DSA	General	Mammography

CARDIOLOGY (CINE-ANGIOGRAPHY)

Angiography and cine-cardiography both require series loadability which makes very high demands on the tube rating (Fig. 4.12b) particularly since high resolution pictures are required which demand small focal spot sizes. Cine-techniques show rapidly moving vascular structures (cardiac walls and vessels) so frame rates of up to 100–200 frames s^{-1} are necessary. Exposure times of 8 ms and run times of 5 to 10 s. Small diameter catheters and stents also require high resolution pictures and focal spot sizes are typically 0.5 mm. The upper limit of focal spot size is 0.8 mm and loadability is very high for these continuous loads. The number of exposures is much higher than for gastrointestinal studies and so requires a much higher tube loading.

COMPUTED TOMOGRAPHY

Since these X-ray tubes are heavily collimated in order to irradiate a thin slice of tissue only a small fraction of the X-rays generated are actually used for imaging. Fast image data processing means that the tube is quickly required to be ready for repeat exposures. Long-term loadability is of prime importance and heat storage capacity and dissipation determines waiting time between slice acquisition. A large mass of graphite (Fig. 4.11c), used to increase heat storage capacity, is not necessarily the best solution since stored heat must be lost quickly. This is most effectively achieved by using an oil cooled sleeve bearing to increase the conductive pathway and large diameter (200 mm) all metal anodes.

MAMMOGRAPHY

The X-ray tubes operate at between 25 and 30 kV_p so the anode heating is not a limiting factor so its mass can be kept low (Fig. 4.11a). The filament rating, however, is critical owing to the space-charge problems. Mammography is covered as a special topic in Chapter 9.

KEYWORDS

automatic exposure control: a radiation detector which monitors exposure and cuts off the X-ray beam

bearing: either ball or sleeve bearing support for the anode

converter: an electronic circuit which converts DC into high frequency alternating voltage

feed-back: the level of the output signal monitored in order to control accuracy

generator (constant potential): a high power generator providing pure DC output

generator (high frequency): a generator using a converter to produce a frequency between 5 and 10 kHz

line frequency: either 50 or 60 Hz

overload: a condition outside the safe operating threshold either electrical or thermal which will damage the X-ray tube

rating: limits imposed on kilovoltage, tube current, and time for operating an X-ray tube

rectification (full wave): both negative and positive AC waveform utilized in the DC output

rectification (half wave): only utilizing the positive AC waveform for the DC output

ripple: residual AC interference on the DC waveform

starter: the electrical circuit driving the anode induction motor

thyristor: a semiconductor switching device used for switching the DC waveform in a converter

Interactions of X- and gamma radiation with matter

5.1 GENERAL INTERACTION WITH MATTER

The section of the electromagnetic spectrum of most concern to radiologists covers visible light, X-radiation and gamma radiation. The visible spectrum concerns the 'end product' which is the image or display. The higher energy X- and gamma radiation are concerned with image formation.

The difference between X- and gamma radiation concerns their origin. X-radiation is produced by the change in energy states of high energy or orbital bound electrons (K or L shells) or by the deceleration of an electron beam (X-ray tube). The energy change during these transformations is accompanied by electromagnetic radiation across a broad X-ray spectrum.

Gamma radiation originates almost exclusively from an atom's nucleus due to nuclear decay processes and appears as discrete energies and not a continuous spectrum. Nuclear decay and its associated radiation will be described in Chapter 15.

X-rays due to the nature of their production have a mix of radiation wavelengths which produces a continuous spectrum. The X-ray spectrum for diagnostic purposes has an energy of 20 to 150 keV; its wavelength can be calculated:

$$\lambda = \frac{1.24}{E} \tag{5.1}$$

where E is in keV and λ in nm, so wavelengths would be 0.062 nm to 0.0082 nm respectively for these energies. These are very short wavelengths compared to visible light which ranges from 400 to 700 nm.

Since gamma radiation occurs as discrete energies it is simpler to use the particulate properties of the photon for demonstrating general interactions with matter. The complexities that arise when considering the continuous spectrum of X-rays will be described later. A general diagram describing gamma photon behavior when penetrating an absorber is shown in Fig. 5.1 where incident photons can be:

- Transmitted through the absorber unchanged
- Totally absorbed
- Scattered from the original direction retaining their original energy
- Scattered from the original direction but losing some of their energy

The arrival of a 'useful' photon at the imaging receptor plane (i.e. film surface) depends therefore

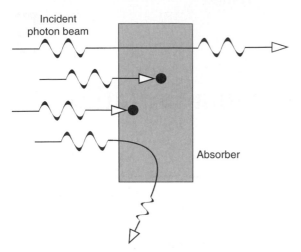

Figure 5.1 *General interactions of X-rays with matter showing transmission through the absorber unchanged; total absorption of the radiation or scatter of the radiation as different angles.*

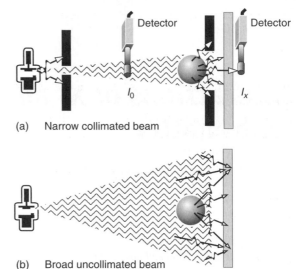

(a)   Narrow collimated beam

(b)   Broad uncollimated beam

Figure 5.2 *Source, absorber, and imaging surface (film or digital) representing (a) narrow- and (b) broad-beam geometry.*

on two factors: photon **absorption** or photon **scatter** from the main beam.

5.1.1 Geometry of attenuation measurements

In some encounters a photon may give up only a portion of its energy to an orbital electron. The remaining energy goes into the creation of a new photon of lower energy than the original. The newly created photon may move off in any direction depending on the energy division among the three particles. Measurements of photon absorption are complicated by the presence of these new or scattered photons.

NARROW BEAM

The set-up shown in Fig. 5.2a is designed to measure the absorption characteristics of a narrow beam of photons. The photons emitted by the X-ray tube source are restricted or collimated to a narrow beam. A second collimator is placed in front of the image surface; in practice this would be the antiscatter grid. An absorber is located within the beam. The example is restricted to photons of diagnostic energies (20 to 200 keV). Secondary photons originating in the absorber by primary photon absorption will be scattered in all directions. Few of these scattered

photons will reach the imaging surface, which will intercept only those photons that pass through the absorber without an interaction. This arrangement is said to have good geometry.

BROAD BEAM

When the imaging surface is not collimated and placed close to the absorber, as in Fig. 5.2b, it will respond to a large fraction of the scattered photons. This arrangement has poor geometry. An imaging surface even with good geometry will receive not only the direct, attenuated beam but also some photons scattered from all points in the absorber. With a broad beam the radiation intensity, if measured, will be greater than that obtained under narrow-beam conditions.

EXPONENTIAL ATTENUATION

Using the geometry arrangement of Fig. 5.2a photon intensity at the detector is I_0 when there is no absorber in the beam. The intensity specifies the rate at which photon energy crosses a unit cross section perpendicular to the beam direction. Intensity is measured as the number N of photons per unit area A (**photon fluence** $\Phi = N/A\ \mathrm{m^{-2}}$) or intensity per unit time t (**photon flux** $\phi = \Phi/t$). For a mono-energetic beam intensity can be expressed in photons $\mathrm{m^2\,s^{-1}}$. As absorbers are introduced, the intensity incident on the detector (I_x) will decrease according to an exponential law:

$$I_x = I_0 e^{-\mu x} \qquad (5.2)$$

where absorber thickness is x and μ is the **linear attenuation coefficient**, a function of the photon energy and the atomic number of the absorber.

Eqn 5.2 is identical in form to the one which describes radioactive decay. The exponential attenuation relationship arises for a reason analogous to that leading to an exponential radioactive decay; the probability of an absorbing event is proportional to the number of photons which pass the point under consideration. The exponential form of eqn 5.2 can be converted to a logarithmic one (natural logarithm as ln). Since

$$\frac{I_x}{I_0} = e^{-\mu x}$$

then

$$\frac{I_0}{I_x} = e^{\mu x} \quad \text{and} \quad \ln I_x = \ln I_0 - \mu x$$

So

$$\ln \frac{I_0}{I_x} = \mu x \qquad (5.3)$$

The overall attenuation of radiation by matter can be readily explained by considering a beam of mono-chromatic (single energy) photons incident on an absorbing material (e.g. aluminum). Figure 5.3 shows 1000 photons having an energy of 200 keV incident on a 1 cm thickness of aluminum. It is found that a certain number are removed from the beam leaving 718 photons transmitted as I_A. These are then incident on the second 1 cm layer; the same fraction ($0.718 \times 718 = 516$) is transmitted as I_B. This is the process of attenuation and is dependent on the absorber material and photon energy. The process of general radiation attenuation follows the exponential form described in eqn 5.2. The value for μ, the linear attenuation coefficient of aluminum, can be obtained from the experiment conducted in Fig. 5.3. For the values 718 and 516 observed the attenuation coefficient μ for 1 cm aluminum and a photon energy of 200 keV is

$$\ln \left(\frac{718}{516} \right) = 33.0 \, \text{m}^{-1} \quad \text{or} \quad 0.33 \, \text{cm}^{-1}$$

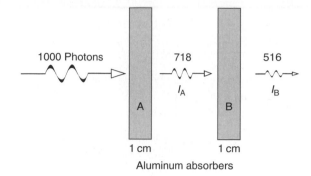

Figure 5.3 *The fractional absorption of radiation through material for a photon energy of 200 keV, this is explained in the text.*

Box 5.1 investigates photon transmission through an absorber. The **logarithmic** difference between the transmitted photons is directly proportional to the difference in thickness x.

The graph in Fig. 5.4a shows the attenuation of a mono-energetic beam as a simple exponential. The main factors to be remembered with transmission of radiation are:

- The intensity is not halved as the thickness is doubled but decreases exponentially with thickness.
- The fraction absorbed depends on the photon energy.
- The linear attenuation coefficient is energy and material Z dependent.

Both linear Fig. 5.4a and semi-logarithmic plots Fig. 5.4b are shown; the straight line semi-logarithmic plot has obvious advantages. The two curves (A) and (B) in Fig. 5.4 show different rates of absorption that could be due to different photon energies or different absorber properties. For a given material a constant fraction is attenuated for equal added thicknesses of absorber.

Box 5.1 uses the basic formula outlined above for overall photon attenuation and calculates the attenuation for two thicknesses of material A and B: where B doubles the absorber thickness. The worked example shows that:

- The fractional decrease in photon intensity is constant:

$$1000 \rightarrow 718 \; (\approx 72\%)$$
$$718 \rightarrow 516 \; (\approx 72\%).$$

Box 5.1 Linear attenuation properties (see Fig. 5.3)

Incident photon intensity is $I_0 = 1000$
Transmission through A is $I_A = 718$
Transmission through B is $I_B = 516$

The difference between I_A and I_B is constant but not directly proportional to the difference in thickness x_A and x_B. Consider:

$$I_A = I_0 e^{-\mu x_A} \quad \text{and} \quad I_B = I_0 e^{\mu x_B}$$

Taking log values:

$$\ln I_A = -\mu x_A \quad \text{and} \quad \ln I_B = -\mu x_B$$

Then

$$\ln I_A - \ln I_B = \mu(x_B - x_A)$$

Since the dimensions are in centimeters the value for the linear attenuation coefficient at 200 keV is $6.57 - 6.24 = 0.33\,\text{cm}^{-1}$.

Calculating μ for aluminum at 200 keV

The density of aluminum $2700\,\text{kg}\,\text{m}^{-3}$ and the HVL at 200 keV is 2.1 cm (0.021 m). The linear attenuation coefficient μ (in meters) is

$$\frac{0.693}{0.021} = 33.0\,\text{m}^{-1}$$

The mass attenuation coefficient μ/ρ is

$$\frac{33.0}{2700} = 0.0122\,\text{m}^2\,\text{kg}^{-1}$$

Note. Divide by 100 to convert to cm^{-1} and multiply by 10 to convert to $\text{cm}^2\,\text{g}^{-1}$.

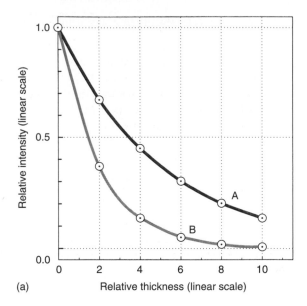

(a)

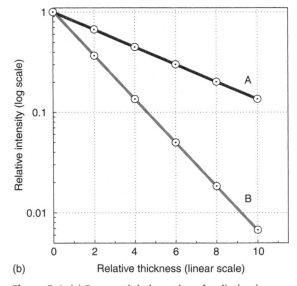

(b)

Figure 5.4 *(a) Exponential absorption of radiation in an absorber for two photon beam energies using a linear scale. (b) Using a log scale on the y-axis will give straight lines (semi-log plot).*

- The difference in the $\log_n$ of the transmitted intensities is proportional to the difference in thickness of the material.

The critical parameters used in the equation which affect the attenuation of radiation in matter are:

- The **thickness** of the material x
- The **linear attenuation coefficient** μ

The linear attenuation coefficient itself is influenced by:

- Atomic number, Z
- Material density, ρ
- Photon energy, E

THICKNESS OF THE MATERIAL X

Attenuation increases with the material (tissue) thickness, but the change in transmission of the photons (penetration) is not linearly dependent on the thickness, i.e. doubling the thickness does not halve the transmission but for a mono-energetic beam the fractional decrease is constant for equal thicknesses.

5.2 PHOTON LINEAR ATTENUATION AND ABSORPTION COEFFICIENTS

The processes of X-ray interaction with matter all involve attenuation, since the intensity of the X-ray beam is reduced (or 'attenuated') as a result. Some of these processes result in complete absorption of an X-ray quantum (photoelectric event), and some in partial or no absorption (scattering). Used in this sense, the term 'absorption' implies that energy is transferred to the atoms of the absorber from the X-rays. The important attenuation processes involving diagnostic energies (20 to 200 keV) are:

- Photoelectric absorption which shows both attenuation and usually complete absorption
- Compton scatter producing attenuation and partial absorption

Therefore the total linear attenuation coefficient μ is applied to the overall attenuation of X-rays by both these processes and describes the probability of a particular event occurring at all (i.e. photoelectric absorption or Compton scatter). Each process has its own linear attenuation coefficient and linear absorption coefficient μ_{ab}.

The family of attenuation and absorption coefficients, important for diagnostic radiology are:

- Linear attenuation coefficient
- Linear absorption coefficient
- Linear scatter coefficient

LINEAR ATTENUATION COEFFICIENT μ

Linear attenuation coefficient μ relates to attenuation of wave or beam of particles along the medium's path attributable to all processes (absorption and scattering). The unit is the reciprocal meter m^{-1}. The value of μ decreases with photon energy. Since μ has greater differences at high keV they are used preferentially

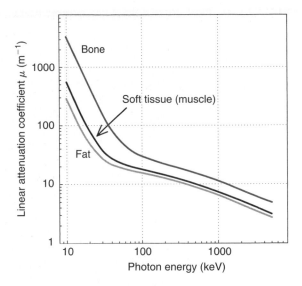

Figure 5.5 *Linear attenuation coefficient μ for soft tissue, fat, and bone.*

for computing the Hounsfield number. So the total attenuation of the photon beam (μ_{tot}) at diagnostic X-ray energies is the sum of photoelectric absorption μ_{en} and μ_{scat} Compton scatter events so: $\mu_{tot} = \mu_{en} + \mu_{scat}$. These are plotted in Fig. 5.5 for a range of diagnostic photon energies.

LINEAR ABSORPTION COEFFICIENT μ_{en}

Linear absorption coefficient μ_{en} is the part of the linear attenuation coefficient that is attributable to absorption by the photoelectric effect (sometimes given the symbol μ_{τ}). The unit is the reciprocal meter m^{-1}. Figure 5.6 shows the absorption component is always less than the overall attenuation, which includes scatter.

LINEAR SCATTER COEFFICIENT μ_{scat}

The Compton scattering process results in beam attenuation and in energy loss. The linear scattering coefficient decreases steadily with increasing energy: high energy radiation is less scattered than lower energy radiation. Not only the amount of energy transferred to the recoil electron increases with increasing incident photon energy but an increasing proportion of the total beam energy is taken by the recoil electron. Consequently at higher energies the energy of the scattered photon is a smaller fraction of the total. A 30 keV photon scattered at a 90° angle

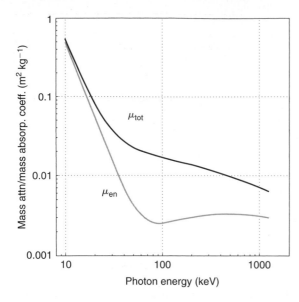

Figure 5.6 *Linear absorption μ_{en} and scatter components for water.*

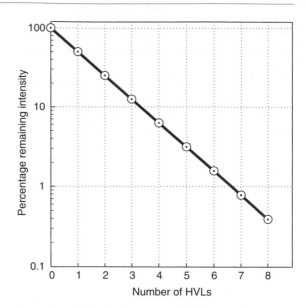

Figure 5.7 *Half-value layers n and intensity reduction using the function ½^n. After four HVLs the intensity has been reduced to ≈6% of the original.*

retains 97% of its energy; a 100 keV retains 91%; a 1 MeV retains 67% and a 10 MeV retains only 9%.

$$\mu_{total} = \mu_{en} + \mu_{scat} \tag{5.4}$$

HALF-VALUE LAYER

The linear attenuation coefficient μ for a particular tissue at a particular energy is a measure of the ability of the tissue to remove photons from a beam of X-rays. It is the fraction of photons (X- or gamma radiation) removed from a beam per unit thickness of absorber (m^{-1}). From the general exponential relationship $I_x = I_0 e^{-\mu x}$ the thickness x absorbing half the radiation is the half-value layer (HVL) where

$$\frac{I_x}{I_0} = 0.5 = e^{-x \times HVL} \tag{5.5}$$

Since $e^{-0.693} = 0.5$ then $\mu \times HVL = 0.693$. So,

$$\mu = \frac{0.693}{HVL} \tag{5.6}$$

This simple relationship is plotted in Fig. 5.7 for intensity versus absorber HVL. The influence on the incident beam of a certain number of half-value layers can

be calculated from ½^n where n is the number of half-value layers.

The accurate determination of half-value layer can be calculated from the formula

$$HVL = \frac{x_1 \times \ln\left(\frac{2y_2}{y_0}\right) - x_2 \times \ln\left(\frac{2y_1}{y_0}\right)}{\ln\left(\frac{y_2}{y_1}\right)} \tag{5.7}$$

where y_0 is the incident radiation intensity measured without absorber, y_1 the intensity measured after x_1 mm filtration added, and y_2 the intensity measured after x_2 mm filtration added. The radiation intensity can be given in mR or mGy. Only a rough indication can be obtained from semi-log graph paper. This formula can be incorporated into spreadsheets and can form part of a full quality control program. Box 5.2 gives an example of its use in mammography.

Table 5.1 gives the values for linear and mass attenuation coefficients for water over the diagnostic photon energies together with the half-value layer computed from eqn 5.7. Since water closely approximates to soft tissue its HVL gives an indication of X-ray attenuation through the body.

Figure 5.8 shows the half-value thickness for lead over the diagnostic energy range. The K edge at 88 keV improves its shielding capabilities for nuclear medicine

Box 5.2 Example of the use of eqn 5.7

A mammography unit gives the following readings:

Measurement with no absorber = 718 (y_0)
Measurement with 0.1 mm aluminum = 583 (y_1)
Measurement with 0.5 mm aluminum = 275 (y_2)

Therefore the half-value layer (HVL) is given by

$$HVL = \frac{0.1 \times \ln\left(\frac{2 \times 275}{718}\right) - 0.5 \times \ln\left(\frac{2 \times 583}{718}\right)}{\ln\left(\frac{275}{583}\right)}$$

Or,

$$HVL = \frac{-0.02665 - 0.2424}{-0.7514} = 0.358 \, mm$$

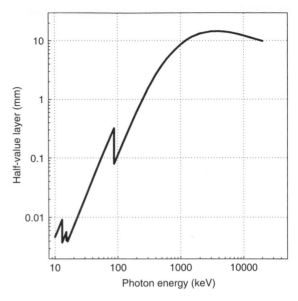

Figure 5.8 *The half-value layer for lead over a wide photon energy range showing a major abrupt change at the K edge. The absorption efficiency of a lead protective apron can markedly improve in this region. The half-value layer (HVL) for 80 keV is 0.5 mm but for 100 keV it is only 0.1 mm.*

Table 5.1 *Linear attenuation coefficients, half-value layers, mass attenuation and mass absorption coefficients for water over the diagnostic energy range 20–200 keV.*

keV	μ (m^{-1})	HVL (mm)	μ/ρ (m^2 kg^{-1})	μ_{en}/ρ (m^2 kg^{-1})
20	80.9600	8.5598	8.096E−02	5.503E−02
30	37.5600	18.4505	3.756E−02	1.557E−02
40	26.8300	25.8293	2.683E−02	6.947E−03
50	22.6900	30.5421	2.269E−02	4.223E−03
60	20.5900	33.6571	2.059E−02	3.190E−03
80	18.3700	37.7246	1.837E−02	2.597E−03
100	17.0700	40.5975	1.707E−02	2.546E−03
150	15.0500	46.0465	1.505E−02	2.764E−03
200	13.7000	50.5839	1.370E−02	2.967E−03

where gamma radiation from ^{99m}Tc (140 keV) and ^{131}I (364 keV) fall after the K edge and so less lead is required.

MEAN FREE PATH

The photon's mean free path, mfp, is the average distance that a photon travels in the absorber before undergoing an interaction:

$$mfp = \frac{1}{\mu} = \frac{1}{\frac{0.693}{HVL}} = 1.44 \times HVL \qquad (5.8)$$

5.3 PHOTON MASS ATTENUATION AND ABSORPTION COEFFICIENTS

The total mass attenuation coefficient is the fraction of radiation removed from the beam (gamma or X-radiation) of unit cross-sectional area in a medium of unit mass. The linear attenuation coefficient μ has units of m^{-1} (or the non-SI value cm^{-1}) whereas the mass attenuation coefficient μ/ρ has units of m^2 kg^{-1} (or the non-SI value cm^2 g^{-1}).

5.3.1 Mass attenuation coefficient μ/ρ

The probability of an interaction between an X-ray quantum and a medium containing N atoms per unit volume is proportional to N. However, since the density (ρ) of a substance is defined as the mass of a unit volume this is proportional to the number of atoms per unit volume. The total mass attenuation coefficient is the quotient of linear attenuation coefficient and material density μ/ρ and is the fraction of the X-rays removed from an X-ray beam of unit

Table 5.2 *Comparison of linear (μ) and mass attenuation coefficients (μ/ρ) at the same keV.*

State	μ (m^{-1})	ρ	μ/ρ (m^2 kg^{-1})
Ice	0.196	0.917	0.214
Water	0.214	1	0.214
Steam	1.2×10^{-4}	5.9×10^{-4}	0.214
Coefficient (at 150 keV)			
Muscle	0.0150	1.00	0.015
Fat	0.0135	0.91	0.015
Bone	0.0277	1.85	0.015

cross-sectional area in a medium of unit mass. The mass attenuation coefficient is independent of the state of the absorber. As an example, water exists in three states, gas (water vapor), liquid and solid (ice), each having three different densities so the linear attenuation coefficient will be different for each state. Since the mass attenuation coefficient removes density differences the value for μ/ρ for each state will be the same. This is shown in Table 5.2.

The linear attenuation coefficient is, however, retained in CT where the differences between physical states are important to separate pathology. The probability of an interaction leading to photon absorption depends on the atomic composition of the absorber and not its state such as density or chemical form. Because of this independence from density, mass attenuation coefficients are more generally used than are the linear values.

The attenuation characteristics of materials (μ) with reference to their density (ρ) in kg m^{-3} are calculated in Box 5.3 allowing comparison between μ and μ/ρ. Photoelectric and scatter each have their own coefficients as mass absorption coefficient and mass scatter coefficient and are combined in the mass attenuation coefficient μ/ρ.

Figure 5.9 plots the mass attenuation coefficient for bone, soft tissue and fat and when compared to the linear attenuation coefficient in Fig. 5.5 it can be seen that when density differences are eliminated attenuation differences are reduced.

The mass attenuation coefficient provides a means of comparing the stopping power of different materials independent of the state of the material; however, the linear attenuation coefficient is more useful in radiology where organ thickness rather than masses are considered.

Box 5.3 Attenuation characteristics of materials with reference to their densities

Comparing the units of the two attenuation coefficients μ and μ/ρ reveals the magnitude of the difference. μ has SI units of m^{-1} (or cm^{-1}); μ/ρ has SI units of m^2 kg^{-1} (or cm^2 g^{-1}).

Lead

The value of μ for a mono-energetic 100 keV photon beam attenuated by lead is approximately 6292 m^{-1} so the value of μ/ρ is obtained by dividing by the density of lead (11 340 kg m^3); the mass attenuation is therefore approximately 0.554 m^2 kg^{-1}.

Aluminum

Similarly, the μ for aluminum at 200 keV is 33.0 m^{-1}. With a density of 2700 kg m^3 the mass attenuation coefficient μ/ρ is 0.01223 m^2 kg^{-1}. Thus the mass attenuation coefficient for aluminum can be plotted alongside lead quite easily on the same semi-log paper whereas plotting μ on the same graph paper would be inconvenient.

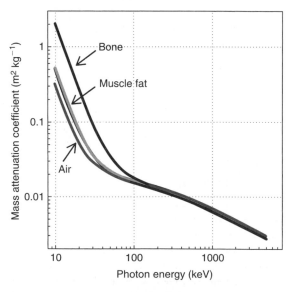

Figure 5.9 *Mass attenuation coefficients for soft tissues.*

5.3.2 Mass energy transfer coefficient μ_{tr}/ρ

In general the main attenuation mechanisms considered here (photoelectric μ_{en} and Compton (incoherent) scatter μ_{scat}) will be operating simultaneously with their probability depending on both photon energy and the atomic number of the absorber. Each process will follow an exponential law with a total attenuation coefficient equal to the sum of their constituent coefficients.

When examining local deposition of energy, the **mass energy transfer coefficient** (μ_{tr}/ρ) is used for diagnostic energies. The same photoelectric and scatter components apply but each must be modified to take into account the energy removed from the primary photon beam but deposited away from the immediate vicinity by penetrating secondary photons (see Fig. 5.10). This includes the average energy emitted as fluorescent (characteristic) radiation when a primary photon undergoes photoelectric absorption. This fraction is assumed lost from the immediate vicinity of the point of primary interaction. However, in soft tissue, at diagnostic photon energies, the characteristic radiation is only a few electron volts, and is easily absorbed.

The mass energy transfer coefficient (μ_{tr}/ρ) represents the energy transferred from the incident photons (X- or gamma radiation) to charged particles in the absorber. The mass energy transfer coefficient can be seen as the escape of secondary photon interactions at the initial photon/atom interaction site. For diagnostic X-ray energies (photon energies below 200 kV) the definition is

$$\frac{\mu_{tr}}{\rho} = f_{pe} + f_{scat} \qquad (5.9)$$

where f_{pe} and f_{scat} represent the average fractions of the photon energy that is transferred to the kinetic energy of the charged particles (electrons) from the photoelectric (characteristic X-rays) and the Compton scattered photon. For the diagnostic energy range the contribution from pair and triplet production is ignored.

5.3.3 Mass energy absorption coefficient μ_{en}/ρ

Charged particles (electrons) from photoelectric and scattering events travel through the absorber and create Bremsstrahlung. The mass transfer coefficient is related as

$$\frac{\mu_{en}}{\rho} = (1 - g)^{\mu_{tr}/\rho} \qquad (5.10)$$

where g represents the average fraction of kinetic energy of secondary charged particles (electrons) produced in photoelectric and Compton interactions and subsequently lost in radiative processes (Bremsstrahlung). In practice since g in eqn 5.10 is very nearly zero at diagnostic energies then

$$\frac{\mu_{en}}{\rho} = \frac{\mu_{tr}}{\rho}$$

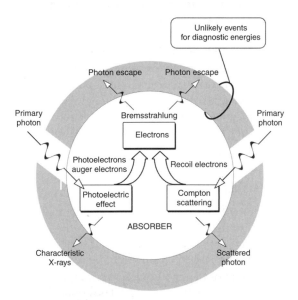

Figure 5.10 *Primary photon interactions showing the components of energy loss with photoelectric effect and Compton scattering. Characteristic (fluorescent) X-rays, Bremsstrahlung and scattered photons from the Compton events (outer area) are very low energy so rarely escape from the point of interaction.*

5.4 INTERACTIONS WITH THE ATOM

The interaction at the atomic level involves collisions with the electrons and nuclei of individual atoms which depend on material density and photon energy. Interactions with the atomic nucleus do not occur at photon energies used in diagnostic imaging so will only be mentioned briefly.

Table 5.3 *The principal K- and L-shell binding energies for elements important to radiology.*

Z	Element	K shell	L shell
6	Carbon	283 eV	Low
7	Nitrogen	409 eV	37 eV
8	Oxygen	542 eV	41 eV
13	Aluminum	1.56 keV	117 eV
15	Phosphorus	2 keV	190 eV
20	Calcium	4 keV	438 eV
29	Copper	8.9 keV	1.1 keV
42	Molybdenum	20.0 keV	2.8 keV
47	Silver	25.5 keV	3.8 keV
50	Tin	29.1 keV	4.4 keV
53	Iodine	33 keV	5 keV
56	Barium	37 keV	6 keV
57	Lanthanum	39.0 keV	62 keV
64	Gadolinium	50.2 keV	8.4 keV
74	Tungsten	69.5 keV	12.0 keV
82	Lead	88 keV	16 keV

ELECTRON INTERACTIONS

The terms 'free' and 'bound' electrons are used when describing photon interactions. Strictly speaking all electrons are held in orbits around a particular nucleus (ignoring conduction electrons in crystalline materials). When describing photon interactions an electron can be considered free when its binding energy is very small compared to the energy of the incident photon. For example, while the M- and N-shell electrons in lead with binding energies of 3.0 and 0.25 eV may be treated as **free**, compared to X-ray diagnostic energies of 60 to 100 keV, the K-shell electrons with a binding energy of 88 keV are certainly **bound**.

Table 5.3 lists some important elements to radiology and their principal K- and L-shell binding energies. For practical purposes the orbital electrons in low Z tissue elements (carbon, nitrogen, and oxygen) that have very small binding energies above the K shell may be regarded as 'free' for the diagnostic X-ray energy range. In higher Z elements (calcium, barium, iodine) the K and L shells are treated as 'bound' and the orbitals above M are 'free' with respect to the X-ray photon energy.

NUCLEAR INTERACTIONS

If the photon energy exceeds 1.022 MeV then nuclear interactions can take place with the formation of a positron and negatron (electron): this is pair

formation. The positron forms a 'positronium' ion with a free electron which then rapidly undergoes mutual annihilation leaving two 0.511 MeV gamma photons. X-ray photon energies do not reach this energy level in diagnostic imaging so pair formation will not be covered further. Positron decay does concern diagnostic imaging, however, and this will be covered in Chapters 15 and 16.

5.4.1 Photoelectric effect

In order to visualize interaction of the X- or gamma radiation with the absorber atoms it is more convenient to consider the particulate **quantum** or **photon** rather than a wave. Each quantum of electromagnetic radiation or **photon** has an energy proportional to its frequency. The constant of proportionality $h = 6.626 \times 10^{-34}$ J Hz^{-1} (or 4.136×10^{-15} eV Hz^{-1}) is **Planck's constant**. The energy of a photon of frequency f is:

$$E = hf \qquad (5.11)$$

The photoelectric reaction plays a very important role in radiology and is encountered in the imaging process and radiation dosimetry. The phenomenon was first studied by Albert Einstein (1879–1955; German/US physicist) who, in 1905, received the Nobel Prize for his work on the photoelectric interactions between light of various wavelengths and metal surfaces which illustrated the particulate (quantum or **photon**) nature of electromagnetic radiation. Although this original work concerned visible light the photoelectric effect in radiology concerns higher energy electromagnetic radiation which is X- and gamma rays.

PHOTOELECTRIC ABSORPTION

For photoelectric absorption the incident photon loses all its energy, with essentially all of it going to one of the orbital electrons, Fig. 5.11. The electron involved will be ejected from the atom with an energy equal to that of the photon, less the energy required to free the electron from its orbital position. The very small amount of energy taken by the recoiling atom is usually neglected. Figure 5.11 shows an interaction by the X-ray photon, of sufficient energy, with the K-shell electron. The photon interacts by transferring all its energy to this K-shell electron which is ejected from the atom as a photoelectron. The kinetic energy

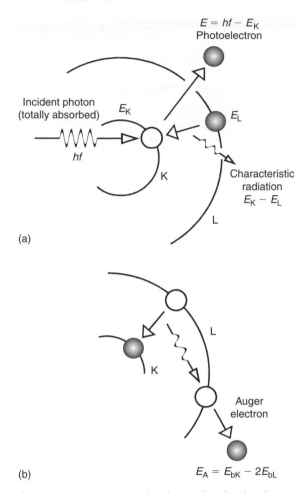

$E = hf - E_K$
Photoelectron

Incident photon
(totally absorbed)

E_K

hf

E_L

K

Characteristic
radiation
$E_K - E_L$

L

(a)

L

K

Auger
electron

(b)

$E_A = E_{bK} - 2E_{bL}$

Figure 5.11 *(a) The photoelectric reaction showing the incident photon ejecting a K-shell electron, which then becomes a photoelectron. The photon energy is entirely absorbed. (b) An Auger electron can be formed instead of characteristic radiation emission. The energy is transferred to and ejecting an L electron.*

of the photoelectron E equals the photon energy hf minus the binding energy of the K or L electron E_B so

$$E = hf - E_B \qquad (5.12)$$

For diagnostic energies the range of the electron is much less than the mean free path of a photon of equal energy. The ejected photoelectron will then expend its energy close to its place of origin, and therefore energy imparted to this electron is energy truly given up to the absorber (radiation dose). The empty K shell is filled by an electron from one of the outer

orbits (L or M). This electron transfer gives a **characteristic X-ray** or an **Auger electron**. Excess photon energy is added to the kinetic energy of the electron.

$$hf = E_B + \frac{1}{2} mv^2 \qquad (5.13)$$

where $\frac{1}{2} mv^2$ is the excess kinetic energy taken up by the electron. The more tightly bound electrons of the atom are the major ones concerned with PE absorption and the most important electron orbit is the K shell. Maximum absorption occurs when the photon equals the K-electron binding energy. This gives rise to the steep K edge in the absorption curves of Fig. 5.12. A list of important K-edge energies is given in Table 5.3. For a photon energy of 100 keV reacting with the K electron of lead which has a binding energy (E_K) of 88 keV the photoelectron energy would be 100 − 88 ($hf − E_K$) or 12 keV. Reacting with the L electron ($E_L = 15$ keV) the photoelectron will have an energy of 85 keV.

The probability of the photoelectric effect increases the closer the energy of the incident photon matches that of the electron. The probability of the photoelectric interaction is directly proportional to the cube of the atomic number (i.e. Z^3) and inversely proportional to the cube of the photon energy $1/E^3$. The overall probability is described as Z^3/E^3. The probability of an interaction between a 30 keV photon and bone (calcium) is $13.8^3/30^3 = 0.097$ while that for soft tissue (where $Z \equiv 7.4$) is $7.4^3/30^3 = 0.015$ therefore photoelectric absorption is nearly ×7 more likely for bone.

The photoelectron energy is absorbed by surrounding atoms. This is the major contribution to radiation dose in tissue. The vacancy or 'hole' left in the orbit is rapidly filled by an electron from a higher (less energy) orbit leading to an electron cascade as these higher orbit vacancies are filled. It is possible to lose energy from this reaction if the characteristic radiation is able to escape; however, for soft tissues this photon energy is so low that it is absorbed.

It is not possible for a photon to give all its energy to a valency or 'free' electron since this process is not able to satisfy both conservation of energy and momentum together. This only happens with tightly bound electrons since the whole atom undergoes recoil enabling the reaction to comply with the conservation of momentum. Figure 5.11a shows the vacated orbit reoccupied by an electron from the adjacent orbit (i.e. L, M, N etc.) at the same time emitting excess energy as characteristic radiation.

In summary, the characteristics of the photoelectric reaction are:

- The photoelectric event is greatest when the photon energy matches the electron binding energy.
- The probability decreases with increase in photon energy as $1/E^3$ and increases with atomic number as Z^3.
- The photoelectric effect (PE) contributes very strongly to attenuation at the lower diagnostic energies.

The PE effect depends on the atomic number Z of the attenuating material; photons whose energy is less than the binding energy will not be absorbed. The probability of a PE reaction increases significantly as the energy of the incident photon approaches the binding energy of the electrons in a shell. Iodine, barium, and rare earth intensifying screens (gadolinium and lanthanum) have K-shell binding energies that are in the diagnostic range to give optimum absorption.

CHARACTERISTIC RADIATION OR FLUORESCENT RADIATION

The photoelectric event shown in Fig. 5.11a results in an electron vacancy which is rapidly filled by a neighboring electron from (in this case) the L-shell emitting radiation in the process, the energy being

$$hf = E_K - E_L \qquad (5.14)$$

The vacancy in the L shell is similarly filled giving an electron cascade producing an emission spectrum of characteristic radiation. The process is exactly the same as in X-ray emission but now the secondary photons are called **fluorescent radiation** because they are excited by a primary photon instead of a bombarding electron. The **fluorescent radiation** that follows photon absorption is nearly a mono-energetic source of X-rays compared to electron bombardment of a target. In the latter case of electron bombardment of tungsten the Bremsstrahlung X-ray production is also accompanied by emission of the same characteristic energies (see the characteristic X-ray peaks in Fig. 5.18, page 131).

The number of characteristic photons is dependent on the number of electron shell vacancies. This is calculated for tungsten in Box 5.4. In the case of a high atomic number absorber the **electron binding energy** is large (88 keV for lead) and the fluorescent radiation is quite penetrating and gives up its energy far from its

Box 5.4 Characteristic radiation and Auger emission

Binding energy for tungsten

K shell	69.5 keV
L shell	12.0 keV
M shell	1.8 keV

Characteristic radiation

The sum of transitions, L to K, M to L etc. is

$$69.5 - 12 = 57.5$$
$$12 - 1.8 = 0.2$$
$$1.8 - 0 = 1.8$$

The total energy is therefore 69.5 keV.

Auger electron energy

From eqn 5.15

$$E_A = E_{bK} - 2E_{bL}$$
$$= 69.5 - 2 \times 12$$
$$= 45.5 \text{ keV}$$

point of origin. Living tissues however are mostly composed of low-Z elements and the **electron binding energy** will be less than 1 keV so these very soft fluorescent radiations will be absorbed very close to the point of emission. The general trend is a rapid increase in photoelectric absorption with atomic number and a rapid decrease as photon energy increases.

AUGER ELECTRONS

(P. Auger, 1899–1993; French physicist) After a photoelectric reaction there is a vacancy in the K shell which is normally filled by an L → K transition with the emission of a K-characteristic X-ray. Alternatively, the energy involved in this transition may be transferred to one of the outer more loosely bound orbitals and these electrons will be ejected from their orbits as Auger electrons. This is a radiationless transition where the characteristic X-ray from the K shell, produced during the photoelectric effect, is energetic enough to eject an electron from the L shell. Figure 5.11b shows that two vacancies are created in the L shell. The kinetic energy of an Auger electron is calculated as

$$E_A = E_{bK} - 2E_{bL} \qquad (5.15)$$

where E_A is the energy of the Auger electron, E_{bK} the binding energy of the inner K shell, and E_{bL} the binding energy of the outer L shell. The binding energy E_{bL} is represented twice in eqn 5.15, once for the transition energy and once to represent the ejected L-shell electron. After an Auger event all the empty orbits will be filled to end the process. Auger events are an important consideration in radiology since they add to tissue dose. The photoelectron is quickly brought to rest by the surrounding atoms of the absorber and its energy is given to them along with energy from any Auger electrons. The Auger electron has more energy than the photoelectron for diagnostic energies in heavy elements (tungsten, lead, etc.); however, soft tissues have binding energies ranging from 0.28 to 0.53 keV (carbon, nitrogen, and oxygen) so the photoelectron would approximate to the incident photon energy.

ABSORPTION EDGES (K EDGE)

Figure 5.12 illustrates the attenuation coefficient in a lead absorber over the region where the energy of the incident photons may be equal to the binding energy of one of the orbital electrons. As the photon energy increases, the absorption coefficient, primarily due to photoelectric interactions, decreases until an abrupt increase in absorption occurs at about 13.0 keV. As the photon energy continues to increase, other sharp breaks appear at 15.2 and 15.9 keV. These signify resonance with the L-shell orbital electrons. The absorption coefficient then continues to decrease smoothly until a final discontinuity is seen at 88 keV. Here resonance between the photon energy and the K-shell electron binding energy removes a significant proportion of the photons seen as a sharp increase in absorption on the curve, which is the **K edge**.

The abrupt increases are due to resonant absorption when the energy of the incoming photon equals the energy required to free a particular orbital electron from its nucleus. A photon with less energy is unable to achieve this. The energies where this abrupt absorption happens are called **absorption edges**. The three low-energy edges seen for lead, in Fig. 5.12, are due to ejection of electrons from sublevels in the L-shell orbit. The single edge at 88 keV comes from the removal of a K electron, the nearest orbit to the nucleus. M, N, and still higher-order edges from

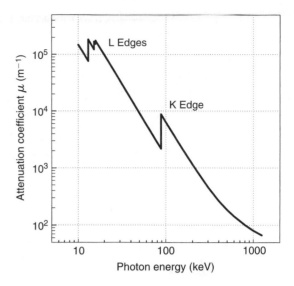

Figure 5.12 *Relative energies of the absorption edges and characteristic emission lines of lead.*

orbits more distant from the nucleus exist but they occur at very low energies where detection is difficult. Characteristic X-ray emission energies involving any particular electron are always less than the absorption edge energy. A characteristic X-ray photon is emitted when an electron drops from one bound state to another. In Fig. 5.12 the edge at 88 keV represents an ejection from the K shell. The Kα emission lines at 73 to 75 keV are the result of L to K transitions, the Kβ lines are from M to K transitions, and so on. These energy bands are unique for the element and can be used for non-destructive elemental analysis. Any orbital vacancy created by photon absorption will be subsequently filled from outer orbits, just as in the case of the generation of characteristic X-rays following electron impact.

For K electrons the absorption can increase by more than ×5. L-shell electrons also show absorption edges as seen in Fig. 5.13. The element tin, on a weight for weight basis, is a better absorber between the energies 29 to 88 keV despite having a lower atomic number (for Sn, $Z = 34$; for Pb, $Z = 88$). This would suggest that tin is a better shielding material than lead at diagnostic energies, but cost must be taken into consideration. Important elements whose K edges appear within the diagnostic energy range are:

- X-ray filters (e.g. molybdenum, rhodium, erbium)
- Intensifying screen materials (e.g. tungsten, gadolinium)

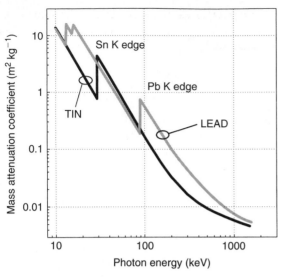

Figure 5.13 *Mass attenuation coefficient for lead and tin over the diagnostic energies. There is greater absorption for tin over the range 30 to 88 keV due to its K edge.*

- Scintillation detectors (iodine, cesium)
- Contrast enhancing agents (barium, iodine)

5.4.2 Radiation scattering

The general picture of attenuation in Fig. 5.1 shows another process as well as absorption which can be responsible for preventing photons from reaching a target area (image receptor plane such as film). This is photon scattering and mostly involves electrons in the outer orbits. The scattered photon can assume any angle from >0° to 180°.

COHERENT OR ELASTIC SCATTERING

When an X-ray or gamma photon is incident on an atom then scattering can take place either:

- From the bound electrons (Rayleigh scattering:) providing that the electrons do not receive sufficient energy to eject them from the atom
- From free or loosely bound electrons (Thomson scattering)

They are both examples of coherent or elastic scattering, in which the incident photon undergoes a change in direction without a change in energy. This is the only type of interaction between X-rays and matter in which no energy is transferred and no ionization of the target atom occurs. The diagram in Fig. 5.14a illustrates this.

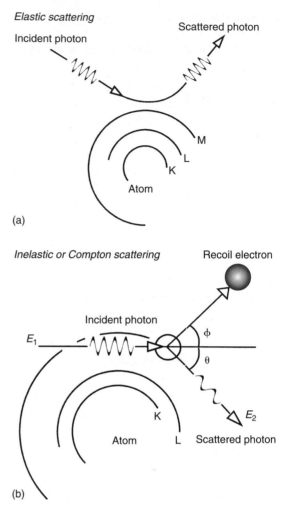

(a)

(b)

Figure 5.14 *(a) Elastic or coherent scattering involving the atom as a whole. (b) The Compton event showing the incident photon sharing its energy between the recoil electron and scattered photon.*

RAYLEIGH SCATTERING

Rayleigh scattering (Lord Rayleigh, 1842–1919; UK physicist) involves the interaction of a photon with closely bound electrons. The photon causes resonance with the electron and as the photon passes in a close proximity to the atom it causes the bound electrons to vibrate or excite, removing energy from the beam; the atom recoils, scattering the photon in the forward direction with very little energy loss. There is negligible photon attenuation and this scattering occurs with low energy incident radiation and with high atomic number absorber materials where the number of bound electrons is greatest. The probability is proportional to Z^2/E. As photon energy increases Rayleigh scattering is gradually replaced by inelastic or Compton scattering when electrons are removed from their bound states.

THOMSON SCATTERING

Thomson scattering (J.J. Thomson, 1856–1940; UK physicist) can occur when the incident photon interacts with a free electron and radiation of a lower energy is emitted in all directions. It is independent of incident photon energy. Only about 10% of interactions involve elastic scattering, both Rayleigh and Thomson, in diagnostic radiology.

COMPTON (INELASTIC) SCATTERING

This occurs if the incident photon interacts with an outer or unbound orbital electron shown in Fig. 5.14b. The electron has a binding energy which is negligibly small when compared with the photon energy. All electrons in soft tissue can be considered to be free electrons and in calcium (bone), all but the two K-shell electrons can be considered as free (18 out of 20 electrons per atom). Material electron density (in electrons per gram) can be calculated from the formula:

$$N \times \frac{Z}{A} \qquad (5.16)$$

where N is Avogadro's number (6.023×10^{23}), Z the atomic number (proton number) and A the atomic mass.

Material density ρ describes the packing density of atoms in a material. A Compton event depends on the probability of the photon encountering an electron. This can be estimated as the number of electrons per cm^3 which is the product of the density and the number of electrons per gram. The number of electrons per cm^3 is the product of density and number per gram so:

$$\text{electrons per cm}^3 = \text{density (g cm}^{-3}) \\ \times \text{electrons per g} \qquad (5.17)$$

Absorber material characteristics such as atomic number do not enter into the Compton equation since the **probability** of Compton interactions increases with the **electron density** of material. It is practically independent of atomic number Z. The probability for Compton scatter decreases slightly over the diagnostic energy range but it is much less than the decrease for the photoelectric effect. The probability of a Compton interaction is influenced strongly by electron density and to a certain extent by energy following the relationship:

$$\frac{\text{electron density}}{E} \qquad (5.18)$$

Scatter is dependent on the number of free electrons per unit volume and Table 5.4 lists the atomic number, atomic mass and electron densities of some important substances and tissues calculated from eqn 5.17. The number of electrons per gram shows a difference between dense materials (bone, lead etc.) and less dense materials (water, soft tissue). The greatest electron density is given by hydrogen (6×10^{23} electrons per gram) so substances containing a lot of hydrogen will have more electrons and cause greater scatter (i.e. water, soft tissues).

PHOTON ENERGY LOSS

The Compton process can be understood by considering the photon as a particle (quantum) with energy hf.

Table 5.4 *The electron densities of important materials in radiology.*

Element	Z_{eff}	A	Electrons g^{-1} ($\times 10^{23}$)	Density	Ratio, Z:A	Electrons cm^{-3}
Air	7.6	15.3	3.01	0.00129	0.49	3.80×10^{20}
Water	7.4	13.7	3.34	1	0.54	3.34×10^{23}
Muscle	7.5	14.5	3.36	1	0.51	3.36×10^{23}
Fat	5.9	10.2	3.48	0.91	0.57	3.16×10^{23}
Bone	13.8	27.7	3.00	1.85	0.49	5.55×10^{23}
Iodine	53.0	127.0	2.51	4.9	0.41	12.3×10^{23}
Barium	56.0	137.0	2.46	3.51	0.40	8.60×10^{23}
Lead	82.0	208.0	2.37	11.3	0.39	26.7×10^{23}

The momentum (mass × velocity) of a photon is mc moving at the velocity of light, so

$$mc = \frac{hf}{c} \qquad (5.19)$$

The incident photon collides with an outer valency electron with energy E_1 and momentum hf/c. The electron recoils accepting a fraction of the photon energy. The geometry involved is shown in Fig. 5.14b where the electron is scattered at an angle ϕ having gained kinetic energy from the incident photon. The scattered photon E_2 emerges at angle θ with a lower energy than the incident photon E_1. Conservation of energy and momentum yields the classic Compton equation that describes the **photon wavelength** shift:

$$\lambda_2 - \lambda_1 = \frac{h}{mc} \times (1 - \cos\theta) \qquad (5.20)$$

The constant h/mc is the Compton wavelength and can be expressed in terms of **photon energy** instead of wavelength by substituting the rest mass of the electron m (0.511 MeV). Eqn 5.20 then becomes

$$\frac{1}{E_2} - \frac{1}{E_1} = \frac{1}{511} \times (1 - \cos\theta) \qquad (5.21)$$

Rearranging gives

$$E_2 = \frac{1}{1 + \left(\frac{E_1}{0.511}\right) - (1 - \cos\theta)} \qquad (5.22)$$

In contrast, the difference in wavelength $\lambda_2 - \lambda_1$ described in eqn 5.20 depends upon h, m, c and the angle θ. Wavelength of the incident X-ray beam does not play a part, so, unlike energy, Compton scatter is independent of the incident wavelength, only the **wavelength difference** plays a role. It can be seen from eqns 5.21 and 5.22 that energy division between the Compton electron and the scattered photon depends on the incident photon energy E_1. At low energy the scattered photon retains a large fraction of the available energy; at higher energies there is a larger energy loss for the same scattering angle; the recoil electron receives an increased fraction. Figure 5.15a identifies the overall scattering coefficient and the energy shared between the scattered photon and electron.

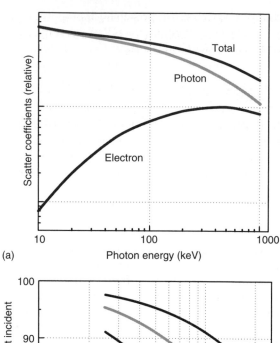

(a)

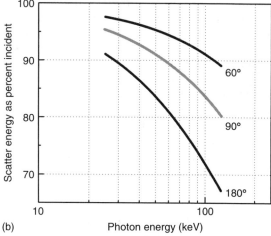

(b)

Figure 5.15 *(a) The proportion of incident energy shared between scattered photon (mass scattering coefficient) and electron (mass absorption coefficient) making up the total attenuation. (b) The energy of the scattered photon as a percentage of the incident energy for the diagnostic photon energy range for 60°, 90°, and 120° scatter angles.*

THE MASS ABSORPTION COEFFICIENT

This determines the fraction of energy absorbed per unit mass and is defined as the fraction of beam energy absorbed per unit mass of absorber. It represents the average energy transferred to the electron. The higher the energy of the photon the greater the energy loss of the scattered photon and increasing energy of the recoil electron as shown in Fig. 5.15a. From this graph the mass attenuation coefficient (total event) decreases with photon energy but the mass absorption coefficient (electron energy) increases with energy up to about 1 MeV.

THE MASS SCATTERING COEFFICIENT

This is a measure of the average fraction of total beam energy remaining after a scatter event and from Fig. 5.15a this photon component is seen to decrease with energy. Curves for the mass absorption coefficient and mass scattering coefficient cross at about 1.5 MeV.

SCATTER ANGLE

Figure 5.15b plots energy loss for scattering angles 60°, 90°, and 180° over the diagnostic energy range showing greater energy loss for the scattered photon with increased photon energy and scatter angle. Calculations are given in Box 5.5.

SCATTER DIRECTION

The direction of the scattered radiation also depends on the energy of the incident beam. The proportions are exaggerated in Fig. 5.16 but show that as the photon energy increases a forward angle of scatter is favored. The length of the radius indicates the probability of a photon being scattered in that direction and a forward angle is slightly favored in the diagnostic range as energy increases. The larger the angle of scatter the greater loss of photon energy to the electron, so the scattered photon will have a low energy. At low scatter angles (forward scatter) a greater proportion of the photon energy is retained. Scattered photons degrade image quality since they do not represent attenuating values in the path of the beam.

5.4.3 Pair formation

INTERACTION WITH THE NUCLEUS

If the photon energy equals or exceeds 1.022 MeV then it has sufficient energy to overcome nuclear electrostatic forces and the photon can be absorbed resulting in the formation of two particles of equal mass, a **positron** and an **electron**; this is **pair formation**. This pair formation event has only academic interest in diagnostic imaging since photon energies approaching 1 MeV are rarely used.

Box 5.5 Compton scatter energy loss

Referring to Fig. 5.15, calculate the percentage energy loss at a scatter angle of 60° for a 30 keV and 100 keV photon. The basic equation (eqn 5.15) is

$$E' = \frac{E}{\left[1 + \left(\frac{E}{511}\right) \times (1 - \cos\theta)\right]}$$

For 30 keV the scattered photon energy is

$$\frac{30}{\left[1 + \left(\frac{30}{511}\right) \times (1 - 0.5)\right]} = 29\,\text{keV} \quad (97\%)$$

For 100 keV the scattered photon energy is

$$\frac{100}{\left[1 + \left(\frac{100}{511}\right) \times (1 - 0.5)\right]} = 91\,\text{keV} \quad (91\%)$$

Conclusion. Higher energy photons lose more energy to the recoil electron during Compton interactions (Fig. 5.15a and b).

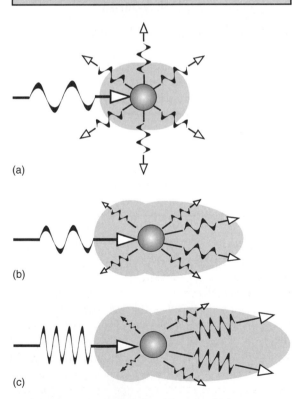

(a)

(b)

(c)

Figure 5.16 *Scatter direction with energy (**a**) low energy (20 to 30 keV) (**b**) medium energy (50 to 80 keV) (**c**) high energy (>100 keV).*

POSITRON EMISSION TOMOGRAPHY

Positron emission tomography is an example where a radionuclide decays by positron emission $(\beta+)$ which then undergoes annihilation with a free electron. This can be treated as the complementary event to pair formation: energy converted to mass (X-ray photon producing positron and electron) or mass converted to energy (positron/electron undergoing annihilation to gamma radiation energy); these events are an excellent illustration of Einstein's famous formula $E = mc^2$ detailed in Box 5.6.

5.4.4 Overall effects

The linear attenuation coefficient for a particular tissue at a particular energy is a measure of the ability of that tissue to remove photons from a beam of X-rays. The removal is due to the processes of:

- Photoelectric absorption; absorption coefficient
- Scattering (both coherent and Compton) and Compton attenuation coefficient

The linear attenuation coefficient μ is the sum of the photoelectric absorption coefficient (τ), the scatter coefficient (σ). Where appropriate the pair production coefficient (π) should be included but this is rarely experienced in diagnostic radiology and so is omitted here. The overall value μ_{tot} represents a combination

of all three processes: $\mu_{tot} = \mu_\tau + \mu_\sigma$. Where μ_τ and μ_σ are the relevant attenuation coefficients: μ_σ is shared between coherent and Compton scatter.

The graphs in Fig. 5.17 show the percentage contributions to μ for soft tissue and bone for each process over the diagnostic energy range. As the photon energy increases the relative importance of the PE decreases and the curve flattens. The probability of a Compton interaction is small but its relative importance as an

---

Box 5.6 Calculation for mass–energy relationship

Rest mass of electron/positron $= 9.1 \times 10^{-31}$ kg

Total mass $m = 1.82 \times 10^{-30}$ kg
Speed of light $c = 3 \times 10^8$ m s^{-1}

$$c^2 = 9 \times 10^{16} \text{m s}^{-1}$$
$$E = mc^2 = (1.82 \times 10^{-30}) \times (9 \times 10^{16}) \text{ J}$$
$$= 1.63 \times 10^{-13} \text{J}$$

Since $1\,\text{J} = 6.24 \times 10^{18}$ eV then energy can be expressed as $(1.63 \times 10^{-13}) \times (6.24 \times 10^{18})$ eV $= 1.022$ MeV.

This appears as two 180° opposed gamma photons having 0.511 MeV each.

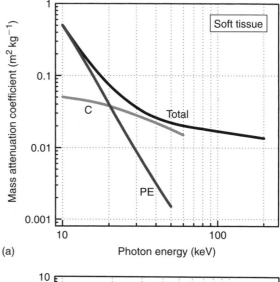

(a)

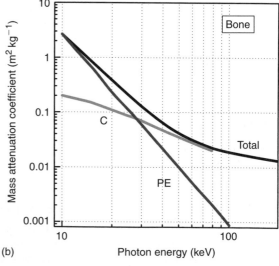

(b)

Figure 5.17 (a) The mass attenuation curves for soft tissue and (b) bone. The photoelectric and Compton components (PE and C respectively) make up the total attenuation process.

attenuating process increases as that of the photo-electric process decreases with energy.

The contribution of coherent scattering to the attenuation process is very small and relatively constant over the diagnostic range. Table 5.5 summarizes the important points associated with photon interactions with the atom in diagnostic imaging.

5.5 HETEROGENEOUS (POLY-ENERGETIC) X-RAY PHOTON BEAMS

In practice X-ray photon beams are not mono-energetic. Poly-energetic beams are inevitable from X-ray tubes since the Bremsstrahlung spectrum shows a continuous distribution from zero up to the maximum energy of the exciting electrons. Any external X-ray beam will be subject to some inherent filtration as it passes through the tube window and perhaps other materials such as cooling oil. Inherent filtration can be reduced by making the window as thin as possible and by using a material of low atomic number to reduce photoelectric absorption. Beryllium is the material of choice for low-absorption windows, stainless steel or titanium are used in diagnostic tubes. The low energy photons of 'soft energy' components of an X-ray beam are undesirable and filters are placed in the beam to remove them. Soft tissue and bone additionally remove the low-energy spectrum components and thus harden the beam further. Figure 5.18 shows two X-ray spectra, before (A) and after (B) entering a patient's body. The added filtration to the

beam in (A) restricts low energy photon energies to about 20 keV. After passing through the patient's body these low energy photons are removed increasing the lower end of the spectrum to about 30 keV.

The amount and type of added filtration introduced for beam hardening depends on the nature of the primary beam and the amount of hardening desired. For a beam of about $200\,kV_p$, as found in

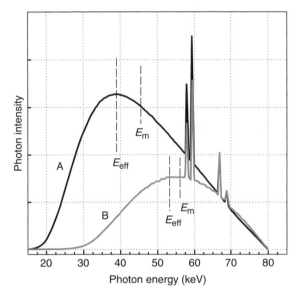

Figure 5.18 *Entrance (**A**) and exit (**B**) 80 kV$_p$ X-ray spectra showing mean photon energy (E$_m$) and an effective energy (E$_{eff}$); the latter is estimated from the HVLs and the graph in Fig. 5.19.*

Table 5.5 *Summary of photon interactions with the atom in diagnostic radiology.*

Interaction	Factors	Process
Photon absorption Photoelectric	$\tau \propto \dfrac{Z^3}{E^3}$	Photon interacts with bound electron. Electron ejected. Orbital vacancy filled producing characteristic radiation or Auger electron
Photon scattering Compton, Inelastic, incoherent	$\sigma \propto \dfrac{electron\ density}{E}$	Photon interacts with free electron. Energy shared between electron and scattered photon. Percentage energy loss increases with energy and scatter angle.
Rayleigh/Thomson, Elastic, coherent	$\mu_e \propto \dfrac{Z^2}{E}$	No absorption or energy loss. Interaction involves free electron or entire atom. Constitutes about 10% of reactions at diagnostic energies.

computed tomography (CT), the added filtration commonly consists of 0.2 to 0.5 mm of copper followed by 0.2 to 0.5 mm of aluminum and perhaps 1 to 3 mm of carbon in the form of dense plastic.

The copper filter will harden the beam by its strong photoelectric absorption of low energy photons. At the same time a strong copper **fluorescent radiation** will be produced by the absorption of photons at energies above the copper absorption edges. The copper fluorescent emissions will be absorbed in the aluminum, whose still lower-energy fluorescent emissions will be absorbed by the carbon. Carbon fluorescence occurs at such a low energy that it will be strongly absorbed even in air. The absorber sequence Cu–Al–C is important, since any reversal of the filter order will reduce the effectiveness of the combination.

EFFECTIVE BEAM ENERGY

The linear attenuation coefficient μ is a general term describing attenuation of a collimated beam of X- or gamma rays passing through an absorbing medium due to both absorption and scattering. In order to simplify attenuation calculations a mono-energetic beam is commonly used; however X-rays are poly-energetic so an **effective beam energy** is assumed. This would approximate to any answer obtained by integration over the entire X-ray spectrum being studied. The effective energy of an X-ray beam can be determined by comparing the measured HVL value with values obtained from mono-energetic beams.

Figure 5.19 shows the HVL for aluminum plotted over the range 10 to 400 keV. The HVL value for a standard kV_p is carefully measured (usually using 80 kV_p for a conventional unit or 30 kV_p for mammography). The HVL result, obtained from these X-ray spectra, is identified on the y-axis of this graph and the effective beam energy read off from the x-axis.

Although effective energy is a useful specification of beam quality, its limitations must be clearly understood. Two beams with equal values of HVL are equal only in terms of the absorption measurements used in making the HVL determinations. Two hetero-energetic beams with identical values of HVL may have quite different spectral distributions and may be unequally effective in a particular application.

The effective energy (E_{eff}) and mean energy (E_m) are identified in Fig. 5.18, where two X-ray spectra (A) and (B) are shown; the entrance (A) and exit (B)

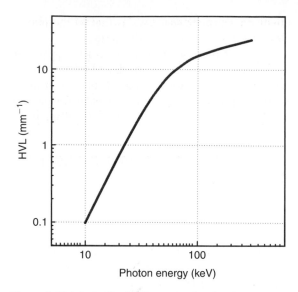

Figure 5.19 *The half-value layer plot for aluminum over the diagnostic photon energy range. This graph can be used to estimate the effective energy of an X-ray beam.*

spectra from a patient study. The HVL for (A) is measured as 3.6 mm Al and for (B) as 7.2 mm Al. From the graph in Fig. 5.19 the HVL values give an E_{eff} of 35 and 50 keV respectively. The calculated mean energies are 46 and 56 keV, respectively. The peak kV of 80 keV is unaltered.

BEAM QUALITY

The spectral distribution or beam quality produced by an X-ray tube is complex and not easy to determine with precision. An approximation of beam quality can be specified by quoting the peak voltage at which the radiation was generated, kV_p, and the half-value layer (HVL), of the useful beam after it has passed through any prior filtration. The HVL is obtained using absorbers appropriate to the beam energy (commonly aluminum) then constructing an attenuation curve (Fig. 5.4) or calculated from the formula in eqn 5.7. The absorbing materials commonly used for HVL measurements in diagnostic radiology for X-ray filtration (Al, Cu) and X-ray shielding (Pb) are given in Table 5.6.

HOMOGENEITY AND BEAM HARDENING

Attenuation of a mono-energetic beam of photons (gamma radiation) follows simple rules but a

Table 5.6 *Recommended filters for determinations of the half-value layer.*

Element	K edge (keV)	Useful range (keV)
Aluminum	1.6	50–150
Copper	8.9	200–400
Lead	88.0	400–upward

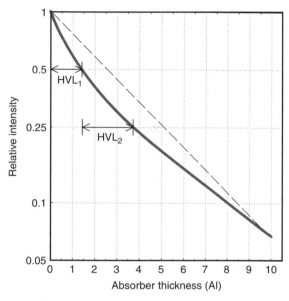

Figure 5.20 *A poly-energetic absorption curve (gray line) for determining homogeneity coefficient. The dotted line represents absorption given by a mono-energetic beam.*

poly-energetic X-ray beam loses lower energies more quickly than the higher ones. Although there is an overall reduction in the number of photons the average energy is higher than that of the incident beam. The beam is 'harder' and the attenuation coefficient will now be smaller. The graph in Fig. 5.20 shows the nonlinear change in photon absorption with absorber thickness, where two values of HVL (1 and 2) can be obtained. The addition of absorbers for making an HVL determination will harden the beam by an amount which depends on its spectral distribution. A useful measure of this distribution is obtained by continuing the absorption measurements and comparing the second HVL_2 with the first HVL_1, so a homogeneity coefficient can be defined as

$$\frac{HVL_1}{HVL_2} \qquad (5.23)$$

A value of 0.8 or more, from eqn 5.23, denotes a homogeneous beam; poor beam homogeneity would give values of about 0.6 to 0.7.

ATTENUATION BY PATIENT

The X-ray beam undergoes further filtration by the patient tissue mass, hardening the beam still further. The exit beam emanating from the patient is therefore different from the entrance beam. Low energy X-rays are removed by the patient's tissue without contributing to the image formation. These unnecessarily contribute to patient dose. The low energy photons are removed from the exit spectrum shown in Fig. 5.18.

PATIENT SIMULATION

For many dose measurements a patient phantom can be substituted for the real thing. Simple body phantoms can be either 30 cm diameter water filled plastic containers, solid PMMA cylinders of the same dimension or, when taking rough measurements, a 1 mm sheet of copper is an acceptable substitute.

5.6 SUBJECT CONTRAST

Differential attenuation of photons in body tissue produces **subject contrast** which is directly responsible for the image information. The factors which affect the individual attenuation coefficients (for photoelectric, μ_{pe}, and scatter, μ_{scat}) in $\mu_{tot} = \mu_{pe} + \mu_{scat}$ will influence beam penetration. All the processes included in the equation lead to the attenuation of radiation as it passes through matter. Only some of the reactions lead to total or partial absorption of radiation. Low energy photons are readily absorbed in the top layers of soft tissue, so they do not contribute to image formation. These photons must be removed by beam fixed filtration, since they increase patient dose unnecessarily.

Figure 5.5 has already shown the overall variation in μ over the diagnostic energy range for equal thicknesses of tissues. The sharp change observed in the curve for bone is due to the rapid change in the probability of a photoelectric effect (proportional to E^3), which is the major process of attenuation in bone ($Z \approx$ 13). For fat ($Z \approx 6$) and muscle ($Z \approx 7.5$) it is seen that the linear attenuation coefficient decreases as E

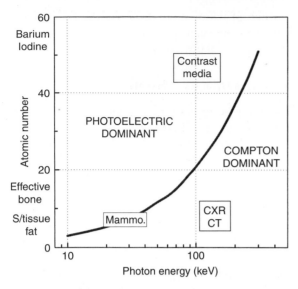

Figure 5.21 *PE and Compton probability plotted on log–log scales for photon energy and effective atomic number Z$_{eff}$ of the absorber. The shaded area represents a general soft-tissue range.*

increases, but the change is not so great since, in these low density materials, the photoelectric effect is less important and the principal process of attenuation is scattering (Compton effect). This is less dependent on photon energy and almost independent of atomic number. The densities of the three materials are also different (bone = 1920 kg m^{-3}; muscle = 1060 kg m^{-3}; fat = 950 kg m^{-3}) so further differences in attenuation coefficient persist even at high photon energies, where the difference in atomic number is unimportant.

Figure 5.21 plots the probability of photoelectric and Compton interactions for soft tissue represented by the shaded block (Z_{eff} up to ≈ 7.5). Photoelectric events are only common at low photon energies (30 kV); most common diagnostic investigations rely to a greater extent on Compton interactions. At higher diagnostic energies (100 kV) the photoelectric effect is minimal and attenuation relies almost entirely on Compton scattering. For equal tissue thicknesses attenuation will now depend on the electron density cm^{-3}. High kV chest radiographs take advantage of differences in the number of electrons cm^{-3} to give subject contrast. Attenuation increases linearly with an increase in density. Table 5.4 lists some important materials, their density, electron density and the ratio atomic number to atomic mass (Z:A).

5.6.1 Effect of absorber characteristics on contrast

The value of the linear attenuation coefficient depends on:

- Density (ρ)
- Atomic number (Z)
- Radiation quality (filtration and energy E)

The linear attenuation coefficients of the physiologically important bone (trabecular and compact), muscle (soft tissue), and fat also vary with radiation quality and this influences subject contrast (which is independent of the imaging process which is considered separately as **image contrast**).

In practical terms the decrease in μ with increasing energy means that as the X-ray kV increases the amount of transmission increases, although *the change* in transmission is greatest at low photon energies. Since mammography wishes to image differences between very similar soft tissues it uses low energy X-rays to accentuate tissue detail (between 26 and 28 keV). The differences in μ seen in Fig. 5.5 between the three tissues fat, soft tissue, and bone are greatest between energies of 10 to 30 keV.

Transmitted photons are responsible for exposing the film image and the image density obviously increases with photon number. The relative intensity of photons transmitted through 10 cm of soft tissue is the inverse of the graph in Fig. 5.5; a rapid increase is seen up to about 60 keV then the transmitted photon intensity only increases slowly. From this it is obvious that if the contrast is to be seen the linear attenuation coefficients of the materials comprising the patient are the important factors in determining the final contrast recorded in the image itself (ignoring at this stage the contrast characteristics of the image surface itself).

In Fig. 5.22 two tissues have been identified; each having a linear attenuation coefficient μ_1 and μ_2 and differing thicknesses x_1 and x_2. The incident X-ray intensity is I_0 and the emerging intensities are I_1 and I_2. So from eqn 5.2 the following relationship holds:

$$I_1 = I_0 \times e^{-(\mu_1 x_1)} \tag{5.24}$$

$$I_2 = I_0 \times e^{-(\mu_2 x_2)} \tag{5.25}$$

The fraction of the X-ray beam I_0 transmitted through thickness x_2 is $e^{-(\mu_2 x_2)}$ and the fraction transmitted

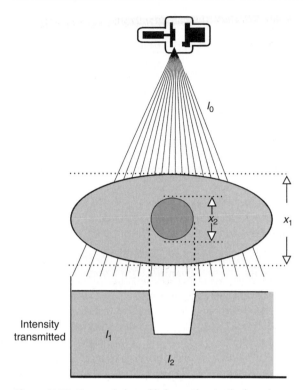

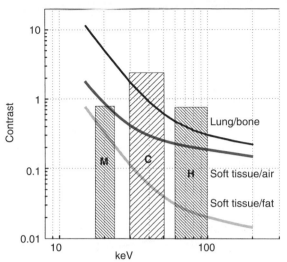

Figure 5.23 *The differences in attenuation coefficient between lung/bone, soft tissue/air and soft tissue/fat over the diagnostic energy range. The effective kilovoltage ranges for mammography (M), conventional radiography (C), and high kV investigations (H) are identified by hatched areas.*

Figure 5.22 *Transmission of information to the imaging surface. x_1 represents soft tissue and x_2 represents hard tissue (bone). The 'blackening' or image density is represented by I_1 and I_2 for these two tissue types.*

through $x_1 - x_2$ is $e^{-\mu_1(x_1-x_2)}$. The overall transmitted fraction I_2/I_0 is $e^{-\mu_2 x_2} \times e^{-\mu_1(x_1-x_2)}$ which becomes $I_2 = I_0 \times e^{-[\mu_1 x_1 - (\mu_2-\mu_1)x_2]}$ from eqns 5.24 and 5.25. The difference between transmitted intensities shown in Fig. 5.22 is just the difference between the attenuation coefficients: $\mu_2 - \mu_1$. Contrast differences between various tissues are plotted in Fig. 5.23 where lung tissue is taken to be approximately 25% of muscle as $0.25\mu_{soft\ tissue}$. Since μ_{air} is insignificant over clinical dimensions $\mu_{soft\ tissue} - \mu_{air} \approx \mu_{soft\ tissue}$. The observed contrast is proportional to the difference in linear coefficients for bone/muscle and for muscle/fat. It can be seen that the contrast in other cases decreases with increase in photon energy but that the change is much more marked for bone/muscle contrast than it is for muscle/fat contrast. It should be noted, however, that, for equal thicknesses, the bone/muscle contrast is always greater than the muscle/fat contrast because of the greater difference in density (both ρ and Z).

As the photon energy increases (when the Compton effect predominates) the contrast differences between bone/soft tissue are less marked. This explains the virtue of high kilovoltage chest radiography when the ribs become more transparent, while lung parenchyma retains its detail. At low photon energies the contrast differences between soft tissues and fat are more marked; the reason for low kilovoltage mammography and soft tissue radiography in general.

5.6.2 Effect of scatter on contrast

The set of graphs in Fig. 5.24a, b, and c indicate the importance of scatter when considering subject contrast. Although the proportion of scatter is most at low energies the amount of scatter leaving the tissue volume is small due to tissue absorption. The scatter component reaches a maximum at about 80 keV and then declines as scatter probability decreases. Tissue characteristics and X-ray photon energy determine the degree of photoelectric absorption that will occur within the tissue volume. Contrast agents such as barium and iodine increase subject contrast because of their high atomic number (Z^3) and their K-edge absorption falls within diagnostic imaging energies.

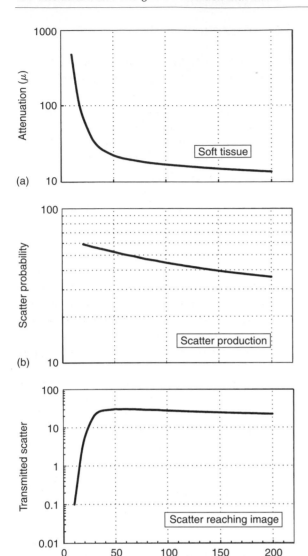

Figure 5.24 *(a) Attenuation coefficient for soft tissue and (b) the probability of scatter production with photon energy are combined in (c) giving an indication of the scattered radiation component in the exit beam. The y-axes are log scale.*

Air is a negative contrast agent since it attenuates less than tissue.

5.7 RADIATION DOSE

Radiation intensity (photons and particles) is measured as the number N of photons/particles per unit area A (m^2); this is the photon fluence in the case of

Table 5.7 *Units of radiation intensity.*

Quantity	Symbol	Definition	SI units
Photon fluence	Φ (phi)	N/A	Photons m^{-2}
Photon flux	ϕ (lower case phi)	Φ per second	Photons m^{-2} s^{-1}
Energy fluence	Ψ (psi)	ΦE	MeV or J m^{-2}
Energy flux	ψ (lower case psi)	Ψ per second	MeV or J m^{-2} s^{-1}

Table 5.8 *Quantities related to the source, field, and patient.*

Source related quantity	Field related quantities	Patient related quantities
Radiation quality (X-ray spectrum, kV$_p$, HVL)	Exposure	Incident air kerma (without backscatter)
Linear energy transfer (LET)	Air kerma (free in air) Air kerma–area product	Entrance air kerma (with backscatter)
	Specific gamma ray constant	Absorbed dose

X-rays and gamma radiation. The photon flux is the fluence per unit time (s^{-1}). The energy fluence for a mono-energetic beam is the product of the fluence and the energy E (joules or MeV). The energy flux is the energy fluence per unit time. These quantities are used in radiation dosimetry. Table 5.7 summarizes the quantities.

A 1 R incident X-ray exposure (8.7 mGy) with an effective energy of 30 keV has a fluence of 1.3×10^{10} photons cm^{-2}.

Table 5.8 shows how the source (beam) quality, field related environmental and patient related dose quantities are divided and measured. A significant proportion of the scattered radiation from a patient occurs in a backward direction; this is **backscatter** and is an important quantity for radiation protection. Backscatter can be excluded from patient surface measurements by recording the dose at a distance from the body surface. Measurements taken at the surface will include a percentage of backscatter so when comparing doses it is important to define the geometry of measurements.

Table 5.9 *Conversion values.*

Measurement	Value
Coulomb	6.24×10^{18} electrons
Electron charge	1.602×10^{-19} C
	$1\,eV = 1.602 \times 10^{-19}\,J$
Roentgen	$2.58 \times 10^{-4}\,C\,kg^{-1}$
Milligray (mGy)	$2.9452 \times 10^{-5}\,C\,kg^{-1}$
	or $29.452\,\mu C\,kg^{-1}$
Roentgen	$8.7\,mGy$

Air kerma–area product is defined as the absorbed dose to air averaged over the area of the X-ray beam in a plane perpendicular to the beam axis multiplied by the area of the beam in the same plane. It is commonly measured in $cGy\,cm^2$, $mGy\,cm^2$ or $Gy\,cm^2$ and since the ion chamber is fixed close to the X-ray housing radiation backscattered from the patient is excluded.

Under broad beam conditions a detector will receive not only direct attenuated beam but also some photons scattered from all points in the absorber. With a broad beam the radiation intensity detected will be greater than that obtained under narrow-beam conditions. The use of narrow-beam attenuation constants will lead to an overestimate of the effectiveness of shielding.

This **build-up factor** is defined as

$$\frac{\text{intensity with broad beam conditions}}{\text{intensity calculated from narrow beam conditions}}$$

Build-up depends on many factors:

- Composition of the absorber
- Size of the absorber
- Energy of the radiation
- Geometry of surrounding material

Calculations can be made for some simple geometrical arrangements but best values of build-up are obtained from the actual operating conditions. Both backscatter and build-up factors emphasize that dose measurement requires very careful design and standardization if dose values are to be compared or reproducibility achieved.

Since values for exposure, kerma, and absorbed dose are expressed in a variety of ways throughout Europe, America, and Asia, Table 5.9 lists the conversion factors used when moving from non-SI to SI values.

5.7.1 Exposure

Traditionally, radiation (X-rays, gamma radiation) has been measured by the amount of ionization produced in air; this was the **exposure** (symbol X). The special unit of exposure was called the roentgen (R), named after Wilhelm Roentgen (Röntgen).

Radiation exposure (X) is the ratio of the total electric charge (Q) which is the sum of all the electronic charges of either sign produced in air when all the electrons released by the ionizing events from a small volume of air of mass m are absorbed. So that

$$X = \frac{Q}{m} \qquad (5.26)$$

Equal numbers of positive and negative charges are produced in any ionization event, since each electron ejected from one atom leaves a positive charged ion. Only the total charge of one sign is considered (e.g. electrons) in this definition.

Exposure has SI units of coulomb per kilogram $(C\,kg^{-1})$ and only applies to air, and no other medium and is measured with an air-filled ion chamber. It has an exact relationship to the roentgen and gray as: $1\,R = 2.58 \times 10^{-4}\,C\,kg^{-1}$ and $2.9542 \times 10^{-2}\,C\,kg^{-1}$ of air, respectively. The roentgen is no longer used in radiation protection but there are many instruments which give readings in roentgen (R) or roentgen per hour $(R\,h^{-1})$. Box 5.7 shows conversion factors for these two quantities. The definition of exposure does not specify any time over which the radiation exposure must be received. The total amount of ionization produced in air is related to the **energy absorbed** from the beam. The energy absorbed from $1\,C\,kg^{-1}$ is calculated in Box 5.8. It is evident that temperature rise is not responsible for radiation damage since this is far too small. Rates of energy deposition (fluence and flux, as described above) are of considerable practical importance when calculating the effect of radiation exposure, since these give exposure rate, energy fluence and fluence rate or flux density. Box 5.9 shows that a very small charge is produced, and consequently sensitive equipment is necessary to record these events.

The average atomic number of air is 7.6 and is close to that of muscle at 7.5 (see Table 5.4), so that the mass attenuation and absorption coefficients (30.2) of air and muscle are very similar. This means that the energy absorbed from an X-ray beam by a given mass of air is almost identical to that absorbed

Box 5.7 Conversion factors for roentgen to gray

Since
$$1 \text{ roentgen (R)} = 2.58 \times 10^{-4} \text{C kg}^{-1}$$
and
$$1 \text{ gray (Gy)} = 2.9542 \times 10^{-2} \text{C kg}^{-1} \text{ of air}$$
Then

$$1R = \frac{2.58 \times 10^{-4}}{2.9542 \times 10^{-2}}$$
$$= 8.733328 \text{ mGy} \quad \text{or} \quad \sim 8.7 \text{ mGy}$$

So, for conversion purposes
$$1 R = 8.7 \text{ mGy}$$
$$1 \text{ mR} = 8.7 \text{ μGy}$$
and
$$1 \text{ Gy} = 115 \text{ R}$$
$$1 \text{ mGy} = 115 \text{ mR}$$
$$1 \text{ μGy} = 115 \text{ μR}$$

Box 5.8 Energy given by 1 C kg^{-1} exposure in air

The energy absorbed from 1 C kg^{-1} exposure given that the ionization for air is approximately 33.8 eV per ion pair. From Table 5.9 the charge on the electron is 1.602×10^{-19} C and the energy of 1 eV is 1.6×10^{-19} J. The energy produced is $33.8 \times (1.6 \times 10^{-19}) = 5.4 \times 10^{-18}$ J. An ion pair represents a charge of 1.6×10^{-19} C so the energy absorbed is

$$\frac{5.4 \times 10^{-18}}{1.6 \times 10^{-19}} = 33.8 \text{ J kg}^{-1}$$

Temperature increase with radiation exposure

Consider the temperature rise due to an exposure to 10 Gy. Since $10 \text{ Gy} = 10 \text{ J kg}^{-1}$ and the specific heat for water is $4190 \text{ J kg}^{-1} \text{ K}^{-1}$, the temperature rise is therefore

$$\frac{10}{4190} = 2.386 \times 10^{-3} \text{ K}$$

The temperature increase in 1 cm^3 water for a 10 Gy exposure is 0.002386°C.

Box 5.9 The charge produced

The average energy to produce ionization in air is 34 eV. So from Table 5.9, a 60 keV X-ray photon, fully absorbed in air, produces about 1765 ionizing events: a total charge of 2.8×10^{-16} C. The remainder of the energy of the absorbed photon produces excitation of the atom and heat.

by the same mass of muscle. Exposure measured in air is related to the energy absorbed both in air and muscle, so air is an important medium for radiation dosimetry and the absorbed dose in tissue can be calculated from the exposure measurement in air.

This works well for diagnostic energies and allows direct and accurate measurements, providing the geometry remains constant. Other types of dosimetry methods are used clinically for relative measurements such as thermoluminescence or film dosimeters.

MILLIAMPERE SECONDS

The output intensity of an X-ray machine is measured by an ion chamber and expressed as mGy or μGy per unit time (second). An X-ray exposure is commonly measured in terms of X-ray tube current (milliamps) and duration (seconds) as the product (milliampere second or mAs). Since 1 mA is 1 mC s^{-1} then mAs is equivalent to $1 \text{ mC s}^{-1} \times \text{seconds} = 1$ millicoulomb (mC). The dose in mGy from an X-ray exposure under specified operating conditions (kV$_p$, source/image distance with a known X-ray beam filtration) can be approximately estimated from the formula

$$0.5 \times \frac{V^2 E}{d^2}$$

where V is the voltage in kilovolts, d is the source to image distance, and E is the exposure in mAs. Using this formula the calculation in Box 5.10 illustrates the benefits of high kV$_p$ imaging.

5.7.2 Kerma

The term exposure is being replaced in radiation dosimetry by **kerma** (K) which stands for **kinetic**

Box 5.10 An illustration of the benefits of high kV$_p$ imaging

A high energy chest X-radiograph having a source-to-image distance (SID) of 2 m at 110 kV$_p$ at 2 mAs gives a surface dose of

$$0.5 \times \frac{110^2 \times 2}{200^2} = 0.30 \, \text{mGy}$$

Similar radiography but using 70 kV$_p$ requires an increase in mAs of $(70/110)^4$. For the same SID the dose is now 0.73 mGy; an increase of $\times 2\frac{1}{2}$.

energy released per unit **mass** and must specify the material concerned. This term differs from exposure because **kerma** measures the **removal of energy** from the photon beam by ionization creating secondary electrons. The term kerma refers to the kinetic energy released per unit mass of absorber and is basically a measure of the kinetic energy of charged particles produced in an absorbing medium by X-ray photons in the case of diagnostic radiology. When the absorbing medium is air, the term **air kerma** or **kerma in air** is used (K_{air}). The unit of kerma is the joule per kilogram and it is given the special name gray (Gy) so 1 Gy = 1 J kg^{-1}.

For X- and gamma-ray energies up to 1 MeV, the interactions which take place between the radiation and the particles of air are nearly the same for both exposure measurement and air kerma measurement.

As already seen in Sections 5.3.2 and 5.3.3 energy transfer by photon radiation to the medium of air takes place indirectly, in two steps: First, charge carriers (electrons) are released through interactions between photons and the atoms of the air (with the photoelectric effect and the Compton effect dominating in the case of X-radiation). Along their paths, electrons transfer energy to the air. For energies above those seen in diagnostic radiology, a fraction of the initial kinetic energy of the electrons is transformed into Bremsstrahlung and is not deposited in the vicinity of the electron paths; this can be discounted for photon energies between 20 and 200 keV.

The subsequent transference of energy from the primary ionizing particle to the medium itself is represented by the dose. The kerma decreases continuously with increasing depth in the absorbing medium, whereas the absorbed dose increases with depth. The kerma has not proved to be of much practical value in radiobiology, and its main use is in clarifying the steps involved in energy deposition.

For X- and gamma rays, kerma can be calculated from the mass energy absorption coefficient of the material μ_{en}/ρ and the energy fluence, so that $K = \Psi \, (\mu_{en}/\rho)$. From Table 5.7 the SI units for energy fluence are J m^{-2}, and the SI units of the mass energy absorption coefficient are m^2 kg^{-1}, so the product, kerma, has units of J kg^{-1}.

The difference between kerma and dose for air is that kerma is defined using the **mass energy transfer coefficient**, μ_{tr}/ρ, whereas dose is defined using the **mass energy absorption coefficient** μ_{en}/ρ or μ_{ab}/ρ. At diagnostic energies (20 to 200 keV) **kerma in air** and **dose in air** (D_{air}) can be treated as equal. Ion pairs generated in each kilogram of air (exposure X) multiplied by the energy required to form one ion pair (W) is equal to the energy removed from the beam (kerma). Thus

$$X \, (\text{C kg}^{-1}) \times W \, (\text{J C}^{-1}) = K_{air} \, (\text{J kg}^{-1})$$
$$\equiv D_{air} \, (\text{J kg}^{-1})$$

As seen from Box 5.8 the energy to form one ion pair in air is close to 34 J C^{-1} (34 eV per ion pair) for diagnostic radiation energies and over a wide range of biological materials. Since 1 Gy = 1 J kg^{-1} then:

- Dose$_{(air)}$ (in Gy) = $34E$ (C kg^{-1})
- Dose$_{(air)}$ (in Gy) = $100 \times (2.58 \times 10^{-4}) \times 34E$ (in R) = $0.88E$ (where 1 R = 8.76426 mGy)

Converting a dose in air to dose in an absorber (i.e. patient), then for the same incident photon flux the energy absorbed per unit mass of absorber depends only on the mass absorption coefficient of the medium. Hence

$$\frac{\text{Dose}_{(tissue)}}{\text{Dose}_{(air)}} = \frac{\left(\dfrac{\mu_{en}}{\rho}\right)_{tissue}}{\left(\dfrac{\mu_{en}}{\rho}\right)_{air}}$$

The subscript 'en' distinguishes **mass energy absorption coefficient** from the mass attenuation coefficient. The **mass energy transfer coefficient** and mass energy absorption coefficient are interchangeable at diagnostic energies and the values of μ_{en}/ρ are readily obtained from tables to convert a known dose in air

Table 5.10 *f-Factors over the diagnostic energy range* $(m^2\,kg^{-1})$.

keV	Bone	Muscle	Fat	Air
10	134.3057	35.7103	19.8139	33.8500
15	149.0962	35.6987	19.5262	33.8500
20	157.8164	35.6278	19.4146	33.8500
30	164.4014	35.6090	20.0281	33.8500
40	156.1530	35.7362	21.9666	33.8500
50	136.4581	36.0081	25.0243	33.8500
60	111.3309	36.3290	28.3285	33.8500
80	75.0981	36.7922	33.1569	33.8500
100	56.0467	37.0627	35.5440	33.8500
150	41.1520	37.2296	37.2839	33.8500
200	37.9292	37.2705	37.6505	33.8500

to the corresponding dose in tissue. This factor is sometimes given as μ_{ab}/ρ.

THE *f*-FACTOR

The deduction of absorbed dose in grays from the exposure in air (coulomb kg^{-1}) is possible since $C\,kg^{-1}$ represents the same amount of energy absorbed from the beam, by air, regardless of radiation energy or quality. An energy input of about 34 eV from the X-ray beam is required to form an ion pair. This ionization energy is directly linked to total energy absorption so exposure values measured in air $C\,kg^{-1}$ can be converted to expected exposure in tissue (grays) e.g. soft tissue or bone. Values of *f*-factors are listed in Table 5.10 for a range of keV values.

CONVERSION FACTOR

The mass attenuation coefficient describes all interactions which lead to the attenuation of photons in matter: photoelectric, elastic and Compton. The mass energy absorption coefficient (μ_{en}/ρ), where μ_{en} is the linear absorption coefficient (sometimes given as μ_{ab}), only concerns photoelectric absorption since this is responsible for tissue radiation dose:

absorbed energy per kg tissue = beam energy
$$\times\ \mu_{en}/\rho = E(\mu_{en}/\rho)$$

The *f*-factor is then defined as

$$\frac{\text{absorbed energy per kilogram of tissue}}{\text{absorbed energy per kilogram of air}} \quad (5.27)$$

Box 5.11 Calculation of the *f*-factor for soft tissue at 60keV

$$\left(\frac{\mu_{en}}{\rho}\right)_{air} = 3.004 \times 10^{-3}\ m^2\,kg^{-1}$$

For soft tissue

$$\left(\frac{\mu_{en}}{\rho}\right)_{tissue} = 3.224 \times 10^{-3}\ m^2\,kg^{-1}$$

So the *f*-factor is

$$\frac{33.85 \times (3.224 \times 10^{-3})}{3.004 \times 10^{-3}} = 36.33$$

For bone

$$\left(\frac{\mu_{en}}{\rho}\right)_{tissue} = 9.888 \times 10^{-3}\ m^2\,kg^{-1}$$

So, the *f*-factor is

$$\frac{33.85 \times (9.888 \times 10^{-3})}{3.004 \times 10^{-3}} = 111.33$$

The *f*-factors for three tissue types and air are plotted in Fig. 5.25.

Using a conversion factor expresses eqn 5.27 in grays:

$$f = 34 \times \frac{\frac{\mu_{en}}{\rho(\text{tissue})}}{\frac{\mu_{en}}{\rho(\text{air})}} \quad (5.28)$$

This is the factor f (in grays) which converts $C\ kg^{-1}$ exposure in air to exposure in tissue (grays). So an exposure of $1\,C\,kg^{-1}$ gives an absorbed dose of 33.85 Gy. Box 5.11 uses eqn 5.28 for calculating *f*-factors for soft tissue and bone at 60 keV.

SOFT TISSUE DOSE

The graph for *f*-conversion factors in Fig. 5.25 shows that across the diagnostic energy range the exposure in air is very close to the exposure in soft tissue. There is also a close correlation between soft tissue and water so that water makes an excellent substitute for soft tissue when carrying out dose measurements.

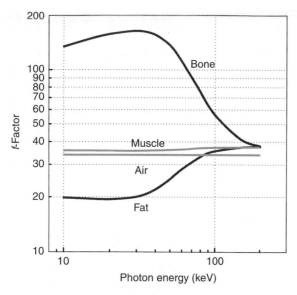

Figure 5.25 *The conversion of dose in air to dose in tissue is plotted across the diagnostic energy range.*

BONE DOSE

This is a very different case. At diagnostic energies the *f*-factors are much higher than for soft tissue. Bone has a higher atomic number (Z = about 13) and the absorption coefficient for bone increases rapidly towards the lower energy end due to increasing photo-electric dominance.

5.7.3 Absorbed dose

The distinction between kerma and dose is slight for the relatively low X-ray energies used in diagnostic radiology. The absorbed dose in any material (water, soft tissue etc.) is the ratio E/m where E is the energy absorbed in a unit mass m of material. The unit is the joule per kilogram which is equal to one gray (1 Gy). The gray replaces the obsolete unit the rad, which is $100\,\text{erg}\,\text{g}^{-1}$ or $10\,\text{mGy}$. The SI units for exposure, kerma and absorbed dose are given in Table 5.11.

Absorbed dose is currently taken as the best physical indicator of biological response. Because of this, absorbed dose to water closely resembles soft tissue and is the quantity commonly used to specify the amount of radiation in diagnostic radiology. Absorbed dose has the further advantage that it is directly measurable in a variety of ways. For volumes which are large compared to the track length, the kerma and

Table 5.11 *Units of radiation exposure and absorbed dose.*

Quantity	Symbol	SI unit	Non-SI
Exposure	X	coulomb per kg (C kg^{-1})	roentgen (R, mR)
Kerma	K or Gy	J kg^{-1}	roentgen (R, mR)
Absorbed dose	Gy	J kg^{-1}	rad (0.01 J kg^{-1}) mrad, μrad

absorbed dose are virtually identical, especially since absorbed dose also includes energy deposition within the volume by electrons set in motion outside the volume. This tends to balance the energy deposited outside the volume by those electrons starting inside the volume.

KEYWORDS

absorbed dose: the gray (Gy) $1\,\text{J}\,\text{kg}^{-1}$ equivalent to 100 rads

absorption coefficient: photoelectric absorption

attenuation coefficient: combined attenuation due to photoelectric and scatter effects. Measured as μm^{-1} (or cm^{-1})

Auger electron: electron ejected from the K or L shell as an alternative to characteristic radiation emission

binding energy: the energy associated with an orbital electron. High for K-shell electrons and low for L, M-, and N-shell electrons

characteristic radiation: electromagnetic radiation emitted when electrons fill orbital vacancies

Compton scatter: an interaction between an incident photon and a 'free' electron. The photon loses energy

elastic scattering: an interaction between an incident photon and the atomic field. There is no loss of energy

electron cascade: filling vacancies in electron orbits (normally K- or L-shell vacancies) by electrons in higher (less energetic) orbits. Accompanied by characteristic radiation and Auger electrons

excitation: energy imparted to an atom without ionization

f-**factor**: used for converting exposure in air to exposure in tissue

free electron: in low Z materials (tissue) any electron outside the K shell

inelastic scattering: see Compton scattering

ionization: loss of an orbital electron from an atom forming a charged ion, e.g. Na^+ or Cl^-

K edge: the abrupt increase in photon absorption when the incident photon energy equals the K-orbit binding energy

mass absorption coefficient: the equivalent of the linear absorption coefficient. It is the fraction of energy contained in the beam (gamma or X-radiation) which is absorbed per unit mass of the medium when a unit area is irradiated

mass attenuation coefficient: the quotient of linear attenuation coefficient and material density (ρ)

pair production: the interaction of a photon with an energy exceeding 1.2 MeV with the atomic nucleus to produce a positron and an electron

photoelectric effect: the complete absorption of a photon by interaction with a bound (K- or L-shell) electron

photoelectron: electron ejected from the K or L shell as the result of a photoelectric reaction

recoil electron: the path taken by the free electron after a Compton interaction

scattered photon: the path taken by the incident photon after a Compton interaction

Interaction of radiation with matter: detectors

6.1 RADIATION DETECTION

The detection of X- or gamma radiation requires the exploitation of their interaction with matter described in Chapter 5 to produce signals proportional to the radiation energy absorbed. Three basic reactions in the absorber provide signals for the measurement of radiation energy or activity:

- **Chemical**: where radiation causes atomic or molecular excitation of electrons. The prime example is the interaction of film emulsion with X-radiation, gamma radiation or light.
- **Ionization**: where atoms lose electrons and become current carrying ions. This reaction forms the basis of gas and semiconductor detectors.
- **Luminescence** (light production): where valency electrons in a crystalline material gain energy from radiation and enter a higher conduction band, from where they eventually move to a lower energy orbit and emit photons in the UV/visible part of the spectrum.

Although these detector materials can be used for detecting most ionizing radiation (alpha, beta, gamma and X-rays) they are commonly used as photon detectors in radiology so they will be described in their role as photon (X- or gamma radiation) detectors in this chapter. The type of detector employed in radiology depends on the application: whether as a non-imaging or imaging detector.

Non-imaging applications include personnel dosimetry badges, radiation monitoring equipment, isotope dose calibrators or organ uptake probes (i.e. thyroid). These detectors either integrate the radiation signal producing a sum measurement of the total exposure ($Gy \, min^{-1}$ or h^{-1}) or measure the activity as individual photon counts. Activity measurement, which would be required for laboratory estimations (small sample activity) would register individual events of a particular energy. Larger activity measurements can also be provided, again as integrated measurements but this time expressed as becquerels (Bq) or disintegrations per second.

Imaging applications would use large area detectors (film, image plate) or many small detectors as a group (CT gas detectors) or large single crystal detectors (nuclear medicine gamma cameras) in order to give positional information for image construction.

Efficiency and sensitivity of a radiation detector depends on geometry as well as its ability to absorb radiation. These characteristics will be discussed after the various methods for radiation detection have been described.

6.2 FILM AS A DETECTOR

Photographic effects are widely used as detectors for X- and gamma radiation. Chapter 7 deals with photochemical reactions in more detail. Photon interactions rely on either photoelectric or Compton events to release electrons which then activate the silver halide crystal in the film emulsion.

Both the silver halide and gelatin in the emulsion play an integral part in the photochemical action. The X- or gamma photon ionizes the silver halide (AgBr) into silver and bromine ions. The bromine ion is absorbed by the gelatin and the silver ion migrates to a sensitive region in the crystal. The developing stage, in the subsequent photographic processing, reduces the silver ions to metallic silver whose density is proportional to the initial radiation exposure. This effect can be used to measure radiation dose (film density being proportional to radiation dose) or form a radiographic image.

FILM SENSITIVITY

The film as an X- or gamma ray detector varies in sensitivity across the photon energy range (Fig. 6.1). Unlike 'tissue equivalent' detectors (see later) AgBr has two K edges that fall within the diagnostic range of photon energies (Ag is 25.5 and Br is 13 keV). Film response (sensitivity) to photon energy decreases at energies lower than 40 keV, due to these K edges as shown by the shaded curve in Fig. 6.1.

A typical X-ray film emulsion contains mixed silver halide (Ag(I)Br) and has a density of $1.84 \times 10^{-2} \, \text{kg m}^{-3}$. The mass absorption coefficient at 60 keV

is typically $0.44 \, \text{m}^2 \text{kg}^{-1}$ so the linear attenuation coefficient is $8.1 \times 10^{-2} \, \text{m}^{-1}$ which gives a quantum efficiency value of $1 - e^{-0.0081}$ or slightly less than 1%.

Film is used as a detector for measuring personal radiation dose but suffers since it is not tissue equivalent. This will be discussed later.

6.3 GAS DETECTORS

GAS IONIZATION

Only a small amount of energy is required to ionize gas. About 30 eV will produce an ion pair. Ion production is proportional to energy absorbed; the charge C (in C kg^{-1}) is:

$$C = \frac{Q}{m} \qquad (6.1)$$

where Q is the number of ion pairs and m is mass of chamber gas. Gas detectors rely on the ionization of gas atoms and the collection of the induced charge by electrodes as shown diagrammatically in Fig. 6.2a. A high voltage is applied across the electrodes in order to collect the free electrons and gas ions caused by the ionizing event. The signal current is extremely small so amplification is necessary.

GAS DETECTOR VOLTAGE

Gas detector action depends on the applied electrode voltage. The following regions can be identified in Fig. 6.2b:

- The **ionization** region. The first plateau. This is found in the ionization chamber. There is very little change in signal output for change in applied voltage over this range.
- The **proportional** region is found at a higher voltage where the ions are accelerated to cause secondary ionization by collision. This is gas amplification and signal strength is proportional to the energy of the primary radiation and applied voltage. It is energy sensitive.
- The **Geiger** region is the second plateau and gives maximum useful gas amplification where each ionization event saturates the chamber with ions giving a peak signal for all energies. It simply registers an ionization event caused by alpha, beta, X- or gamma radiation as a single electrical pulse.

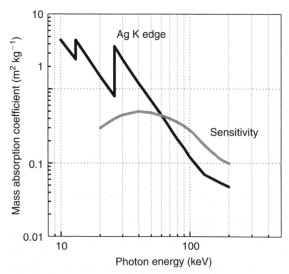

Figure 6.1 *Variation of AgBr mass absorption coefficient with photon energy and general film sensitivity with keV.*

6.3.1 Ionization detector

The ionization chamber is the simplest form of gas detector and uses the simple design illustrated in Fig. 6.3a. The region between the plates is filled with air or inert gas. Air requires an average energy of 34 eV to produce an ion pair so for a 100 keV photon approximately 3000 ions or electrons are formed.

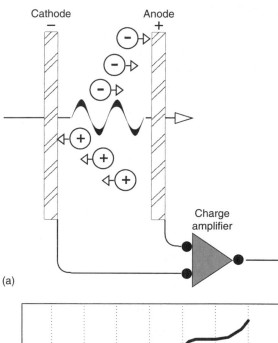

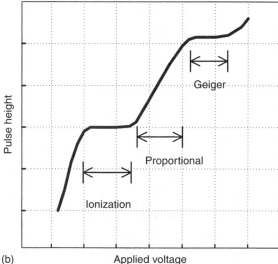

(a)

(b)

Figure 6.2 *(a) Simple gas detector design showing an ionization event giving positive gas ions and electrons. (b) Increasing the applied voltage alters the characteristic of a gas detector into three regions described in the text.*

Signals from an ion chamber are very small and need considerable amplification before a useful signal is produced. The amplitude of the signal depends on the number of ions formed and is independent of the applied voltage between the plates. The applied voltage does, however, influence the speed of ion collection. The ion chamber has a very slow response and consequently the ion chamber is not used for pulse or event counting. Owing to its slow response radiation energy deposited in the chamber is integrated to give a steady reading of **radiation dose/dose rate** (mGy or mGy s^{-1}) or medium level **radionuclide activity** in disintegrations per second: kBq, MBq. Radiation level is measured as a current which is dependent on both source activity or X-ray intensity and energy of the radiation.

DOSE CALIBRATOR

This design uses a 'well' or 're-entrant' design where a central hollow electrode holds a radioactive sample to be measured (Fig. 6.3a). Maximum efficiency is achieved by capturing the majority of emissions in a 4π geometry which has been described in Chapter 1. In order to increase efficiency still further a dense gas filling is used, either nitrogen, argon or xenon under pressure: ($>$10 atmospheres). The ion chamber does not have a linear response to energy. This is shown in Fig. 6.3b and corrections for different gamma energies must be applied for each radioactive sample counted.

XENON GAS ION CHAMBER

These are found in some older CT machines as multiple detectors. They are manufactured as a single channel divided into many hundreds (700–800) of separate individual chambers with electrodes. The width of each detector is about 1 mm, their depth anything up to 20 cm. The xenon gas is under pressure to increase density and so efficiency, which is of the order of 50–60%. Table 6.1 shows the considerable pressure necessary to increase gas density and so improve the detector efficiency.

SURVEY OR MONITORING ION-CHAMBER

These instruments have a simple construction consisting of flat electrodes and are commonly used in radiology for measuring total dose or dose rates during patient examinations (dose–area product meter) or for quality control measurements (HVL, X-ray room dose rates).

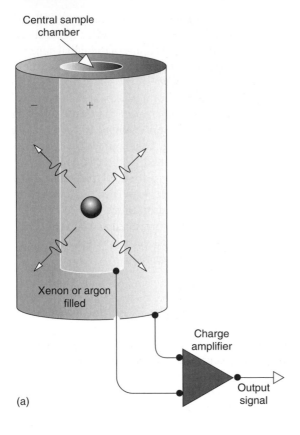

(a)

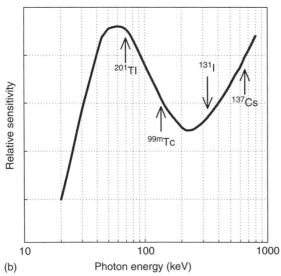

(b)

Table 6.1 *Xenon density and pressure.*

Pressure (atm)	Density (g cm^{-3})
10	0.056
20	0.121
40	0.26

Box 6.1 Ionization current (using eqn 6.1)

1 cm^3 of air weighs 1.3×10^{-6} kg at NTP

A 350 cm^3 chamber holds 4.55×10^{-4} kg

Since the energy deposited per ion pair is approximately 34 J C^{-1}, then 7.5 µGy h^{-1} will give

$$\frac{7.5}{34} = 0.22\,\mu\text{Ci kg}^{-1}\,\text{h}^{-1}$$

Exposure,

$$C = \frac{Q}{M}$$

and charge

$$Q = C \times m$$

Therefore the current is

$$\frac{(2.2 \times 10^{-7}) \times (4.55 \times 10^{-4})}{3600}\text{ amps}$$
$$= 2.78 \times 10^{-14}\text{ amp}$$
$$= 0.0278\text{ picoamp}$$

Note. Factors which increase current density are:

- Xenon density is ×5 that of air (Table 6.1).
- Pressurized gas gives a higher density.

The electrodes are made from air equivalent material (plastic) and air is the detector gas. The chamber can be calibrated in either radiation dose (µGy, mGy) or dose rate (µGy or mGy min^{-1}). The sensitivity of a survey/monitoring ion chamber is related to gas volume or the size of the chamber itself but very small (thimble) ion chambers are valuable for sampling radiation dose in small volumes (simulated tissue depth dose).

The very small current given by the ionization event is amplified electronically to give a useful signal. Typical signal currents are shown in Box 6.1 for an air chamber. The tiny signals require good cabling

Figure 6.3 *(a) Isotope dose calibrator with almost 4π geometry filled with pressurized gas. (b) The change in response with photon energy for a dose calibrator. Common isotope gamma energies are marked on the curve. Corrections are applied to the readings which allow for this.*

and connectors; cable movement can induce noise signals that spoil measurements.

SUMMARY OF ION CHAMBER DETECTORS

These have the following advantages and disadvantages:

Advantages

- Walls can be made tissue equivalent
- All radiation types can be measured
- Can be calibrated for any energy (isotope)

Disadvantages

- Small signal currents need very sensitive (expensive) electronic amplification
- Has restricted sensitivity

6.3.2 Proportional counter

The common gas ion chamber is not fast enough to distinguish individual photon events. Its signal is a result of integrating the many photon interactions happening within its volume. As a consequence this signal is a slowly changing voltage which is proportional to activity level. In order to record individual photon events the detector response time must be improved which can be achieved by increasing the applied voltage to about 1000 V. The resulting larger electric field accelerates the electrons in the chamber so their increased kinetic energy can produce secondary ionization (Townsend avalanche) producing about 10^3 to 10^5 secondary events per original ionization event providing event amplification. The chamber is operated so that the number of secondary events is **proportional** to the number of primary events; this is the origin of the detector's name. Proportional chambers are found as large area radiation monitors (Fig. 6.4) and as CT detectors. Both counters use xenon to improve efficiency. The high voltage is between 1000 and 2000 V. Since the sensitivity varies with applied voltage, proportional chambers need very stable power supplies.

Operating voltages depend upon the fill gas which is normally an inert gas such as nitrogen or argon. Krypton and xenon are used for higher energies and higher efficiencies. Gas pressure increases the density of the detector which improves quantum efficiency. Table 6.2 lists some common gas fills for proportional chambers. Butane offers a cheap high density gas but requires frequent replenishment.

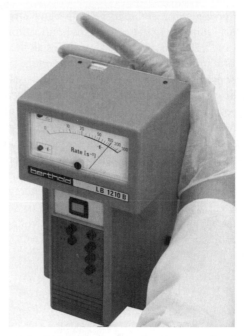

Figure 6.4 *Photograph of proportional counter showing large surface area (courtesy of Berthold Inc.).*

Table 6.2 *Ion chamber gases.*

Gas	Density (kg m^{-3} at 20°C)	Application
Air	1.293	X-ray dosimeters
Nitrogen	1.250	Dose calibrators
Argon	1.784	Dose calibrators
Xenon	5.500	Alpha, beta, gamma radiation and CT
Butane	5.560	Alpha and beta radiation measurement

A typical large surface area contamination monitor operating at proportional region is xenon filled with a 100 cm^2 to 200 cm^2 surface detector area with a 6 mg cm^{-2} titanium foil window. Detection sensitivity would be of the order of 3 to 5 Bq cm^{-2} for common isotopes (^{125}I and ^{99m}Tc).

6.3.3 Geiger detector

H.W. Geiger (1882–1945; German physicist) discovered that if the electric field in an ion chamber is increased still further then secondary avalanches can occur giving considerable increase in signal strength for each ionizing event and gas amplification can reach 10^{10}. There is no proportionality as all incident radiation produces the same saturated voltage signal. The construction, shown in Fig. 6.5a, consists of a cylindrical outer electrode with an inner electrode composed of a thin wire which serves to concentrate the electric field. The operating voltage is much higher (900 to 1200 V) which increases gas amplification considerably. An ion cascade due to energetic collisions gives a very strong signal for each ionization event. The Geiger detector is insensitive to energy, due to the cascade effect and also insensitive to supply voltage variations since the operating voltage is chosen to be in the center of the plateau.

The discharge produced by an ionization event must be quenched so that the detector returns to its original state, ready for the next event. The Geiger–Müller (GM) tube is inactive until quenching is complete; this **dead time** can be hundreds of microseconds long, so limiting it for high count rates. Chemicals are added to the detector gas in order to quench ion avalanche so that after each ionization the ion cascade quickly stops; this improves the long count dead time. The most common additive is bromine and these tubes can be operated at a lower voltage. GM counters are sensitive to most types of radiation providing the entrance window is thin enough (mica in the case of low alpha or beta radiation). GM counters are excellent cheap contamination monitors or radiation leakage detectors, having peak sensitivity in the diagnostic energy range (Fig. 6.5b). Their response can be dampened electronically so that radiation levels can be measured in μGy h^{-1} or mGy h^{-1}.

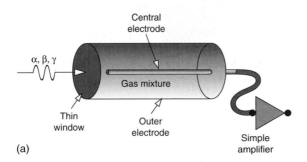

(a)

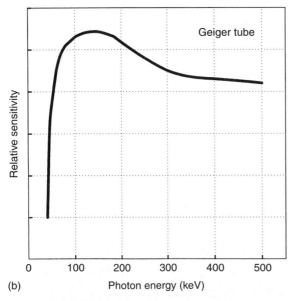

(b)

Figure 6.5 *(a) Basic design for Geiger counter showing a cylindrical outer electrode and a central wire electrode. (b) The energy response curve for a Geiger counter which peaks over the diagnostic range.*

6.4 LUMINESCENCE DETECTORS

Roentgen accidentally observed the first interaction of X-rays with matter when activating a luminescent phosphor near his workbench. Luminescent phosphors still occupy an essential place in diagnostic imaging.

Gamma or X-radiation interacts with the phosphor or scintillator producing a light event whose intensity is proportional to the photon energy deposited. Light production can be instantaneous or delayed and the duration of the light signal can be measured in nano-seconds (10^{-9} s) or tenths of seconds (10^{-1} s). Properties of a good scintillator are:

• Transparency to emitted light
• Large light output
• High photon absorption for gamma and X-rays
• Available in large sizes

Figure 6.6 shows the electron bands involved in the general phenomenon of luminescence. Its name is given to a wide range of phenomena which result in light being produced after stimulation by either photons or charged particles (electrons).

The incident photon energy is deposited in the outer valency orbits which causes electrons to jump through the forbidden zone into the conduction zone.

At a certain time after this photon event the electrons fall back into the valency band emitting radiation in the form of light.

If impurity traps are present in the forbidden zone the electrons can be caught; their fate then depends on other factors. The term luminescence covers three major phosphor types that are commonly found in radiology and used for both imaging and radiation dose measurement such as counters or storage devices. These are:

- Phosphorescence
- Fluorescence
- Thermoluminescence

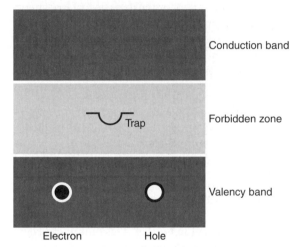

Conduction band

Forbidden zone

Trap

Valency band

Electron   Hole

Figure 6.6 *Electron bands and the forbidden zone with impurity traps. The valency band shows the presence of an electron and the absence (hole).*

DOPING

Phosphor sensitivity is improved by doping the pure phosphor material (e.g. NaI, CsI) with impurity atoms. Examples of doped crystals, commonly used in radiology, would be NaI:Tl, CsI:Na and Gd_2O_2S:Tb.

The doping materials are responsible for trapping centers in the forbidden zone which give the phosphor its unique properties (light spectrum and wavelength).

6.4.1 Phosphorescence

This is shown diagrammatically in Fig. 6.7. Radiation ejects electrons from the valency band into the conduction band from where they attempt to return again to the valency band but are caught by trap defects in the forbidden zone. They eventually leave these traps falling into the vacant 'holes' in the valency band and in so doing they emit light. Light output can continue for some time after stimulation by radiation since electrons from the traps are periodically excited into the conduction band. Summarizing Fig. 6.7; the reactions are:

(a) The phosphor has **empty** traps near the top of the forbidden zone and X-ray photons eject electrons from the valency band into the conduction band.

(b) After the photon event electrons in the conduction band fall into empty traps in the forbidden zone.

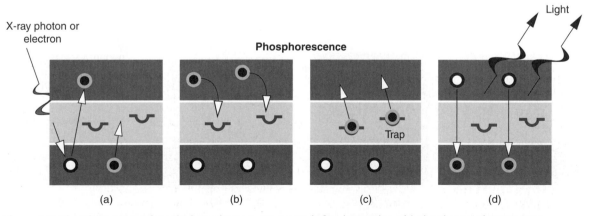

X-ray photon or electron

Phosphorescence

Light

Trap

(a)   (b)   (c)   (d)

Figure 6.7 *Phosphorescence where the impurity traps are empty before interaction with the photon. The sequences (a), (b), (c), (d) are described in the text.*

(c) Intrinsic energy supplied by the crystal again lifts some trapped electrons into the conduction band.

(d) Electrons then fall from the conduction band into vacancies in the valency band (holes) emitting a broad continuous light spectrum. The time between (c) and (d) determines the period of emission (10^{-4} to many seconds).

Phosphorescent materials are ideal for video monitor screens or image intensifier output screens yielding a continuous spectrum.

6.4.2 Fluorescence

This is illustrated in Fig. 6.8 where light output stops immediately after photon irradiation; in practice a finite dead time (afterglow) does exist but this is very short and measured in nano-seconds. Summarizing the reactions associated with fluorescence in Fig. 6.8:

(a) The phosphor has full traps near the top of the forbidden zone.

(b) X-ray photons eject electrons from the valency band into the conduction band.

(c) After the photon event the trapped electrons fill holes in the valency band emitting a light pulse (10^{-8} to 10^{-9}s) which has a narrow spectrum.

(d) Electrons from the conduction band then fall into the empty traps in the forbidden zone.

The simplest model for an inorganic scintillator involves crystal impurities and lattice defects providing energy levels in the normally forbidden region.

Electrons from the conduction band may enter these centers but there are alternative events that may occur leading to information loss and so reducing the conversion efficiency of the detector.

The **conversion efficiency** for inorganic scintillators can be improved by impurity activation (doping). The added impurity probably occupies interstitial positions in the crystal lattice functioning as luminescence activators. Thallium is a common impurity added in concentrations of 0.8 to 2.0%.

A common fluorescent detector material is sodium iodide which has high density ($3.76\,\mathrm{g\,cm^{-3}}$) and, owing to the high atomic number, Z, of iodine (which is 53), has a high photoelectric event absorption coefficient suited for the detection of low energy X-rays and gamma rays. Cesium iodide is also found as a scintillation material in radiology. The common applications for fluorescent detectors (scintillators) that are found throughout radiology are:

- Intensifying screens in film cassettes
- Scintillation crystals in conjunction with photomultiplier light detectors in nuclear medicine, uptake probes and CT detectors
- Cesium iodide on the face of image intensifiers

6.4.3 Thermoluminescence

This is represented in Fig. 6.9. Thermoluminescence differs from the previous examples of phosphorescence and fluorescence because the energy obtained from the radiation exposure is stored indefinitely within the crystal matrix and the output signal (light)

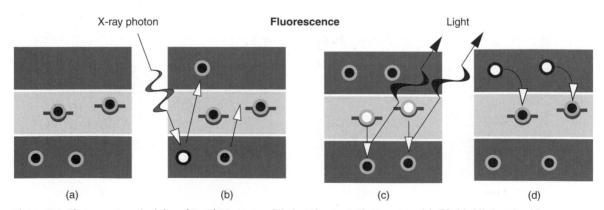

Figure 6.8 *Fluorescence principles where the traps are filled at the start. The sequence (a), (b), (c), (d) described in the text.*

is only emitted when the trapped electrons are dislodged by infrared energy (heat or infrared laser).

Since the light output is directly proportional to radiation energy input thermoluminescent materials are used as dosimeters and, on a larger scale, phosphor imaging plates. Lithium fluoride, a thermoluminescent material, has an effective atomic number similar to air and soft tissue, showing only a small variation in response to photon energy. It therefore shows **tissue equivalence** making it a valuable radiation dosimeter.

Summarizing the events shown in Fig. 6.9 the series of reactions for thermoluminescence are:

(a) The phosphor has empty traps in the forbidden zone at different energy levels and during X-ray interaction electrons are ejected from the valency band into the conduction band.
(b) These electrons then fall into the empty traps where they can stay indefinitely.
(c) Energy (heat) is required to eject the trapped electrons once again into the conduction band.
(d) They fall back into the valency band emitting a broad light spectrum whose intensity is equivalent to the original radiation exposure in (a).

6.5 PRACTICAL DETECTORS

A list of practical detectors using luminescent materials and found in radiology is given in Table 6.3.

6.5.1 Intensifying screens

Thin sheets of plastic impregnated with fluorescent phosphor are incorporated into film cassettes that are used in plain film radiography. They convert X-radiation into visible light which then exposes the film. A large increase in quantum efficiency is obtained and a radiograph can be obtained at a very low patient dose. The general construction is shown in Fig. 6.10a where the intensifying screen consists of phosphor particles bonded within a thin plastic sheet supported on a plastic base. A reflective layer directs the light forward. In order to improve efficiency a dual emulsion film is commonly used sandwiched between

Table 6.3 *Summary of luminescent detectors.*

Scintillator	Application
Fluorescence	
NaI:Tl	Scintillator for nuclear medicine
CsI:Tl	Scintillator for CT
$CaWO_4$	Intensifying screen
Gd_2O_2S:Tb	Intensifying screen
Phosphorescence	
ZnS complex (P4)	Video monitor
ZnCdS:Ag (P20)	Image intensifier
Thermoluminescence	
LiF	Dosimeter
BaF(X) where X = F, I or Br	Image plate

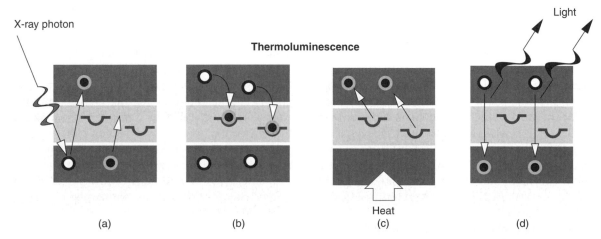

Figure 6.9 *Thermoluminescence principles where the traps are scattered at different energy levels in the forbidden zone. The sequence (a), (b), (c), (d) is described in the text.*

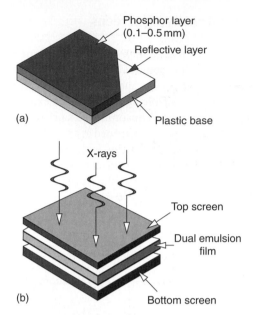

Figure 6.10 (**a**) *Construction of an intensifying screen containing a scintillation phosphor.* (**b**) *A dual emulsion film sandwiched between two intensifying screens to increase efficiency.*

two intensifying screens; this general arrangement is shown in Fig. 6.10b.

Common phosphor materials used for these fluorescent screens are rare earth materials containing gadolinium and lanthanum; other phosphors use yttrium tantalate or tungstate. All the phosphor materials are doped with impurity elements (e.g. terbium, thulium) in order to improve their light output. Intensifying screens are discussed further in Chapter 7.

6.5.2 Scintillation detectors

These are commonly found in nuclear medicine where they are used in gamma cameras and single crystal detectors for uptake studies. Sodium iodide is the scintillator of choice owing to its high quantum efficiency. Photoelectric events within the crystal can be selected by the electronic circuits so eliminating counts due to scatter. The photoelectron output is about 4 to 12 for NaI:Tl and 1 to 3 for CsI:Tl. Some plastics are also used as very fast scintillation devices but are not usually seen in radiology.

Scintillation phosphors produce a brief pulse of light for each gamma photon detected; the light output from sodium iodide is in the ultraviolet spectrum.

The light pulse is detected and converted into an electrical signal by a **photomultiplier** tube. This can multiply the initial light signal by 10^6 or more. Figure 6.11 shows a complete scintillation detector system with its photomultiplier tube (PMT), amplifier, power supply and count display for photopeak events. The photomultiplier consists of a photocathode which produces electrons from the light pulse given by the scintillator (usually NaI:Tl) which is in optical contact with its face.

A dynode chain having an increasing positive voltage further multiplies the electrons, achieving in excess of 10^6 multiplication. A very stable high voltage supply to the photomultiplier is essential. The high input impedance (charge) amplifier, shown in the diagram, feeds a pulse height analyzer which sorts the pulses into a storage device depending on their amplitude. In this way scatter events can be discarded and only photo events recorded.

GAMMA SPECTRUM (SEE ALSO ENERGY RESOLUTION)

An ideal scintillation detector (crystal with PMT) converts all the energy of the gamma ray into an electrical signal directly proportional to the gamma energy.

A theoretical spectrum shown in Fig. 6.12a for ^{137}Cs identifies the basic gamma spectrum components. The Compton process shares the incident photon energy between the scattered photon and the recoil electron; the latter decides the intensity of the light output. This depends on whether the collision gives a 180° scatter event (maximum energy deposited) or smaller angle scattering (20° 30° 45° etc.). The variation in the Compton interactions gives the long Compton scatter spectrum ending abruptly at the Compton edge (180° scatter). The Compton distribution, or Compton valley, represents energy lost in the crystal due to photon scattering events. Only the energy of the recoil electron is transferred to the scintillation crystal; the scattered photon either escapes or is absorbed producing a secondary event. The maximum electron energy which would be given by a 180° scatter can be calculated from eqn 5.22. For a gamma energy of 662 keV the scatter photon energy would be

$$\frac{662}{1 + (1.295 \times 2)} = 184\,keV$$

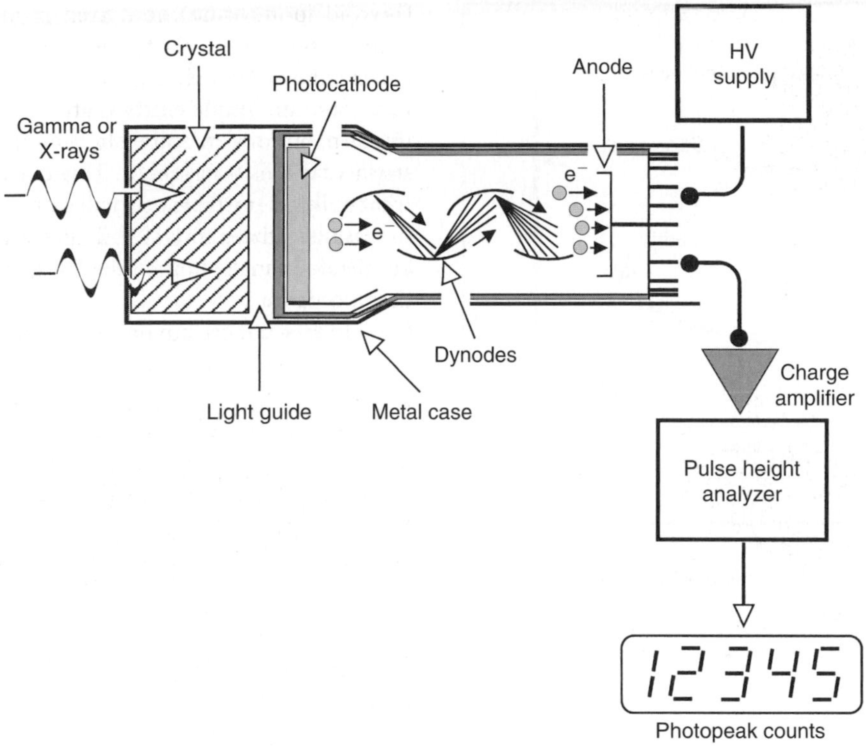

Figure 6.11 *Scintillation detector with PM tube and the associated electronic circuits: a stable high voltage, a high input impedance amplifier and a pulse height analyzer. The latter discriminates between signal amplitudes. The final output is shown as a counter display.*

The electron energy is therefore the incident minus the scattered energy 662 − 184 which is 478 keV; this value defines the Compton edge in Fig. 6.12a. Beyond the Compton edge is a Compton plateau which leads to the **photopeak** representing the energy imparted by the photoelectron, in this case 662 keV given by the single gamma photon from the ^{137}Cs decay. Multiple gamma photons would give a multi-photopeak spectrum.

A real gamma spectrum from ^{137}Cs obtained using a typical single NaI:Tl detector is shown in Fig. 6.12b. Due to statistical fluctuations (caused by thermal effects, non-uniform scintillator response, for example) the photopeak is represented not as a line spectrum but as a distribution. The magnitude of the photopeak distribution is expressed as the **energy resolution**.

ENERGY RESOLUTION

This is measured as the **full width at half maximum** (FWHM) obtained by measuring the width of the

photopeak at half its height (identified by the horizontal dotted line in Fig. 6.12b); the values for the width are 634 and 690 keV, in this example, so the resolution is

$$\frac{690 - 634}{662} = 0.08 \text{ or } 8\%$$

The best energy resolution is about 7% for a 662 keV ^{137}Cs gamma using a 7.5 × 7. 5 cm (3 × 3″) crystal. Energy resolution is slightly worse for smaller crystal detectors. A gamma camera would have an energy resolution of 10 to 14%. Energy response of the scintillator becomes nonlinear for gamma energies below 200 keV due to light output variation (about 5%).

Compton scattering causes only a fraction of the deposited energy being recorded since scatter events can escape from the crystal leaving an **escape peak**. This is commonly seen for characteristic X-rays of iodine in an NaI detector. **Backscatter** from the lead shield surrounding the detector can also re-enter the crystal causing interference peaks in the Compton part of the spectrum seen in the spectrum of Fig. 6.12b.

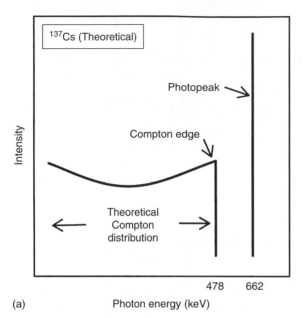

(a)

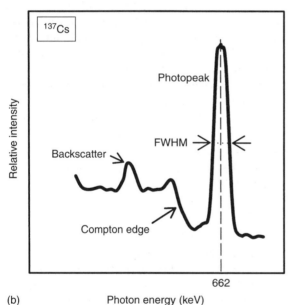

(b)

Figure 6.12 *(a) A gamma spectrum given by a perfect (theoretical) scintillator identifying the Compton event distribution and the photopeak for a gamma photon with a photopeak energy of 662 keV from ^{137}Cs. The Compton edge represents the maximum scatter energy. (b) The same spectrum but obtained from a practical NaI:Tl scintillator detector.*

THE SODIUM IODIDE DETECTOR NaI:Tl

This is the most common scintillator providing very large detector crystals for both portable machines

(thyroid monitoring) and fixed multiple detectors (whole-body counters). Large thin crystals are used for imaging radionuclide distribution in nuclear medicine. Sodium iodide emits short wavelength light in the near UV and require photomultipliers that are sensitive to this wavelength. This makes them somewhat bulky as portable or small detectors.

Cesium iodide emits visible light and can therefore be operated with a photodiode. The entire detector can then occupy a very small volume. They are used in CT scanners and certain portable radiation detectors.

6.5.3 Thermoluminescence dosimeter

The number of materials which exhibit the phenomenon of thermoluminescence is considerable but only a limited number find use in radiology. The important properties of a practical thermoluminescent phosphor are photon energy response shown in Fig. 6.13a and the main trapping center should allow light emission at around 200°C shown as the glow curve in Fig. 6.13b. The material should emit light preferably in or near the blue region of the spectrum. A list of suitable thermoluminescent materials is given in Table 6.4.

A **personal dosimeter** should absorb radiation with the same sensitivity as soft tissue; these are normally lithium based phosphors in the form of small disks or pellets. The calcium based material is less noisy at low dose rates and is ideal for monitoring low-dose rate areas in laboratories or radiology X-ray rooms. Their dose range is considerable when compared to film dosimeters.

IMAGE PLATE

The principles of thermoluminescence are utilized in the construction of the image plate, which has a similar construction to the intensifying screen shown in Fig. 6.10a. This uses a different compound from those used in dosimetry but are, in effect, large area thermoluminescence dosimeters which carry spatial (image) information. The thermoluminescent material is commonly a barium fluorohalide of the type BaFX:Eu^{2+} where X is the halide atom Cl, Br or I. Under X-ray exposure the europium ion changes from the divalent to the trivalent state Eu$^{2+} \rightarrow$ Eu^{3+}. On stimulation by light (laser) of a particular wavelength the trivalent state returns to its original divalent state releasing short wavelength light. This is described further in Chapter 7.

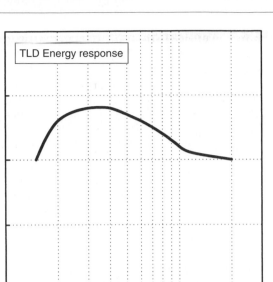

(a)

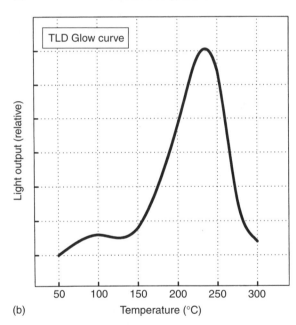

(b)

Figure 6.13 *(a) The photon energy response of a thermoluminescent detector. (b) The glow curve showing the optimum temperature for maximum light emission.*

6.6 SEMICONDUCTOR DETECTORS

The principle of the semiconductor detector has been described in Chapter 2. The depletion layer provides an excellent radiation detector, behaving very much like a parallel plate ionization chamber

Table 6.4 *Thermoluminescence dosimeter used for radiation monitoring.*

Phosphor	Application	Dose range (Gy)
LiF	Personal monitoring	10^{-5} to 10^3
$CaSO_4$:Tm	Environmental monitoring	10^{-7} to 10^2
CaF_2:Dy	Environmental monitoring	10^{-6} to 10^4
$Li_2B_4O_7$:Mn	Tissue equivalent	10^{-3} to 10^3

since electrons are generated as a result of ionizing interactions.

6.6.1 Operation

The semiconductor detector resembles an ionization chamber because it also has ionization events within the sensitive volume of the detector which is converted into a voltage pulse that is then amplified and then enters counting circuits. The amount of energy necessary to create an electron–hole pair is only about 3 eV compared to 34 eV for a gas ionization detector. Since many more charge carrying pairs are created for each keV absorbed, counting statistics are much improved. The size of the voltage pulse is proportional to the energy deposited in the detector. Compared with an ionization chamber, the voltage pulse is larger and the amplitude is photon energy sensitive. The rise time of the pulse is shorter because the ionization events are swept out of the sensitive volume more rapidly.

SIGNAL

If a charged particle, X- or gamma ray loses energy within the depletion region, electrons are raised from the valence band to the conduction band; here they migrate toward the positive n-type region layer. The holes migrate toward the negative terminal as if they were positively charged particles (see Chapter 2). The migration of positive holes in the valence band constitutes a current similar to that provided by electrons moving in the conducting band to the positive terminal. In fact, electrons released from the valence band together with the positive holes left behind constitute the ion pairs for a semiconductor detector.

NOISE

With a potential difference applied across a semiconductor, a current is present even without exposure to ionizing radiation. This current is the sum of a **bulk current** depending on the semiconductor resistance, the number of electron–hole pairs produced by thermal excitation and a charge leakage current at the surface of the semiconductor. The sum of these currents produces intrinsic noise which interferes with the signal current produced by radiation events within the detector. This total bulk current is reduced by introducing a p–n junction. The p–n junction reduces the bulk current in silicon to an acceptable level at room temperature but even with a p–n junction the bulk current in a germanium detector is far too great at room temperature. Consequently, germanium semiconductor detectors must be operated at reduced temperature, usually maintained at the temperature of liquid nitrogen ($-190°C$). The intrinsic noise in these detectors increases markedly with volume so larger volume semiconductor detectors need some form of cooling.

ENERGY

The range of pulse heights produced by the absorption of a given amount of energy is much narrower for a semiconductor detector than for a gas-filled ionization chamber or scintillation detector and so the energy resolution of the semiconductor detector is much better. The limiting factor for achieving maximum resolution with a semiconductor detector is the preamplifier itself rather than the detector.

6.6.2 Properties

The efficiency of semiconductor detectors is nearly 100% for particulate radiations and relatively high for low-energy X- and gamma rays. Semiconductor detectors exhibit many desirable properties:

- A response that varies linearly with exposure
- Independent of radiation type
- A negligible absorption of energy in the entrance window of the detector
- Excellent energy resolution
- The formation of pulses with fast rise times
- Small size

They are used for direct detection of X- or gamma rays. These detectors also respond very well to visible light and near infrared so they can be used as silicon photodiodes in conjunction with a scintillation crystal. The most recent application is as photodetectors in direct radiography flat panel detectors (Chapter 12).

6.6.3 Application

SMALL DETECTORS

Small semiconductor diode radiation detectors are simple, robust and do not need cooling. They are used in some kV_p meters and for measuring radiation doses in specific locations. Cadmium telluride is a semiconductor material manufactured in the form of small probes for measuring local activity. It gives good energy resolution and can resolve separate gamma energies.

Typical performance characteristics for X- and gamma radiation are:

- A range from $1\,\mu Gy$ to over $16\,Gy$
- A linear response with dose rate from $5\,\mu Gy\,h^{-1}$ to $3\,Gy\,h^{-1}$
- Can be calibrated better than 5%
- Rapid response time ($\approx 1\,\mu s$)
- Stable over a wide temperature range (-20 to $+80°C$)
- Not hydroscopic

However, since the mean atomic number of silicon is very different from that of air, there is variation in detector sensitivity with photon energy and they are not **tissue equivalent**.

Silicon diode detectors are used in electronic personal monitors. They give an immediate reading of the dose rate or cumulative dose and have data storage so that readings can be downloaded as a permanent dose record. The direct reading allows the worker to be aware of their immediate radiation environment.

LARGE DETECTORS

Semiconductor detectors using 'hyper-pure' germanium are used for gamma and X-ray spectrometry. They give superior resolution but require liquid nitrogen cooling (when operational). Hyper-pure germanium detectors show energy resolutions typically less than 1% for the diagnostic energy range: 1 keV at 122 keV (0.8%) and 2 keV at 1.33 MeV (0.15%). This FWHM figure is compared to a good sodium iodide detector resolution in Fig. 6.14. For X- and gamma spectroscopy larger germanium detectors are used but must be cooled to liquid nitrogen temperatures ($-190°C$) during operation to reduce noise.

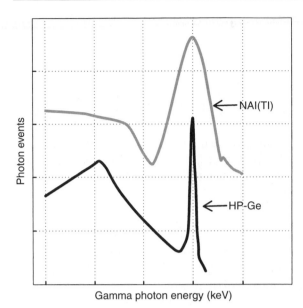

Figure 6.14 *An NaI:Tl spectrum with an energy resolution of 8 to 9% and a semiconductor (Ge) spectrum with an energy resolution of <1% compared.*

6.7 PHOTOCONDUCTIVE DETECTORS

The single most important photoconductor used as an X-ray detector in diagnostic radiology is amorphous selenium (a-Se). Unlike crystalline selenium which is a semiconductor, amorphous selenium has a very high electrical resistance but on exposure to light or ionizing radiation it becomes a photoconductor.

6.7.1 Operation

Amorphous selenium may be sensitized to X-ray radiation by applying an electric charge to its surface. When exposed to light or X-rays, the selenium plate acts as a photoconductor, generating electron–electron hole pairs which can move freely under influence of the applied electric field. This results in local discharging of the plate in areas exposed to X-rays. X-ray imaging exploits the photoconductive properties of selenium. The receptor is typically a 125 µm layer of amorphous selenium evenly deposited on an aluminum backing plate. Unlike other X-ray imaging devices the photoconductive selenium detector converts incident X-radiation directly into an electrical

signal which can be read directly after exposure; there is normally only a few seconds' delay for readout.

PREPARATION

Prior to radiographic exposure, the surface of the selenium is given a uniform positive charge. The selenium plate is kept under light-tight conditions (sealed cassette) so maintaining the charge until the X-ray exposure. However, there is a very small dark current and the surface charge leaks away with a $T_{\frac{1}{2}}$ of just over 1 h.

EXPOSURE

When the plate is exposed to X-rays, the energy absorbed from the incident photons creates electrons and holes within the bulk of the material. These charge carriers migrate towards the surfaces of the selenium layer under the influence of the internal electric field. The surface ion pattern forms a latent or **charge image** by discharging the original uniform distribution. This discharge is proportional to the radiation intensity and results in a latent charge image. In the next step the remaining charge pattern is either electrically scanned, or the charge image read by an underlying thin-film transistor matrix; each transistor has a charge collector for this purpose. Figure 6.15 shows the basic arrangement. A more detailed description is given in Chapter 12.

THE DIGITAL IMAGE

The selenium detector is more susceptible to humidity and temperature variations than the storage phosphor detector and therefore requires extensive protection from the environment.

6.7.2 Properties

The sensitivity of the selenium receptor depends upon the X-ray absorption efficiency of the selenium layer, the surface charge neutralized per unit energy absorbed. The efficiency is quite high at low photon energies due to the density ($4810\,kg\,m^{-3}$) and thickness of the plate and having a $Z = 34$ but the efficiency falls off rapidly as the photon energy increases. The K edge and fluorescent yield of selenium (12.66 keV and 0.56, respectively) are fairly low and the energy absorption efficiency does not show the large changes in efficiency associated with the K edge of materials of higher atomic number.

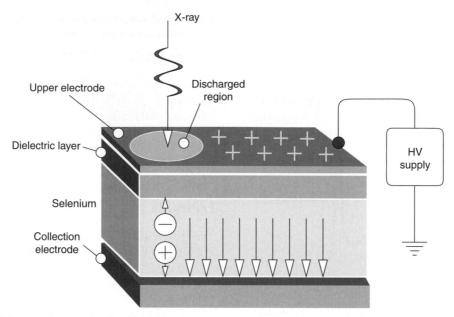

Figure 6.15 *Selenium photoconductive detector.*

6.7.3 Applications

Selenium was first used in xeroradiography. The main application for this was mammography although it also found a use in extremity radiography. Its only advantage was its high contrast sensitivity due to inherent edge enhancement: low contrast detail was very poor. Xeroradiography has disappeared into the mists of radiographic history but selenium has remained as an electronic detector in the field of digital imaging. It made its reappearance as a chest unit (Philips Thorotrast) where the charge image was read out by miniature electrodes. The most recent application has been a direct radiography flat panel detector. These are described in Chapter 12.

6.8 EFFICIENCY AND SENSITIVITY

If the detector is treated as a simple absorber it is clear from Fig. 5.1 that:

- Not every photon will interact within the detector and will be transmitted unchanged.
- Some photons will be totally absorbed by the detector.
- Some photons will scatter outside the detector volume.

The effectiveness as a detector will depend on both its linear attenuation coefficient μ, thickness x and the proportion of the photon beam that the detector surface will intersect and be absorbed within the detector volume. A further measure of a detector's efficiency, not represented in the diagram, concerns those photons that are totally absorbed and their ability to give a useful signal allowing for the detector's dead time or speed of response and ability to discriminate between a photon event and noise.

A detector's response to radiation is measured in terms of both its efficiency and sensitivity. Efficiency can be separated into three types:

- **Geometric efficiency:** the area or volume of the detector intercepting the radiation
- **Intrinsic efficiency:** the absorbing power of the detector for the particular energy radiation
- **Extrinsic efficiency:** which can be identified as the usefulness of the detector signal itself; its light output and light collection (e.g. photomultiplier assembly)

The sensitivity of a detector is a term used here for describing its response relative to photon energy and comparing it to the response given by tissue. This is a measure of its tissue equivalence and is valuable information when using a detection device for measuring radiation dose and relating detector dose measurement to real tissue dose.

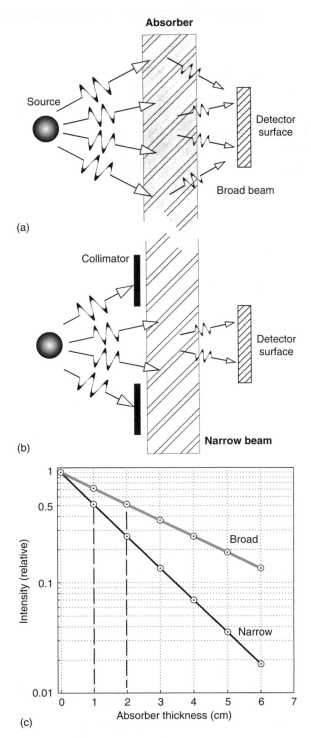

(a)

(b)

(c)

Figure 6.16 *(a) Broad-beam geometry where scatter events can interfere with detection. (b) Narrow-beam geometry using beam collimation. (c) Half-value layer for broad- and narrow-beam geometry. The HVL for the narrow beam is 1 cm whereas the HVL for the broad beam is 2 cm.*

6.8.1 Detector efficiency

BROAD- AND NARROW-BEAM GEOMETRY

Figure 6.16a and b compare the performance of broad- and narrow-beam geometry (X or gamma radiation) on a detector surface. In Fig. 6.16a an uncollimated broad beam allows scattered radiation (whose source originates outside the detector field of view) to reach the detector surface so more radiation reaches the detector than would occur with a narrow-beam geometry. A narrow beam in Fig. 6.16b is obtained by using collimators which closely restrict beam dimensions. Collimators are commonly constructed from sheet lead, 2 to 3 mm thick depending on photon energy. A narrow beam ensures that only radiation transmitted in a narrow conic section will be counted. This will be mainly primary radiation with only a small scatter component. Broad-beam geometry allows a far greater proportion of scattered radiation to enter the detector's field of view. Narrow-beam geometry is also improved by positioning the source further from the collimator, making the angle subtended by the detector surface still smaller.

Figure 6.16c shows that when the half-value layer of two identical source activities is measured, different values are obtained for the broad- and narrow-beam geometry. The broad beam appears to have a higher HVL due to the greater proportion of scattered radiation reaching the detector surface. The narrow-beam HVL measurement collects fewer of these scattered photons so gives a smaller value. Broad- and narrow-beam geometries have important implications in radiology:

- HVLs measured under broad-beam conditions are useful for calculating room shielding requirements.
- Narrow-beam geometry is important when considering patient examinations.

X-ray field sizes should always be collimated to cover the area of interest so both patient exposure is reduced and scattered radiation reaching the detector surface (film or image intensifier) is reduced. HVL measurements of X-ray equipment should always use narrow-beam geometry.

GEOMETRICAL EFFICIENCY

For a point source radiation is emitted isotropically (that is, over a spherical surface) Figure 6.17a shows that it is determined by two parameters: the effective

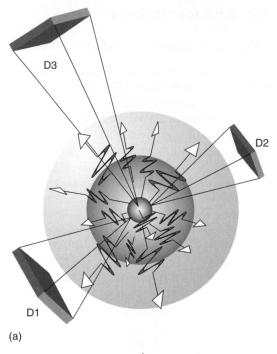

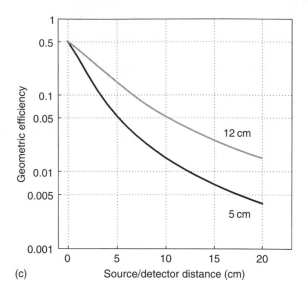

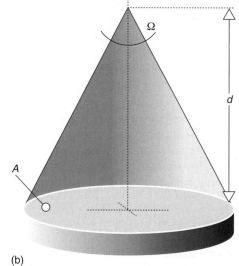

(c)

(a)

(b)

Figure 6.17 (a) 4π geometry given by an isometric source. Two detectors, D1 and D3, have the same size but the third detector, D2, is smaller. (b) 2π geometry given by a flat detector subtending the solid angle Ω. (c) The 2π geometrical efficiency for two detectors of 12 cm and 6 cm diameter.

area of the detector (D1, D2, D3) intercepting the beam and the source to detector distance. The geometry is represented diagrammatically in Fig. 6.17b and the general expression for counting an isotropic source can be stated as

$$\frac{\text{photons reaching detector}}{\text{photons emitted from source} \times 4\pi}.$$

For a large detector (D1) there will be more incident photons striking the detector surface than for a smaller

detector (D2) and a similar sized detector D3 at a greater distance will intersect fewer photons so size and distance define the solid angle (Ω) subtended by the flat detector, relative to the source:

$$\Omega = \frac{A}{d^2}$$

where A is the detector area and Ω is in steradians. For a sphere, $\Omega = 4\pi$ or 12.56 and a spherical detector would capture all the radiation; this is referred to as 4π geometry. When the source is on the surface of a flat detector, $\Omega = 2\pi$ or 6.28 steradians; this is 2π geometry and gives 50% geometrical efficiency representing a flat surface detector (e.g. gamma camera).

4π GEOMETRY

An isotropic source emits radiation over a spherical surface of 4π steradians and true 4π detectors would give a geometrical efficiency of 100% so detector efficiency E_G when counting a geometrical source is measured as

$$E_G = \frac{\Omega}{4\pi} \times 100\%$$

Very few detectors approach anywhere near 4π geometry in radiology. The exception is the dose calibrator where accurate measurement of radioactivity is necessary for patient radiopharmaceutical injections. The detector used is a hollow cylinder which allows the sample to be placed in the center of the detecting volume (gas); the design shown in Fig. 6.3a.

2π GEOMETRY

If the radiation source is placed on a large flat detector (e.g. a gamma camera crystal) so that the radiation over a hemisphere is subtended by the detector then this will have 50% geometrical efficiency and show 2π geometry. Clearly, from Fig. 6.17b, a large area detector and a short distance are desirable making Ω large but practical limitations are imposed by the detector encapsulation and shielding, for example.

A practical formula for calculating geometrical efficiency E_G for a point source with 2π detector geometry is

$$E_G = 0.5 \times \left(1 - \frac{h}{\sqrt{h^2 + d^2}}\right)$$

where these parameters are identified in Fig. 6.17b. This function is plotted in Fig. 6.17c for two sizes of detector, both show 2π efficiency (50%) with the source on the detector surface (0 cm) but the larger detector (12 cm) maintains a higher geometrical efficiency than the smaller (5 cm) at distance from the source. At a point 5 cm from the source the smaller detector intersects only 5% of the radiation whereas the larger detector intersects approximately 12%.

6.8.2 Detector intrinsic efficiency

QUANTUM EFFICIENCY

The ability to absorb incident photons is a measure of detector quantum efficiency and is the fraction of incident photons that are absorbed by the detector. It should not be confused with detective quantum efficiency (DQE) described in Chapter 8. Detector quantum efficiency (E_Q) is measured as

$$E_Q = 1 - e^{-\mu x_d}$$

where μ is the linear attenuation coefficient and x_d the detector thickness. Since μ is dependent on photon energy, there are three parameters influencing quantum efficiency:

1 Linear attenuation coefficient of the detector material
2 Detector thickness
3 Photon energy

Overall detector quantum efficiency is also modified by the shielding material surrounding the detector volume such as the input window (aluminum, glass, titanium etc.) and any collimation or grids which would also absorb incident radiation, so E_Q is modified so that

$$E_Q = e^{-\mu x_w} \times (1 - e^{-\mu x_d})$$

where μx_w is the attenuation coefficient and thickness of the covering material.

6.8.3 Detector extrinsic efficiency

CONVERSION EFFICIENCY

Photons absorbed by the detector must contribute to a measurable signal, either electrical or light. The conversion efficiency E_C compares the available photon energy with the energy absorbed in the detector. If all the photon energy is utilized (provides a signal) there will be a conversion efficiency of 1.0, but some energy of the incident photon is carried by secondary photons which can scatter outside the detector volume reducing E_C to a value less than 1.0. Compton interactions do not contribute a useful signal but they may end in a photoelectric event which does contribute.

Conversion efficiencies of gas detectors may be quite high particularly if gas amplification takes place

(Geiger counter). The quantum efficiency of a gas detector is, however, low so a measure of total efficiency is required; this is simply

$$E_T = E_Q \times E_C$$

Box 6.2 gives some worked examples of total efficiency, comparing various detector types.

DEAD TIME

The intrinsic efficiency of a detector decreases with increasing count rate due to the inability to handle high count rates. Consequently there is pulse pile-up due to dead time τ which can be expressed as

$$\tau = \frac{\text{detected signals}}{\text{total incident photons}}$$

The effect of dead time on detector response is shown graphically in Fig. 6.18. The value differs considerably between the different types of counter.

The largest dead times are shown by gas detectors where the presence of ionization events from previous interactions blocks further signals until these events are neutralized; some gas detectors (Geiger counters) having long dead times (300 μs) but scintillation detectors have very short dead times (0.22 μs). If a detector with dead time τ indicates a count rate of N then the true count rate N_T is

$$N_T = \frac{N}{1 - N\tau}$$

For slow count rates dead-time correction is negligible but as Fig. 6.18 shows, at higher count rates significant loss of information is possible. For a Geiger counter with a dead time of 300 μs which indicates a count rate of 1000 cps, the true count rate would be

$$N_T = \frac{1000}{1 - (1000 \times 0.0003)} = 1428$$

so for this count rate a Geiger counter would underestimate the count rate by nearly 50%. On the other hand a scintillation detector with a much shorter dead time of 0.22 μs and an indicated count rate of 100 000 cps would give an under-estimation of only 2%.

Box 6.2 Total efficiency of detectors

$$E_T = E_Q \times E_C$$

Gas detector with gas amplification

If E_Q is 0.01 and E_C is 1.0 then E_T is 1%.

Scintillation detector (NaI:Tl)

If E_Q is 0.8 and E_C is 0.5 then E_T is 40%.

Intensifying screens (two thicknesses and different materials)

For screen 1, if E_Q is 0.4 and E_C is 0.5 then E_T is 20%.

For screen 2, if E_Q is 0.25 and E_C 0.8 then E_T is 20%.

Although the two screens give identical total efficiencies the first screen is thicker, giving it a higher E_Q, but it has poorer resolution than the second screen, which has a thinner screen but higher E_C.

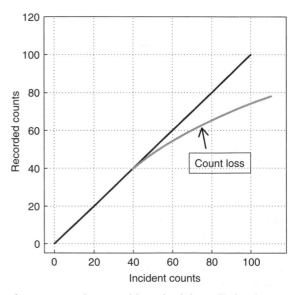

Figure 6.18 *A detector with no dead time will give the same detected counts as incident counts for all count rates (straight line). A nonlinear response will be seen when fast count events are not resolved and detected counts are less than incident counts above a certain count rate.*

ENERGY RESOLUTION

Detectors that are able to give individual photon event signals such as the proportional counter, the scintillation detector and the semiconductor detector are photon energy sensitive, that is the pulse height is proportional to photon energy. A pulse height discriminator as shown in Fig. 6.11 enables a photon energy spectrum to be generated. The energy resolution, as a percentage, is measured as FWHM.

Scintillation detectors give a typical energy resolution of about 8 to 9% already seen in Fig. 6.14. This figure includes crystal and photomultiplier resolution. Non-uniformity in crystal response is due to dispersion within the crystal giving loss of useful light. Spectrometers resolving power is poorer at lower energies so ^{137}Cs (662 keV) is commonly used as a standard for resolution measurements.

The **intrinsic peak efficiency** of an energy sensitive detector is the fraction of gamma photons represented within the photopeak distribution. Electrical noise in the photomultiplier amplifier chain also contributes to loss of resolution.

The proportional counter gives a similar energy resolution but the semiconductor detector typically gives resolution figures of <1% across the energy range but since its density is lower than the scintillation crystals its efficiency is much lower, being about 20 to 30% that of NaI:Tl.

6.8.4 Sensitivity

The absorbed dose has already been defined in Chapter 5. Detector sensitivity is determined by comparing the mass absorption coefficient of the detector material with that of air which is a measure of the energy (radiation dose) absorbed by the detector material per unit of absorbed dose in air (μ_{ab}/ρ for air).

Relative sensitivity or response is measured by comparing this value with the detector's own absorption coefficient (μ_{ab}/ρ for the detector). If these two absorption coefficients are the same for the diagnostic energy range then the detector will have the same sensitivity. Figure 6.19 shows that soft tissue and air have similar sensitivity or response over the diagnostic range. So radiation dose measured by an air ion detector will be representative of tissue radiation dose. Detector materials that have a mean atomic number close to soft tissue will show **tissue equivalence**.

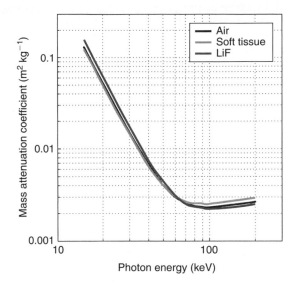

Figure 6.19 *Mass absorption coefficient for air, soft tissue, and LiF over the diagnostic energy range showing tissue equivalence.*

The value of the effective atomic number Z_{eff} for soft tissue is 7.64; for air, 7.78; and for water, 7.51; air and water are therefore tissue equivalent (see Fig. 6.19). Lithium fluoride, used as a personal radiation dosimeter has a Z value of 8.31 and is also treated as tissue equivalent. Film emulsion, however, has a mean Z value exceeding 35.0 so would have a significantly different sensitivity response to radiation (including K-edge differences) and would not be tissue equivalent.

KEYWORDS

2π geometry: relating to a flat detector surface e.g. a gamma camera

4π geometry: relating to a volume detector e.g. dose calibrator

becquerel: a measure of radionuclide activity in disintegrations per second (1 dps = 1 Bq)

broad beam: an uncollimated radiation beam (X-rays or gamma)

Compton edge: the edge of the gamma spectrum representing 180° scatter

dead time: the speed of response of a detector for counting individual events. Usually measured at a 20% count loss

efficiency (conversion): the efficiency of signal (e.g. light) production in a detector

efficiency (geometrical): the fraction of the isotropic emission collected by the detector surface

efficiency (quantum): a measure of photon absorption

energy resolution: measured as FWHM of the photopeak

luminescence: a general property of some inorganic crystals and plastics involving electron transition between valency and conduction bands

narrow beam: a collimated radiation beam

photomultiplier: a light sensitive device for amplifying very small light signals

photopeak: the part of the gamma spectrum which identifies the photoelectric event. This represents the peak gamma energy

scintillator: a crystalline or liquid compound which exhibits luminescence

sensitivity: the response of a detector to different photon energies

tissue equivalent: having the same sensitivity to photon energy as soft tissue

Photography and the film image

7.1 THE PHOTOGRAPHIC PRINCIPLE

Film is the most common hard copy used in radiology. Although departments are striving to introduce a film-less service with all the theoretical benefits of low cost and security, the demand for an easily portable, high quality image will maintain film as the display medium of choice for the next few years.

The film emulsion has been successively refined for radiology and is used in X-ray imaging with and without screens, video recording, cine recording and film records from image plates.

7.1.1 The film emulsion

A film emulsion is a mixture of silver halides suspended in gelatin. The silver halide is the light sensitive compound and the gelatin acts both as a supporting material and takes part in the photo chemistry.

SILVER HALIDES

Silver chloride (AgCl), bromide (AgBr) and iodide (AgI) are used in various mixtures to alter the sensitivity of the film. The order of light sensitivity is:

AgBr greater than **AgCl** greater than **AgI**

They have a cuboid crystal structure shown in Fig. 7.1a and are formed by reacting silver nitrate with alkali halides:

$$AgNO_3 + (KBr \text{ or } NaCl \text{ or } KI)$$
$$\rightarrow AgBr \text{ or } AgCl \text{ or } AgI$$

PHOTOSENSITIVITY

This increases with the amount of added silver iodide but rarely exceeds 8% of the silver bromide content. In preparing the silver halide the silver iodide crystallizes first forming nuclei for the silver bromide which then forms the larger crystals (grains).

GELATIN

This is the suspending medium for the photochemical mix during the formation of the silver halides (described above). It also separates the crystals or grains. Various control parameters at this stage influence **grain size**. After grain formation the suspension of silver halides in gelatin undergoes a series of ripening processes which introduces a small proportion of silver sulfide from free sulfur present in the gelatin. These Ag_2S crystal defects act as an important **sensitivity centers** in the silver halide crystal and have significant effects on the speed of the film. Their average concentration is about 1:1 000 000. Greater concentration will increase background darkening or emulsion fog. Modern emulsion uses purified gelatin with controlled amounts of sensitizers (sulfur) added during the course of preparation.

EMULSION CONSTRUCTION

Overall formation of the film emulsion involves:

* Reacting alkali halides with silver nitrate in the gelatin

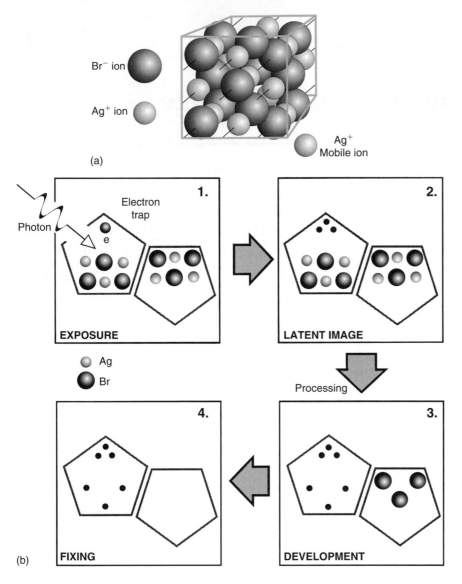

Figure 7.1 (a) The construction of the AgBr crystal showing the cuboid structure and positioning of silver and bromine atoms in the compound; a mobile interstitial silver ion is within the crystal structure. (b) The photographic action (1, 2) of light exposure and latent image formation. After development (3) silver atoms are separated in the exposed crystals. The fixed image (4) has remaining silver halide removed (see description in the text).

- Physical ripening: emulsion stirring to increase grain size
- Chemical or after-ripening: sensitive-center formation
- Additional compounds: optical sensitizers (see below), stabilizers to maintain properties through aging, hardening agents to protect the emulsion surface

OPTICAL SENSITIZERS

The emulsion in its first stage of manufacture is only sensitive to the blue/ultraviolet part of the light spectrum. Small quantities of optical sensitizers are added to increase sensitivity to the green/yellow/red end of the spectrum.

7.1.2 The photochemical process

The silver halide crystal in its pure form consists of alternate atoms of silver and bromine arranged in a cuboid lattice (Fig. 7.1a). **Interstitial silver ions** can move within the crystal lattice towards negative electron traps which are positively charged. The lattice silver and bromine atoms are fixed. Individual silver halide crystals within the emulsion contain:

- Interstitial silver ions which are mobile and positively charged
- A number of electron traps, defects or sensitivity centers, usually in the form of silver sulfide, which are formed from sulfur in the gelatin during the ripening process (Fig. 7.1b)

EXPOSURE TO LIGHT

When the emulsion is exposed to light the photon excites a bromine atom in the crystal, which loses an electron (Fig. 7.1b). The liberated electron is trapped in the crystal defect. The free bromine, which is formed, escapes into the gelatin and is held there. Neighboring unexposed crystals are unaffected.

All the free electrons produced by light photons are trapped in these centers. The positive charged interstitial silver ions are then attracted to these increasingly negative defect centers neutralized by the accumulated negative charges and become silver atoms.

Thus the sensitivity sites become concentrations of silver atoms which are potential **development centers** carrying information in the form of a **latent image**; Stage 1 in Fig. 7.1b shows these interstitial silver atoms joining the electron trap and forming a complete latent image.

DEVELOPING

This process magnifies the latent image by reducing the remaining AgBr in the exposed crystal to silver and giving the developed image as Stage 2 in Fig. 7.1b. Developers usually contain ring compounds of hydroquinone, amitol or metol. The reaction is:

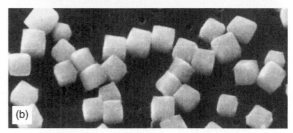

Original developer   *Oxidized developer*

The AgBr in this reaction is the exposed or activated silver halide which is reduced to silver, leaving the developer in an oxidized state which is no longer active. Latent image silver atoms cause the entire silver halide crystal or grain to be reduced to silver so when the emulsion has been completely developed

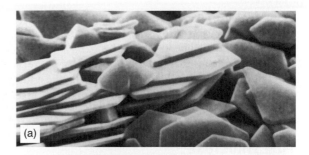

Figure 7.2 *Two crystal formations, flat T-grain and cuboid found in current radiography emulsions.*

it will consist of:

- Silver halide crystals reduced completely to silver atoms representing amplified latent image information
- Unexposed and unaltered silver halide crystals

This is the developed image: Stage 3 in Fig. 7.1b.

FIXING

After development the silver halide emulsion is desensitized by fixing the image, this is the final Stage 4 in Fig. 7.1b. The fixer compound is ammonium thiosulfate $(NH_4)_2S_2O_3$ which removes the unexposed, unaltered silver halide as a soluble complex:

$$Ag^+Br^- + (S_2O_3)^{2-} \rightarrow Ag(S_2O_3)^- + Br^-$$

The silver thiosulfate complex is carried out of the emulsion when the film is thoroughly washed with clean water. This complex is still light sensitive and will slowly decompose leaving a silver deposit on the film image in poorly washed films which is the main cause of darkening and consequent deterioration of archived films.

GRAIN (CRYSTAL) SIZE

An enlarged picture of silver halide grains is shown in Fig. 7.2. The grain affects the film image in four ways:

1. Large grain sizes increase **film sensitivity** because more silver atoms are produced from each light photon.

2 **Resolution** is degraded by large grain sizes because the large area will intercept more photons, fine image detail will be lost.

3 The **contrast** of the film is influenced by the variety of grain sizes: mixed grain size will give a low contrast; single grain size will give a high contrast.

4 Large grains are visible as **mottle** on the final image.

FILM STRUCTURE

Films used for radiography usually consist of a polyester base onto which the silver halide emulsion is spread. **Single-** or **double-sided** emulsion layers can be provided for different applications. Figure 7.3a shows a four layer single-sided emulsion and a seven layer double emulsion film. The four layers of a single emulsion film are:

• The supporting polyester **base**
• The **sub-coating** which ensures the emulsion adheres to the film base
• The halide **emulsion** itself
• The **protective coating** which protects emulsion from mechanical damage

The single-emulsion film is used for recording high definition images such as mammographs or electronic displays (cathode ray tube (CRT) or laser imagers). Double-sided film is designed for cassettes that have dual intensifying screens. It increases efficiency but has poorer resolution.

The polyester base offers important properties:

• Strength and tear resistant
• Waterproof
• Dimensional stability and flatness
• Non-flammable
• Good aging properties for archiving

Conventional **screen film** has a thin emulsion layer designed for automatic processing. The thinner emulsion gives:

• Shorter development and fixing times
• More efficient washing (removing practically all of the resident chemicals)
• Rapid drying

Non-screen film has thicker emulsion which is more sensitive to X-radiation. It is sometimes used for very high resolution work (bone imaging) and should not be used in automatic processors, since this will damage its thicker emulsion layer.

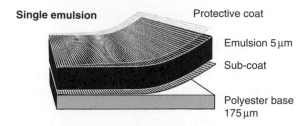
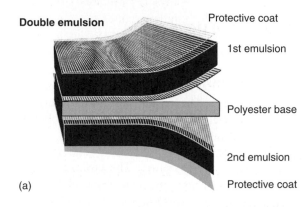
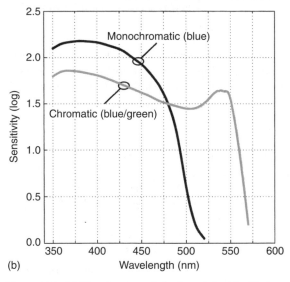

(a)

(b)

Figure 7.3 *(a) Film structure of single and double sided emulsions. Only the film base and emulsion are shown; the two coatings are omitted for clarity. (b) Film response to different light wavelengths for monochromatic (blue) and orthochromatic (green) light.*

OPTICAL SENSITIZERS

These are added to film emulsion in order to extend the sensitivity to longer wavelength light, so that the film type can be manufactured closely matching the light output from intensifying screen phosphors used in the cassette. The spectral sensitivity for two film types, **monochromatic** (blue) and **orthochromatic** (blue/green) are shown in Fig. 7.3b.

MONOCHROMATIC FILM

The natural sensitivity of silver halide emulsion, without sensitizer, is for the UV and blue part of the light spectrum. This film type is used for blue emitting intensifying screens i.e. tungstate, lanthanum, barium or yttrium based screens.

ORTHOCHROMATIC

The film response is extended into the green portion of the spectrum by adding optical sensitizers to the film emulsion. Rare-earth gadolinium intensifying screens require orthochromatic film since they emit green light. Mixed screens of lanthanum and gadolinium use the full sensitivity of ortho-film by supplying both green and blue light; this increases sensitivity.

PANCHROMATIC

This film type is sensitive to the entire visible spectrum and is not commonly met in radiology except in cine fluorography which uses commercial panchromatic 35 mm cine film.

FILM STORAGE

As unexposed film ages certain chemical and thermal changes occur in the emulsion which increase background fog levels. Ideal storage conditions for unexposed film are a maximum temperature of 20°C with a relative humidity of 50%. Cold storage can lengthen the useful life of a film which can have significant effects in hot climates. Exposed but unprocessed film deteriorates gradually, losing low contrast detail, unless placed in cold storage.

If either unexposed or exposed film is kept in a cassette its sensitivity to background radiation will be increased considerably (due to light emission from the intensifying screen) and its fog level will increase over time. Cassettes loaded with film for immediate use should be shielded from X-ray scatter or placed at some distance from the X-ray machine.

Exposed and processed film is stable and providing it has been processed properly (adequately fixed and washed) and stored under the same conditions as unexposed film it should retain its image detail for two to three decades before low contrast information is lost.

SUMMARY

- Film emulsion consists of AgBr + AgI in gelatin. AgBr is the major ingredient.
- AgI enhances sensitivity (8% maximum concentration).
- A gelatin base keeps silver halide as separate crystals. Small sulfur impurities in gelatin form silver sulfide sensitivity centers or defects which increases sensitivity.
- Gelatin acts as a bromine receptor.
- Emulsion ripening: increases grain size and sensitivity.
- Exposure to light forms free electrons: $hf \rightarrow Br^- \rightarrow Br + e^-$
- Sensitivity centers absorb the free electrons forming regions of negative charge within the exposed crystal.
- Mobile silver ions migrate to these negative sensitivity centers where they are neutralized and form silver atoms.
- Defects holding the silver atoms contain latent image information and become development centers.
- Developing amplifies the latent image by reducing all the remaining AgBr in the silver halide grain to silver.
- Fixing removes unexposed silver halide as a soluble complex.
- Grain size affects sensitivity; large grains are more sensitive (contrast) but reduce resolution (graininess).
- Mixed grain size has greater latitude (low contrast).

7.2 FILM SENSITOMETRY

Film was originally constructed for recording changes in light intensity (L.J. Daguerre, 1789–1851; French physicist and inventor, and W.H. Fox-Talbot, 1800–77; British scientist). The relative sensitivity of film to light and X-rays is shown in Fig. 7.4. It is shown to have a sensitivity to very low light levels but is relatively insensitive to X-ray exposure, although it does have a useful linear response to X- and gamma radiation exposure which is utilized for measuring radiation dose as a film dosimeter. Film's most sensitive

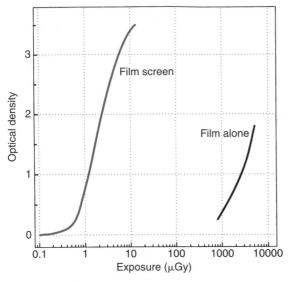

Figure 7.4 *Film's high sensitivity for light as compared to the low sensitivity for X-ray photons. However, the X-ray response is linear which is useful for measuring radiation dose.*

region is in the blue spectrum; optical sensitizers extend the response toward green as already described.

INTENSIFYING SCREENS

In order to improve the efficiency for recording X-ray information a phosphor intensifying screen which converts X-rays to light is interposed between the X-ray beam and film. The screen is a phosphor scintillator and converts high energy X-ray photons into lower energy visible light photons; the light wavelength depends on the phosphor type.

7.2.1 Film characteristics

The **characteristic curves** plotting film response (or density) against exposure, shown in Fig. 7.4, compare the sensitivities between an X-ray exposure made with and without intensifying screens. A significant increase in sensitivity is obvious when screens are used and the film exposed to light, but only a section of the curve retains linearity.

Although Röntgen first observed the effect of X-rays when they reacted with a phosphor (barium platino-cyanide), the introduction of practical phosphor intensifying screens to radiography was made in 1896 by T.A. Edison (1847–1931; American inventor).

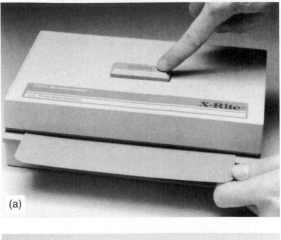

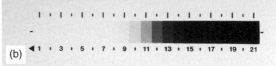

Figure 7.5 *(a) A light sensitometer with a carefully calibrated illuminated gray scale exposing a strip of film (courtesy X-Rite). (b) A sensitometric gray scale obtained from a calibrated sensitometer directly exposing film to either blue or green light.*

His intensifying screens were responsible for increased sensitivity and a significant reduction in patient dose during radiological investigations.

LIGHT SENSITOMETRY

Film characteristics are best obtained by illuminating the film with a calibrated gray scale from a **sensitometer**, Fig. 7.5a. If the gray-scale densities are plotted against exposure then a film **characteristic curve** is obtained. The characteristic curve for a film obtained from a light sensitometer is shown in Fig. 7.5b. The different steps are measured using a calibrated spot **densitometer** shown in Fig. 7.6a. The characteristic curve obtained under these conditions is shown as a sigma shaped curve in Fig. 7.6b. The densitometer calculates each optical density (OD) as:

$$OD = \log_{10} \frac{I_0}{I} \qquad (7.1)$$

where I_0 is the reference intensity of the incident light source and I the intensity through the exposed section of the film (wedge step). If the log relative exposure level is plotted on the x-axis and the resultant optical density (D) plotted on the y-axis then a characteristic

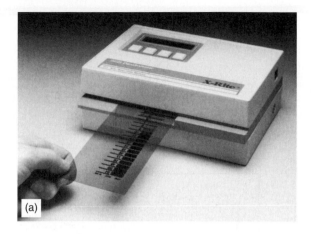

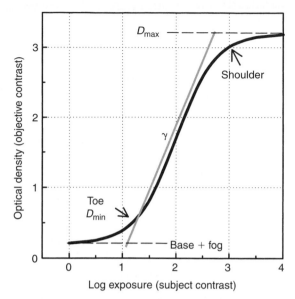

Figure 7.7 *The component parts of the film characteristic curve showing the minimum optical density (D$_{min}$) and a base/fog level. The maximum optical density (D$_{max}$) occurs at the shoulder region of the sigmoid curve. The slope (gamma) of the straight section of the curve is a measure of latitude or dynamic range.*

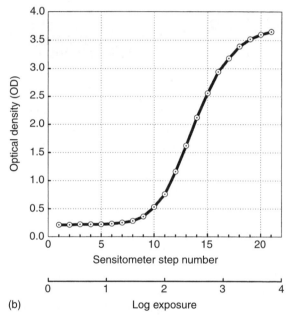

Figure 7.6 *(a) A densitometer reading the exposed and developed gray scale test strip (courtesy X-Rite). (b) The characteristic curve generated by the densitometer showing the response of a film to light, plotting log exposure against optical density.*

curve is obtained which describes the film quantitative response to light and reveals many important film qualities.

An early name for the characteristic curve was the H & D curve after F. Hurter (1844–98; Swiss) and V.C. Driffield (1848–1915; American). The curve is now commonly called the *D/*log *E* curve. Figure 7.7 shows the distinguishing parts:

- The **fog level** is a density reading of the background noise caused mainly by thermal effects; it can also result from high radiation background levels (unshielded storage conditions).
- The **threshold value** marks the lowest exposure that gives a density value above the fog level.
- The **toe** region is the low exposure nonlinear portion of the curve seen in the radiograph in denser tissue: bone, heart shadow and diaphragm.
- The straight line or **slope** of the curve describes the most important property of the film since it carries most information about soft tissue detail as seen in the lung fields and most clearly in mammography. The steeper this portion of the curve the more **contrast** will the film image have.
- The **shoulder** region enters another nonlinear response where all the film grains have been saturated and maximum density is seen (black); hollow regions of the anatomy (gut) and gas (pneumothorax) are radiographic examples.

X-RAY SENSITOMETRY

The response of X-ray film alone can be investigated with a light sensitometer which exposes the film to an illuminated, exactly calibrated, step wedge. Figure 7.5(b) shows the gray scale obtained when the film is developed. In order to measure the response of a **film-screen** combination to radiation it is necessary to expose it to a graded radiation intensity. This is commonly achieved by using an X-ray source and a stepped aluminum wedge but this is not ideal since the X-ray beam undergoes non-uniform filtration through the increasing thicknesses of aluminum. This can be solved to some extent by hardening the beam with added filtration but a more consistent X-ray exposure is made when (for a fixed value of kV and mAs) a lead screen is moved a fixed series of distances over the cassette creating a stepped series of exposures. At the end of the exposure sequence the first strip has seen the most radiation and the last strip has seen one exposure. Beam quality remains constant throughout this method.

As with light sensitometry, exposure is represented on the x-axis of the characteristic curve as the radiation intensity per unit time:

$$E = I \times t \qquad (7.2)$$

The value E is usually a relative measure of exposure. Optical density is directly related to X-radiation exposure E from eqn 7.2 measured in mAs ($I \times t$). Under film-screen conditions **optical density** is proportional to **exposure** as measured by the product of X-ray tube current and time (**mAs**) in the above equation. Optical density is a logarithmic product of transmitted intensities (eqn 7.1). When using an X-ray exposure on a film-screen combination, the exposure values on the characteristic curve are represented by a logarithmic quantity $\log_{10} E$ which encompasses a wide range of exposure levels representing the exponential absorption of radiation. The characteristic curve is therefore a plot of **density** versus relative **log exposure**; this is a representative measure of subject contrast whereas optical density is an objective measure.

7.2.2 Film optical density (OD)

OPTICAL DENSITY

If I_0 is the light intensity of the film viewing box and I is the intensity transmitted by an area of exposed film then its optical density is described by eqn 7.1. Allocating a value of 1000 for I_0 and 100 for I then the film's optical density is $\log_{10} 1000/100$ or 1.0. An optical density equal to 1.0 represents a medium gray level.

The optical density measurement is independent of the incident (viewing box) intensity. Table 7.1 gives

Table 7.1 *Optical density and log intensity.*

Fraction transmitted	$\log_{10}$ value	Optical density
1.0	log 1.0	0.0
0.5	log 0.5	0.3
0.1	log 10	1.0
0.01	log 100	2.0
0.001	log 1000	3.0
0.0001	log 10 000	4.0

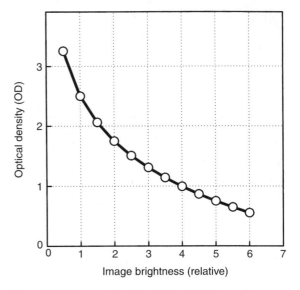

Figure 7.8 *The logarithmic relationship between image brightness and film optical density.*

examples of the logarithmic scale of light intensity transmitted through a gray-scale film image and Fig. 7.8 plots image brightness against optical density showing the logarithmic response.

The response of the eye to different light intensities is also logarithmic so the objective measurement of density agrees with the subjective assessment by the eye. This table shows that an increase in density of 0.3 reduces the transmitted light intensity by half.

Useful densities seen in radiographs range between 0.2 and 2.0. Lung areas where little absorption has taken place are between 2.5 and 3.0; densities higher than this carry little information. Denser areas of the mediastinum are between 0.2 and 1.0.

7.2.3 Exposure latitude

Figure 7.9a and b shows two characteristic curves. Film (a) is a high contrast film requiring only a narrow

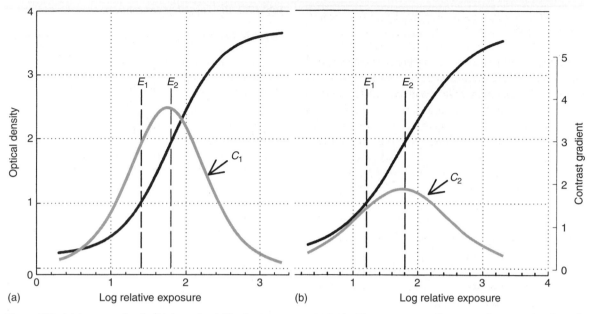

Figure 7.9 *(a) An example of a high contrast film having narrow latitude. The contrast gradient curve has a peak value of 2.5 (right hand y-axis). Points E₁ and E₂ are used in Box 7.1. (b) A low contrast film having a wider latitude. The contrast gradient peak value is 1.6.*

exposure range to achieve this optical density difference whereas the film in (b) requires an increased exposure range. The film in (a) has a steeper straight line or slope and so will give more rapid density changes for a given narrow range of exposures.

The film in (b) has a longer slope and has less contrast than film (a) for the same exposure; it has a wider **latitude** than (a).

The slope of the straight portion of the characteristic curve gives a measure of the film contrast (see Fig. 7.7). The steeper this slope the greater the range of optical densities for a small change in exposure levels. This slope is measured as the gamma (γ) and can be defined:

$$\gamma = \frac{D_2 - D_1}{\log E_2 - \log E_1} \qquad (7.3)$$

The measures D_1 and D_2 used in eqn 7.3 are the film densities obtained from exposures E_1 and E_2 represented in Fig. 7.9a and b. A large value of γ has a high contrast useful for imaging a narrow range of tissue densities and so accentuating any small differences between normal and abnormal states e.g. mammography. Film (b) with a wider latitude (smaller γ) is useful for imaging mixed tissue types with a broader range of attenuation coefficients such as chest radiography.

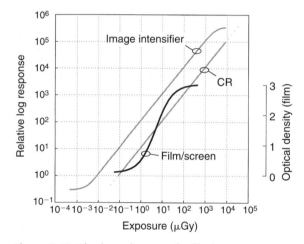

Figure 7.10 *The dynamic range of a film/screen system compared to an image intensifier and computed radiography (CR) or image plate.*

So high contrast film will image small differences in tissue attenuation while low contrast (wide latitude) film will image a wider variety of tissue densities. Film latitude is therefore a measure of the film's **dynamic range**. The dynamic range of a film/screen response is very restrictive when compared to other X-ray imaging technologies. Figure 7.10 superimposes the sigma curve response of a film-screen with the linear

Box 7.1 Contrast differences in Fig. 7.9

Calculations are for the same density difference, ΔD, of $D_2 - D_1 = 2 - 1 = 1$.

High contrast film (Fig. 7.9a) requires an exposure difference $\Delta \log E$: $\log E_1$ of 1.4 and $\log E_2$ of 1.8:

$$\gamma = \frac{\Delta D}{\Delta \log E} = \frac{1}{0.4} = 2.5$$

where γ is the contrast.

Low contrast film (Fig. 7.9b) requires an exposure $\log E_1$ of 1.2 and $\log E_2$ of 1.8, so

$$\gamma = \frac{\Delta D}{\Delta \log E} = \frac{1}{0.6} = 1.66$$

Therefore the high contrast film gives a contrast range of almost $\times 1.5$ that of the low contrast film.

The contrast gradient peaks C_1 and C_2 in Fig. 7.9a and b reflect these calculated values (right hand y-axis).

Table 7.2 *Divisions of image contrast.*

Subject contrast
- Kilovoltage
- Attenuation coefficient (μ)
- Scatter (tissue thickness x)
- Beam filtration

Radiographic contrast
- Film type (emulsion, grain size)
- Film gamma (γ)
- Film processor (developer temperature, processing time)
- Screen type (rare earth etc.)
- Grid type

Objective contrast
Optical density

Subjective contrast
- Film viewer
- Light color
- Masking

responses of an image intensifier and an image plate (computer radiography (CR)). The useful range of a film-screen is about 1.5 orders of magnitude while the image intensifier and CR show a useful range exceeding 4 orders of magnitude. Quite low exposure levels therefore will yield an image which would not be recorded by a film-screen system.

CONTRAST GRADIENT CURVE

This gives the film contrast value for all parts of the characteristic curve by taking the contrast differential of the slope. Its peak value corresponds to the center of the characteristic curve.

Contrast gradient curves (C1 and C2) indicate the magnitude of film contrast in Fig. 7.9 (a) and (b). The first characteristic curve is steep so has a larger peak value for C1. The second curve has a wider latitude and a smaller peak contrast value C2. The peak values of C1 and C2 correspond to the γ values calculated in Box 7.1 (allowing for rounding errors).

FILM AND VISUAL CONTRAST

The film gamma, or slope, is a measure of film contrast; a typical value being about 3. Since contrast

difference C is $D_2 - D_1$ this can be rewritten from eqn 7.3 as:

$$C = \gamma(\log E_1 - \log E_2) \qquad (7.4)$$

Visual contrast between two light intensities I_1 and I_2 is appreciated as a logarithmic scale:

$$\text{visual contrast} = \log I_2 - \log I_1 \qquad (7.5)$$

Since the two exposures E_1 and E_2 were obtained from two X-ray intensities the visual contrast can be expressed as

$$\text{visual contrast} = \gamma(\log I_2 - \log I_1) \qquad (7.6)$$

This demonstrates that film contrast has a similar logarithmic response to visual contrast.

Table 7.2 lists the four major types of contrast which influence image quality: subject, radiographic, objective and subjective contrast. These all influence the visibility of low contrast detail in a diagnostic image.

From the characteristic curves shown in Fig. 7.9a and b the x-axis represents log exposure values $\Delta \log E$ and is influenced by **subject contrast**, in other words those factors which control the exit radiation dose (kV, μ, thickness etc.), and ΔD (y-axis) represents **objective contrast**, the quantitative measure of film optical density.

Box 7.2 Film sensitivity and speed

Film sensitivity

The film in Fig. 7.9a requires an exposure level of 1.4 to obtain an OD of 1.0 and an exposure of 1.8 for an OD of 2.0. The $\Delta \log E = 0.4$. The anti-log of this is $10^{0.4} = 2.5$ so an OD of 2.0 for this film will require $\times 2.5$ increased exposure over OD 1.0 (e.g. from 20 to 50 mAs).

Film speed

Films A and B in Fig. 7.11 require an exposure $\log E_A$ of 1.6 and $\log E_B$ of 2.0 for the same reference density (OD = 1.0). The difference, $\log E_B - \log E_A = 0.4$. Converting from log values: $10^{0.4} = 2.5$. So film A is $\times 2.5$ faster than film B.

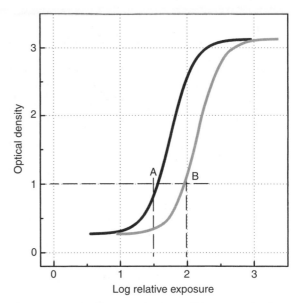

Figure 7.11 *The films A and B have different speeds; film A is more sensitive, or faster, than B.*

7.2.4 Sensitivity (film speed)

Figure 7.11 shows two characteristic curves, A and B, having identical gammas but the curve for film B is displaced further to the right since film A responds to lower exposure levels: it is more sensitive than film B; it is a **faster** film.

Fast films will be displaced to the left, slow films to the right on the x-axis. A mid-point density value of 1.0 is usually chosen to measure relative film speeds. Box 7.2 calculates the increased exposure necessary for higher film densities and film speed. The faster film in Fig. 7.11 will require less radiation to achieve the same optical densities as the slower film.

7.2.5 Film processing

DEVELOPING TIME AND DEVELOPER TEMPERATURE

The characteristic curve changes for different developer times and temperatures. The change for developing temperature is shown in Fig. 7.12a. Both the slope (contrast) and position of the curve (speed) alter along with an increase in the level of base + fog. There are optimal conditions for each film type and in order to maximize film contrast and speed the manufacturer's recommended temperatures and processor timing should be adhered to. Most daylight film processors have their timing fixed to suit either 90 s or 3 min processing cycles but the temperature can be easily adjusted; the optimal setting is typically between 33°C and 36°C.

Higher developer temperature increases film contrast sensitivity (speed); as a consequence X-ray exposure can be reduced so the patient **radiation exposure** is similarly reduced. This is a most important factor particularly in mammography and pediatric examinations where patient dose must be held at minimum levels. There is a limit to these increases, however, since the graph in Fig. 7.12b shows that base + fog levels increase significantly if temperature is increased excessively.

QUANTIFICATION OF FILM RESPONSE

To produce a characteristic curve a series of film densities is produced by known exposures (already described in Section 7.2.1). These can be a series of stepped exposures on the film using a sensitometer as shown in Fig. 7.5; a similar exposure scale can be obtained from X-rays using an aluminum wedge placed on the film cassette. This is X-ray sensitometry, described previously, and although it provides an easy method for judging film response, it suffers from inaccuracies due to X-ray spectrum filtration by the individual aluminum steps.

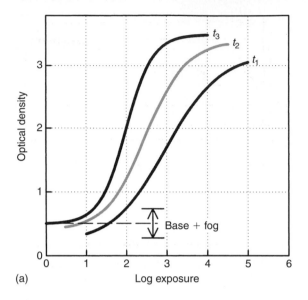

(a)

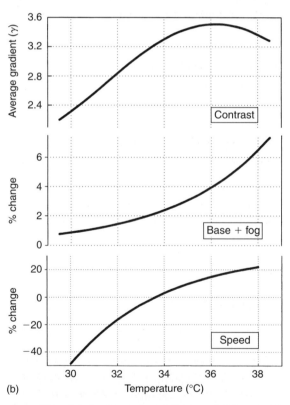

(b)

Figure 7.12 *(a) The change in the characteristic curve with developing conditions; as the developer temperature is increased from* t_1 *to* t_3 *the characteristic curve becomes steeper and displaced to the left (speed increased). (b) The variation of film contrast, base + fog and speed (sensitivity) with developer temperature.*

Box 7.3 Sensitometry results (Fig. 7.13a)

Base + fog (BF): 0.20

D_{min}:	Step 6	$\text{Log } E_{min}$	0.90
D_1:	OD 1.0 + BF: Step 12	$\text{Log } E_1$	1.80
D_2:	OD 2.0 + BF: Step 14	$\text{Log } E_2$	2.1

Speed index = D_1 = 1.80
Contrast index = $D_2 - D_{min}$ = 1.2

$$\text{Average gradient } (\gamma) \quad \frac{D_2 - D_1}{\log E_2 - \log E_1} = 3.3$$

Note: Calculations may vary between manufacturers of printing densitometers.

PRACTICAL SENSITOMETRY

Figure 7.13a is a characteristic $D/\log E$ curve similar to the ones already given in Fig. 7.9a and b. This curve was obtained by using a 21 step (0 to 20) density wedge using a light sensitometer.

The sensitometer is a stable light source illuminating an optical step wedge. Blue or green light is used, depending on film type. Each step on the wedge represents a log $E/2$ or 0.15 incremental change in light intensity (exposure) which spans the typical density range of a radiographic film. The 21 steps will therefore cover a log E range from 0 to 3.

The curve obtained from a sensitometry step wedge can be used routinely for testing film processing quality for the same film type or the differences between different film types under identical processing conditions. The following parameters can be measured from the curve shown in Fig. 7.13a:

- Base + fog or the gross fog
- Maximum density or D_{max}
- The speed index (SI)
- The contrast index (CI)
- The average gradient (γ)

The calculations in Box 7.3 explain how these measurements are obtained from the characteristic curve of Fig. 7.13a. The precise calculations differ between manufacturers but the speed index and contrast index are useful warning measures for changes in film processor performance such as developer chemical changes or temperature conditions, providing that one manufacturer's instrument is used.

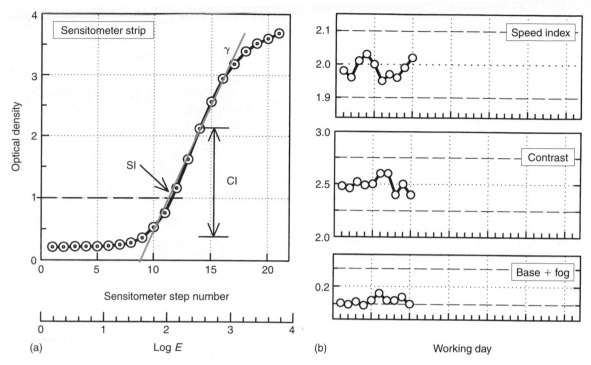

Figure 7.13 (*a*) *A characteristic curve obtained from the sensitometric strip shown in Fig. 7.7a. The speed index and contrast index range are indicated.* (*b*) *Quality control sheet used for daily routine film processor checking.*

The sensitometric strip can be read either automatically when the results are produced on a printout or the strip can be analyzed manually. Both methods rely on a **densitometer** which is an illuminated photoelectric cell calibrated directly in optical density units.

Figure 7.13b is an example of a quality control sheet for a film processor plotting the values for SI, CI and base + fog on a daily monitoring routine.

SUMMARY

- **Characteristic curve**: is a plot of density against log exposure.
- **Density**: represents objective contrast and is a quantitative measurement.
- **Exposure**: is influenced by subject contrast (attenuation coefficient, kV, filtration etc.).
- **Gamma**: the slope of the characteristic curve is a measure of film contrast (a component of radiographic contrast) and is inversely proportional to latitude.
- **Sensitivity**: is measured as film speed.

7.3 INTENSIFYING SCREENS

Film responds to light far more efficiently than X-rays so phosphor intensifying screens are interposed between the X-ray beam and the film emulsion in the cassette. Phosphors emit light due to **luminescence** where short wavelength radiation is absorbed and longer wavelengths are emitted (ultraviolet and visible). Two kinds of luminescence play an important role in intensifying screens:

- **Fluorescence**: light emission stops when the exciting radiation ceases.
- **Phosphorescence**: light emission continues for a time after the exciting radiation has stopped giving afterglow. This is an undesirable property for intensifying phosphor screens and substances are added during manufacture to quench phosphorescence.

An X-ray film alone absorbs about 1 to 2% of the incident beam but intensifying screens using elements that have *Z* values from 57 to 74 are effective absorbers of X-radiation (30 to 50%).

7.3.1 Phosphor materials

An early phosphor material used for intensifying screens was calcium tungstate, but this has been superseded by other materials such as complex compounds of yttrium and rare-earth elements lanthanum and gadolinium. The increased attenuation coefficients for these elements (K edges) and peak light production are important parameters which contribute to their efficiency. Table 7.3 lists the properties of these phosphor compounds.

The screen phosphor absorption over a range of X-ray energies is shown in Fig. 7.14. The K edges for lanthanum, gadolinium, and tungsten occur within the diagnostic energy band from 20 to 120 kV which change their quantum efficiency with photon energy as shown in Table 7.3.

Table 7.3 *Common intensifying screen phosphors.*

Phosphor	Fluorescence wavelength (nm)	K edge (keV)
$CaWO_4$	Main peak 420	69.5 (W)
Gd_2O_2S:Tb	545	50.2 (Gd)
La_2OBr:Tb	360, 475	38.8 (La)
$YTaO_4$	320	17 (Y)
$YTaO_4$:Nb	410	67.4 (Ta)

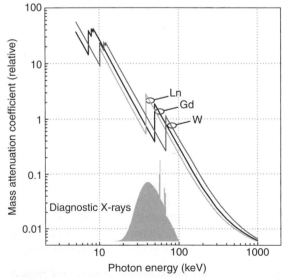

Figure 7.14 *Relative absorption curves for lanthanum, gadolinium and tungsten showing the position of the K edges.*

IDEAL PROPERTIES

The ideal phosphor for intensifying screens should have the following properties:

- A single line emission: the light spectrum should not be too broad. The film can then be designed to respond to a specific wavelength reducing light scatter within the phosphor.
- A medium energy K edge, so that higher energies (primary beam) are absorbed more efficiently than lower energies (scattered radiation).
- Long-wavelength light which gives more light photons for each X-ray photon.
- High conversion efficiency of X-ray to light photons.

CALCIUM TUNGSTATE

This was an early choice for phosphor screens. Its light emission is in the UV/blue part of the spectrum (Table 7.3) which complements the blue sensitivity of silver halide in the basic film. It has a continuous spectrum, which is a disadvantage, having a maximum peak at 420 to 450 nm. Pigment added to the calcium tungstate phosphor reduces light scatter within the intensifying screen but this also affects overall light output. Calcium tungstate has rapidly been replaced by rare-earth phosphor materials which are up to five times more efficient (Table 7.4).

RARE-EARTH MATERIALS

Table 7.4 lists intensifying screen phosphors based on the rare-earth elements lanthanum and gadolinium along with other compounds using yttrium tungstate and tantalate.

These intensifying phosphors are a precise mixture of phosphor and activator material. The activators give peaks or emission lines to the fluorescent spectrum; common doping materials used as activators are:

- Europium (Eu)
- Thulium (Tm)
- Terbium (Tb)

Table 7.4 *Relative phosphor intensification factors for selected kV_p values.*

Screen	40 kV_p	60 kV_p	80 kV_p	100 kV_p
$CaWO_4$	33	38	41	44
LaOBr:Tb	34	36	44	51
Gd_2O_2S:Tb	31	34	44	55
$YTaO_4$	33	42	44	50

Calcium tungstate has no added activator and gives a continuous spectrum. The spectra for current phosphors and calcium tungstate are compared in Fig. 7.15a, b and c.

LANTHANUM PHOSPHORS

Lanthanum oxybromide (LaOBr) doped with terbium was one of the first rare-earth phosphors to be used for intensifying screen material. Its great advantage was that it emitted blue light which matched available film stock still being used for calcium tungstate screens.

Lanthanum gives two light emissions at 360 nm and 475 nm. The spectrum shown in Fig. 7.15a compares its relative light output with calcium tungstate.

GADOLINIUM PHOSPHORS

Gadolinium oxysulfide doped with either terbium or europium is a more efficient phosphor than lanthanum and gives greater light output. Although several small peaks are seen in the spectrum a single dominant peak occurs at 540 nm which corresponds to the green part of the visible spectrum; calcium tungstate is shown

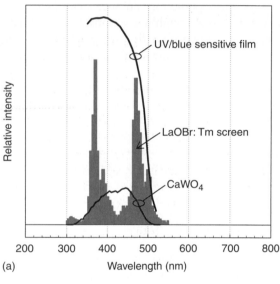

(a)

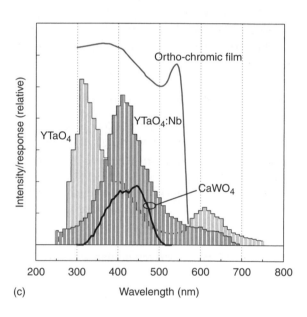

(c)

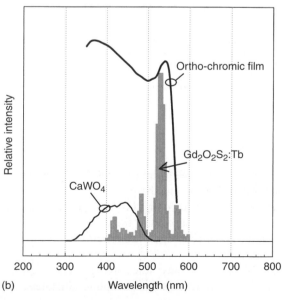

(b)

Figure 7.15 *(a) Lanthanum (b) gadolinium and (c) yttrium tantalate light spectra compared to CaWO$_4$. The CaWO$_4$ shows an inefficient broad wavelength spectrum compared to the spectral peaks of La, Gd, and YTaO$_4$.*

Table 7.5 *Absorption efficiency of screens; composed of 100 mg cm^{-2} phosphors.*

Phosphor	Absorption (percent)	Conversion efficiency
CaWO$_4$	26.7	5
YTaO$_4$	27.0	20
Gd$_2$O$_2$S	37.7	15
LaOBr	41.5	13

here for comparison (Fig. 7.15b). Gadolinium is more sensitive than both calcium tungstate or lanthanum and as a consequence is the most common phosphor material used in film-screen radiology. Table 7.5 shows the relative absorption for differing X-ray energies and phosphor type. The overall **intrinsic efficiency** for the phosphor is a combined figure for both absorption and conversion efficiency. An yttrium/tantalum phosphor compound has recently been introduced with emissions in the ultraviolet. Spectra from two yttrium phosphors, one pure and the other doped with niobium are shown in Fig. 7.15c. Since UV is easily absorbed in the polyester film base, print-through and halation are both greatly reduced (see Fig. 7.17 on p. 184).

Lanthanum and gadolinium are sometimes mixed to produce a comprehensive intensifying screen combining the benefits of both K edges giving increased absorption from 40 to 100 kV and light output in the blue and green spectrum: this increases film sensitivity.

7.3.2 Phosphor properties

Most rare-earth phosphors offer advantages over calcium tungstate (CaWO$_4$) for two reasons:

- Higher absorption efficiency
- Greater conversion efficiency

Compared with calcium tungstate, such phosphors as gadolinium oxysulfide and lanthanum oxybromide have greater absorption per unit thickness (absorption efficiency) of X-ray photons in the energy range used in diagnostic radiology (Fig. 7.14) so screens composed of these phosphors are more efficient and more X-ray photons are available for image formation. Since more X-ray photons are absorbed by screens that contain gadolinium or lanthanum phosphors, the light output of these screens can be increased considerably without significant sacrifice of image quality.

The X-ray absorption efficiency of a phosphor increases sharply at the K edge of the predominant heavy element present. The K edge of lanthanum at 38 keV gives lanthanum oxybromide an absorption advantage over calcium tungstate in the middle of the diagnostic kilovoltage range and the gadolinium K edge at 50 keV makes gadolinium oxysulfide better in the higher kilovoltage. When absorption efficiency is expressed as a percentage versus mass per unit area of phosphor, gadolinium, lanthanum, and barium phosphors have a greater absorption efficiency than calcium tungstate (Table 7.5). The mass per unit area of phosphor coating mix in most screens is about 100 mg cm^{-2}, with a range of about 80 to 140 mg cm^{-2}.

Rare-earth phosphors produce more light photons for each X-ray photon absorbed, so they have a greater **conversion efficiency** of X-ray photon to light photon which amplifies the X-ray image information.

Gadolinium oxysulfide and lanthanum oxybromide have both higher absorption efficiency and greater conversion efficiency so the speed advantage of screens composed of each of these rare-earth phosphors results from both absorption and conversion mechanisms; the yttrium oxysulfide speed advantage is exclusively the result of greater conversion efficiency.

The effect of aging on phosphor materials is unclear. Lanthanum oxybromide is hygroscopic and is stabilized during manufacture to prevent moisture absorption and deterioration with prolonged use.

Some of the specific properties that should be considered in evaluating screen/film combinations are:

- Speed
- Sharpness
- Contrast
- Mottle
- Clinical usefulness

These parameters are interrelated.

SPEED

The speed of a screen-film combination is important in reducing motion unsharpness. Increased speed of any screen-film combination can reduce motion unsharpness and also allow the use of an X-ray tube with a smaller focal spot, thus decreasing geometric unsharpness.

The speed of any intensifying screen can be increased by increasing phosphor thickness, so increasing absorption efficiency and light output. A reflective layer can be added to the screen base, thus increasing the amount of light reaching the film. Unfortunately, in both cases, sharpness will be degraded because of the resultant increased light diffusion.

The speed of a screen-film combination is the **reciprocal of the exposure** required to yield a given density. The speed of a system depends on the number and the energy of X-ray photons absorbed, the number of light photons produced by the absorbed X-ray photons, the number of light photons reaching the film, the sensitivity of the film to the light photons, and the film processing conditions.

As a generator's kilovoltage is lowered, the X-ray absorption efficiency of the screen increases. On the other hand, with a lower kilovoltage, the X-ray energy from a radiographic tube is less and the light output per absorbed photon in the screen also decreases. These effects are thus inversely related, and the resultant speed of the system will depend on the relative importance of each factor as well as the location of the K edges of the phosphors being used.

The effect of the phosphor absorption edge on the resultant light output is of considerable importance. From a practical point of view however, the use of broad X-ray spectra and clinically realistic exposure factors is more meaningful.

Because of the many variables involved, most investigators do not measure the speed of a screen-film combination in absolute values – they normalize it to a known reference system. A selective comparison of the relative speeds of several rare-earth screen-film combinations using clinically realistic exposure factors is shown in Fig. 7.16a. The speed of a reference system consisting of a pair of par-speed screens and XRP film was taken as unity.

Gadolinium oxysulfide exhibits a decreased relative speed at lower kilovoltages, thus reducing their speed advantage in those examinations performed at low kilovoltage. Other phosphors, such as yttrium oxysulfide and lanthanum oxybromide, maintained their relative speed at the lower energy levels.

Since speeds of different screen materials are energy dependent, it is to be expected that different amounts of scatter will produce different speed characteristics. Thus, the relative speed of a particular screen-film combination will vary with the kilovoltage used, the part being radiographed and its overall scatter characteristics, the grid used, the amount of collimation, and the amount of filtration.

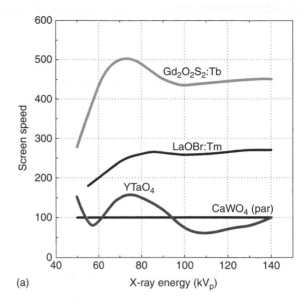

(a)

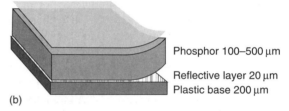

(b)

Figure 7.16 (*a*) *The change of sensitivity (speed) with X-ray energy for three screen types. Par-speed is 100, medium speed from 200 to 300 and fast screens above 400.*
(*b*) *Screen construction showing waterproof protective layer, the phosphor layer and supporting layers. There is an absorbing or reflective layer depending on application (detail or speed).*

THE PHOSPHOR LIGHT SPECTRUM

Depending on the phosphor material and the activator being used, the spectral emission from the screen can be ultraviolet, blue or can extend into the green region of the spectrum (Fig. 7.15). Screens that produce blue light are designed to be used with film that is sensitive to blue and ultraviolet light. Screens that produce green light are designed for use with orthochromatic film, which has an expanded range of sensitivity.

If a blue-sensitive film is used with predominantly green-emitting screens, there will be a significant loss of speed because only a portion of the light output of these screens is in the ultraviolet and the blue portion of the light spectrum. If an equally fast orthochromatic film is used with blue-emitting screens, the speed will be equal or greater because orthochromatic film is sensitive not only to green light but also to ultraviolet and blue light; since there is some green light emitted by yttrium oxysulfide, the speed of a system using screens with this phosphor can be increased by about 40% if the screens are used with an equally fast film extended to cover the green spectrum.

SHARPNESS

Modulation transfer function (MTF) curves can be used to evaluate loss of resolution (blurring) resulting from light diffusion in a particular screen/film combination (see Chapter 8).

With any given screen, absorption can be increased by increasing the amount of phosphor. A thicker phosphor layer, however, results in more light diffusion in the screen and therefore less sharpness. A pair of screens composed of an efficient rare-earth phosphor can be thinner than other screens and maintain similar absorption characteristics resulting in essentially the same speed for both systems but improved sharpness for the rare-earth system.

Sharpness can be increased by adding a dye to an intensifying screen to decrease light diffusion within the screen. The addition of dye, however, also decreases speed. Furthermore, the light produced by one screen that passes through the film base results in 'crossover' exposure of the opposite emulsion and degrades sharpness. Films with improved 'crossover' characteristics are now available; unfortunately, the resulting improvement in sharpness of some of these systems is accompanied by a loss in speed. Intensifying screens that emit primarily in the **ultraviolet** region produce sharper radiographs than might otherwise be predicted because more of the ultraviolet light emitted by one screen is absorbed in the film emulsion next to it, resulting in a considerable improvement in the crossover characteristics. Screen sharpness also depends on phosphor particle size, screen thickness, and characteristics of the reflective layer.

CONTRAST

The contrast of a radiographic image is determined primarily by the type of film, the processing conditions, the type of object being radiographed, and the radiographic technique used and is determined only secondarily by the screen characteristics. Scattered X-ray photons have a lower energy than primary X-ray photons. Since some rare-earth screens lose part of their speed advantage at the lower energy ranges, they are relatively less sensitive to scattered photons. These rare-earth screens will therefore exhibit higher contrast.

Contrast is expressed here as the slope of the curve at an optical density of 1.0 above base and fog of the respective characteristic curves.

MOTTLE

Radiographic mottle is the result of the random statistical variation of X-ray photons absorbed in the screen, the inhomogeneous crystal structure in the screen, and film graininess. The contributions of screen inhomogeneity and film graininess are usually insignificant compared with quantum fluctuation, which is a function of the number of X-ray quanta used to record the image.

The visualized radiographic mottle also depends on the ability of the system to record mottle. Therefore, light diffusion (as measured by the modulation transfer function), contrast, and perhaps film density are important in the imaging of mottle. For example, the speed of a system can be increased by increasing the X-ray absorption of the intensifying screens. If all other factors remain the same and speed is increased by making the phosphor material thicker, the resultant radiographic mottle is reduced. The reason for this is that the system cannot record the mottle as well because there is more lateral spreading of light in the thicker screen. If, however, speed is increased by using a faster film, the composite MTF will not change significantly, but mottle will increase because fewer quanta are required to form an image of the same radiographic density. Increasing the contrast of a film will also increase the visualized mottle. Although rare-earth screens typically have an increased absorption efficiency, which gives increased system speed without sacrifice in mottle properties or MTF, an additional speed increase results from increased efficiency in converting X-ray energy to light. Hence, fewer X-ray photons are required to produce an image and more mottle might be expected. This can be compensated for, however, by the use of slower films with these screens.

There is no universally accepted method for evaluating mottle. One may use the Wiener power spectrum, autocorrelation function (see Chapter 8).

7.3.3 Practical intensifying screens

CONSTRUCTION

The construction of a phosphor screen (Fig. 7.16b) consists of four layers:

- A **polyester support** which is made from plastic (0.2 mm). A thin light-absorbing layer can also be present on which the phosphor is deposited.
- A **phosphor coating** which is the uniform layer of phosphor crystals in a binder substance sometimes containing pigment. The thickness of this layer 0.1 to 0.5 mm is critical to the speed and resolution of the intensifying screen.
- A **protective layer** on top prevents build-up of static electricity, abrasion and is waterproof so allowing cleaning.
- A **reflective layer** is usually made from titanium dioxide, but in high detail screens this layer is replaced with an absorbing layer.

LIGHT OUTPUT

Knowing the wavelength of the emitted light (Table 7.3) and the conversion efficiency of the phosphor (Table 7.5) then the number of light photons generated by the phosphor can be calculated. This is demonstrated in Box 7.4 showing that the rare earth phosphors can give four to five times more light than $CaWO_4$.

INTENSIFICATION FACTOR

If a film is exposed to give the same density with and without screens then intensifying screen properties can be compared as:

$$\text{intensification factor} = \frac{\text{exposure without screens}}{\text{exposure with screens}}$$

This is a measure of screen speed. The three general categories for screen speed in conventional radiology are:

- Speed 25: slow, high resolution detail screens
- Speed 100: medium speed (par-speed)
- Speed 200–400: fast/very fast, low patient dose examinations, e.g. lumbar spine

X-RADIATION ENERGY

The K edge of the phosphor element determines absorption already seen in Fig. 7.14. The overall

---

Box 7.4 Conversion efficiency of intensifying phosphors

The ability of the intensifying screen to convert X-ray photons to light photons can be calculated for any particular phosphor type if the light output is known. For a photon energy of 60 keV.

Calcium tungstate emits most light at 430 nm with approximately 5% efficiency

$$= \frac{1240}{\text{wavelength}} = \frac{1240}{430} = 3 \, \text{eV}$$

$$\text{Light output} = \frac{60000 \times 0.05}{3} = 1000 \text{ photons.}$$

Lanthanum oxy-bromide emits two peaks at 360 nm (3.4 eV) and 475 nm (2.6 eV) with approximately 20% efficiency.

$$\text{Light output} = \frac{60000 \times 0.2}{0.5(3.4 + 2.6)} = 4000 \text{ photons}$$

Gadolinium oxy-sulfide emits light at a major peak of 530 nm (2.3 eV) also with approximately 20% efficiency.

---

sensitivity (light output) also varies with energy. The set of graphs in Fig. 7.16b for three screen speeds shows that the sensitivity for each screen peaks at about 70 to 80 keV. The calcium tungstate par-response (speed 100) is shown as reference.

EFFICIENCY

Screen efficiency is the product of absorption and conversion efficiency. Major factors playing a part are:

- **Phosphor type** (conventional or rare earth): a higher atomic number increases absorption and conversion efficiency influences light output.
- **Phosphor thickness**: X-ray absorption increases with increased thickness; light output also increases but resolution decreases substantially so there is a compromise between speed/sensitivity and resolution. Light reaching the film is also reduced due to internal absorption.
- **Phosphor crystal size**: in the same way as thickness for larger phosphor grain size increases fluorescent emission. High speed screens have larger crystal sizes.

- Phosphor **pigments** used in conventional screens (calcium tungstate) reduce lateral spreading thus improving resolution but also block some light emission.
- Photon energy is an important factor influencing overall screen efficiency (see Table 7.4 and Fig. 7.16a).

SCREEN THICKNESS

The absorption of X-rays by the screens depends on the X-ray energy. Low energy X-rays are absorbed mostly by the front screens, so a mammography cassette needs only one screen. At higher energies the X-rays are equally absorbed by a twin screen cassette. High detail screens give the best resolution and use thin screens. The increased efficiency of the rare-earth phosphors gives improved efficiency even with thin phosphor thickness. These screens have below-par (<100) speed. Low dose fast screens are more efficient and give the lowest patient dose. They have thicker phosphor layers and absorb more X-radiation but their resolution and low contrast detail are compromised. They can also give significant image mottle since they require fewer X-ray photons (quantum noise). These features are less important in some investigations (lumbar spine, pregnant patients) since screens with speeds from 200 to 800 require very low X-ray exposure so the patient dose is correspondingly smaller.

FILM-SCREEN ARTIFACTS

Image unsharpness is made up of geometric unsharpness (focal spot and source, object, film distances), movement unsharpness and radiographic unsharpness. Film-intensifying screen contact is a major contributor to radiographic unsharpness. The three main factors are illustrated in Fig. 7.17a, b, and c. Crossover or print-through effects (a) are caused by light penetrating across the film base and scattering into the opposite emulsion; pigmentation is added to the polyester layer to prevent this.

Halation is caused by reflection (b) and this is prevented by applying a black absorbing layer. Separation of the intensifying screen (c) from the film surface by dust or grit causes major distortion so the screens should be cleaned regularly. A too thick protective layer can also add to this type of distortion.

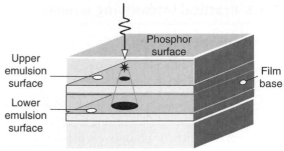

(a) Print-through

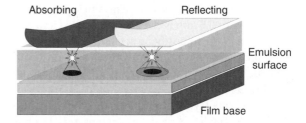

(b) Halation

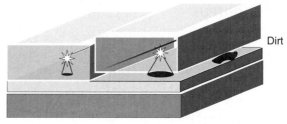

(c) Separation

Figure 7.17 *Film-screen artifacts: (**a**) print-through, (**b**) halation, (**c**) separation.*

SUMMARY

- Intensifying screen: a scintillation phosphor that converts X-rays to light.
- Phosphor materials: the early phosphor, calcium tungstate (5% efficient), has been replaced by rare-earth compounds lanthanum and gadolinium (nearly 20% efficient).
- Light spectrum: lanthanum blue, uses monochromatic film; gadolinium green, uses orthochromatic film.
- Intensification factor is a measure of screen speed and ranges from 25 (detail) up to 400 (low dose).
- Screen thickness influences screen speed.
- Radiographic contrast is influenced by film gamma and intensifying screen type.

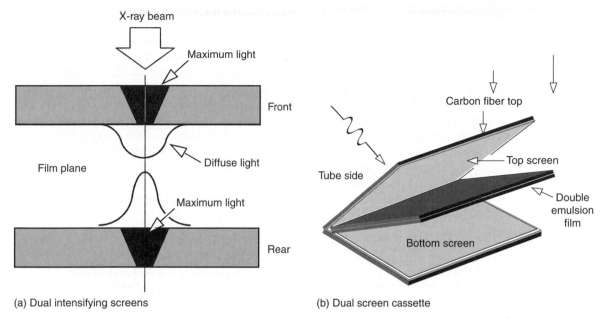

(a) Dual intensifying screens

(b) Dual screen cassette

Figure 7.18 *(**a**) Screen thickness and the diffusion of light. (**b**) A typical cassette design for a double emulsion film. The entrance face is made from carbon fiber for minimum losses.*

7.3.4 Cassette design

A number of designs are offered by manufacturers but they all combine the following basic components.

DUAL SCREEN CASSETTES

For a dual screen cassette, used at conventional kilovoltages ($\approx 60\,kV$ and above), the front screen stops contributing useful light to the film at quite low densities but the rear screens continue to contribute useful light. The dual screen cassette is the most common design in radiology and gives a significant increase in quantum efficiency.

SINGLE SCREEN CASSETTES

At lower kilovoltages (mammography) light output comes almost entirely from just below the screen surface so light from the front screen is quickly absorbed and does not reach the film. This is shown in Fig. 7.18a where the light from the front screen undergoes diffusion giving a blurred image but the rear screen contributes surface light and a sharper image. Figure 7.18b shows the design for a typical dual screen cassette where the X-ray beam passes through the top screen

exposing the first emulsion layer while other X-rays are absorbed in the bottom screen when the second emulsion is exposed; quantum efficiency is thereby increased quite considerably.

Different screen thicknesses in dual screen cassettes are used depending on the investigation. In some instances screen asymmetry is an advantage:

- For low kilovoltage work thin front and rear screens are most efficient.
- For medium kilovoltage work an advantage can be achieved by having thin front screens and thicker rear screens (screen asymmetry).
- For high kilovoltage work (fluoroscopy and chest) a medium thickness front screen and maximum thickness rear screen would be the best choice.

MAMMOGRAPHY

This poses a special problem since all the light is produced in the first few microns of the screen surface. A single emulsion film is used and a single thin screen applied. The X-ray beam is directed through the back of the film where some of the low energy photons interact with the emulsion; the rest of the photons interact with the surface of the phosphor so exposing the emulsion.

RADIATION DOSE REDUCTION

Patient dose reduction can be significant with the careful application of fast screens to X-ray investigations. The fastest screens are reserved for those studies where maximum detail is not required: some barium/iodine contrast studies and dorsal/lateral and pelvic studies fall into this category. Table 7.6 demonstrates the magnitude of dose reduction possible by increasing screen speed from par-speed which is given as reference. For studies requiring a wide gray-scale capability such as chest radiography and mammography, quantum mottle becomes a serious objection to increasing screen speed further above 200; valuable diagnostic detail could be lost.

7.4 FILM PROCESSORS

The diagram of an automatic film processor commonly found in diagnostic radiology departments is shown in Fig. 7.19. There are three baths containing developer, fixer, and water (used as the film washing bath). The chemicals in the developer and fixer are gradually exhausted so a method of replenishment is necessary. The temperature of the developer is critical and influences image quality; its influence on film speed, contrast, and film fog have been seen already in Fig. 7.12.

Table 7.6 *Dose reduction using faster screens.*

Investigation	Par-speed (mGy)	Fast (mGy)
Lumbar spine	22.0	7.0
AP abdomen	14.8	7.3
AP pelvis	11.2	6.0
IV urogram	4.0	1.5
Mammography	5 to 10	0.12 to 0.2

REPLENISHMENT

The developer activity gradually diminishes so concentrated developer solution is added from time to time to the tank so maintaining effectiveness. Replenishment can be continued for some days before the tank requires complete emptying and renewal. The replenishment cycle is controlled by monitoring film throughput. Exhausted fixer goes into a silver recovery unit so that the soluble silver compound is decomposed to give pure silver which is recovered before the fixer is disposed via the drain. Table 7.7 lists the parameters and performance of a common processor.

7.4.1 Silver recovery

The silver content of radiography films varies between 3000 and 6000 g $1000\,\mathrm{m}^{-2}$ depending on film type. A surface area of $1000\,\mathrm{m}^{-2}$ is equivalent to 6000 films of size $14'' \times 17''$ or 36×43 cm.

Scrap processed film contains about 7 to 26 g silver per kilogram. The limit of silver concentration in fixer is 4 to 6 g L^{-1} before replacement. Most regulations require that the silver recovery effluent for discharge to the public sewer should be less than 0.2 g silver per liter. Three methods are available for silver recovery.

Table 7.7 *Typical film processor specifications.*

	Developer	Fixer
Temperature	32°C to 37°C	
Tank capacity	20 L	20 L
Film treated (m²)	400 ml m^{-2}	600 ml m^{-2}
Processor speed	92 cm min^{-1}	(2 min)
	46 cm min^{-1}	(4 min)
Capacity	240 films/hour	
	120 films/hour	

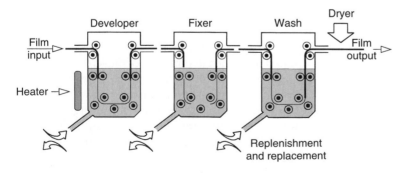

Figure 7.19 *The basic components of a film processor showing separate tanks holding developer, fixer, and washing water. Developer and fixer are replenished continuously.*

ELECTROLYTE METHOD

Uses a carbon anode and stainless steel cathode: $Ag^+ + e^- \rightarrow Ag$ precipitated on cathode. A good recovery is possible and the fixer can be reused. The current density of the equipment is critical; too high and silver sulfide is formed, too low and efficiency is lowered. The optimum pH is 5. This is the common method for silver recovery attached to automatic processors in radiology departments.

METAL REPLACEMENT

This uses steel wool to precipitate silver. The iron goes into solution and the fixer cannot be reused. It is 98% efficient.

CHEMICAL METHOD

This uses sodium sulfide to precipitate silver sulfide from solution. It removes 100% of the silver but produces hydrogen sulfide which is hazardous.

8

The analog image: film and video

8.1 VISION

There are two light sensitive receptors in the eye: the cones and the rods. The cones (~6.5 million in each eye) are primarily used for photopic or daylight vision. Cones see fine detail and are color sensitive (maximal sensitivity 550 nm: yellow–green). Each cone is directly connected to the brain. The rods are used for poor light conditions (scotopic vision), each eye having about 120 million. Several rods share their signals along a common nerve fiber, unlike the cones, and are most sensitive to 510 nm or blue–green. If a typical clinical radiograph is considered that is recorded on film the clinician is mainly concerned with:

- The ability to see small detail, e.g. hairline fractures, micro-calcifications
- The recognition of low contrast differences that may indicate pathology, e.g. pneumothorax, breast cancer, TB lesions
- The image quality (signal-to-noise ratio) sufficiently high to inspire confidence in the diagnostic accuracy

The human eye has limitations in resolution and contrast levels that must also be considered when viewing diagnostic information in a radiograph. The critical factors are:

- Image brightness level
- Low contrast differences within the image
- Image detail

8.1.1 Visual sensitivity

LUMINANCE

The units commonly used to describe light intensities depend on the source. For example, when measuring the amount of light emanating from a view box or a video monitor the luminance is measured in SI units of candela m^{-2} (or nits in the m.k.s. system). A table of values is given in Table 8.1 comparing SI and non-SI values.

Table 8.2 shows the range of luminance intensity that the human eye is exposed to in the environment, showing that the dynamic range of the eye is about $1:10^6$.

ILLUMINANCE

When measuring the illumination of objects in a room such as the light level at a desk top, or light level incident on a video screen (glare), the illuminance is

Table 8.1 *Units for luminance and illuminance.*

Luminance	
SI unit	1 candela m^{-2} (cd m^{-2})
Non-SI unit	1 lambert = cd cm^{-2}
Conversion factor	1 millilambert = 3.183 cd m^{-2}
Non-SI unit	1 foot lambert = cd ft
Conversion factor	1 nit = $\frac{1}{3.426}$ ft lambert
Illuminance	
SI unit	1 lux = 1 lumen m^{-2}

Table 8.2 *Approximate luminance levels.*

Object	Luminance (cd m^{-2})
White surface – sunlight	3×10^4
Viewing, light box	2×10^3
White level video screen	200
Reading light	30
Black level video screen	0.1
White surface — moonlight	0.03

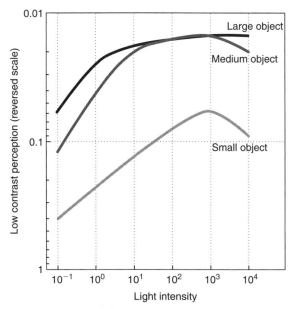

Figure 8.1 *The loss of visible contrast with intensity of illumination. Low contrast difference is toward the top of the y-axis.*

measured in SI units of lux. The old units were foot candles or lumen m^{-2}.

The effect of object brightness on visible contrast differences is shown in Fig. 8.1 where the ability to see low contrast differences increases toward the top of the y-axis. Loss of visual contrast occurs at high and low illumination levels. Peak sensitivity occurs at levels equivalent to radiograph viewing boxes and video screens; levels are listed in Table 8.2.

8.1.2 Visual contrast

The eye has a very large dynamic range achieved by adapting to a given luminance level. In order to show a video monitor which is operating in the range of 0.1 to 100 cd m^{-2} the eye must adapt to a lower level of illumination than it would when viewing a hard-copy text in bright daylight.

Visual contrast sensitivity is described in terms of the log difference between intensities. Visual contrast C between two intensities I_a and I_b would have a contrast difference of

$$C = \log I_a - \log I_b \qquad (8.1)$$

An eye that is adapted to the average light intensity of a video screen can accept a brightness range of about 1:30 (30 dB) so a gray-scale range of about 35 shades can be appreciated.

The signal amplitudes that are visible are evaluated logarithmically in compliance with Weber's law, which states that visible differences in light intensity are separated by fixed logarithmic values. The signal dynamic range of 30 dB is resolvable in contrast differences of about 1 dB; this has a significant influence on the eye's spatial resolution. A wider range of contrasts can be distinguished if the image is digitally 'windowed' which selects a narrow range of image data for display (discussed further with computed tomography).

INTEGRATION TIME

This is the time taken by the eye to accumulate visual information and varies according to viewing conditions. It depends on the state of adaptation to lighting conditions and intensity of the light stimulus. Integration time has values from 100 to 300 ms in the dark adapted (scotopic) eye and 15 to 100 ms in the light adapted eye (photopic). More detail cannot be extracted from the image by extending viewing time so optimum image quality (contrast, density) is essential if visual detail is to be distinguished particularly in moving (real time) fluoroscopic images.

8.1.3 Visual resolution

LINE PAIRS

A common method for measuring visible resolution uses a line pairs grating as illustrated in Fig. 8.2. The

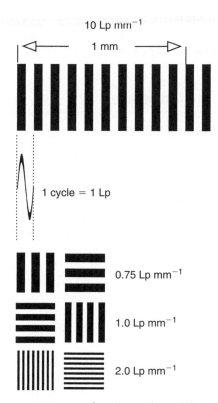

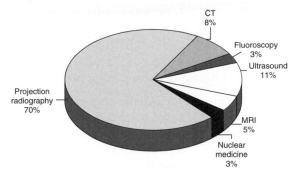

Figure 8.3 *Pie chart showing percentage of diagnostic imaging techniques. Projection X-ray imaging (film-screen, digital radiography) still occupies the major workload of any general hospital.*

Figure 8.2 *A 10 Lp mm^{-1} grating. A line pair is equivalent to 1 cycle mm^{-1}. Line pair patterns in radiology sometimes take the form of blocks as shown here which test resolution in both the x- and y-axes.*

grating has bars, one black and one white which represents one line pair. A line pair (Lp) is equivalent to 1 cycle. The grating shown in the diagram has 10 black and white line pairs over a 1 mm distance; gratings are available for radiography having line spacings up to 20 Lp mm^{-1}. The resolution limit is reached when the system will just resolve two lines spaced $1/x$ mm apart; this will represent x Lp mm^{-1}. A 0.5 mm line separation would be represented by 2 Lp mm^{-1} (each line pair covers 0.5 mm) and 0.1 mm line spacing would be 10 Lp mm^{-1}. Five line pairs per millimeter (5 Lp mm^{-1}) would be represented by 10 black and white bars on the film image; each bar being 0.1 mm thick. This is the typical resolving power of a conventional radiograph, correctly exposed and developed.

Maximum visual resolution, determined by the cones, is just about 30 Lp mm^{-1} under optimal conditions. Doubling the distance reduces this figure to

15 line pairs. Resolution in a film-screen system is limited by the intensifying screen and varies from 3 to 8 Lp mm^{-1} depending on screen type (speed and phosphor). Resolution is sometimes expressed in larger units of line pairs per centimeter (Lp cm^{-1}) (nuclear medicine).

8.2 IMAGE DETECTOR SURFACE

The separate factors and devices making up the radiographic image have been described earlier in Chapter 7 identifying the film-screen detector as the most common form of analog image.

The pie chart in Fig. 8.3 identifies that projection radiography, that is, plain film and full field computer radiography or digital radiography, still dominates the diagnostic imaging scene.

IMAGE QUALITY

There are three major parameters that describe image quality:

- **Resolution** is influenced by the machine itself (X-ray tube), movement (patient) and recording medium (film, image plate, video, computer digitization).
- **Contrast** is also influenced by system performance but also by the physical attributes of the different tissues, kilovoltage, and detector sensitivity. The dynamic range of a recording medium (film,

video display) decides the contrast range that can be represented.

- **Noise** is a component of all images, and is introduced either by quantum effects (photon density), mottle, film graininess or electronic noise.

Several factors also play an important role in forming the radiographic image sensitivity (speed). Acceptable image quality depends on the absorption efficiency of the image detector and its response (blackening or light output).

DIAGNOSTIC QUALITY

Image quality varies in the separate disciplines of radiology (i.e. conventional X-ray, nuclear medicine, ultrasound etc.); all show limitations in resolution, contrast, and noise. This does not detract, however, from their diagnostic usefulness. An image acceptable as diagnostic quality in nuclear medicine and ultrasound would be rejected as sub-standard in conventional radiology.

The diagnostic quality of an image is a subjective measurement and indicates the ability to demonstrate an abnormality. An inherently photon-poor imaging system (nuclear medicine) is equally able to give a diagnostic quality image as well as a high resolution system where increased photon density gives finer pathological detail (chest radiograph or mammography). This can be demonstrated by ranking the contrast and resolution capabilities of the common imaging procedures from 1 (poor) to 3 (excellent) in Table 8.3. Nuclear medicine and ultrasound, in spite of their intrinsic poor image quality, give adequate diagnostic information.

Improvements in display performance (increased resolution and contrast) would probably not influence this ranking since image quality is limited by other factors (quantum noise). So increasing the resolution of

nuclear medicine displays from $1\,\text{Lp}\,\text{cm}^{-1}$ to $4\,\text{Lp}\,\text{cm}^{-1}$ will have no effect if the gamma camera imaging device can only resolve $2\,\text{Lp}\,\text{cm}^{-1}$.

8.2.1 The film image

FILM SPEED (SENSITIVITY)

It has already been shown that film alone is a very insensitive medium for X-ray imaging; radiographic film is specially designed to be used in combination with intensifying screens. The list in Table 8.4 compares the performance of X-ray film with conventional 35 mm black and white camera film. Generally, X-ray film offers a much higher contrast for a reduced resolution. Film resolution is usually limited, in radiology, by other factors than the film itself (intensifying screens).

CONTRAST

The contrast offered by the film emulsion has been discussed in Chapter 7. Peak contrast is measured as the film's gamma and this is shown to be high in radiological film compared to conventional film stock (Table 8.4). The dynamic range can be tailored to the application: film used for video screen recording has a wide latitude (large dynamic range) while mammography film has a narrow dynamic range so that close tissue characteristics can be separated.

RESOLUTION

Conventional radiographic film can resolve 5 to $8\,\text{Lp}\,\text{mm}^{-1}$ and this is sufficient for most detailed conventional examinations. Since mammography demands a higher resolving power film resolution is increased although it is not a limiting factor even in this examination since the intensifying screens

Table 8.3 *Ranking diagnostic image quality.*

Image	Resolution	Contrast	Noise
Mammogram	3	3	3
Chest film	2	2	2
Extremity film	3	2	2
CT	2	3	3
MRI	2	3	2
Ultrasound	2	1	1
Nuclear medicine	1	1	1

Table 8.4 *Medical and conventional film compared.*

Performance	Medical X-ray film	Conventional B/W film
Speed (ASA/DIN)	60/19° to 80/20°	100/21°
Contrast	2.5 to 3.0	0.7 to 0.9
Tonal value	black	mid-gray/black
Grain size	2.0 to 2.3 μm	0.6 to 0.8 μm
Resolution	$40\,\text{Lp}\,\text{mm}^{-1}$	70 to $120\,\text{Lp}\,\text{mm}^{-1}$

themselves have a poorer resolving power and these are the limiting factor.

8.2.2 Intensifying phosphors

The mechanism causing phosphorescence (described in Chapter 6) is found in several types of imaging devices in radiology:

- Intensifying screens in film cassettes
- Image intensifier input and output screens
- Large single crystal detectors for nuclear medicine gamma cameras
- Image plates used in computed radiology

The first three phosphor imaging devices translate X- or gamma radiation directly into light photons, but the image plate requires a secondary energy source (infrared laser) in order to release stored energy in the form of light which can then be used for image formation.

PHOSPHOR MATERIALS

Intensifying screens predominantly use rare-earth phosphors containing gadolinium or lanthanum but newer materials containing yttrium offer improved efficiency. Image intensifier tubes use sodium doped cesium iodide (CsI:Na), since this material has a good absorption for X-ray photons and its needle-like crystal structure reduces light scatter which maintains resolution. Image plates use complex barium fluorohalide compounds.

SENSITIVITY

In all cases the light output varies according to X-ray intensity and energy so the continuous X-ray spectrum gives a range of light intensities. Phosphor detectors are most commonly seen as intensifying screens in film-screen cassettes and conventional radiology uses a double emulsion film sandwiched between two intensifying screens whose thickness is chosen for the particular investigation. Screen thickness (from 100 to 500 μm) is normally quoted as a weight per unit area: 100 to 165 mg cm^{-2} is a typical range. Sensitivity increases with thickness due to improved absorption but resolution becomes poorer.

In general, intensifying screens contribute 97% to film blackening; the X-radiation itself contributing only 3%. The increased sensitivity achieved by using intensifying screens decreases patient radiation dose by a factor of 15 to 20 and the consequent shorter exposure times reduce movement unsharpness.

RESOLUTION

Radiographic unsharpness is introduced by all phosphor screens since the light production occurs at some depth within the phosphor depending on the photon energy (Fig. 8.4a). As the X-ray photon energy increases it penetrates further into the phosphor causing diffusion of the deeper light event so there is a significant geometrical broadening when it reaches the film emulsion at the phosphor surface. As a consequence conventional film screens have a typical resolution of 5 to 8 Lp mm^{-1}. Image plates can also

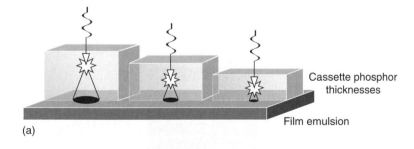

(a)

Cassette phosphor thicknesses

Film emulsion

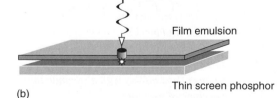

X-ray beam

Film emulsion

Thin screen phosphor

(b)

Figure 8.4 *(a) An image phosphor surface (intensifying screen or image plate) showing shallow and deep light events depending on photon energy. These cause radiographic unsharpness. (b) Thinner phosphors are used for mammography.*

be treated as intensifying phosphors but they store information using thermoluminescence principles; their light emission occurs at depth within the phosphor so degrading image resolution which is typically $5\,\mathrm{Lp\,mm^{-1}}$.

Light diffusion can be controlled by using thinner phosphor screens (Fig. 8.4b) but sensitivity is greatly reduced since only a fraction of the beam is absorbed. Low keV photons react at the surface so the light event undergoes minimal diffusion giving a sharp film image (usually 10 to $15\,\mathrm{Lp\,mm^{-1}}$ for single screen mammography). For this reason the beam enters the film back so photon interaction occurs near the film emulsion.

SUMMARY

In general, intensifying screens:

- Increase radiographic unsharpness
- Reduce movement unsharpness
- Reduce patient dose

The properties of an intensifying screen are influenced by:

- Phosphor compound (density and light conversion efficiency)
- Phosphor thickness ($\mathrm{mg\,cm^{-2}}$)
- Proportion of light diffusion
- Phosphor grain size
- Phosphor transparency
- Radiation energy

Screen resolution can be increased by having:

- A thin phosphor
- Small phosphor crystals
- A light absorbent layer on the phosphor base preventing reflection
- A very thin protective layer

Optimum phosphor performance is obtained by:

- Maximum absorption
- Maximum X-ray to light conversion efficiency
- Matching phosphor light wavelength to film sensitivity

8.2.3 The video image

The principles of television using a scanning electron beam were simultaneously developed by L. de Forest (1873–1961; American physicist) and A.D. Blumlein (1903–42; British engineer). The television or video display is an analog image but, unlike film, breaks up image information into a sequence of scan lines which degrade the original X-ray image data, particularly resolution.

VIDEO WAVEFORM

The basic video waveform is shown in Fig. 8.5a for a single scan line with black and white levels and

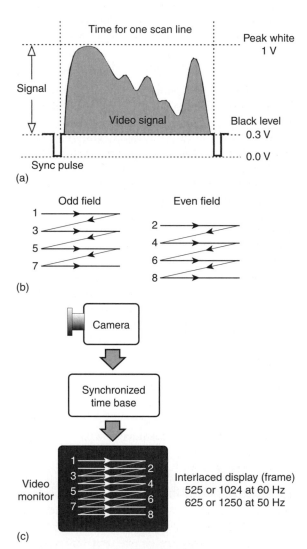

Figure 8.5 *(a) A single video scan line showing the extreme signal levels associated with black and white and the synchronization pulses for end of line. (b) Video interlacing pattern showing odd and even fields combined to form a video frame. (c) Camera and display with a common time base giving a synchronized scan rate.*

synchronization pulses which indicate the 'end-of-line'. The time per scan line will differ according to the video standard.

The scanning pattern is identical between camera and display maintaining overall synchronization.

INTERLACING

In the early development stages of television the requirement for high speed electronics was reduced by employing a method of scan-line interlacing. Half the image was transmitted at a time as alternate fields (odd then even-line numbers); combining each field gave a complete interlaced frame at 25 or 30 frames per second, depending on the supply frequency (50 or 60 Hz). Domestic television is still broadcast in an interlaced format. Since 25 or 30 frames s^{-1} (fps) are adequate, it is only necessary to transmit this rate so the complete line count (525 or 625) is transmitted in two halves, odd lines then even lines, as shown in Fig. 8.5b. The interlacing patterns shown in Fig. 8.5b have odd and even line fields at 50 or 60 fields per second which are combined to give a complete video picture frame at 25 or 30 frames per second. Frequency restrictions in domestic television are not a serious problem in radiological imaging; non-interlaced high resolution displays having increased scan lines and line densities greater than 1000 have become standard. The line scanning for a video system (as transmitted or using a closed circuit) is synchronized between camera and display with a common time base, shown in Fig. 8.5c.

BANDWIDTH

The frequency necessary to transmit video display data is the product of the display resolution, the number of scan lines in the display and the frame rate. Box 8.1 gives some examples.

LINE STANDARDS

The number of horizontal scanning lines used for domestic television has 525 lines in the Americas and Japan and 625 lines in Europe. For moving pictures it is necessary to display a frame rate which takes advantage of vision persistence and high enough to prevent flicker. Figure 8.6a shows the sensitivity of the eye to frame frequency and flicker.

For historical reasons the frame rate is dictated by the mains line frequency; 525 lines uses a frame rate of 60 fps, 625 lines uses 50 fps. Increasing scan line

numbers (up to 2000 to 3000 in some high definition displays) require a much higher frame rate in order to prevent flicker problems.

VIDEO STANDARDS FOR RADIOLOGY

In order to achieve acceptable sharpness video displays in radiology have a higher resolution standard than those offered by domestic television. Original radiology display systems used domestic television standards but most recent video displays now utilize high definition line standards of 1024, 1249, and 2048 lines using a non-interlaced format.

Box 8.1 Video bandwidth

Video bandwidth can be calculated from the formula: $r \times s \times f$ where r equals the resolution along the line (normally symmetrical with the line standard), s = line standard and f = frames per second, this is 30 fps (USA) and 25 fps (Europe). So video bandwidth for the USA is

$$500 \times 512 \times 30 = 7.6 \,\text{MHz}$$

and for Europe is

$$600 \times 625 \times 25 = 9.3 \,\text{MHz}$$

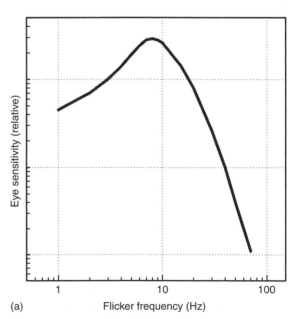

(a)

Figure 8.6 *(a) Flicker sensitivity of the human eye peaks at about 10 Hz but is still apparent at 20 Hz.*

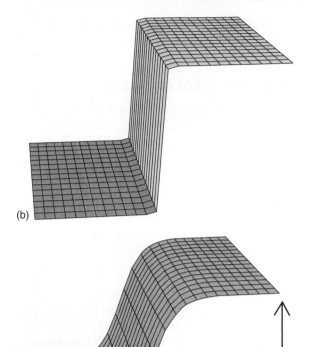

(b)

(c)

Figure 8.6 *(Contd) (**b**) A sharp change across an image boundary (tissue difference) giving optimum visibility. (**c**) The overall effect of unsharpness which smoothes the boundaries reducing both resolution and contrast difference. Visible contrast is lost as* d *increases although* h *is the same.*

These display systems use 70 to 100 frames per second eliminating flicker. High definition radiology displays can use 3000 scan lines in order to give film-like image quality.

Video and film image resolution is compared in Table 8.5. A good chest radiograph can achieve 5 Lp mm^{-1} and a detail screen about 8 Lp mm^{-1}. The best film resolution is given in mammography where 15 to 20 Lp mm^{-1} is routinely obtained. High resolution, progressive scan (non-interlaced) 2000 to 3000 scan line monitors can achieve in excess of 5 Lp mm^{-1} but film-screen is still able to offer the best image quality in terms of resolution.

Table 8.5 *Resolution of film and video compared.*

Analog image	Resolution (Lp mm^{-1})
Film	
Chest (35 × 43 cm)	5
Mammography (24 × 18 cm)	20
Video (scan lines)	
1024	3.0
1249	3.5

8.3 IMAGE QUALITY FACTORS

The three factors which define image quality are:

- Resolution
- Contrast
- Noise

All images, whether analog, video or digital can be analyzed using these parameters. Image quality should be able to reproduce faithfully the machine's capabilities, i.e. its own potential resolution (focal spot size), contrast (attenuation coefficients), and noise (dictated by the photon density). An image system which is unable to record all the X-ray image information will miss important diagnostic detail; conversely, an image that exceeds the performance figures of the machine will only serve to emphasize noise.

8.3.1 Resolution

Figure 8.6b shows an image density change as a step which can represent contrast between two structures or fine detail (resolution). Image spatial resolution in the radiographic image is influenced by two factors which degrade resolution giving overall 'image unsharpness'; this is shown in Fig. 8.6c. The ability to distinguish a step change in image density depends on the magnitude of the change h and the distance d over which the change occurs.

Although the intensity change across the boundaries are the same in Fig. 8.6c the sharp boundary in the top step is easily visible whereas the gradual intensity change in the bottom step becomes less visible as distance d increases although the height h remains the same. Objects having a gradual change must be larger in order to be visible. The combined unsharpness of a radiograph is made up from geometric unsharpness,

Table 8.6 *Parameters applying to all detector surfaces.*

Old term	New (universal) term
Focus to film distance (FFD)	
Source to image distance (SID)	Focus to image distance (FID)
Focus to object distance (FOD)	Focus to object distance (FOD)
Object to film distance (OFD)	Object to image distance (OID)

movement or kinetic unsharpness and radiographic unsharpness (i.e. film-screen):

- **Geometrical unsharpness** U_g is influenced by distances between X-ray tube, patient and image surface as well as X-ray focal spot size.
- **Movement unsharpness** U_m is due simply to patient and organ movement.
- **Radiographic unsharpness** U_r causes image blurring due to poor film-screen contact and diffusion of light within the phosphor material.

The total unsharpness U_{total} is then the geometrical mean of these values:

$$U_{total} = \sqrt{U_g + U_m + U_r} \qquad (8.2)$$

GEOMETRICAL UNSHARPNESS

There are three parameters which influence geometrical unsharpness in film projection radiography:

- Focus to film distance (FFD), which is the same as source to image distance (SID)
- Object to film distance (OFD)
- Focal spot size (FS)

Since the introduction of digital radiography and electronic flat panel detectors the naming of these parameters has been changed to a more universal form substituting 'image' for 'film'. Even film imaging relies on intensifying screens as the primary image converter before the light reaches the film emulsion (Table 8.6).

Figure 8.7a to c shows the relationship between these parameters and **penumbra** size which causes edge smoothing and consequent loss of resolution. The central area, called the **umbra**, has this shadow penumbra whose size is determined by geometrical factors; this is similar to a light penumbra described in Chapter 2.

Loss of image detail is primarily caused by the X-ray tube focal spot size, however the focal spot size itself is a trade-off between image sharpness and tube heat dissipation. The point source in Fig. 8.7a gives the sharpest image with no geometrical unsharpness regardless of beam distances. However, X-ray tubes do not have a point source; the target always has finite dimensions as shown in (b). Optimum resolution is therefore achieved by keeping the FS small, the FID large, and the object to image distance (OID) small.

Table 8.7 shows the relationships between the different geometrical parameters which cause unsharpness. They can be related with geometrical unsharpness as:

$$U_g = \frac{FS \times OID}{FID - OID} \qquad (8.3)$$

So a large focal spot (FS) and increased distance between object and imaging detector surface OID increases unsharpness, conversely increasing the distance between X-ray tube and image surface (FID) decreases unsharpness.

8.3.2 Image distortion

MAGNIFICATION

This does not depend upon the position of the object relative to the centre of the beam, but only upon the object/image distance (OID) and the focal spot/image distance (FID) although Fig. 8.7c does demonstrate outline distortion for volume objects. For a point source focal spot magnification M:

$$M = \frac{FID}{FID - OID} \qquad (8.4)$$

The most important practical consequence of the above expression for radiography is the fact that the magnification factor, M, varies as OID is changed and if the object is on the detector surface (OID = 0) magnification is unity, as OID increases then the divisor decreases, so increasing magnification. Eqn 8.4 shows that increasing the distance between object and image surface will magnify the image but this is incompatible with minimum geometrical unsharpness so the focal spot size is reduced, e.g. from 0.4 to 0.1 mm in mammography.

Magnification also leads to image distortion since anatomy or pathology further away from the detector is magnified compared to the same size objects close to the detector, so that all radiographs give a

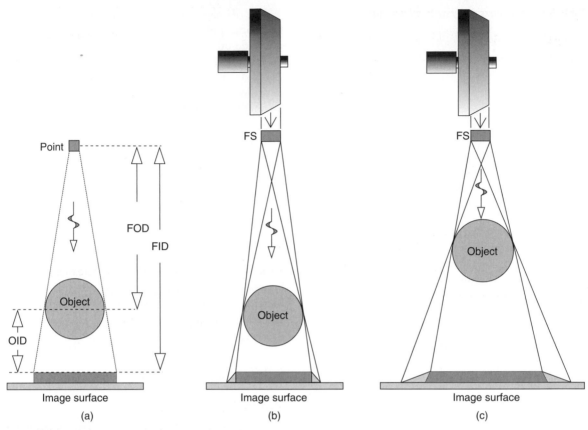

Figure 8.7 (*a*) For a small (point) focal spot giving no geometrical unsharpness. (*b*) A broad focal spot causes a penumbra to be formed which results in sloping edges and unsharpness. A chest unit minimizes the unsharpness by maintaining a large FFD. (*c*) Magnification views require a reduction in the focal spot size.

Table 8.7 *Parameter change.*

	Increase unsharpness	**Decrease unsharpness**
Focal spot	Large	Small
FID	Small	Large
OID	Large	Small

distorted image compared to the true shape of the object being imaged. This effect is minimal in most cases and may be reduced by increasing the FID.

However, the focal spot (FS) has a finite size, usually 0.6 to 2.0 mm for conventional radiography and 0.1 to 0.4 mm for mammography and this projects unsharpness at the detector surface (**geometrical unsharpness** U_g) and degrading image resolution:

$$U_g = \frac{FS \times OID}{FID - OID} \qquad (8.5)$$

The graph in Fig. 8.8a shows how the FID affects image unsharpness in chest radiography. For an FID of 2 m unsharpness is negligible even for a 2 mm focal spot size, which is necessary in order to comply with X-ray tube loading (see Chapter 3).

Geometrical unsharpness is an important source of image degradation in mammography since consistent image quality is necessary across the full tissue depth from 0 to 50 mm within a compressed breast. Figure 8.8b plots unsharpness obtained from 0.1 mm and 0.4 mm focal spot sizes.

8.3.3 Detector

Radiographic unsharpness is caused almost entirely by the intensifying screen. This can be single (in the case of mammography) or double (conventional screen-film radiology). Single screens used in detail

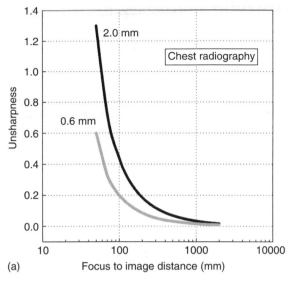

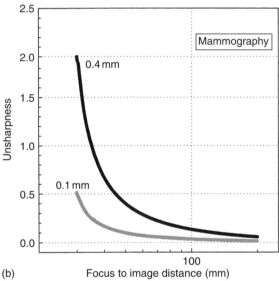

(b)

Figure 8.8 *Image unsharpness for focus to image surface distances (FID) used in (**a**) chest and (**b**) mammography.*

radiography and mammography give the highest resolution since light diffusion is minimal (see Chapter 7). Grid stops may be visible when using static grids (chest radiography) either as lines on the film or moiré fringes on a video display.

Eqn 8.5 can be restated as

$$U_g = \frac{1}{M \times FS \times (M-1)}$$

where M is the magnification value from eqn 8.4. In this form the overall image unsharpness can be

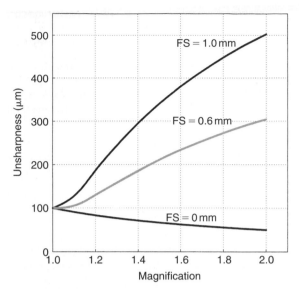

Figure 8.9 *Detector unsharpness calculated from eqn 8.6 for focal spot sizes of 0 (point source), 0.6 and 1.0 mm. The detector unsharpness is constant at 100 μm.*

expressed by combining the intrinsic **detector unsharpness**.

Radiography film, on its own and without intensifying screens, has a very high resolution approaching 50 Lp mm^{-1}. However, intensifying phosphor screens reduce this figure to 2 to 5 Lp mm^{-1} for conventional work and 15 to 20 Lp mm^{-1} for mammography, since they have an intrinsic detector unsharpness U_D caused by phosphor grain size (intensifying screens in film-screen imaging or computed radiography image plates), and photodetector size (direct radiography digital detectors). The formula can be modified to include this:

$$U_g = \frac{1}{M} \sqrt{(M-1)^2 \times FS^2 + U_D^2} \qquad (8.6)$$

Figure 8.9 plots the overall unsharpness, using eqn 8.6, for three focal spot sizes and the same detector unsharpness of 100 μm. The focal spot size remains the significant factor responsible for image unsharpness during magnification.

CHEST RADIOGRAPHY

A large FID is commonly used in chest radiography and Box 8.2 gives a worked example showing the

Box 8.2   Image resolution FS and FFD

Focal spot size (eqn 8.6)

The fixed FDD in mammography is 60 cm and the focal spot is 0.4 mm. If the center of the breast is 3 cm from the film plane (ODD) then

$$U_g = \frac{0.4 \times 3}{60 - 3} = 0.02 \, \text{mm}$$

For ×2 magnification the ODD is increased to 30 cm and the focal spot changed to 0.1 mm. To maintain sharpness $U_g = 0.1$ mm.
   Conclusion. In order to resolve micro-calcifications of ≈130 μm a smaller focal spot is essential.

Focus to film distance (chest radiography)

Using a focal spot of 1.2 mm, an FDD of 1 m and a chest depth 25 cm (mid-lung field ODD 12.5 cm). For surface lesions, $U_g = 0.4$ mm. Mid-field lesions give U_g of 0.17 mm. For an FDD of 2 m surface lesions are shown with a U_g of 0.17 mm and mid-field lesions with a U_g of 0.08 mm.
   Conclusion. At an FDD of 2 m lesions are shown sharply at all volume depths.

benefits of large focus to film distances. The examples given demonstrate that the large FID employed in chest radiology reduces the importance of focal spot size and its effect on determining image resolution but focal spot sizes are critical for closer FIDs such as those used in mammography.

Figure 8.10a illustrates how a large FID overcomes differing resolution with depth. The 2 m FID used in a chest unit allows image detail to be retained throughout the depth of the lung fields, whereas shorter FIDs cause unsharpness.

At large FIDs the beam intensity is much reduced due the inverse square law and since the exposure timing is also short the tube rating must be high. Figure 8.10b shows the setup for mammography, having a shorter FID (65 cm). Breast compression is an important method for reducing unsharpness with depth.

MOVEMENT UNSHARPNESS U_M

A major factor is patient or organ movement and Fig. 8.10c shows how a sharp edge can be degraded by patient or organ movement. Machine movement or vibration can also play a significant part. Movement unsharpness is kept small by using high kilovoltage.

Due to the increased efficiency of X-ray production at high kilovoltages a reduction in mAs can be made giving a faster exposure time for the same tube current. Faster intensifying screens can also be used.

Cardiac movement and large vessel movement in chest radiography are examples of movement unsharpness. It is necessary to give an exposure time of 0.01 s to overcome movement and maintain a 1 Lp mm^{-1} resolution in the final image. Movement can also be controlled if respiration or EKG signals are used to gate image data acquisition but this requires digital data acquisition that will be described in subsequent chapters.

8.3.4   Contrast

Image contrast is measured in practice by viewing specific test patterns; examples are shown in Fig. 8.11. The strict definition of contrast (the difference between two areas as ΔC) varies depending on conditions:

- **Subject contrast**, which concerns beam intensity differences within the subject (patient), is described as

$$\Delta C = I_2 - I_1 \qquad (8.7)$$

- **Radiographic contrast**, which concerns an image density difference, is

$$\Delta C = \frac{D_2 - D_1}{D_1} \qquad (8.8)$$

- **Film contrast**, which relates film exposure to density, is

$$\gamma = \frac{D_2 - D_1}{\log E_2 - \log E_1} \qquad (8.9)$$

- **Visual contrast**, the perception of the image, concerns itself with intensities in the same way as subject contrast but using a logarithmic scale in eqn 8.5:

$$\Delta C = \log I_2 - \log I_1 \qquad (8.10)$$

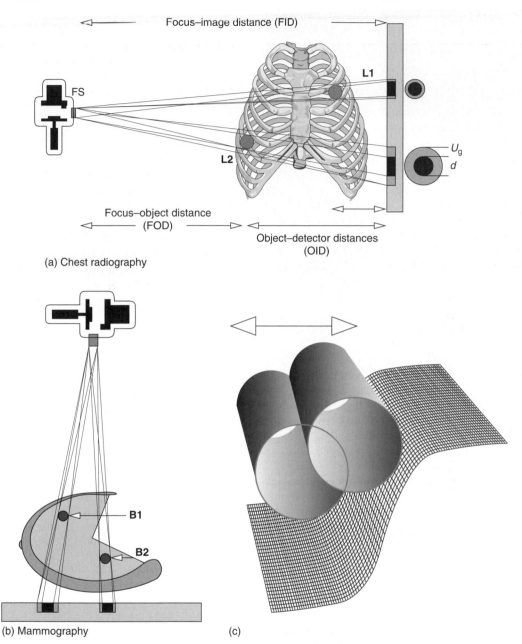

Figure 8.10 *(a) The critical dimension of the FID used in chest radiography. Lesion L1 is recorded with a small penumbra but a short FID causes lesion L2 to lose sharpness. Changing FID from 1 to 2 m allows both L1 and L2 to be recorded with minimum penumbra. (b) Mammography uses a shorter FID so compression is needed to visualize B1 and B2 with equal clairty. (c) An example of movement unsharpness given by a beating vessel which destroys the sharp boundary that would otherwise be given by a static vessel.*

The difference between intensities (I_1 and I_2) is given by an absolute difference (subject and visual contrast). As an example of eqn 8.7 intensity contrasts: $100 - 20 = 80$ and $25 - 5 = 20$ whereas radiographic and film contrast are **relative** differences; if the above values now relate to D_1 and D_2 as in eqns 8.8 and 8.9 then the relative contrasts will be the same, i.e. 4.0. So the contrast between signal and background is

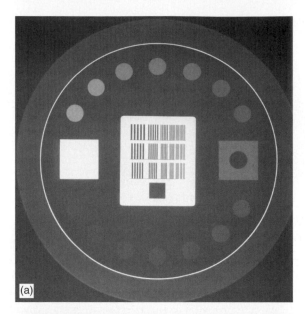

(a)

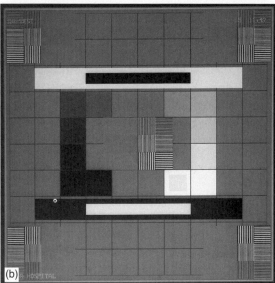

(b)

Figure 8.11 *Contrast and resolution test patterns for both (a) film display and (b) equipment performance such as CT or DSA. These low contrast images are also used for quantifying contrast.*

calculated differently depending on whether we are considering intensities or image densities.

SUBJECT AND VISUAL CONTRAST

Substituting I_a and I_b for I_1 and I_2 in eqn 8.10 then the difference in subject contrast C between two intensities is simply $C = I_a - I_b$ but since the eye has

---

Box 8.3 Derivation of visual contrast parameters

Rearrange eqns 8.11 to remove the negative sign. Since

$$\frac{I_a}{I_0} = e^{-\mu_a x} \quad \text{then} \quad \frac{I_0}{I_a} = e^{\mu_a x}$$

Taking common logs:

$$\log \frac{I_0}{I_a} = \log(e^{\mu_a x})$$
$$= \log e \times \mu_a x$$
$$= 0.4343 \mu_a x$$

(since $\log_{10} e = 0.4343$).

Then from the general equation (eqn 8.12)

$$C = (\log I_0 - 0.4343\mu_a x) - (\log I_0 + 0.4343\mu_b x)$$
$$= 0.4343x \times (\mu_b - \mu_a)$$

which is eqn 8.13.

---

a logarithmic response (Weber's law) the visual contrast difference is

$$C = \log I_a - \log I_b$$

Applying the exponential law formula derived in Chapter 2 to the incident beam I_0:

$$I_a = I_0 e^{-\mu_a x} \quad \text{and} \quad I_b = I_0 e^{-\mu_b x} \quad (8.11)$$

The two tissues of thickness x have attenuation coefficients of μ_a and μ_b. Visual contrast C_v can now be expressed as

$$C_v = \log(I_0 e^{-\mu_a x}) - \log(I_0 e^{-\mu_b x})$$

Box 8.3 shows that this can be simplified since

$$I_a = \log I_0 - 0.4343\mu_a x \quad (8.12)$$

So the visual contrast varies as

$$C = 0.4343x \times (\mu_a - \mu_b) \quad (8.13)$$

which indicates that contrast increases with tissue thickness x (giving more attenuation) and with the increasing difference in the attenuation coefficients $\mu_a - \mu_b$.

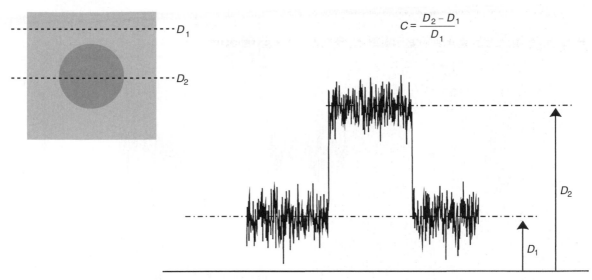

$$C = \frac{D_2 - D_1}{D_1}$$

Figure 8.12 *A profile through a dual density image (upper sketch) demonstrating radiographic contrast measurement using D1 as the background mean value and D2 as the signal mean value. Noise is superimposed on both the background and object.*

SUBJECT CONTRAST

This has been described in Chapter 5 and in general concerns interaction of X-rays with matter, X-ray beam quality together with machine and tissue characteristics. In detail these are:

- Tissue thickness x (in mm or cm)
- Tissue density (kg L^{-1} or kg m^{-3})
- Tissue electron density
- Tissue effective atomic number Z_{eff}
- Tissue attenuation coefficient μ
- X-ray energy (in keV)
- X-ray filtration (spectrum quality)
- Scatter within the tissue

SUBJECT CONTRAST AND KILOVOLTAGE

The effect of atomic number on photoelectric absorption and electron density on Compton scattering has already been described in Chapter 5. As X-ray energy (keV) increases subject contrast becomes more dependent on electron density as the probability of Compton reactions increases.

RADIOGRAPHIC CONTRAST

This concerns image forming properties of the detector which are:

- Film and screen characteristics

- Detector performance (image intensifier, gamma camera etc.)
- Scatter rejection (collimator and grids)

Figure 8.12 illustrates radiographic contrast as an intensity profile taken through two densities on the film, D_1 and D_2. The profile is a step change complete with image noise. The densities are measured as the mean level of the noise variation.

OBJECTIVE CONTRAST

This is a quantitative measure of the optical density of the image. This has been described in Chapter 7 in conjunction with the film characteristic curve and depends on image density difference (film, video) or the windowing level (CT or DSA).

SUBJECTIVE CONTRAST

This depends on image viewing conditions and covers all external factors:

- Room viewing conditions (background lighting, viewing distance)
- View box characteristics (intensity, light color)
- Magnification and minification

The two test phantoms in Fig. 8.11 are used for measuring the low contrast capability of a film-screen and

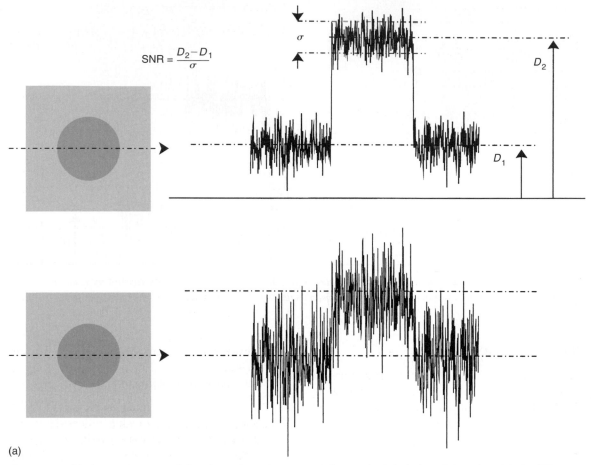

(a)

Figure 8.13 *(a) The measurement of signal-to-noise ratio compares the standard deviation of the noise with the difference between background and signal amplitude. The upper profile has a higher SNR than the lower where the central object is less visible.*

a video display and the low contrast measurement of a CT machine.

8.3.5 Image noise

SIGNAL-TO-NOISE RATIO (SNR)

This is illustrated in Fig. 8.13a. The noise component of the signal is the standard deviation (σ) of the signal level D_2. The signal strength ΔS is first measured:

$$\Delta S = D_2 - D_1 \qquad (8.14)$$

where D_2 is the target intensity and D_1 the background intensity (as before), measured by taking a

profile through the object. The standard deviation (σ) of the noise is measured and the signal-to-noise ratio is then calculated as

$$SNR = \frac{\Delta S}{\sigma} \qquad (8.15)$$

The SNR should be as high as possible (keeping σ small) in order to achieve good low contrast recording and Fig. 8.13b to e explores the problem of lesion visibility in the presence of noise. The examples show that for a given background noise lesion visibility is achieved by increasing either signal levels or lesion size. The best solution, however, is to decrease the noise itself.

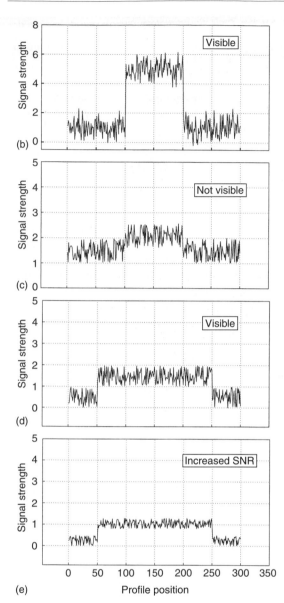

Figure 8.13 (*Contd*) (**b**) *and* (**c**) *show that signal strength is an important parameter in a noisy image and although a larger lesion is more visible,* (**d**) *noise reduction in* (**e**) *(increasing SNR) improves this lesion's visibility.*

QUANTUM NOISE

When a screen-film is exposed to a uniform X-ray exposure the film density, on processing, shows microscopic fluctuations. This is **mottle** and varies according to three major parameters:

- Graininess of the film (this is not usually a problem)

Table 8.8 *The properties of analog images.*

Film/screen	Resolution (Lp mm^{-1})	Noise	Dose (mGy)
CaWO$_4$			
High speed	4.5	31	5.0
Universal	5.6	26	13.0
Detail	8.0	24	24.0
Gd$_2$O$_2$S:Tb			
High speed	4.7	26	2.0
Universal	5.5	24	3.0
Detail	7.5	22	8.0
Mammography	11.0	20	3.0
Cut film	5.0*	30*	1.0
Cine film	5.0*	High	Low

*Limited by image intensifier.

- Phosphor thickness (sensitivity)
- X-ray photon density

These random fluctuations become more obvious if the photon number is small: this causes quantum noise or mottle on the image. Since this depends on photon density quantum noise is inversely proportion to patient dose. Quantum noise is influenced by:

- Fast intensifying screens using far fewer X-ray photons for image formation so $\sqrt{N}$ becomes significant. This stage in image formation and loss of photon density is called the quantum sink.
- Enlargement of the radiograph by altering the object to film distance decreases photon density and increases noise.
- Patient dose; increased photon density increases patient dose.

Quantum noise reduces the level of low contrast detectability and will affect resolution since it reduces the sharpness of intensity change.

A typical radiographic density would be 1×10^5 photons mm^{-2}. Quantum noise at this level would be minimal but noise is most evident on nuclear medicine images where densities are of the order of 12 to 15 photons mm^{-2}. The performance of intensifier screens and film is given in Table 8.8. The relative noise figures and sensitivity in terms of dose are given.

DYNAMIC RANGE

The need to represent a wide range of anatomical detail on a film image is an important diagnostic

Box 8.4 Dynamic ranges required

The overall attenuation of a beam through a patient is

$$I_{out} = I_{in}e^{-\mu x}$$

The dynamic range required to register full attenuation information is I_{in}/I_{out}, where $I_{in} = 1.0$.

Example A

For mammography, where $E_{eff} = 20\,keV$, $x = 5\,cm$, and $\mu = 0.7613$, the dynamic range is

$$\frac{1}{e^{-(0.7613 \times 5)}} = 50{:}1$$

Example B

For the abdomen, where $E_{eff} = 60\,keV$, $x = 20\,cm$, and $\mu = 0.2046$, the dynamic range is 60:1.

Example C

For the chest, where $E_{eff} = 125\,keV$, $x = 30\,cm$, and $\mu = 0.160$, the dynamic range is 120:1.

The film latitude must match these dynamic ranges to capture the entire contrast range. A typical film dynamic range is from 10:1 to 100:1 depending on film latitude. Image plate displays have a very wide dynamic range of about 10 000:1.

Table 8.9 *Projection radiology: typical spatial resolution.*

Image type	Best resolution (Lp mm^{-1})
35 mm Camera film (fine grain)	100 to 200
Film/screen (mammography)	15 to 20
Film/screen (conventional)	2 to 10
Computed radiography (CR)	5 to 8
Direct radiography (DR)	5

definition video displays (1024 and 1250 lines) and consequently these units have SNR values at least ×2 higher (1:2000 and up to 1:6000). Since fluoroscopy uses low X-ray exposures the video signal is small so the dynamic range is an important parameter.

Table 8.8 lists the performance figures for several radiographic studies using film screen or film by itself. Table 8.9 compares the high contrast resolution obtainable in commercial 35 mm photography and routine projection radiography using film screen, computed radiography (image plate) and flat panel direct radiography (DR) using full field solid detectors and a TFT detector array.

8.4 SCATTER AND GRIDS

The influence of scatter on contrast is simplistically demonstrated in Fig. 8.14a where areas outside D_1 and D_2 contribute scattered photons so significantly decreasing subject contrast. This scatter within the patient appears on the image detector as a misplaced event, adding to image noise.

8.4.1 Scatter to primary ratio

The scatter component S degrades maximum subject contrast C giving a final scatter contrast C_S. So

$$C_S = \frac{\Delta D}{D_1 + S} \qquad (8.16)$$

Box 8.5 shows that this is equivalent to

$$C_S = \frac{C}{1 + R} \qquad (8.17)$$

where R is the scatter to primary ratio. The values given in Fig. 8.14a are recalculated in Box 8.5. The

requirement; the wider the range the greater the image information. The dynamic range of the signal itself is the ratio of X-ray intensity with no attenuation to X-ray intensity at maximum tissue attenuation. A calculation for dynamic range in Box 8.4 shows the dynamic range of radiographic film as 1:100 which covers an optical density of about 0.5 to 2.5. The video dynamic range is the maximum video signal (typically 1 V) divided by the RMS of the noise. Noise values are typically 1 mV, so the dynamic range of an image intensifier video system is given by the system SNR and a dynamic range of 1:1000 would be expected.

The SNR decreases with video bandwidth so very high quality components are essential with high

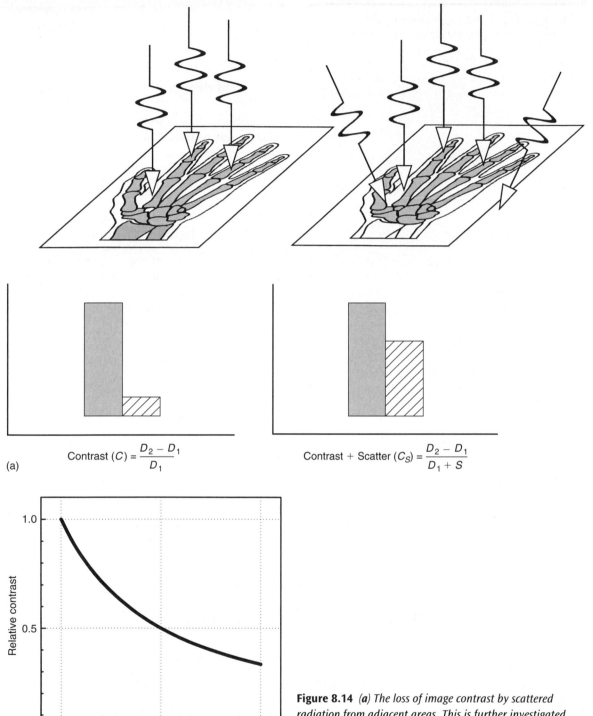

(a)

$$\text{Contrast } (C) = \frac{D_2 - D_1}{D_1}$$

$$\text{Contrast + Scatter } (C_S) = \frac{D_2 - D_1}{D_1 + S}$$

(b)

Relative contrast

Scatter to primary ratio

Figure 8.14 (*a*) *The loss of image contrast by scattered radiation from adjacent areas. This is further investigated in Box 8.5.* (*b*) *The scatter to primary ratio influencing image contrast. A scatter to primary ratio of 1.0 reduces contrast by 50%.*

Box 8.5 Scatter component and scatter to primary ratio

If the values for D_1, D_2, and S are 12, 3, and 2, respectively, then for contrast without scatter, C:

$$C = \frac{D_2 - D_1}{D_1} = 3.0$$

For contrast with scatter (C_S):

$$C_S = \frac{(D_2 + S) - (D_1 + S)}{D_1 + S}$$

Since $(D_2 + S) - (D_1 + S) = D_2 - D_1$ then

$$C_S = \frac{D_2 - D_1}{D_1 + S} = 1.8$$

Introducing the scatter : primary ratio R (2:3), then

$$C_S = \frac{C}{1 + R} = \frac{3}{1.666} = 1.8$$

scatter to primary ratio is plotted against contrast degradation in Fig. 8.14b and shows that when this ratio has a value of 1:1 then contrast is reduced by 50%.

Chapter 5 has already shown that the probability of Compton scatter is highest at low photon energies but the greatest proportion of low energy scatter is absorbed within the patient. So the amount of scatter reaching the imaging surface increases with energy, peaking at about 80 kV; since the scatter is in the forward direction it travels toward the film.

Tissue type also influences scatter production since the probability of a scatter event (σ/ρ) is proportional to electron density but inversely proportional to energy, so

$$\frac{\sigma}{\rho} \propto \frac{\text{electron density}}{\text{photon density}} \quad (8.18)$$

Various factors also reduce the effect of scatter on the image. The intensifying screen phosphor sensitivity is much less for low energy scatter photons and K-edge filtration precisely shapes the X-ray spectrum reducing the intensity of higher energy photons from the X-ray beam that are not required (e.g. mammography) so reducing the amount of scattered radiation reaching the film.

8.4.2 Grid design

The problem of separating scatter from primary radiation was addressed by Bucky in 1913 when he introduced a grating or grid of thin lead strips which collimated the emerging radiation from the patient allowing the unscattered primary beam to reach the film, blocking most of the off-axis scatter radiation which approached the lead strips at an angle. Scatter is significantly reduced by placing a grid between the patient and the film cassette or imaging surface (image intensifier).

FOCUSED OR PARALLEL GRIDS

A focused and parallel grid design is shown in Fig. 8.15a and b. Focused grids follow the sector geometry of the X-ray beam more closely so are more efficient in accepting the primary beam at shorter FIDs. Common focal distances for these grids are 80, 100, 140, and 180 cm for conventional radiology and 60 cm for mammography.

If larger FIDs are used than those recommended then the X-ray beam is cut off at the image periphery. Off-center beams also give image artifacts. This is discussed later. Parallel grids have their lead strips arranged in a parallel fashion (they are not focused). Since the X-ray beam radiates at an increasing oblique angle toward the edge of the grid there will be increasing cut-off with a parallel design so they are only suitable for FIDs exceeding 2 m when the X-ray beam itself approximates to parallel lines; this is the case in chest radiography where static high ratio parallel grids are used.

LEAD STRIP THICKNESS, *d*

The grid has very thin strips of metal sandwiched between radiolucent material (plastic or carbon fiber) which forms a composite grating (Fig. 8.16a). Metals used in the construction of grids are lead ($Z = 82$), tungsten ($Z = 74$), and tantalum ($Z = 73$); lead is the most common material. The quantity of lead ($g\,cm^{-2}$) of a grid is a measure of its contrast improvement capability since this is a rough measure

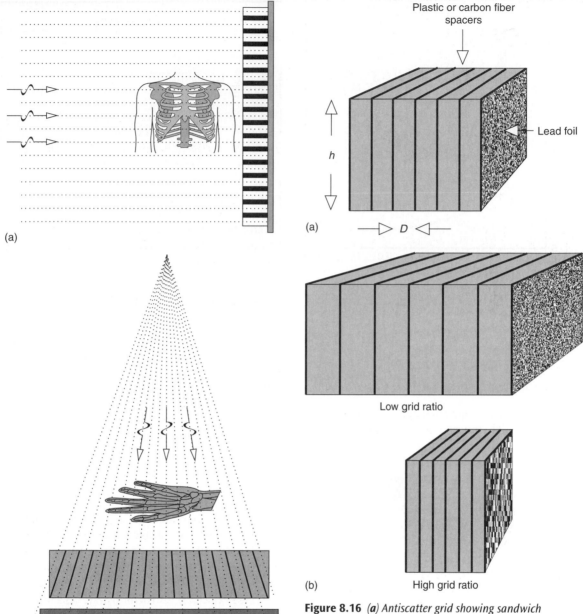

(a)

(b)

Figure 8.15 *(a) The design and operation of focused and (b) parallel antiscatter grids. The focused grid gives increased efficiency since it mimics the beam geometry.*

(a)

Plastic or carbon fiber spacers

h

Lead foil

D

Low grid ratio

(b)

High grid ratio

Figure 8.16 *(a) Antiscatter grid showing sandwich construction with lead strips with interspace material (thickness D). The grid assembly has a height h and it is protected by a thin plastic or metal cover. (b) The difference in interspace gap between a low and high ratio grid.*

of lead-strip density per unit area of grid surface. Thick lead strips, however, remove a significant proportion of the primary radiation which is required for image formation so the lead strips should be thin enough to stop scattered radiation at the intended kV_p at the same time blocking minimal primary beam photons. Typical thicknesses for general radiology are between 0.036 and 0.07 mm; thinner strips can be obtained by using tungsten or tantalum. Example dimensions are given in Fig. 8.16b for a low and high ratio grid.

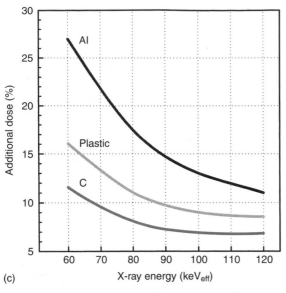

(c)

Figure 8.16 *(Contd) (c) Dose reduction over the diagnostic X-ray range by using carbon fiber (C) instead of aluminum (Al) or plastic (P) spaced grids.*

INTERSPACE MATERIAL THICKNESS, *D*

The lead strips are supported and separated by low density material, transparent to X-rays. This can be aluminum in the finer grids (high strip density) but is more usually paper, plastic or, more recently, carbon fiber; the thickness is normally limited to 0.150 mm.

The interspace material will remove a small proportion of the primary beam so its density should be as low as possible particularly in low dose investigations such as mammography and pediatric studies. Figure 8.16c shows the percentage dose reduction that can be achieved by using carbon fiber instead of aluminum or plastic/paper. The carbon fiber interspace material achieves dose reduction by up to 30% depending on kilovoltage and grid ratio.

LINE DENSITY, LINES cm^{-1}

Very thin lead strips or lamellae stop less primary radiation and in high ratio grids line density is increased by decreasing the strip thickness d. This is calculated as

$$\frac{10}{D + d} \qquad (8.19)$$

Box 8.6 Grid specifications

Grid parameters that are used are strip thickness (d), interspace thickness (D), and grid height (h). These give the grid ratio, r:

	r	d	D	h
Grid A	8:1	0.07	0.18	1.4
Grid B	12:1	0.035	0.10	2.1
Grid C	3.5:1	0.035	0.28	1.0

Line density is $10/(d + D)$ lines per cm.

Transmission of primary radiation $T_{p} = D/(d + D)$ percent.

Grid A (conventional)
Line density = 40 lines cm^{-2}
Transmission = 72%
Grid B (chest X-ray)
Line density = 74 lines cm^{-2}
Transmission = 74%
Grid C (mammography)
Line density = 32 lines cm^{-2}
Transmission = 88%

Common line densities are 22 to 77 lines cm^{-1}. High line density grids are less selective than low line density at higher kV$_p$. Box 8.6 calculates the different line densities and X-ray transmission for three grid types: conventional (A), high resolution (B) and mammography (C).

These calculations demonstrate that primary transmission is typically 75% for common grid types and increases to over 80% for mammography where it is important to reduce patient radiation dose by utilizing the maximum proportion of primary beam.

MOVING AND STATIONARY GRIDS

Although the use of antiscatter grids in diagnostic radiology prevents scattered radiation reaching the film surface one of the disadvantages is that the shadows of the metal strips can be seen on the resulting image. A moving grid (developed by Potter in 1920 and called the Potter Bucky diaphragm) eliminates the grid patterns on the image.

These were introduced first as a spring operated device but modern Potter Bucky diaphragms are now motor driven giving a more uniform oscillating movement during exposure. They can produce a stroboscopic artifact with very short exposure times.

Fluoroscopy has a lower visual resolution than film so stationary grids are used. Very fast exposures of about 20 ms (high kilovoltage chest X-ray) also use stationary grids since grid movement would be too slow. It is important to have effective grid movement in mammography since this procedure has the highest resolution.

MULTI-LINE GRIDS

Advances in the manufacture of grids have produced line densities up to 60 to 70 lines cm^{-1}. The advantages are that these grids can be stationary since 70 lines cm^{-1} can only be detected by magnifying the image. Image contrast is similar to a moving 40 lines cm^{-1} grid.

CROSS GRIDS

These consist of two focused grids lying on top of one another. Crossed grids give a high reduction of scattered radiation in both x and y planes but beam alignment must be exactly perpendicular if they are not to introduce artifacts.

8.4.3 Grid specifications

Various parameters are used for describing grid performance. These are:

- Grid ratio
- Line density
- Grid factor/Bucky factor
- Contrast improvement factor
- Selectivity

Figure 8.17a to d shows the general grid construction and the dimensions that take part in the various specifications. Grid performance, in general, can be described in terms of contrast improvement factor (CIF) and exposure (or radiation dose) increase factor (grid factor). Both are strongly dependent on exposure conditions (e.g. kV_p, field size, tissue type).

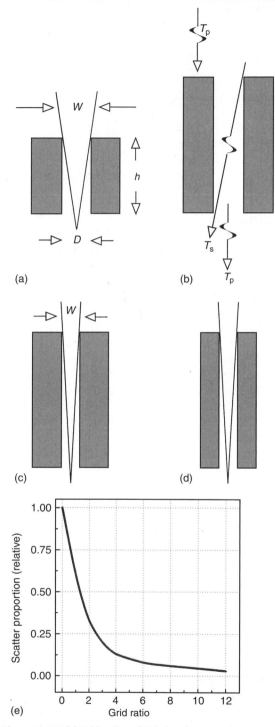

Figure 8.17 (**a**) Grid ratios of 5:1 showing acceptance angle and (**b**) identifying primary and scattered beams. (**c**) 15:1 ratio grid demonstrating that reducing the thickness of the lead foil in (**d**) does not alter the grid ratio. (**e**) Plot of scatter reduction reaching image with increasing grid ratio.

Table 8.10 *Grid specifications.*

Term	Definition		Typical value
Grid ratio	$\dfrac{h}{D}$		12:1 5:1
Line density	$\dfrac{1}{d+D}$ lines cm^{-1}		28 to 60 lines cm^{-1}
General specification	Small field		Pb 12/40
	Large field		Pb 5/28
	Mammography		Pb 3/28
	Fluoroscopy		Pb 12/36

GRID RATIO, *r*

This is the ratio between grid height h and interspace distance D so that

$$r = \frac{h}{D} \tag{8.20}$$

Common values are 3.5:1 or 5:1 for mammography, 15:1 up to 20:1 for conventional radiography, and 30:1 to 40:1 for high kilovoltage chest radiography. The ratio for both grids Fig. 8.17a and b is 5:1; the height and spacer thickness have been altered proportionately. The grid ratio for (c) and (d) is 15:1, the thickness of the lead strip has not altered this but the proportion of available primary radiation T_p would have increased due to the thinner lead septa. The width W of the acceptance angle θ is related to h and D as

$$\tan \theta = \frac{D}{h} \tag{8.21}$$

Grid ratio determines the scatter to primary ratio that reaches the image detector. High ratio grids pass less scatter and give better image contrast components but need more careful alignment with beam geometry. The graph in Fig. 8.17e shows the reduction of scatter transmission as the grid ratio is increased, for the same kilovoltage. Both axes are logarithmic so the straight-line relationship shows that scatter reduction follows a square law relationship. The grid ratio and line density are used for describing grids in terms of ratio and density. The combination is shown in Table 8.10.

The parameters associated with radiation incident on the grid I_0 and transmitted by the grid, identified in Fig. 8.17b, are defined as:

- The primary radiation transmitted through the grid, T_p
- The scattered radiation transmitted through the grid, T_s
- The total radiation transmitted through the grid, $T_t = T_p + T_s$

The fractional transmission for a grid can be simply measured by noting the exposure values with and without the grid in place:

$$T_t = \frac{\text{mAs with grid}}{\text{mAs without grid}} \tag{8.22}$$

This value has already been calculated for the grids in Box 8.6 using the various thicknesses of the lead and interspace material but this calculation does not allow for absorption by the interspace material itself.

GRID EXPOSURE FACTOR

This is also known as the grid factor (GF) or Bucky factor. It is a measure of the increased dose required when using a grid.

GF is the exposure multiplication factor in order to achieve the same film blackening when using the grid at the same kV$_p$. It is usually obtained by measuring the transmitted radiation T_t and incident radiation I_0 and is a direct measure of absorption of both primary and secondary radiation by the grid:

$$\text{GF} = \frac{I_0}{T_t} \tag{8.23}$$

The grid factor is an indication of the grid's ability to stop both primary and secondary radiation but decreases with increasing kV$_p$ due to penetration of the lead septa (Fig. 8.18a).

CONTRAST IMPROVEMENT FACTOR

An X-ray grid has only one function and that is to improve the contrast of the X-ray image by preventing scattered radiation reaching the image surface. The effectiveness of this operation is indicated by the contrast improvement factor (CIF):

$$\text{CIF} = \frac{\text{contrast with grid}}{\text{contrast without grid}} \tag{8.24}$$

Two densities are chosen (on an aluminum step wedge) and their differences measured with and without a grid. If the total transmitted radiation were

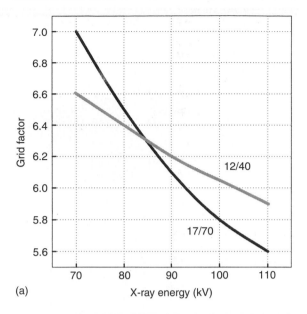

(a)

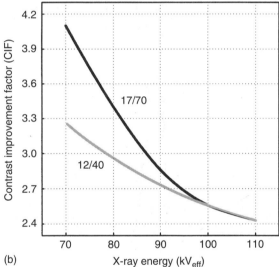

(b)

Figure 8.18 *(a) Grid factor decreasing with increased kilovoltage. (b) CIF factor decreases with increasing kilovoltage. The higher ratio/line number grid has a superior CIF at low energies but this is lost for higher energy X-ray imaging.*

$T_t = T_p + T_s$ then the above equation can be expressed as

$$CIF = \frac{T_p}{T_t} \qquad (8.25)$$

Contrast degrades as the scatter component of T_t increases. A typical grid can improve contrast by a factor of ×3 to ×4 but depends a great deal on size

Table 8.11 *Summary of grid terms, the ratio GF :CIF gives an overall quality factor.*

Grid	CIF	GF	Σ	Quality factor, CIF:GF
General				
8/28	3.3	4.7	5.5	0.70
12/28	3.9	5.7	7.9	0.67
High Contrast				
8/36	2.9	3.9	4.3	0.74
12/36	3.6	5.1	6.4	0.72
Mammography Image intensifier	2.4	3.0	6.2	0.80
12/44	3.6	5.2	6.6	0.70

and tissue type as well as the kV_p being used. The CIF value degrades as kV_p is increased due to penetration of the lead strips (Fig. 8.18b) and a steady decline in contrast is seen.

SELECTIVITY, Σ

This depends on grid ratio and lead strip thickness, it measures transmitted scatter T_s as a percentage of the primary beam T_p reaching the film.

$$\Sigma = \frac{T_p}{T_s} \qquad (8.26)$$

An efficient grid would stop all scattered radiation and pass all the primary so making $\Sigma = \infty$. If 20% of scatter is transmitted then Σ is 5 which would seriously degrade image quality; a more acceptable figure would be a Σ value of 6 to 8. More efficient grids will have still higher values.

Table 8.11 lists a series of grids with various ratio/line density values with their GF, CIF performance figures. These last two parameters can be combined to give a quality factor. Since the CIF value should be large and GF small the quality factor value should be as high as possible.

GRID MISALIGNMENT

Figure 8.19a and b illustrates two common faults that are found when using either parallel or focused grids. The focused grid must be used at a recommended distance from the focal point since bringing the focal spot (X-ray tube) nearer will cause shadowing, seen as thick bars on the image.

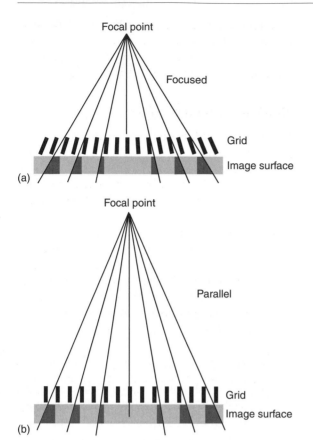

Figure 8.19 *Misalignment for both (**a**) a focused and (**b**) a parallel grid showing how grid shadow is caused by the lead strips.*

Similarly, if the X-ray tube is used too near a parallel grid shadow bars will be seen. High ratio parallel grids are commonly used in high kilovoltage chest radiography; a distance of at least 2 m should be maintained in order to prevent these artifacts.

8.5 IMAGE QUALITY MEASUREMENT

8.5.1 Resolution and contrast

The three-dimensional representation of a point source of radiation on a detector surface is shown in Fig. 8.20a; instead of sharp edges a Gaussian distribution is evident. The dimension of this point source is measured at the half-width mark as full width at half maximum (FWHM). A tenth maximum point is sometimes used with this (Fig. 8.20b).

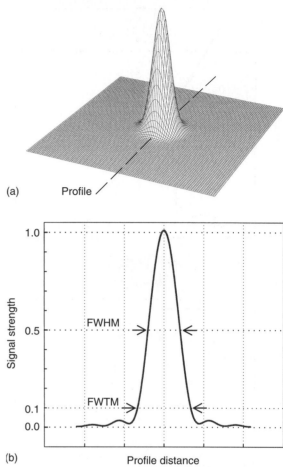

Figure 8.20 *(**a**) A three-dimensional representation of a point source of radiation on an imaging surface showing the Gaussian distribution. (**b**) A profile taken through this source measuring the full width at half maximum (FWHM) and tenth maximum (FWTM).*

RESOLUTION

Two point sources can be used to measure the resolving power of a display. The point sources can theoretically be resolved if the separation is greater than the FWHM of the point spread function (PSF). This is demonstrated in Fig. 8.21. A distance less than the FWHM in (a) displays the points as a single entity. In (b) the point source separation equals the FWHM; this is the threshold point when two separate points can just be resolved. The two point sources in (c) are separated by a distance that is greater than the FWHM, the overall envelope clearly resolves the two separate points.

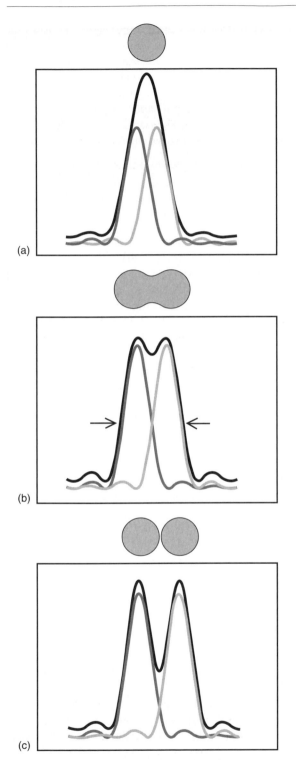

(a)

(b)

(c)

Figure 8.21 *(a) Complete merging of the point sources when their separation is <FWHM. (b) Resolvable points are displayed when distanced by their FWHM value. (c) Points clearly resolved when separation is >FWHM.*

A film-screen can resolve approximately 50 to 100 μm point sources, CT 0.3 mm and MRI 0.7 mm. Ultrasound resolves about 1 mm and nuclear medicine 3 mm, depending on the field of view.

POINT SPREAD FUNCTION

The point spread function (PSF) is the simplest test of spatial resolution in an imaging system. The X-ray image surface (film cassette) is covered with a lead sheet pierced with 10 μm (micron) holes. This size is critical since they must be smaller than the resolution limit of the system.

Sufficient exposure is given to achieve a point image on the film and then a micro-densitometer is used to measure a profile density through the point center. This profile is the PSF. An example is given in Fig. 8.20a and b. In practice it is difficult to measure since a very small point needs to be displayed requiring considerable exposure time under very steady conditions.

The PSF profile in Fig. 8.20b gives a FWHM value. The effect of scatter reaching the image detector (grid or collimator having septa penetration) broadens the 'skirt' or 'tail' of the curve giving a larger value for the full width at tenth maximum (FWTM). Long 'tails' cause spreading beyond the source boundaries which contributes to the total unsharpness (geometrical and radiographic). This is an indication of the radiation penetrating the lead strips in an antiscatter grid or collimator on a gamma camera.

LINE SPREAD FUNCTION

A point spread function has limitations as an image test tool since it only represents discrete points on the image surface. A line source in the form of a 10 μm metal slit (usually made from platinum) provides a measure along a complete axis of the imaging surface as shown in Fig. 8.22. This is measured as the line spread function (LSF).

The LSF is a better measure since it is easier to make a line source using two knife edges with a 10 μm gap. The density of the line profile, recorded by the image, is then read with a microdensitometer as before.

The LSF example in Fig. 8.22 shows a more comprehensive measure of image detector performance. The resolving power of a complete image axis is demonstrated in one measurement.

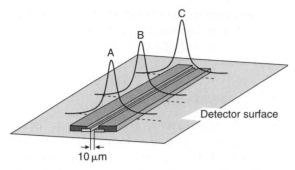

Figure 8.22 *A line source placed on an imaging surface and yielding a series of profiles A, B and C as line spread functions.*

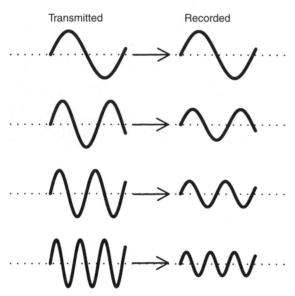

Figure 8.23 *Transmitted signal frequencies and recorded image signals showing loss of signal strength with frequency. The loss of frequency information (resolution) is plotted as the MTF curve.*

8.5.2 Modulation transfer function

A quantitative analysis of an imaging systems resolution capability and the degradation it gives to the image data is given by the modulation transfer function (MTF).

The principle of the MTF is shown in Fig. 8.23 where an input signal, usually in the form of fixed amplitude but varying frequency sine waves is recorded by the imaging medium: film, television monitor, image intensifier, gamma camera etc.

As the frequency of the input signal increases the ability of the recording system to faithfully follow the signal begins to fail. The recording system modulates, or degrades, the signal so that the output amplitude is reduced. The ratio of the output signal amplitude to the input signal amplitude at each frequency is the MTF. The transfer of frequencies from source to the imaging system defines the MTF as

$$\text{MIT} = \frac{\text{recorded signal frequencies}}{\text{original signal frequencies}} \quad (8.27)$$

A perfect system would have an MTF of 1.0 and this value is given by most imaging systems for very low frequency signals. The MTF value then falls off as higher frequencies are recorded.

The MTF is extremely useful since it allows the resolving power of each image component to be quantified, e.g. intensifying screen, film, and the combination of both. A complete fluoroscopy imaging chain can be studied: the image intensifier input phosphor, the photocathode, the output screen, the video camera, and the final video display, so that weak points can be identified and corrected.

DERIVATION OF THE MTF

Individual readings are taken from the line spread function at fixed intervals shown in Fig. 8.24a. The formula which is used for calculating the MTF involves a Fourier analysis (Chapter 1, Section 1.12.2). The resolution of each factor in the LSF can be described in terms of spatial frequency response and those frequency dependent variations (amplitude losses) are combined in the modulation transfer function. The following MTF equation which extracts the frequency components from the LSF uses the Fourier transform:

$$\frac{\sum_{j=1}^{m} L(x_j, z) \times (\cos 2\pi v x_j - i \sin 2\pi v x_j)}{\sum_{j=1}^{m} L(x_j, z)} \quad (8.28)$$

where $L(x_j, z)$ represents m individual line spread values at Δx sampling interval using a spatial frequency of $v \, \text{Lp mm}^{-1}$ shown taken from the readings in the figure.

The MTF is easily calculated by digitizing the PSF or LSF measurements and using eqn 8.28. The individual MTFs for film A and intensifying screen B are shown in Fig. 8.24b and c. Multiplying the individual

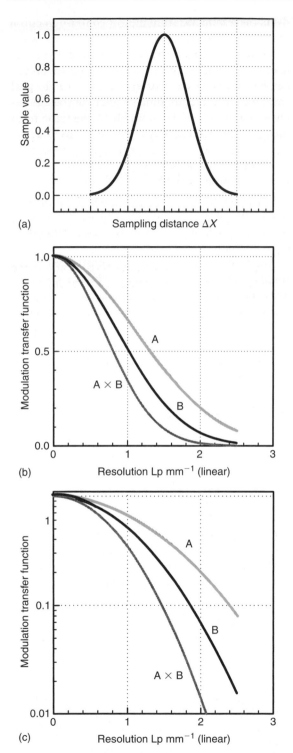

(a)

(b)

(c)

Figure 8.24 *(a) The LSF used as a data source for computing the MTF. (b) The MTF plotted on linear axes and (c) the MTF values plotted on a log scale for the same two film-screen systems.*

MTFs gives the expected MTF of the final display $A \times B$ shown in the linear–linear and semi-log of the same MTF data in Fig. 8.24b and c.

An imaging system having perfect reproduction of its transmitted frequencies gives an MTF value of 1.0. However, all imaging systems show a limitation; the limit of visual detail is normally taken at an MTF of 0.1 (10%) which is the **cut-off frequency**. Others quote the resolution limitation to be nearer 4%. The area under the MTF curve, up to the cut-off frequency, gives a value of the overall system resolution. Manufacturers sometimes quote 50%, 10%, and 2% values.

WIENER SPECTRUM

Noise can be measured quantitatively by using the Wiener spectrum which plots the noise of a system as a function of its frequency content; high and low frequency noise can be readily identified. It is generally agreed that the frequency range of 0.2 to 1 Lp mm^{-1} is relevant to radiology since these frequencies are easy visible and their effect noticed. For film-screen systems the relationship between the MTF and the Wiener spectrum, WS, is

$$\mathrm{WS} = \frac{G^2}{n} \times \mathrm{MTF}^2 \qquad (8.29)$$

where n is the number of photons absorbed and G is the film gamma. For a given X-ray exposure the film gamma (contrast) is proportional to the Wiener spectrum. A change in the speed (sensitivity) alters n since noise increases with sensitivity.

The Wiener spectrum shown in Fig. 8.25 shows a typical noise spectrum from a film-screen combination. The background noise is predominantly low frequency, identified as film grain and phosphor structure. High frequency noise is increased when detail (thin) intensifying screens are used and is related to poor photon absorption (quantum efficiency).

CONTRAST DETAIL DIAGRAM

The results from the low contrast phantom shown in Fig. 8.11 can be expressed as a contrast detail diagram (CDD) in Fig. 8.26a which indicates the threshold contrast needed to detect an object as a function of its diameter. Contrast detail analysis is a graphic representation which relates the minimum (threshold) contrast necessary to visualize an object of a certain size in a noisy image. The basic components of a contrast

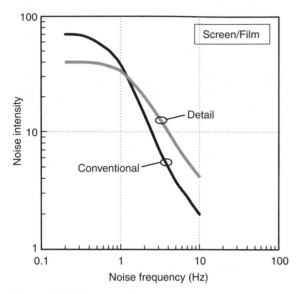

Figure 8.25 *Wiener spectrum.*

detail curve obtained from the low contrast phantom are shown in Fig. 8.26a.

Contrast is displayed on the *y*-axis and object size on the *x*-axis. The curve shows that larger objects can be seen more easily at low contrast levels while smaller objects require much higher contrast differences before they become visible in the same noisy image. This has already been demonstrated in Fig. 8.13b to e when discussing signal-to-noise ratio. The contrast detail curve in Fig. 8.26a starts at the upper left corner at an object size which is the resolution limit of the system and declines asymptotically. Above the curve the conditions (image noise) satisfy visibility of the object; below the curve conditions prevent visibility.

Contrast detail curves are constructed using results obtained from a group of observers, viewing a test image containing a set of precisely sized objects and varying contrast levels. The test image is obtained

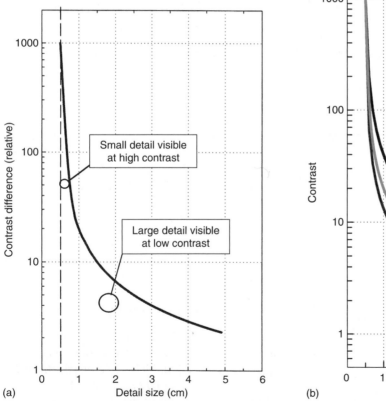

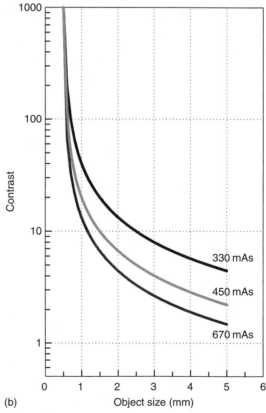

Figure 8.26 *(a) Contrast detail diagram showing small object size visible at high contrast levels but as the object detail loses contrast then these are only visible if their sizes increase. Contrast levels above the curve are not visible. (b) Contrast detail improvement with increasing exposure levels (mAs) allowing smaller low contrast objects to be seen at 670 mAs.*

from an imaging system under different conditions (kV_p, mAs, screen types, film types, etc.). Figure 8.26b gives an example of a set of contrast detail curves obtained for two exposure (mAs) settings.

DETECTIVE QUANTUM EFFICIENCY (DQE)

The DQE of an imaging system describes the system accuracy of response to information (emerging X-ray beam, gamma radiation, light etc.). Signal-to-noise ratios vary at every stage of image production and will increase overall. If the SNR variation in the photon beam (subject contrast) is SNR_{in} and the SNR of the detection process (radiographic contrast in the intensifying screen, image intensifier phosphor or image plate, etc.) is SNR_{out} then the DQE compares input and output SNR as

$$DQE = \left(\frac{SNR_{out}}{SNR_{in}} \right)^2 \qquad (8.30)$$

The SNR of an incident photon flux N is $\sqrt{N}$ which is due to quantum noise variations. The SNR of the detector is dependent on absorbed photon number N_{ab}, its noise being $\sqrt{N_{ab}}$. The value of N_{ab} is closely dependent on photon absorption which is influenced by both μ and screen thickness. Conversion efficiency (e.g. light production) is also crucial.

The DQE for film (Fig. 8.27a) shows how critical film processing is so that optimum film density between 1 and 2 is maintained for the image density likely to represent pathology in the image. The comparison between film-screen and image phosphor plate DQE values in Fig. 8.27b indicates the change of DQE value with system resolution since in order to improve resolution the phosphor screen thickness must be reduced, increasing noise and so reducing SNR_{out}. The limiting spatial resolution for CR at present is $5\,Lp\,mm^{-1}$ compared to film-screens which can extend to $15\,Lp\,mm^{-1}$; the smallest detail resolvable with present film-screens (mammography) is about $130\,\mu m$.

8.5.3 Total image quality assessment: ROC curves

Receiver operating characteristic (ROC) curves provide an objective assessment of an imaging chain, whether it be a simple string such as

film-screen → film processor → film quality

or a more complex string such as

image plate → image digitization → data manipulation → color video display

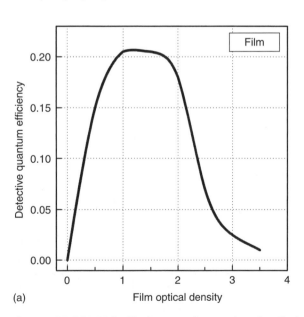

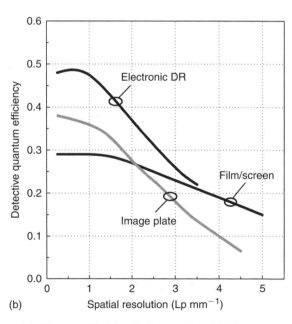

(a)   Film optical density

(b)   Spatial resolution (Lp mm⁻¹)

Figure 8.27 *(**a**) DQE for film has a maximum value when the image detail has an optical density between 1 and 2. Film processing quality is important in order to maintain this. (**b**) The decrease with resolution of DQE for film/screen and image plate exposed to 50 μGy. The performance of a typical DR selenium detector is also compared.*

Table 8.12 *Results table.*

Test result	Master+	Copy−	Total
Positive test image	TP	FP	TP + FP
Negative test image	FN	TN	FN + TN
Total	TP + FN	FP + TN	TP + FN + FP + TN

It enables display sensitivity, specificity and overall accuracy of a particular display system to be compared with another system so that decisions can be made regarding the success or improvement that the new system may give and a measure of its diagnostic sensitivity and specificity.

SENSITIVITY AND SPECIFICITY

The final test for any display system is its clinical success for detecting disease. This is purely subjective and depends not only on the quality (resolution, contrast, noise) of the image but also the viewing conditions and the skill of the observer in discriminating between a true and a false uptake or lesion on the display.

Detecting a positive lesion (true positive) or reporting a negative finding (true negative) becomes more difficult as either contrast or size diminishes. A procedure for estimating the accuracy of visual image analysis considers also the reporting of mistaken lesions (false positive) and missed lesions (false negative) and gives a measure of **sensitivity**, which is the ability to detect abnormality and **specificity** or the ability to report a negative finding or detect a normal result. A 2 × 2 table format for this analysis is shown in Table 8.12.

Applying this test to an imaging system requires a series of images to be recorded which contain lesions/objects of varying size and contrast. These are either radio-opaque objects in the case of X-ray images or radio-active sources in the case of nuclear medicine. They can also be computer derived 'lesions'. Certain images in the series are completely clear and contain no lesions. A noisy image background is present to a fixed degree in all the images. About 100 images make up the series and these are given to a panel of observers for judging. Tables 8.13 and 8.14 show how the results would be set out comparing the known lesion number (master copy) with the reported lesion number (test result).

Table 8.13 *Series total of 200 images with a 50% incidence.*

Test result	Master+	Copy−	Total
Positive test image	75	30	105
Negative test image	25	70	95
Total	100	100	200

From eqns 8.31, 8.32, and 8.33, the sensitivity = 75/100 = 75%; the specificity = 70/100 = 70%; and the accuracy = 145/200 = 72.5%.

Table 8.14 *The second series of 200 images, with a 10% incidence.*

Test result	Master+	Copy−	Total
Positive test image	10	30	40
Negative test image	10	150	160
Total	20	180	200

From eqns 8.31, 8.32, and 8.33, the sensitivity = 10/20 = 50%; the specificity = 150/180 = 83%; and the accuracy = 40/200 = 20%.

The results from the table give three measurements:

- **Sensitivity**

$$\frac{TP}{TP + FN} \tag{8.31}$$

- **Selectivity**

$$\frac{TN}{TN + FP} \tag{8.32}$$

- **Overall accuracy**

$$\frac{TP + TN}{grand\ total} \tag{8.33}$$

where TP = true positive, TN = true negative, FP = false positive, and FN = false negative. For a dual series of 200 images, one with a 50% incidence of lesions and the other with a 10% incidence the results shown in Tables 8.13 and 8.14 were obtained. These two examples demonstrate the real effect of disease incidence in the population being studied on the sensitivity and specificity of a test. A high incidence of disease (or a high number of lesions in the image) gives a test with a higher sensitivity than a population with a low incidence of disease (lower number of lesions in the image data set). The specificity shows the opposite effect.

Table 8.15 *Sensitivity and specificity for two tests (A and B) in nuclear medicine and computed tomography.*

Investigation	Sensitivity (%)	Specificity (%)
Test A	80	60
Test B	90	90

THE DIAGNOSTIC IMAGE

If two investigations (test A and test B) are performed on the same patient then the separate sensitivity and specificity figures for each test can be combined to give improved accuracy. For instance the sensitivity/specificity for a nuclear medicine and CT investigation are known to give the precision given in Table 8.15. Then the combined sensitivity/specificity figures for the first case when:

- A and/or B are positive,
- A and B are negative

are

combined sensitivity

$$= \frac{\text{sensitivity A} + (100 - \text{sensitivity A}) \times \text{sensitivity B}}{100}$$

and

$$\text{combined specificity} = \frac{\text{specificity A} \times \text{specificity B}}{100}$$

The combined sensitivity/specificity figures for the second case when:

- A and B are positive
- A and/or B are negative

are

$$\text{combined sensitivity} = \frac{\text{sensitivity A} \times \text{sensitivity B}}{100}$$

and

combined specificity

$$= \frac{\text{specificity A} + (100 - \text{specificity A}) \times \text{specificity B}}{100}$$

For the combined nuclear medicine and CT investigations the first case will present a sensitivity of 98% and a specificity of 54% and the second case will present a sensitivity of 72% and a specificity of 96%. So combining the results from carefully chosen investigations markedly improves overall sensitivity and specificity.

A test with a high sensitivity is good for detecting disease in a population where the incidence of disease is low: it will give few false negatives. This will exclude disease which should be the object with screening tests. A test with a high specificity is good for detecting the absence of disease in (say) a patient group where there is a high probability of the disease since there are few false positives so preventing unnecessary treatment, particularly if the treatment carries its own risk. Double viewing the same images from one investigation (mammography) will similarly improve sensitivity and specificity in a population with low disease incidence and improve significantly on the figures demonstrated in the second group having only 10% disease.

THE RECEIVER OPERATING CHARACTERISTIC CURVE

This plots the true positive fraction (TPF) of an observer response against the false positive fraction (FPF). It allows a quantitative comparison between imaging systems (CT, MRI, film radiology etc.) for detecting various pathology.

A typical ROC curve is shown in Fig. 8.28a. The TPF, on the y-axis, is the percentage of patients correctly identified as having positive findings. The FPF score is the percentage of patients who were called positive but were really normal. A move towards the right is a less sensitive diagnostic test. A move towards the left denotes a more sensitive test, i.e. increase in specificity but decrease in sensitivity. The upper right corner shows a 100% sensitivity and 0% specificity, i.e. all the findings deemed abnormal. The lower left corner shows 0% sensitivity but 100% specificity: all the findings are normal.

Since FPF is 1 − specificity, reversing the values on the x-axis directly converts it to specificity (Fig. 8.28b). In order to judge effectiveness of a new film-screen, video or digital imaging system for the improvement (if any) in sensitivity, a series of test images (usually 100) containing objects with a range of contrast, corresponding to a range of detection difficulty, are viewed by a group of observers who report their confidence at detecting the object. Roughly half the cases in the image set have no objects. A ranking/scoring system from 1 to 5 would be:

1 *Definitely normal* (only obvious normals scored) where false positive rate would be high and the false negative low

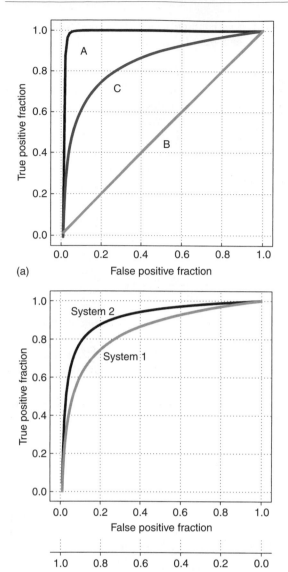

(a)

(b)

Figure 8.28 *(a) A set of ROC curves. Curve A would be given by a perfect system, curve B by a system giving a purely random result (50:50) and curve C by a practical display system offering diagnostic advantages. (b) A set of two curves from two separate display systems showing that display system 2 has a superior performance to display system 1 for detecting a particular pathology.*

2 *Probably normal* (probably no lesion)
3 *Maybe normal* (do not know)
4 *Probably abnormal* (probably a lesion)
5 *Definitely abnormal* (only obvious lesions scored) where the false positive rate would be low and false negative would be high

The ROC curve shown in Fig. 8.28b shows such a result and demonstrates quite convincingly that system 2 has a better detection performance than system 1.

8.6 HARD-COPY DEVICES

The eventual film record from a clinical study can originate from three sources:

- Cassette with intensifying screens
- A video screen through a system of lenses
- A laser imager

The first has been described in Chapter 7 and is the simplest method of recording X-ray images. The second and third methods require electronic handling of the image information to produce a video signal which is then transferred to either a cathode ray tube (CRT) screen or laser optical system which eventually produces the light which exposes the film.

8.6.1 Video film formatter

This method uses a CRT. The image is directed by a series of mirrors and lenses onto a film surface. Since it can provide single or multiple images on a single sheet of film it is often referred to as a multi-format camera. It can handle low or high resolution video signals (512/625 or 1024/1249 lines). Each image contains the full complement of scan lines so resolution is unaffected even for small images. Since a video camera is commonly restricted to an 8 × 10 film size it is not possible to hold more than about six images on each film for routine clinical inspection and the CRT screen must be optically flat to give perfectly rectangular film images without rounded verticals. These cameras have mostly been replaced by more versatile laser imagers.

8.6.2 Laser imager

The main action of a laser imager is to capture the incoming digitized video signal which then modulates a laser beam scanning a film surface. Several machines (CT, MRI, nuclear medicine etc.) can share a single laser imager.

The diagram in Fig. 8.29a identifies the major component parts of a laser imager. The critical design concerns the prism and mirror scanning

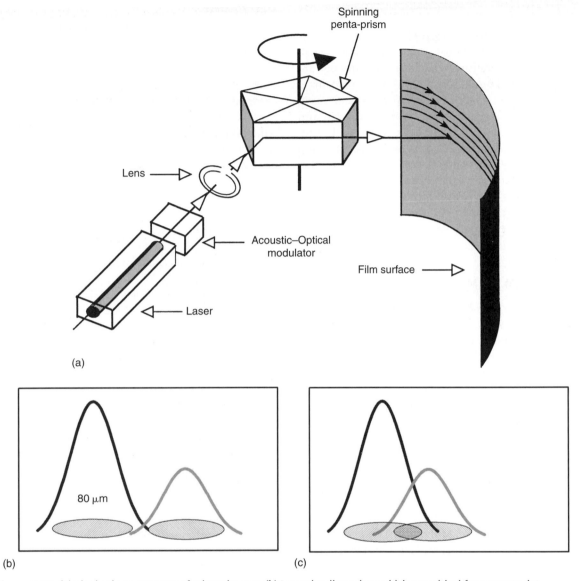

(a)

(b)　　　　　　　　　　　　　　　　　　(c)

Figure 8.29 *(a) The basic components of a laser imager. (b) Laser dot dimensions which are critical for accurate dot placement. (c) Overlapping dot placement degrades image quality.*

assembly which moves the modulated laser beam over the film surface. The film scanning is achieved by a constantly rotating prism in the laser light beam which traces a path on the film which is held in a semi-circular drum. At the end of each scan line the beam is shifted down until the entire sheet of film has been exposed.

SIZE OF IMAGE

The laser scans a 14 × 17 inch film producing an area of 4096 × 5120 pixels; a total of 21 million pixels.

This would accommodate about twenty 1024 × 1024 images from a CT, MRI etc. Each line of pixels (4096) is exposed in approximately 3.8 ms so the time required to expose the complete film area is about 20 s. The He–Ne laser produces red light (630 nm) so special red-sensitive film is necessary. Dry laser imagers which do not rely on photographic principles use opaque carbon or silver based film stock. The laser removes small areas of this opaque material forming an image equal to or superior than the quality of a wet (photographic) laser film imager.

GRAY SCALE

The exposure density of each pixel is determined by the signal strength at that point. The image signal modulates the intensity of the laser beam through an acoustic optical modulator (AOM) which contains a crystal transducer. An electrical signal is converted into an acoustic signal which changes the refractive index of the crystal scattering the light at different angles from the main beam, so reducing the main beam intensity. The scatter intensity depends on the size of the acoustic signal. The main beam passes through a small slot which blocks the scattered light from reaching the film surface. The AOM operates with a 12 bit resolution.

LASER BEAM DIAMETER

The size of the laser dot which exposes the film is critical for producing good spatial resolution (Fig. 8.29b) and misplacement of the spot leads to lost image detail (Fig. 8.29c). The laser beam passes through a lens system which gives a typical beam diameter of $85\,\mu m$ giving an image matrix size of typically 4096×5120 pixels, representing 12 pixels mm^{-1}.

A line error deviation of 3% requires a laser beam placement accuracy of $\pm 1.3\,\mu m$. The mechanical precision is therefore very high and vibration must be prevented over the exposure 20 s exposure time. Look-up tables within the digital control can give a truly linear or various nonlinear scales.

The disadvantage of the laser imager is the fixed image matrix size. Multiple images would share the total 4096×5120 matrix. High definition (1024/1249 line) video images in multi-format (4×5 image set) would only just be faithfully recorded. Specifications for a typical laser imager are given in Table 8.16.

Table 8.16 *Laser imager specifications.*

Laser type	Helium/neon
Film	Red sensitive
Film sizes (inches)	8×10, 11×14, 14×17
Modulation depth (gray scale)	12 bits
Pixels on 14″ × 17″ film	4096×5120
Processor cycle	48 to 60 s
Number of inputs	4

KEYWORDS

anisoplanasy: resolution varying over the tube face

Bucky factor: exposure increase factor when using a grid

contrast detail diagram: graphic display comparing contrast and resolution

contrast improvement factor: improvement of contrast when grid is used

contrast: film: the slope of the characteristic curve: film gamma

contrast: image: relative measure of density differences

contrast: subject: absolute measure of intensity differences

contrast: visual: absolute measure of log intensity differences

detective quantum efficiency (DQE): comparison of input and output signal-to-noise ratios

dynamic range: range of exposure levels that can be displayed or recorded

film speed: film sensitivity measured for an optical density of 1

grid factor: increase in exposure when grid is used (see also, Bucky factor)

grid line density: number of lead strips in an antiscatter grid per centimeter

grid ratio: ratio of grid height to interspace distance

illuminance: reflected light intensity, in lux

interlacing: a method for reducing the bandwidth necessary to give a video display. Fields are interlaced to give each frame

line pairs: resolution measurement using a grating of paired light and dark lines

line spread function: a count profile taken through a line strip on a display

line standard: the standard number of video lines in a display, i.e. 525, 625,1024, 1249 etc

luminance: the light intensity given by a source measured in candela

modulation transfer function (MTF): a complete description of the display resolution. Derived from the PSF or LSF

Nyquist frequency: the minimum frequency at which a signal must be sampled to prevent signal distortion

phosphor: a compound exhibiting luminescence

point spread function (PSF): the count profile through a displayed point source

quantum mottle: random noise exhibited by a display system

resolution: spatial: the minimum distance required by a display to resolve two point sources

resolution: temporal: the ability to separate to events in time

selectivity: ratio of transmission of primary and scatter radiation

signal-to-noise ratio (SNR): the displayed signal divided by the standard deviation of signal noise

spatial non-uniformity: irregular response to radiation across the input field of view

unsharpness: geometric: penumbra associated with an edge or point source due to geometrical factors: focal spot or source to object or source to detector distances

unsharpness: movement: display penumbra due to movement

unsharpness: radiographic: display penumbra due to image detector properties

vignetting: reduced energy transfer on the periphery of the field of view

9

Basic projection X-ray imaging systems

Projection imaging refers to the acquisition of a two-dimensional image of the patient's three-dimensional anatomy. Projection imaging delivers a great deal of information compression, because anatomy that spans the entire thickness of the patient is presented in one image. A single chest radiograph can reveal important diagnostic information concerning the lungs, the spine, the ribs, and the heart, because the radiographic shadows of these structures are superimposed on the image. Of course, a disadvantage is that, by using just one radiograph, the position along the trajectory of the X-ray beam of a specific radiographic shadow, such as that of a pulmonary nodule, is not known.

Radiography is a *transmission* imaging procedure. X-rays emerge from the X-ray rube, which is positioned on one side of the patient's body, they then pass through the patient and are detected on the other side of the patient by the film-screen detector.

9.1 CONVENTIONAL IMAGING (60 TO 80 kV$_p$)

Projection radiography using plain film or full-field digital imaging can be regarded as the basic core of radiography, a distinction is made between chest, skeletal and soft-tissue examinations on one hand, and specialized examinations performed on specialized equipment.

Conventional radiography commonly employs X-ray energies between 50 and 80 kV$_p$ but special imaging requirements sometimes utilize the particular properties offered by lower (25 to 40 kV$_p$) and higher (125 to 140 kV$_p$) X-ray photon energies. Lower energies ensure that photoelectric events are dominant, even in soft tissues giving maximum subject contrast. It is very effective for differentiating soft tissue detail but is only practical for tissue thicknesses of a few centimeters; its most important application is mammography.

Fast closed-loop feedback systems for controlling tube voltage and tube current are an essential design point for modern radiology systems. They are provided in constant-potential and most high frequency generators. Both the tube loadability and the focus size are important for this application and a balance must be struck between these two parameters. For this reason double focus X-ray tubes are more commonly used.

9.1.1 Mid-range X-ray tube

Both the tube loadability and the focus size are important for this application and a balance must be struck between these two parameters. For this reason double focus X-ray tubes are more commonly used. Figure 9.1a shows a typical anode construction for general use and Table 9.1 lists typical parameters for low, medium and high loadability X-ray tubes. Skeletal and abdominal radiography require added image contrast and detail given by a lower kV technique. Tube voltages are typically in the region of 50 to 85 kV; the most common range is between 60 and 75 kV. This is needed in order to provide sufficient low contrast detail in the radiograph. The higher kV$_p$ values are almost exclusively used for regions with high X-ray attenuation, such as oblique projections of the abdomen or lateral projections of the spine. Low kV_p values, between 40 and 60 kV, are used for examinations of the extremities and joints.

The range between 65 and 70 kV, which is used for urography and examinations involving the bones of the trunk, is coupled with the requirement for a format length of 43 cm at a source-image distance of 100 cm, and a small focus. Depending on the type of examination, it is important to determine whether the loadability of the tube, and hence the shortness of the exposure, have the higher priority, or whether it should be the smallness of the focus, and hence the reduced geometric unsharpness. At a source–image distance (FID) of 100 cm, the geometric magnification may be ×1.2 or more, so that the focus size can become a limiting factor. Due to this inter-relationship, double-focus tubes are particularly common in this type of application.

The minimum anode angle for coverage of a format length of 43 cm at 100 cm can be calculated as 13°. As a heavy tube load should be available to reduce exposure times and movement unsharpness to the minimum, a loadability of 50 or even 100 kW is required.

At reduced FIDs there is a significant distortion of the focal spot at the extremes of the image field. Figure 9.1b illustrates that the level of this distortion is greatest at the cathode end of the tube. Short FIDs should only be used over a restricted field in order to reduce this effect and the region of interest should occupy the anode end of the field where focal spot distortion is not so pronounced.

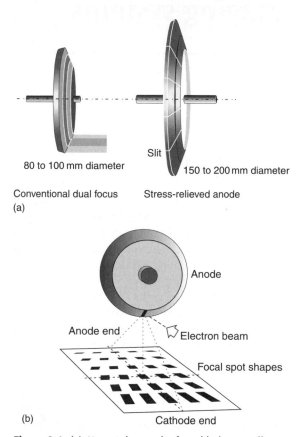

Slit

80 to 100 mm diameter

150 to 200 mm diameter

Conventional dual focus

Stress-relieved anode

(a)

Anode

Anode end

Electron beam

Focal spot shapes

(b)

Cathode end

Figure 9.1 *(a) X-ray tube anodes found in low, medium and high loadability (rating) designs. (b) The focal spot distortion to be expected when selecting a large region of interest at a short source to image distance.*

X-RAY SPECTRUM

The spectrum shape for a filtered X-ray beam from a tungsten anode supplied with a high voltage of 80 kV is shown in Fig. 9.2; characteristic radiation for the K electrons of tungsten at about 59 and 69 keV. A useful K-edge filter material is erbium, which has a K edge at 57.5 keV.

Table 9.1 *Typical specifications for three X-ray tubes used for general work.*

Specification	Low power	Medium power	High power
Maximum voltage	150	150	150
Anode heat capacity	111 kJ	260 kJ	600 kJ
Anode construction	Tungsten/molybdenum	Tungsten/molybdenum	Tungsten/graphite
Focal spot	1 mm	0.3/1.2 mm	0.6/1.2 mm
Target diameter	73 mm	80 mm	
Target angle	16°	12°	12°
Housing heat capacity	880 kJ	1100 kJ	1500 kJ
Cooling	Forced air ventilation	Forced air ventilation	Water
Anode heat dissipation	500 W	740 W	1.47 kW

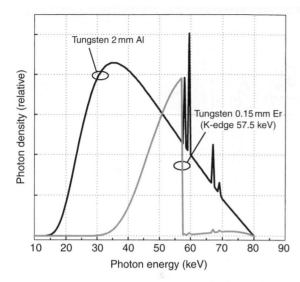

Figure 9.2 *X-ray beam spectra from a tungsten target with 2.5 mm aluminum filtration and 0.15 mm erbium K-edge filter.*

9.1.2 Mid-range generator

The high frequency generator combines the advantages of a constant-potential generator with less cost (about 30% less). This type of generator combines the advantages of the direct-current generator, however, with very small volume and lower costs. The reproducibility and consistency of tube voltage is enhanced by a relatively fast closed loop control circuit, and is virtually independent of changes in both the line voltage and tube current. Additional features include the following:

- Fast tube voltage closed-loop control with about 200 μs response
- Tube voltage independent of changes in tube current and line regulation
- Excellent exposure reproducibility and consistency; maximum variation 5% for X-ray tube voltage, tube current, and exposure time

- Reduced patient dose due to low tube voltage ripple typically 2 to 10%
- Space savings of 60 to 80% relative to conventional generators

High frequency generators produce many X-ray tube voltage pulses per second, depending on the firing frequency of the inverter–high-tension transformer system. The operating frequency of 5 kHz is commonly increased to values above 20 kHz in order to reduce size, eliminate audible hum from the generator and improve generator efficiency.

HIGH FREQUENCY GENERATOR (MULTIPULSE GENERATOR)

Typical specifications for different power rated generators are listed in Table 9.2. High frequency generators produce a string of pulses during each cycle of line voltage. Their number depends on the firing frequency of the inverter system, consequently high frequency generators are sometimes called multipulse generators. The high frequency generator combines the advantages of a constant-potential generator but at less cost (about 30% less).

Figure 9.3 shows the different independent circuits of such a high frequency generator. The selection of a dose reference value (D_{Ref}) for the AEC is more accurate than guessing the milliampere–second reference value required for a specific patient. The D_{Ref} value depends on the recording system sensitivity (film or CR) and desired image quality. Important features are:

- The line supply can be either single phase or 3-phase (220 to 440 V).
- Series oscillator circuit (inverter), which generates a high frequency alternating current from the DC voltage of the intermediate circuit.
- The tube voltage can be switched on and off at any point in time (no delay time).

Table 9.2 *Typical specifications for generators (general work) having different power rating.*

	32 kW	50 kW	65 kW	80 kW
mA at 80 kV	10–400	10–630	10–800	10–1000
Tube (12° angle: 0.6/1.2 mm FS)				
Heat capacity (tube)	150 kJ		212 kJ	
Heat capacity (housing)	930 kJ		1111 kJ	
Heat dissipation		180 W		432 W
Rotor speed	3450		3450 to 10 000 rpm	

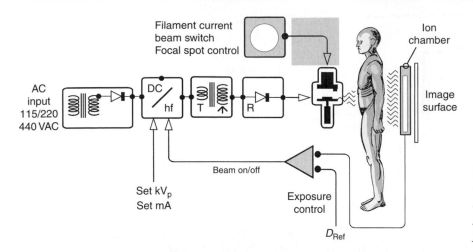

Figure 9.3 *The schematic of a general X-ray system showing high frequency generator and some of the feedback mechanisms.*

- The tube voltage is pre-set as a reference value and is virtually independent of both the tube current and any changes in it.
- The response time for this method of fully electronic voltage closed loop control is approximately 250 μs.
- Extremely compact high-voltage generator accomplished by raising the operating frequency f to between 5 and 20 kHz. This allows reduction of the cross-section A of the core and the number of turns n on the coils ($kV \approx A \times n \times f$).

The response time of the closed loop control circuit depends on the trigger frequency. It is approximately 250 μs, which is slower than that of a direct-current generator but is by far faster than the response time of a conventional generator.

RIPPLE

A figure of <2% variation for tube voltage, tube current and exposure time is a typical specification for high frequency conventional X-ray units. Ripple depends on the technique factors (power), the smoothing capacity C parallel to the X-ray tube, and the value of the voltage U_r of the intermediate DC circuit. The ripple is typically:

- 13% for medium power (30 to 50 kW) in 3-phase, 6-pulse systems
- 4% for high power (50 to 100 kW) in 3-phase, 12-pulse systems
- <1% for high frequency generators of all powers (10 to 20 kHz)

Figure 9.4 shows the spectrum difference when ripple is present; there is a significant decrease in the

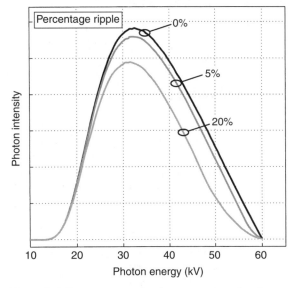

Figure 9.4 *X-ray spectrum for three generators showing 20, 5, and 0% ripple.*

proportion of higher energy photons in the spectrum envelope.

The volume of the generator is about 80% less, the space requirement about 85% less, and the weight about 75% less than the corresponding values of a direct-current generator.

For exposure power up to and including 50 kW the high voltage generator and the X-ray tube can be built into the same housing assembly. This method of construction is called a 'single-tank generator', does not require high voltage cables and is most suitable for mobile X-ray units.

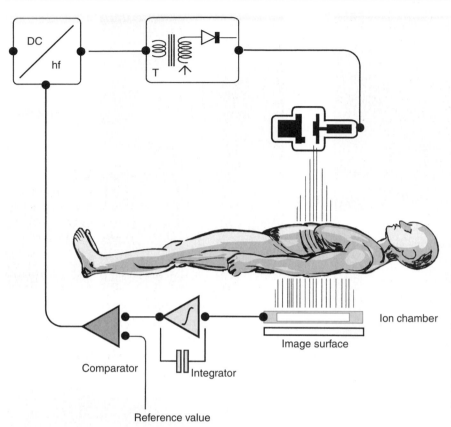

Figure 9.5 *A table mounted automatic exposure control design whose output signal switches the X-ray generator off after a pre-determined exposure has been made. The timing is controlled by the reference value which depends on detector sensitivity (film-screen speed) and dose registered by the ion chamber.*

9.1.3 Automatic exposure control system

In an AEC system for radiology, the selection of a dose reference value (D_{Ref}) is more accurate than guessing the milliampere–second reference value required for a specific patient. D_{Ref} depends on the recording system sensitivity and desired image quality. Figure 9.5 shows the basic circuit diagram of an AEC system.

The region of an object which is of diagnostic interest is called the **dominant**. In the radiograph this is the region which maintains a specific image optical density. The measuring field of the sensor (either ionization chamber or semiconductor radiation detector) coincides with the dominant when positioning the patient's anatomy. Automatic exposure control systems are designed for all types of exposures allowing alignment of the light beam measuring diaphragm and dominant; the collimated X-ray field must coincide with the illuminated area. This technique is applied in conventional Bucky, mammography, and fluoroscopy.

Automatic exposure control systems operate by integrating dose rate (Fig. 9.5). Signal integration is obtained which is proportional to the actual dose accumulated during exposure. A pre-set reference dose value D_{Ref} removes the necessity of guessing the mAs value and allows for the required image density, which is pre-set according to film-screen or image sensor (CR or DR) characteristics. The main types of sensor are used:

- An ionization chamber is placed in front of the image cassette (film or CR).
- A semiconductor detector is placed behind the cassette.

The ionization chamber should be as narrow as possible, and should not create a shadow on the film. A current proportional to the dose rate is created by ionization events in the chamber which is charged to 300 or 1000 V. The magnitude of the ionization current is extremely small (picoampere range 10^{-12}).

The semiconductor radiation detector is placed behind the film cassette or in film changers behind the film-screen combination because it would create a shadow on the film if it were placed otherwise. Its advantage over the ionization chamber is that the

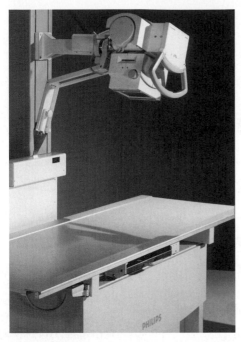

Figure 9.6 *A conventional X-ray unit, suitable for general radiography, whose exposure is controlled by feedback from the ion chamber contained in the center of the table top with the Bucky.*

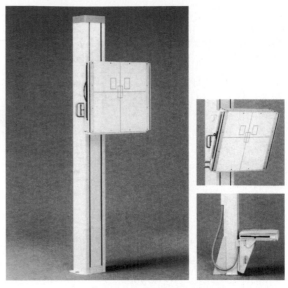

Figure 9.7 *A separate vertical cassette holder (vertical Bucky unit) which can be used for film or digital image detectors. The X-ray unit shown in Figure 9.6 can be part of this vertical Bucky and used for chest radiography etc.*

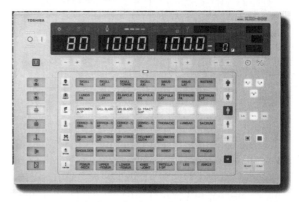

Figure 9.8 *Top of high frequency generator control unit showing pre-set clinical program list.*

dose can be kept at a somewhat lower level due to reduced absorption in front of the film (e.g. mammography, pediatrics). The current of this detector is proportional to the dose rate received behind the cassette and not in the plane of the film. The image optical density is no longer directly proportional to detector current.

mAs SWITCHING

Timing devices are not used any longer in diagnostic equipment with the exception of dental exposures and some mobile X-ray units. This is due to improvements in mAs switching and automatic exposure control systems. Separate timing devices are no longer incorporated into system designs and have been superseded by pulse counting circuits which switch the high frequency generator. Figure 9.5 shows how an exposure control, placed within the table top, switches the high voltage supply to control a pre-set image quality. Figure 9.6 shows a conventional X-ray unit, suitable for general work, with a table mounted cassette holder (for film, CR or full field digital image detectors); the automatic exposure control (AEC) unit is an integral part

of this assembly. Figure 9.7 shows an alternative separate vertical cassette holder (vertical Bucky or grid/cassette unit); the positions of the three ion chambers associated with the AEC are marked on the surface. The layout of an X-ray generator control panel with pre-set exposure programmes is shown in Fig. 9.8.

PERFORMANCE

The contrast and resolution in a radiograph are determined, among other things, by the X-ray generator and its properties. Movement unsharpness or kinetic blurring is influenced by the generator power rating. The dose delivered to the patient by the X-ray unit (D) is calculated by the AEC as a product of the X-ray tube peak value U (kV$_p$), the tube current in mA and exposure time as:

$$D = k_0 \times U^n \times Q \qquad (9.1)$$

The factor k_0 depends on the irradiated object, the tube voltage, the prefiltration at the radiation source, the geometry of the X-ray system, and the image receptor. Since the X-rays are produced as a continuous spectrum the absolute value of the dose (in grays) cannot be calculated by using eqn 9.1. The exponent n is a function of the tube voltage; at 150 kV it is approximately 3.

As the value of the tube voltage is decreased, the value of the exponent increases; thus, at 50 kV it is about 5. The dose is proportional to both the tube current mA and the exposure time, therefore the value Q is the mAs product.

The generator should produce a tube output with low ripple in order to keep the proportion of low-energy radiation as small as possible (Fig. 9.4). The ideal would be direct-current (DC) voltage because of the impact of the exponent n. A moving object (cardiac and vessel movement) can only be sharply imaged with very short exposure times so the mAs product is maintained by increasing tube current (from 100, 200, 400 or even 800 mA) and reducing exposure time (down to a few milliseconds). Organ motion, especially in the heart and the lung, can well amount to a speed of 200 mm s^{-1}. Arterial vessels pulsate similarly, and even more so in pediatric applications. The mAs product decides the appropriate image optical density. After selecting and applying the tube voltage, the tube current is measured and integrated for an exposure time. Once the mAs product reaches its pre-set value for the required image density the tube voltage, and so the radiation delivered is cut off. Feedback for this is obtained from the ion-chamber (automatic exposure control) and pre-set image density factors (Fig. 9.5).

The reproducibility of generator parameters contributes to the consistency of image quality. A tolerance of $\pm 10\%$ in generator performance is barely within acceptable limits for qualitative recording of morphology and organ functions.

OPTICAL DENSITY CORRECTION

Since the proportion of scattered radiation depends on the irradiated volume, more scattered radiation occurs in a thick object. The sensor of the automatic exposure control system measures the total radiation emerging from the object. It includes the scattered radiation, and therefore the reference dose value is reached sooner in the case of thick objects. The film thus exhibits a lower optical density than the pre-set one.

Experienced operators alter the reference dose value D_{Ref} by means of an optical density correction switch depending upon the object to be examined. This switch is graduated in plus and minus exposure points. In organ-programmed exposure techniques this adjustment may already be pre-programmed in the organ key (Fig. 9.8). Preference should be given to organ-programmed operation because the choice of film-screen or digital image sensor is also included.

9.1.4 Mobile X-ray units

GENERAL POINTS

The mobile X-ray unit has been developed for routine bedside radiographic procedures in intensive care, emergency, central X-ray and pediatric departments and in operating theaters. The mobile unit should be able to provide a 24-hour service and deliver image quality fully comparable with those of stationary systems.

DESCRIPTION

The typical small mobile X-ray unit (Fig. 9.9) consists of a chassis with a control console and digital display, and an arm system bearing the high frequency generator, the X-ray tube and the multi-leaf collimator with positioning illumination. The mobile unit can come with or without motor drive. Sealed lead/acid batteries are contained within the body of the unit so that radiographs can be taken independent from a mains supply. A built-in battery charger is included so that the mobile can be plugged into an AC supply when not in use. Table 9.3 lists some typical specifications for two sizes of mobile unit, a small mobile without a battery drive suitable for pediatrics and a larger unit with battery drive for general hospital work. The main disadvantage of mobile X-ray units is the absence of a reliable automatic exposure control although some models can have a semiconductor AEC connected to the generator that operates behind the imaging cassette (film, CR or digital). Dose–area product (DAP) measuring systems should be fitted to the X-ray housing so that patient dose levels can be recorded.

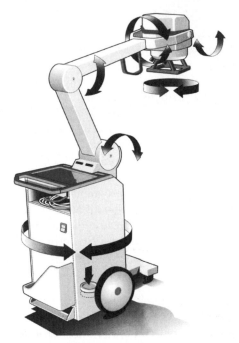

Figure 9.9 *A small mobile X-ray unit showing the considerable maneuverability of the body and arm. The generator is integrated within the X-ray tube housing. The body contains the battery and charger unit. (Courtesy Siemens Inc.)*

Table 9.3 *Typical specifications for a small and large mobile X-ray unit.*

Specification	Small mobile	Heavy duty mobile
Generator power	12.5 kW	30 kW
Maximum current	100 mA	450 mA
kV_p range	50 to 125 kV_p	40 to 133 kV_p
Shortest exposure	3 ms	1 ms
X-ray tube heat storage	90 kJ (122 kHU)	200 kJ (275 kHU)
Focal spot	0.7 mm	0.8 mm
Mobility	Not motorized	Motorized
Weight	200 kg	490 kg

9.2 PEDIATRIC RADIOGRAPHY

Adult patients vary in size, but their variation is minimal compared to the range in pediatric patients. Size differences can range from premature infants, weighing considerably less than 1000 g, to adolescents approaching 70 kg. X-ray imaging systems investigating pediatric patients must be able to cover this very wide range.

AUTOMATIC EXPOSURE CONTROL

Automatic exposure controls are a major problem as many of the available systems are far from ideal for pediatric imaging. They have a relatively large and fixed chamber aperture since they are designed for adults. Their size, shape and position are unable to compensate for the many variations of body size in pediatric patients.

It is a common design to place the ionization chambers of AEC behind the antiscatter grid. Consequently the AEC may be calibrated with grid use so removing the grid, which is frequently necessary with low dose pediatric radiology, is not practical.

Specially designed pediatric AECs consist of small mobile detectors for use behind specially transparent lead-free cassettes. Their position can be carefully selected with respect to the most important region of interest. Since high sensitivity screens (400 or 800 speed) require only a tiny dose at the cassette front the detector behind the cassette must be able to work in the range of a few micrograys which is difficult to maintain with any constancy.

At the present time, when radiographing the pediatric patient, exposure charts are used corresponding to radiographic position and patient's weight (the body index). There is still a great deal of work to be done developing a practical AEC design for pediatrics. This development may take advantage of recent digital detector designs, since the application of direct electronic radiography using full field TFT detectors would lend itself to this problem.

EXPOSURE TIME

Exposure times must be short because pediatric patients are difficult to restrain. These short times are only achieved with powerful generators and tubes with high rating.

The cable length between the high voltage transformer X-ray tube is important since the cable has capacitance so will interfere with fast exposure times giving extended post-peak radiation lasting for 2 ms or more so single tank high frequency generators with minimum cable runs are ideal with grid controlled switching (see grid switching in Chapter 10).

IMAGING SYSTEMS

In non-digital imaging (film or CR), the selection of higher speed screen-film systems has the greatest impact on dose reduction in pediatric radiology. In addition, it allows shorter exposure times that reduce movement unsharpness. The reduced resolution of higher speed screens is comparatively insignificant for the majority of clinical indications. For special purposes (e.g. bone detail) speed classes of 800 can be used.

9.3 LOW KILOVOLTAGE: MAMMOGRAPHY (20 TO 30 kV$_p$)

In the majority of conventional radiographic applications, most contrast to be visualized is that between air, bone, soft tissue and/or liquid. In mammographic examinations low kV X-radiation is required in order to discriminate between very similar soft tissues (fat, parenchyma, etc.).

The mammographic image must show the contrast between different density soft tissue, fat and blood vessels, without the application of contrast media. In addition, micro-calcifications ($\approx$100 μm) must be distinguished. The critical selection of tube kilovoltage is best achieved with the aid of mixed molybdenum/tungsten/rhodium anode targets using a selection of K-edge filters.

The practical X-ray energy range for mammography is between 25 to 30 kV which ensures photoelectric events are dominant. Although the spectrum embraces lower photon energies of $\approx$15 kV these are preferentially absorbed within the tissue. Higher energies ($>$30 kV) do not contribute to image contrast so are not utilized. Higher kV imaging energies relies on Compton interactions which allow a broad range of tissue types (bone and soft tissue) to be represented on the image. Figure 9.10 shows relative contributions from photoelectric and Compton events for mammography (shaded column). The double hatched region is the voltage range 100 to 120 keV which relies almost entirely on Compton reactions for image formation.

9.3.1 Low kV interactions

It has been seen from Chapter 5 that the major factors which emphasize photon absorption differences in tissue (subject contrast) are kilovoltage, linear attenuation coefficient, and tissue thickness. Very similar soft tissues in the breast require low kilovoltage imaging so maximizing photoelectric effects which are most sensitive to even small tissue differences.

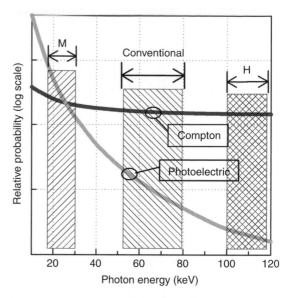

Figure 9.10 *The probability for photoelectric and Compton reactions changes with photon energy. At mammography energies (single hatching) the photoelectric dominates but at high kilovoltages (double hatching) image formation depends on Compton.*

Photoelectric absorption τ is influenced by tissue density, atomic number ($Z \approx 7.4$) and photon energy E. Photoelectric absorption for soft tissue decreases rapidly with increasing energy, this can be seen over the shaded portion of Fig. 9.10. The steep portion of the linear attenuation coefficient curve is predominantly due to photoelectric interactions where:

$$\tau \propto \frac{Z^3}{E^3} \qquad (9.2)$$

TISSUE ABSORPTION

Tissue thickness considerably influences photon transmission at low kilovoltages. The photon transmission for a tissue thickness of 5 cm is plotted in Fig. 9.11 and shows that for photon energies between 20 and 30 kV$_p$ the transmitted photon fraction is between 3 and 35%, being about 20% at practical kilovoltage levels of 28 kV$_{eff}$.

Dense breasts would have even less transmission. Tissue thickness plays a very important part in mammography and tissue (breast) compression significantly improves photon transmission. It also reduces scatter radiation which increases significantly with tissue thickness degrading subject contrast.

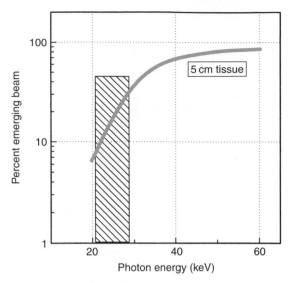

Figure 9.11 *Photon transmission through 5 cm soft tissue. The shaded area identifies the mammography energy range.*

9.3.2 Mammography X-ray systems

In order to achieve the best image quality at low kV, for minimum patient dose, all aspects of machine design must be optimized to give the best quality image for minimum patient radiation dose. Important design points are:

- Efficient generator supply
- X-ray tube construction
- Tissue compression
- Automatic dose control

GENERATOR (HIGH FREQUENCY)

Due to space charge effects adequate tube current is a problem in low kV studies. Low power generators (single-phase or 3-phase) with limited tube current (about 200 mA) overcome this limitation by increasing exposure time to achieve the required mAs value. This has two serious disadvantages, the loss of image resolution due to movement unsharpness and reduced film density due to reciprocity loss.

X-RAY TUBE

The overall design for a mammography X-ray tube is shown in Fig. 9.12a. Cooling problems are not as serious as conventional X-ray tubes; a surrounding oil bath is not necessary since forced air cooling is adequate. A list of X-ray tube specifications is given in Table 9.4 for two common types.

Mammography tube

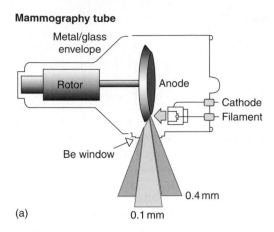

Alternative mammography dual target anodes

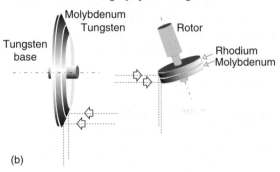

(b)

Figure 9.12 *(a) General X-ray tube design showing very close positioning of cathode and anode. Dual focal spots are achieved here by cathode focusing. The beryllium window has a very low absorption factor for these low kV X-rays. (b) A dual target anode giving both molybdenum and tungsten targets which gives optimum image quality for different breast thicknesses.*

Table 9.4 *Mammography tube specifications.*

Specification	Molybdenum	Tungsten
Anode diameter (mm)	100	100
Target angle	22°	22°
Focal spot (mm)	0.15/0.4	0.1/0.4
Loading (kW)	0.9/6.5	1.3/9.5
Maximum mA at 30 kV	Fine, 26	36
	Broad, 185	250
Heat storage	200 kJ	300 kJ
	(270 kHU)	(400 kHU)

The X-ray tube window must be made from low density material in order to transmit the low energy photons. A glass window would be too dense and be a significant absorber so a beryllium insert is commonly used. Tubes having a metal construction (stainless steel and glass) are now common.

FOCAL SPOT

The mammography X-ray tube gives two focal spot sizes 0.4 mm for surface and 0.1 mm for magnification imaging. The effective dimensions vary across the beam width and Fig. 9.12a shows the focal spot can be quite broad at the edge of the beam near the cathode (chest wall) but improves toward the tube anode (central area of the breast).

ANODE

Anode construction is shown in Fig. 9.12b. The common form of X-ray tube design uses a molybdenum anode to give useful K-edge peaks in the spectrum at 17 keV and 20 keV as shown in Fig. 9.13a, although more efficient X-ray production is obtained from a tungsten anode which is shown for comparison (efficiency for Mo ≈0.09% and ≈0.16% at 20 kV).

X-RAY SPECTRUM

The spectral shapes of molybdenum and tungsten are compared in Fig. 9.13a; both have useful properties. Molybdenum anodes have characteristic radiation at 17 and 20 keV which comprise 19 to 29% of the output intensity giving peak output in the most valuable part of the spectrum. Tungsten, having a higher atomic number, improves X-ray intensity overall.

Table 9.4 shows that a molybdenum target has lower ratings than tungsten but since it provides useful characteristic line spectra it is retained by some manufacturers who provide a twin anode design having targets of both molybdenum and tungsten.

FILTERS (K EDGE)

Beam quality (HVL) incident on the breast depends on the thickness and composition of the compression paddle and the fixed filtration employed. The HVL of a 30 kV X-ray beam should lie within 0.3 to 0.4 mm. Higher HVLs indicate a higher effective kV, which is not useful since it will reduce overall photoelectric effect resulting in loss of image contrast. Employing suitable filters whose K edges fall within the mammography kV range (Rh 23.2, Pd 24.4, Mo 20.0 keV shown in Fig. 9.14a) effectively reduce higher photon energies from the X-ray beam. The use of K-edge filtration on the X-ray spectrum is show in Fig. 9.14b where molybdenum and rhodium give a spectrum shape which restricts the higher energies above the K edge so reducing patient dose.

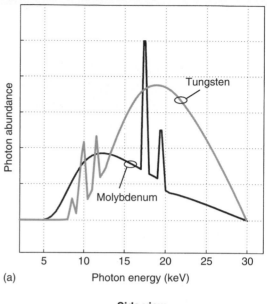

(a)

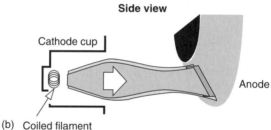

(b) Coiled filament

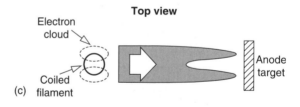

(c) Coiled filament

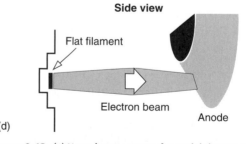

(d)

Figure 9.13 (*a*) *X-ray beam spectra for molybdenum and tungsten targets used in mammography. The characteristic X-rays of molybdenum are a significant part of the spectrum. Tungsten gives more intensity at a higher effective energy.* (***b***) *Cathode assembly with coiled filament giving a broad electron beam with shadowing;* (***c***) *this also gives a 'camel hump profile' generating two focal areas.* (***d***) *The flat filament gives a more tightly focused uniform beam.*

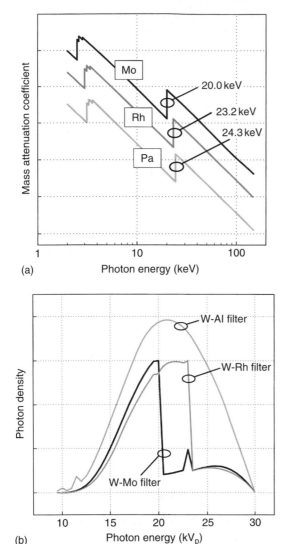

(a)

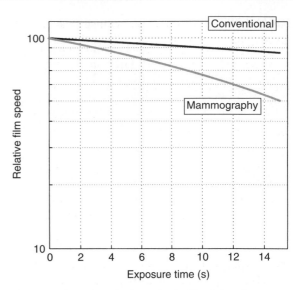

Figure 9.15 *Reciprocity losses in the film image for extended exposure times.*

Figure 9.14 *(a) Attenuation curves for molybdenum, palladium, and rhodium showing their K edges. (b) K-edge filtration using rhodium and molybdenum filters on an X-ray spectrum from a tungsten anode.*

Generator kV plays a minor role in deciding effective energy. So K-edge filtered spectra offer precise energies over a narrow spectrum range and significantly reduce the less useful high kV energies.

CATHODE FILAMENT

Designs for the filament cathode assembly are shown in Fig. 9.13b, c and d. These use either a double wound filament to increase the electron density (b) or a flat ribbon filament (d). Circular filaments at short distances

from the anode can give an unfocussed beam of electrons causing penumbra formation on the target.

Since the electron cloud tends to concentrate on the edges of the filament the cross section of the electron beam is not uniform but has a 'camel's hump' profile shown in Fig. 9.13c. This shape forms two areas of high intensity on the anode surface instead of just one which effectively gives two focal spots side by side. These mutually interfere giving another source of geometrical unsharpness and seriously limiting image resolution. A flat section filament minimizes this problem.

Different focal spot sizes are selected by either a negative bias on the cathode which re-focuses the electrons, or by using dual filaments focused on two target areas.

SPACE CHARGE EFFECT

Space charge problems at low kilovoltages reduce the maximum available tube current regardless of extra filament heating. As a consequence filament design is optimized to give sharp electron beam shapes already seen in Fig. 9.13d. Electrical compensation circuits are necessary for adjusting the filament current when changing low kV_p settings, this overcomes space charge effects on tube current for different kV settings.

RECIPROCITY LOSSES

Figure 9.15 compares loss of film speed due to reciprocity effects in mammography and conventional radiography. For exposure times longer than 2 s reciprocity losses become serious. These losses are not so evident in conventional work. When higher tube currents are required at low values of kV$_p$ the filament must be raised to much higher temperatures to maintain the mA value. This is the rating restriction seen previously (Chapter 4) as the flattened curve at 20, 30, and 40 kV.

At low anode kilovoltages, especially for strongly focused small focal spots (0.1 mm magnification), tube current is essentially space charge limited which can be improved by increasing filament area (double filaments) and decreasing the cathode anode distance. Alternative filament designs have already been seen in Fig. 9.13. Tube current cannot be increased by raising the filament temperature and attempting to increase available electrons. Modern high frequency generators (5 to 10 kHz) are able to deliver tube currents up to 300 mA, allowing much shorter exposures.

Disadvantages
- Conflicts with the practice of high kV to reduce patient dose
- X-ray tube operates inefficiently at low kilovoltages
- High filament current
- Low tube current
- Extended exposure times
- Heel effect for small anode angles
- Image non-uniformity (resolution and contrast)
- Scatter radiation problems
- Intensifying screen low sensitivity
- Primary beam absorption by cassette

Advantages
- Scatter radiation easily absorbed
- Very high resolution
- Good contrast between soft tissues
- Staff radiation dose low

9.3.3 Mammography image quality

Although photoelectric reactions are dominant in mammography some weak Compton scatter is present (Fig. 9.10). Very few of these low energy scatter events reach the film surface since they are easily absorbed within the tissue. This has been discussed in Chapter 5. Scatter photon attenuation over the diagnostic range is very effectively absorbed by tissue at low energies giving only a small scatter component at the film/image surface. The scatter photons reaching the film

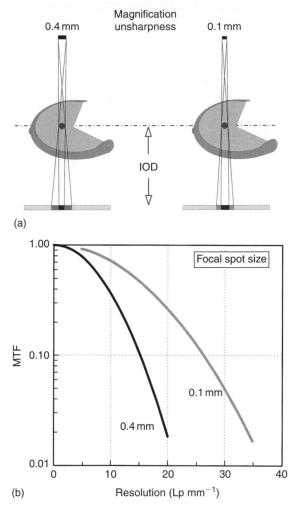

Figure 9.16 (*a*) Geometrical unsharpness for 0.4 mm and 0.1 mm focal spots showing loss of resolution for magnification views (large object to film distance). (*b*) The modulation transfer function curves for 0.4 and 0.1 mm. The 20% cut-off is at 10 and 22 Lp mm^{-1} respectively.

increase above 30 kV as tissue attenuation coefficient plays a less important role.

UNSHARPNESS AND MAGNIFICATION

Magnification is commonly used in mammography to increase resolution for equivocal regions. This is achieved by decreasing FOD. The increased unsharpness can be minimized if the focal spot size is reduced from 0.4 to 0.1 mm. Comparative unsharpness for large and small focal spots is demonstrated in Fig. 9.16a.

The improvement in image resolution can be measured by comparing the MTF for the two focal spot sizes 0.4 mm and 0.1 mm (Fig. 9.16b). Since the anode loading increases for 0.1 mm the tube rating is smaller for magnification views (as seen in Table 9.4 for maximum current (in mA) at 30 kV for fine and

broad focal spots) and fine focus is not used routinely. Box 9.1 estimates the smallest visible detail with a 0.4 mm and 0.1 mm focal spot. Patient dose also increases due to decreased FOD (inverse square law). Focal spot size does not visibly influence resolution with surface contact (non-magnification) imaging.

CASSETTE DESIGN

The cassette design used for mammography is shown in Fig. 9.17. Since the X-ray photon, at low kilovoltages, is preferentially absorbed within the first few micrometers of the screen surface it is important that very close contact is made between the single film emulsion and the screen. In some instances the film and screen are vacuum packed to achieve this. The illustration shows that the X-ray beam is directed through the back of the film, passing first through the emulsion before interacting with the screen surface whose light output then exposes the film.

SCATTER AND GRIDS

Low energy photons are scattered isotropically so the antiscatter grid used in mammography has a low ratio: $h/D = 4$ or 5. Efficiency is improved by using a grid focused to 60 cm with lead septa density of 27 to 50 lines cm^{-1}. Its construction is shown in Fig. 9.18a.

The grid factor (the ratio between incident and transmitted radiation) is kept as low as possible (approximately 2) by using thin septa; these are typically

---

Box 9.1 Unsharpness for mammography

Focus to image distance (FID) = 60 cm
  Object to image distance (OID) = 28 cm (magnification)
  Focal spot (FS) = 0.4 mm. The value s is the resulting penumbra size.

$$\frac{s}{FS} = \frac{OID}{FID - OID}$$

Using eqn 8.3,

$$s = \frac{FS \times OID}{FID - OID}$$
$$= \frac{0.4 \times 280}{600 - 280}$$
$$= 0.35 \text{ mm}$$

The 350 μm penumbra would seriously reduce the ability to see 100 μm micro-calcifications. A focal spot of 0.1 mm reduces this unsharpness to 0.08 mm (80 μm) giving a better performance for magnification imaging. Routine imaging, with little magnification can safely use 0.4 mm focal spots.

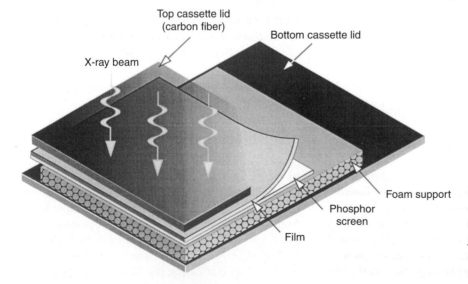

X-ray beam

Top cassette lid (carbon fiber)

Bottom cassette lid

Foam support

Phosphor screen

Film

Figure 9.17 *Film-screen cassette construction showing single emulsion film lying face down onto the intensifying screen phosphor.*

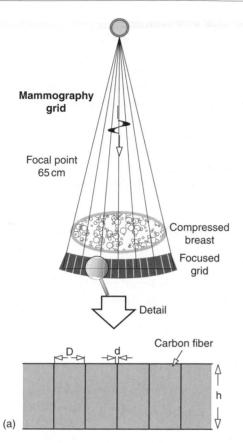

Mammography grid

Focal point 65 cm

Compressed breast

Focused grid

Detail

Carbon fiber

(a)

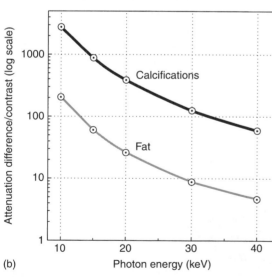

(b)

Figure 9.18 *(a) Focused grid and construction used for mammography showing lead-septa thickness* d, *carbon fiber dividers* D *and carbon fiber top and bottom plates. The height* h *is typically 0.7 to 1.0 mm. (b) The change in subject contrast with kV between soft tissue and fat from the difference in linear attenuation coefficient values.*

<20 μm thick. The grid height h is usually <1 mm. Specifications for two mammography grids are given in Table 9.5 where septa thickness d, grid height h and spacer thickness D are compared.

CONTRAST

Subject contrast can be estimated by subtracting the attenuation coefficients for soft tissue and fat; the result is plotted in Fig. 9.18b. Differences between like tissues can be best distinguished at low photon energies but Fig. 9.11 has already demonstrated that transmission is poor at low energies so a compromise energy must be chosen at about 28 kV giving good transmission while retaining sufficient image contrast for diagnostic quality images. Atomic number Z, tissue density, and thickness all play an important part in subject contrast.

Table 9.6 gives reference values for minimum image detectability for a good quality mammography system (UK Breast Screening Programme). At the present time only film-screen mammography can attain these levels.

THE HEEL EFFECT

This is more pronounced in mammography where small anode angles are used. Figure 9.19a illustrates the heel effect in mammography. The beam intensity decreases quite rapidly toward the anode end of the tube. The focal spot dimensions also vary across the

Table 9.5 *Two grid specifications (in mm).*

Grid	Septa thickness, d	Grid height, h	Spacer thickness, D	Pb (%)
4/27	0.05	1.2	0.32	13.5
5/44	0.016	1.0	0.21	7.0

Table 9.6 *Optimum image quality references for a mammography system.*

Parameter	Minimum reference value
High contrast resolution	10 Lp mm^{-1}
Minimum detectable contrast (5 to 6 mm detail)	1%
Minimum detectable contrast (0.5 mm detail)	5%

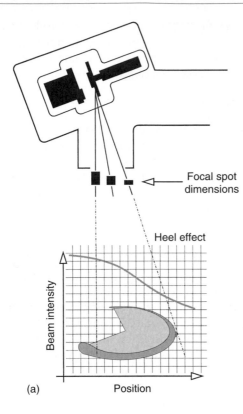

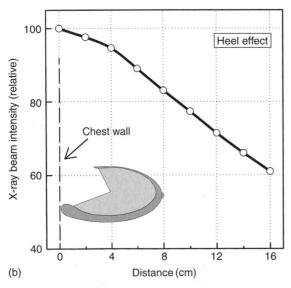

Figure 9.19 *(a) The combined alteration in focal spot dimension and heel effect from the edge of the support plate. The focal spot is larger at the cathode end and decreases toward the anode (compare focal spot distortion in Figure 9.1b). (b) The heel effect for a typical mammography machine operating with a 0.4 mm focal spot.*

field of view giving poorer resolution at the chest wall. The magnitude of the heel effect is plotted in Fig. 9.19b. At the nipple region of the breast the beam intensity has dropped to 60% of maximum but the focal spot dimensions still enable optimum resolution.

In order to reduce the heel effect on the image the tube itself is angled placing the cathode over the chest wall (nearest patient) where greater intensity is needed; the anode is further from the patient.

9.3.4 Patient radiation dose

The high proportion of photoelectric absorption is responsible for potential high patient radiation dose. Absorption of low energy scatter within the tissue also increases dose. This is a problem with low kV imaging and in order to reduce it to optimum levels (lowest dose versus diagnostic quality image), the major factors influencing patient dose must be carefully controlled as:

- Tissue thickness (breast compression)
- X-ray beam quality
- Detector sensitivity

BREAST COMPRESSION

A plastic paddle parallel with the support surface compresses the breast and maintains uniform tissue thickness. This improves image resolution throughout the breast volume by reducing object to image distance (OID) and reducing geometrical unsharpness. Subject contrast is also improved due to scatter reduction within the breast volume.

Tissue compression also significantly lowers patient radiation dose by minimizing photon scatter since it is low energy and would be absorbed. The high fraction of photoelectric absorption by the primary beam is responsible for potential high patient radiation dose in mammography, so photon density must be reduced for minimum radiation dose therefore mammography uses the most sensitive film-screen units for maximum efficiency. Patient dose is also influenced by anode material and filters.

Patient radiation dose is strongly influenced by the choice of grid, cassette, screen and film so that there is efficient capture of all emerging X-ray photons for image formation. Grid septa thickness has already been discussed and efficiency can be further increased by using carbon fiber for all non-metal construction grid and cassette. Film sensitivity can be improved by using longer film processor times and an elevated developer temperature.

ENTRANCE DOSE

The dose at the surface of the patient can be measured directly with a dosimeter. Measurements of surface dose usually assume soft tissue or a soft tissue equivalent material (plastic or water). The beam energy (effective or peak) and the beam's half-value layer (HVL) must be known since low energy photons will be preferentially absorbed in the surface layers.

Any dose measured at the surface of the patient will include a fraction from photons backscattered from deeper tissue layers. This is the backscatter fraction (BSF). This contribution to the entrance dose is not present when simple air readings are taken without a patient or suitable phantom being present in the beam. The terms entrance exposure and entrance surface dose are sometimes used to distinguish measurements made with and without BSF correction respectively. Acceptable maximum values for entrance surface dose are between 5 and 6 mGy for an optical density of 1.5. Recent mammography systems can significantly improve on this value.

MEAN GLANDULAR DOSE

Glandular tissues receive varying doses depending on:

- Depth from the skin entrance site
- Beam quality (kV and filtration)
- Breast thickness
- Breast consistency
- Optical density of the mammogram

The mean glandular dose (MGD) to the standard breast for a standard optical film density allows direct comparison between different mammography systems. It also allows a better estimation of risk to the patient. The standard breast which is used for these measurements comprises a 50:50 mixture of adipose and glandular equivalent material with a superficial adipose layer of 0.5 cm giving an overall thickness of 5 cm which represents the average compressed breast. The mean glandular dose is energy dependent as shown in Fig. 9.20a which is a plot of MGD for effective beam energies from 26 to 34 keV at the stated HVL.

Factors used in the MGD calculation which relates entrance exposure values to the average MGD have been measured by several workers. The breast phantom is exposed for optimum image quality having

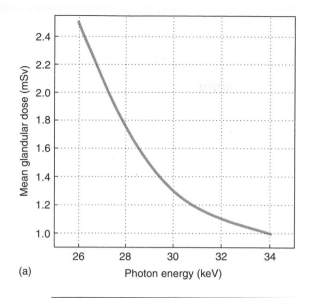

(a)

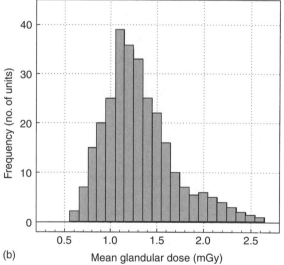

(b)

Figure 9.20 (a) The mean glandular dose decreasing with increasing beam energy (kV). (b) A histogram of the mean glandular dose obtained for a group of breast screening centers showing a mean value of about 1.3 mGy.

a mean background optical density of 1.5. The incident air kerma K is obtained in grays. These factors depend on the X-ray tube target material and the beam HVL. The glandular dose is then obtained for the air kerma value K as:

$$MGD = K \times p \times g \qquad (9.3)$$

Factors p and g are conversion values obtained from tables for the HVL as measured; an example is given in Table 9.7. The MGD to the standard breast should

Table 9.7 *Conversion values* p *and* g *for the mean glandular dose.*

Half-value layer	Conversion factor, *p*	Conversion factor, *g* (mGy Gy^{-1})
0.30	1.10	183
0.35	1.10	208
0.40	1.09	232
0.45	1.09	258
0.50	1.09	285

not exceed 3 mGy and more recent reports suggest 1.3 mGy. Surveys of MGD values using current equipment now give recommendations that values should not exceed 1.3 mGy for the standard breast. Figure 9.20b indicates the range of MGD values published by a number of breast screening centers confirming the new recommended limit of 1.3 mGy. The anode target material also has a significant effect on overall dose to the tissue and Fig. 9.21a shows the level of dose reduction given by various combinations of molybdenum and tungsten targets with K-edge filtration. Table 9.8 lists the maximum and average dose levels that would be expected from modern film-screen mammographic units.

FILM-SCREEN TYPE

The single screen/single emulsion design gives a very high efficiency and superior resolution. Figure 9.16b has shown the potential resolution using 0.4 and 0.1 mm focal spots can exceed 20 Lp mm^{-1}. Mammography film-screens can almost match this giving approximately 20 Lp mm^{-1} as against 5 to 10 Lp mm^{-1} for high detail conventional radiography. Screen materials are almost always rare earth, although these show a reduced sensitivity for low kV photons (Fig. 9.21b).

9.3.4 Automatic exposure controls

The conventional AEC (photo-timer) would use an ionization chamber placed in the primary beam. If used at low kilovoltages it would absorb a significant proportion of X-ray photons so a different procedure is used. A very sensitive balanced detector is placed behind the film cassette; the arrangement is shown in Fig. 9.22a. These are twin detectors in a sandwich design comprising two detectors (D1 and D2) separated by a metal filter. The output signals from D1 and D2 are electrically balanced; detector D2 behind its

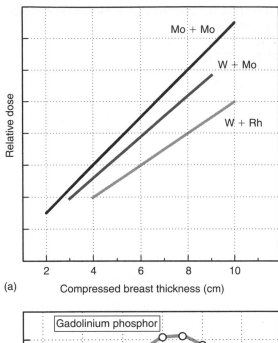

(a)

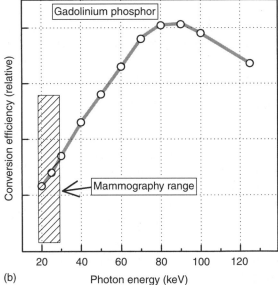

(b)

Figure 9.21 *(a) Breast surface dose increase with tissue thickness for different anode and K-filter combinations. (b) Intensifying screen conversion efficiency variation with photon energy.*

beam hardening filter acts as a reference. Any small change in low kV photon flux caused by a change in breast density influences D1 more than D2 and a signal difference will be given. The magnitude of this difference signal controls the film exposure (mAs value). Information concerning screen and film sensitivity, kilovoltage, and tube current influence this

Table 9.8 *Acceptable mammography radiation dose for a selected film density.*

Measurement	Value
Film density	1.5 Optical density
Entrance surface dose	Between 5 and 6 mGy
Mean glandular dose	
Maximum acceptable	3 mGy
Optimum	1.3 mGy

Table 9.9 *Specification for mammography unit.*

X-ray tube	Current rated >200 mA for short exposure times
Focal spot	0.4 and 0.1 mm
Generator	High frequency with feedback control for kV, mA, and time
FID	60 cm
Filters	Automatic K-edge filter change with kV (Mo, Rh, Al)
AEC	Compensation for kV film screen and breast thickness
Compression	Motor driven (150 N, max.)
Grid	5:1 to 4:1
	27 to 40 lines cm^{-1}

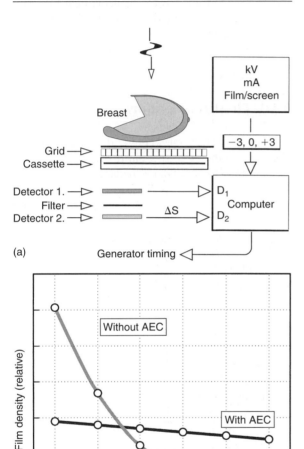

Figure 9.22 *(a) Typical automatic exposure control design for mammography showing balanced detectors placed beneath the film cassette. (b) Graph showing constant image density for increasing breast thicknesses. The image density would sharply decrease without automatic exposure control.*

difference signal to give an optimum exposure value for all variables.

The film density is kept quite constant for a wide range of breast thicknesses. Figure 9.22b shows the difference between exposure levels with and without this automatic exposure device (photo-timer). The controlled range (black line) shows very little variation in film density for a 1 to 6 cm variation in breast thickness. The film density can be varied by the operator; this is the +3, 0, −3 density control in the illustration. Table 9.9 lists the minimum requirements for a mammography unit that would be used for a screening program.

9.3.5 Basic machine design

Figure 9.23 shows the essential features of a modern mammography machine itemized in Table 9.9. The X-ray tube is commonly tilted to angle the X-ray beam which minimizes heel effect problems which are encountered with small focal spot sizes. Tissue compression is obtained by using a thin plastic compression paddle so that the breast has a uniform thickness. This significantly reduces patient dose and improves image quality by reducing geometrical unsharpness (object to film distance minimal). Automatic exposure control is obtained by placing the detector under the support plate, grid, and film cassette; in this way there is no added absorber between the cassette and the X-ray beam. At low kilovoltages even the thin walls of the AEC ionization chamber would offer significant absorption.

The mammogram example shown in Fig. 9.24 has been taken at 27 kV$_p$ with a single emulsion film using a single rare-earth screen. Macro- and

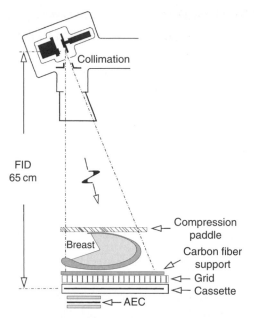

Figure 9.23 *Overall design for a mammography X-ray set showing angled X-ray tube positioned 60 to 65 cm from the image plane, the compression paddle of thin plastic and the automatic exposure device under the cassette.*

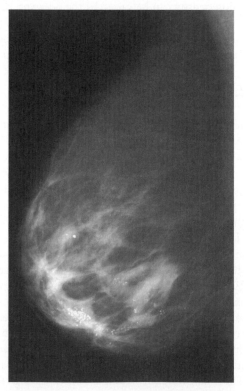

Figure 9.24 *Mammogram showing both soft tissue detail and micro-calcifications.*

micro-calcifications can be seen and small differences between soft tissues can be easily distinguished.

9.4 HIGH KILOVOLTAGE IMAGING

The advantages of high kilovoltage imaging are utilized not only in chest imaging but also in fluoroscopy and computed tomography. By using high kV beam penetration is maximized through thick body parts and since Compton scatter is the major absorption process most tissue types can be evenly represented on the image.

9.4.1 Chest radiography

Good quality chest radiography demands relatively high tube voltages at very short exposure times so X-ray tubes with short-term loadability are required. Since the source–image distance (SID) is relatively long (1.5 to 2 m) the focus size and anode angle are not critical. The majority of chest radiographs are made for examinations of the lungs using a high kV technique (100 to 140 kV_p) with a source–image distance of between 1.5 and 2 m. Very short exposures are needed, in the range of 1 to 5 ms, to prevent movement artifact by the heart and great vessels.

During exposure times used for a lung study, the X-ray tube anode will only rotate one or six complete revolutions, so tube loading is close to the maximum if focal track heating is to be kept within limits.

The use of X-ray photons with energies in excess of 100 kV_p presents several important advantages in diagnostic imaging. High kV is widely used where different tissue types are being imaged (bone, soft tissue or iodine/barium contrast materials). High kV techniques give fast exposure times which freeze motion (movement unsharpness) due to either patient movement (during breath hold) or cardiac motion. The common applications are found in:

- Chest radiography
- Fluoroscopy (gastro-intestinal tract)
- Obstetric pelvis
- Lumbar and dorsal spine investigations
- Computed tomography (CT)
- Digital subtraction angiography (DSA)

Above 70 kV tissue interactions are predominantly Compton and image formation relies on the primary beam being scattered away from the image plane in its passage through the body. A high ratio grid is necessary to block this radiation from reaching the film since unlike low kV imaging it travels in a forward direction.

Since image formation is dependent on Compton scatter the subject contrast depends on electron density and not atomic number and bone appears more transparent. This property is exploited in chest radiography where the rib cage is rendered more transparent.

X-RAY TUBE

The two anode designs shown in Fig. 9.25a and b are for heavy duty use (high loadability). The first has a diameter of 100 mm and graphite backing where heat dissipation is predominantly by radiation. The second anode has a 200 mm diameter designed for a double sleeve bearing where heat loss is by conduction through the bearing itself. These two factors enable the anode to have a very high thermal rating since both these tubes are operated at near maximum

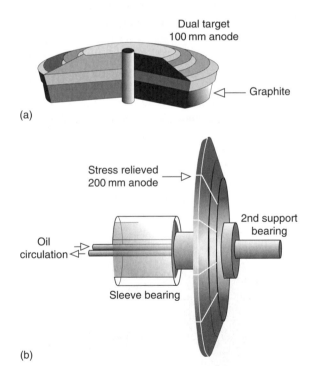

(a)

(b)

Figure 9.25 *(a) Anode design for high voltage uses a dual focus anode between 100 and 200 mm diameter. Graphite increases the radiation surface. (b) A large diameter anode used in dual bearing tubes with sleeve bearings where the majority heat loss is by conduction.*

Table 9.10 *High kV X-ray tube specifications.*

	Chest	Fluoro-DSA	CT
Heat	600 kHU	1.35 kHU	3.5 MHU
Focus	1.2	0.6/1.0	1.6
Power	450 W	2 kW	30 kW

Table 9.11 *X-ray intensity increases as kV^2.*

kV	Current (mA)	mAs	Time (s)
60	200	20	0.1
80	200	11	0.055
100	200	7	0.035
120	200	5	0.025

specification. Table 9.10 lists common specifications for three tube types: chest, fluoro/DSA, and CT.

TUBE RATING

For the short exposure times given in Table 9.11 an anode revolving at 300 rpm will make one revolution in 20 ms; at shorter exposure times only a fraction of the target will be used so the entire electrical energy is dissipated only over a small area. For this reason increasing anode diameter and anode rotation speed can improve the tube's rating. Since these X- ray tubes are operating at near their maximum rating heat dissipation is of prime importance. The focal spot size influences the tube loadability as shown by the family of electrical rating curves in Fig. 9.27c. Increasing anode loadability can be achieved by:

- Large diameter anodes
- Fast rotation speeds
- Ceramic metal housing
- Sleeve bearing instead of ball bearings

FOCAL SPOT SIZE

The size of the focal spot can be larger than those in low kV imaging since the focus to image distance (FID) can be 70 to 200 cm. Chest radiography is the least limited since at an FID of 200 cm a 2 mm focal spot will give an unsharpness of only 0.2 mm using calculations from Box 9.1 and recalculating image unsharpness for an FID of 2 m. Box 9.2 demonstrates that small detail is not lost even with focal spot sizes of 2 mm. Figure 9.26a and b indicates the degree of unsharpness *S* for short and long FIDs and how, in the case of mammography, deep lesions (large values of *d*) resolution can be lost. At an FID of 200 cm the anode angle should be at least 11° for full coverage of the thorax.

X-RAY INTENSITY AND FID

It has been seen in Chapter 3 that increasing the tube kilovoltage increases the intensity of Bremsstrahlung production as the kilovoltage squared. The overall effect on film blackening is further influenced since the proportion of radiation transmitted by the patient (and so reaching the film) is increased and the intensifying

> ### Box 9.2 No loss of detail with a focal spot of 2 mm
>
> For chest radiography at 2 m FID (from Fig. 9.26 and using the same calculations as Box 9.1), if the FID is 200 cm, the OID is 12 cm, and the FS is 2 mm, then the resulting penumbra size, *s*, is
>
> $$\frac{2 \times 120}{2000 - 120} = 0.12 \text{ mm}$$
>
> A focal spot of 2 mm at 2 m will give adequate resolution for chest radiography. In practice the focal spot is typically 1.6 mm which improves the resolution to $\approx 100\ \mu m$.

screen response to higher energy photons is greater. At higher kilovoltages (above 80 kV) film density doubles for every 15 kV. The increased X-ray intensity at high kilovoltages has a valuable practical application: to maintain the same mAs value the exposure time can be greatly reduced typically 20 ms for chest radiography; movement unsharpness is therefore not a problem. Table 9.11 demonstrates how, by increasing kilovoltage but keeping the tube current the same, the required mAs can be achieved by shortening exposure times. This produces anode rating problems (see Fig. 9.27a), however, since only a part of the available target length will be used for these very fast exposure times unless fast anode rotational speeds are used.

9.4.2 High kilovoltage machine design

The important components of the X-ray machine designed for high kV are the grid, which cannot be the usual moving Bucky since exposure speeds can attain 1 ms; much too fast for a mechanically operated Bucky, the X-ray generator which must deliver high current levels and the X-ray tube which needs a high rating.

GRIDS

Low energy oblique scatter in mammography can be stopped by employing a low ratio grid (Pb 3.5/77 or

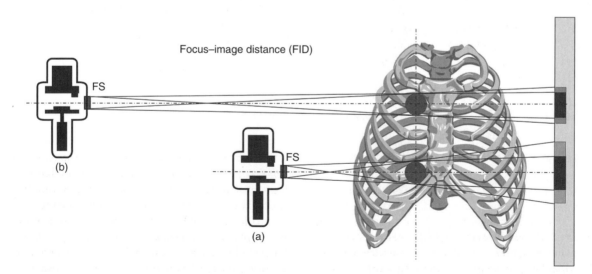

Figure 9.26 *(a) Image unsharpness (S) is a major problem at short focus to image distances (FIDs). (b) Increasing the focus to image distance decreases the unsharpness for the same focal spot size (FS).*

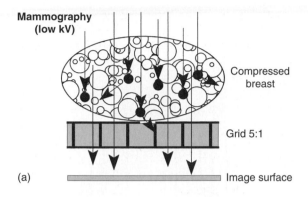

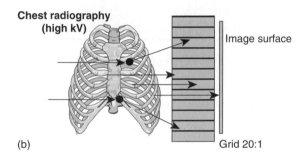

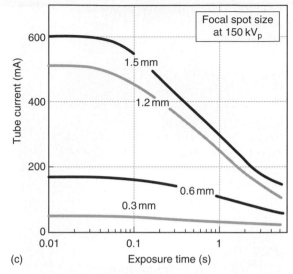

Figure 9.27 (*a*) *Grids used for low kilovoltages have a low ratio of 5:1 since scatter is oblique. (**b**) High kV radiography requires high ratio grids 20:1 to stop the forward scatter. (**c**) The electrical rating for an X-ray tube operating at high kV decreases with focal spot size.*

Pb 5/44) as illustrated in Fig. 9.27a. High ratio grids are necessary to reduce the amount of forward high energy scatter reaching the film in the chest radiograph (Pb 16/44) seen in Fig. 9.27b. These are usually parallel grids since high ratio focused grids are difficult to align. High voltage fluoroscopy uses lower ratio focused grids (Pb 8 or 12/44) which can produce problems with high resolution (1000 × 1000) digital matrices.

A 125 to 133 kV chest radiograph exposure time is about 20 ms using a large FID. A valuable diagnostic property of high kV chest imaging is the easy penetration of the mediastinal regions.

9.4.3 Automatic exposure control

This is provided by an ionization chamber positioned in front of the cassette. This is transparent to the X-ray beam at higher kilovoltages. More than one ion chamber can be used as already seen in Chapter 6. Because of the greater penetration less absorbed radiation and shorter exposure times the patient dose is low in high kV work, typically 20 to 100 μGy for a chest radiograph.

9.4.4 Image quality

SUBJECT CONTRAST

At high kilovoltage this depends on differing electron densities between tissues. It has already been seen that for photoelectric reactions there is a wide contrast between the different tissues (muscle, fat and bone). However, subject contrast due to Compton scatter obeys the approximate rule:

$$\rho \times \frac{\text{electron density}}{\text{kV}} \qquad (9.4)$$

where ρ is tissue density; it is independent of the atomic number Z, soft tissue differences are reduced and also bone will be more transparent allowing features behind to be observed (Fig. 9.28a). Air (as with the photoelectric effect) is virtually transparent and would give a dense black shadow. These points are particularly valuable in high kV chest radiographs where the rib cage is more transparent allowing visibility of the full lung fields. Pneumo-thorax would be a black shadow.

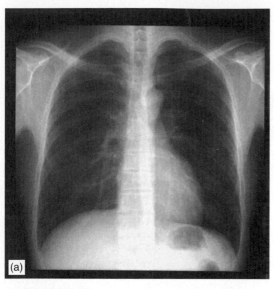

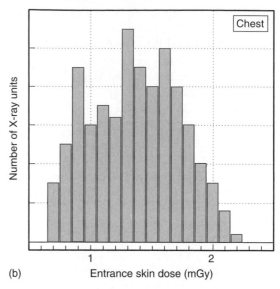

Figure 9.28 (*a*) Chest radiograph (CXR) using 125 kV$_p$ at 5 mAs. The rib cage is relatively transparent allowing a clear view of the lung fields. (*b*) The range of entrance skin doses measured from a large number of chest film units.

Table 9.12 Overall properties of low and high kV techniques.

	Conventional systems (60–80 kV$_p$)	Low kilovoltage (20–30 kV)	High kilovoltage (100–150 kV)
X-ray tube			
Focal spot	0.6/1.2 mm	0.4/0.1 mm	1.6 mm
Anode material	Tungsten/molybdenum	Molybdenum or tungsten	Tungsten with graphite or large diameter
Filament	Single or double	Double	Single
Tube current	800 mA	300 mA (space charge effect)	1000 mA
Anode heat capacity	212 kJ	200 kJ	600 kJ
Exposure time	1 s to 5 ms	Long	5 to 1 ms
Unsharpness			
Geometrical	FID 1 m	FID 60 cm	FID to 200 cm
	FS critical	FS critical	FS not critical
Movement	Present	Present	Not present
		Long exposure times	Very short times
Grid			
Ratio	8, 10, 12	4	12 to 15
Factor	3 to 4	<2	>4
Film			
Emulsion	Double	Single	Double
Contrast	Medium	High	Variable
Intensifying screens			
Number	Double	Single	Double
Film image			
Contrast	Good	High	Low–medium
Resolution (Lp mm^{-1})	3 to 5	20	2
Noise/mottle	Low	Low	Fair–poor
Patient dose			
Organ	Medium	High	Low
Whole body	Low	Low	Low

High kV fluoroscopy using dense iodine or barium contrast materials depends on photoelectric reaction in these high Z materials to give fine details. Very fast exposure times of 10 to 20 ms freeze all involuntary movement; movement unsharpness is almost zero. CT images depend almost entirely on Compton interactions for image formation; very sensitive electronic detectors replace film. These are tightly collimated to remove scatter events in the same way as high ratio grids. Comparisons between low and high kV imaging techniques are summarized in Table 9.12. Photoelectric reactions preferentially occur at low kilovoltages and the primary beam photon is removed entirely. Their probability increases with the atomic number Z of the absorber. Total photon absorption is very effective in producing a high contrast image.

Compton reactions decrease slightly with energy (eqn 9.4) and they are not dependent on absorber Z. Scatter photons are produced that travel at narrow angles to the primary beam and are removed by high ratio antiscatter grids. Compton reactions depend on the electron density in the absorber and are less dependent on photon energy above a certain threshold (≈ 80 kV).

RESOLUTION

Since image formation is dependent on scatter the image resolution is poorer than mammography. A typical resolution limit for double emulsion film-screen chest radiography would be no better than $2\,\mathrm{Lp\,mm^{-1}}$ whereas a good quality single emulsion film mammogram can register $20\,\mathrm{Lp\,mm^{-1}}$.

9.4.5 Patient dose

When comparing entrance surface doses for chest radiography there is a very wide range between analog and digital images. The fastest film-screens used in conjunction with high-kilovoltage systems (140 to 160 $\mathrm{kV_p}$) give about 700 μGy and image phosphor plates return approximately the same value. Large field of view image intensifier units using either digital output or 100 mm cut film cameras give an entrance dose of about 100 μGy. Recent full field digital imaging units can reduce this figure still further. Figure 9.28b indicates typical surface doses from a wide range of chest X-ray units using a mixture of film-screen combinations and using kilovoltages ranging from 110 to 140 $\mathrm{kV_p}$. There is a considerable spread of values over the 1 to 2 mGy range but a fair number of units are capable of doses below 1 mGy.

SUMMARY

The overall properties of low and high kV techniques are shown in Table 9.12.

10

Fluoroscopy

Conventional film radiography is restricted to static patient investigations. If dynamic events need to be studied, i.e. movement of contrast material through blood vessels or the gut, the image must be viewed directly using fluoroscopic methods.

The earliest fluoroscopic systems used phosphor screens when the transmitted X-rays caused scintillations that were viewed directly by the radiologist. The fluorescent screen was backed by lead glass so reducing radiation dose to the eyes. The images were of very poor quality for a number of reasons:

- Poor light output by the fluorescent screen for safe exposure rates
- Low efficiency of the light conversion mechanism of the screen
- Poor spatial resolution

Only a small percentage of the light from the screen was available to the eye owing to a very narrow viewing angle (about 6°) to the light photons. Fluorescent screens also give poor image quality because the visual acuity of the eye is ×10 less at low light levels (see Chapter 8).

Fluorescent screens are no longer used since they gave high radiation dose to the operator and the sensitivity of fluoroscopy is greatly improved by electronic intensification of the X-ray signal using an image intensifier.

10.1 THE IMAGE INTENSIFIER

The general design is shown in Fig. 10.1a. Electronic intensification of the incident X-ray beam is achieved by first converting it to light using a fluorescent input phosphor CsI:Na. The light photons are then converted to photoelectrons using a photocathode. The electrons are accelerated by high voltage electrodes which focus them onto a much smaller fluorescent screen.

The following basic features can be identified in the figure:

- A thin glass or metal (aluminum or titanium) input window
- An input fluorescent screen (CsI:Na)
- A photocathode
- High voltage focusing electrodes
- Output fluorescent screen coupled to a video camera and/or film cameras

The casing or **housing** of the image intensifier is mu-metal (except for the input and output windows) which are surrounded by a layer of lead shielding. Mu-metal is an alloy which is highly permeable to magnetic fields so strongly reducing magnetic interference from Earth's magnetic field and other equipment (MRI machines) which would seriously distort the electronic focusing. A commercially available

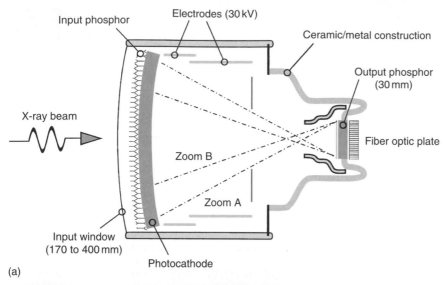

(a)

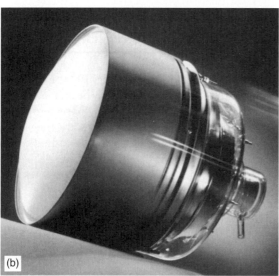

(b)

Figure 10.1 (*a*) *Image intensifier design. A metal window encloses the input phosphor (CsI:Na) and photocathode. Electrons ejected from the photocathode are accelerated by the electrodes E1, E2 and E3 towards the anode (+30 kV) and onto the output screen. (**b**) Full size 40 cm image intensifier showing face plate and metal/glass body.*

image intensifier employing metal construction is shown in Fig. 10.1b; the diameters vary between 15 and 40 cm (6 to 16 inches).

10.1.1 Image intensifier: the input window

The face of the image intensifier is illustrated in Fig. 10.2a. The entrance window is thin metal through which the X-ray beam passes onto a scintillator (CsI:Na); this converts the X-ray energy into light

photons. The light photons interact with an antimony/cesium photocathode material which produces photoelectrons, these are then accelerated by a large potential difference (30 kV) onto a small display screen.

The input window was originally glass in early designs but is now commonly aluminum or titanium which allows approximately 95% transmission for 60 kV X-rays (effective energy); glass provided only 80% transmission. Figure 10.1a shows that the input window of the intensifier has a convex shape; this is the origin of slight pincushion distortion in all image intensifiers.

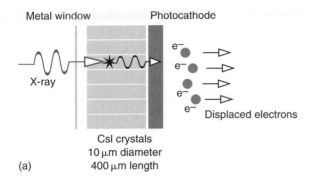

(a)

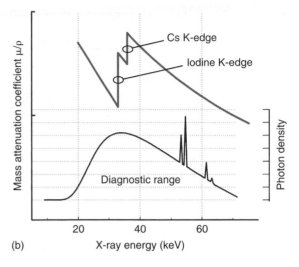

(b)

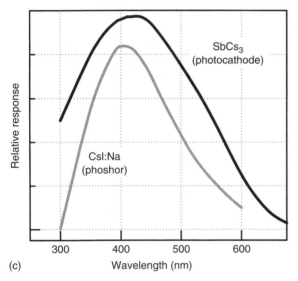

(c)

Figure 10.2 *(a) Input phosphor and photocathode. The X-rays penetrate the input window, undergo photoelectric absorption by the CsI:Na phosphor and the resulting light photons eject a cloud of electrons from the photocathode. (b) Absorption of X-radiation for cesium iodide showing the K edges for iodine and cesium giving optimum absorption over diagnostic photon energies from 30 to 80 keV. (c) The peak sensitivity of the photocathode matches the peak wavelength of light from the cesium iodide phosphor at about 400 to 500 nm.*

THE INPUT PHOSPHOR

Directly behind the window is a phosphor or scintillator which converts the incident X-radiation into visible light. Modern intensifiers use cesium iodide doped with sodium (CsI:Na), deposited as monoclinic columnar crystals on the input window itself.

These crystals form an array of tiny needle elements which collimate the light photons produced by photoelectric interactions within the scintillator crystals. This form of **light collimation** improves spatial resolution by reducing dispersion or **flare** at the phosphor surface.

Overall image quality depends on efficient X-ray absorption by the input phosphor. The CsI:Na phosphor absorbs about 60% of the incident X-ray beam assisted by the favorable position of the K edges of cesium and iodine at 36 and 33 keV respectively which is shown in Fig. 10.2b.

THE PHOTOCATHODE

The photocathode is a layer of a complex cesium antimony compound (CsSb$_3$) directly applied to the surface of the input phosphor and converts light photons from the scintillator into an electron cloud whose flux is proportional to light photon flux. The light spectrum from the cesium iodide phosphor and the photocathode is matched for wavelength as shown in Fig. 10.2c. There is a linear relationship between X-ray intensity at the intensifier face, light production, and electron density from the photocathode.

THE FOCUSING ELECTRODES

The electrons produced by the photocathode are accelerated by a high voltage applied to the internal electrodes identified in Fig. 10.1a as E$_1$, E$_2$, E$_3$ with the anode which carry an increasing voltage level. The electrons, produced by the photocathode, are accelerated towards a cylindrical anode, and focused onto the **output phosphor**. The focusing electrodes act as electrical lenses by modifying the electrostatic field between the photocathode (at earth potential) and the anode which is set at a very high potential, typically 25 to 35 kV.

Altering the voltage levels on the electrodes (electronic switching) controls the **area** of the input screen used by the image intensifier. This provides a **zoom** or **multi-field** facility. A single image intensifier can be electronically switched to give up to three fields of view: e.g. 33 cm (13 inches), 23 cm (9 inches) and 17 cm (7 inches); image resolution improves with decreasing field size.

10.1.2 Image intensifier: output screen

The output screen scintillation phosphor is a few micrometers thick deposited on a glass base which serves as the output window of the intensifier. Figure 10.3 shows a general design for an image intensifier output screen. A complex silver–zinc–cadmium sulfide is frequently used as the scintillator (type P20) although several other compounds are available. Typical output diameters range from 20 to 25 mm, the area being about one hundredth of the input area.

The accelerated electrons, from the photocathode, acquire enough kinetic energy to produce multiple light photons when they bombard the output phosphor. The image produced is an inverted, reversed, and minified version of the light pattern from the input phosphor.

The inner surface of the output phosphor is coated by a layer of very thin aluminum foil which allows electron transmission but prevents the light produced by the phosphor returning to the photocathode where it might release secondary electrons not associated with X-ray transmission causing **veiling glare**.

OUTPUT COUPLING

Some designs of output screen, for dedicated video camera output, have a fiber optic plate which acts as an interface between output screen and video camera tube; this design is shown in Fig. 10.3 and significantly reduces light dispersion at the camera face but it restricts output to a single video camera.

Image intensifiers which share output devices (cine-camera, 100 mm cut-film camera and video camera) use a system of lenses and a split mirror to share the light signal from the output screen. This arrangement is shown in Fig. 10.4 where the output screen is shared between a cine-camera, a 100 mm cut-film camera and video tube.

In most fluoroscopic systems the output from the image intensifier passes through a two lens system serving a film recording device and video camera. The first and second lens transmit the image as a parallel beam to the video camera. A rotating split mirror intersects the parallel beam directing light to either a cut-film or cine-camera for a permanent record. The lens system reduces the light output from the image intensifier and the light intensity is reduced for each imaging device added to the output. In practice only one film camera would be used and this would receive about 70% of the available light.

A dedicated video output for digital systems (digital fluorography (DF)) uses a direct fiber optic link between the image intensifier and camera, this would capture 100% of the available light and film records would be taken as video or digital images.

10.2 SPECIFICATIONS

The magnitude of signal amplification given by an image intensifier depends on the transparency of the input window (glass or metal) and the conversion efficiency of the input phosphor, photocathode and output phosphor. Figure 10.5 identifies the losses incurred by converting X-ray information into a visible image using a

phosphor $\rightarrow$ photocathode $\rightarrow$ phosphor system

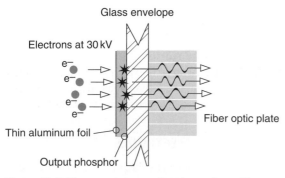

Figure 10.3 *The output screen of an image intensifier designed for a dedicated video output showing the fiber optic plate which is in contact with the screen and video camera face.*

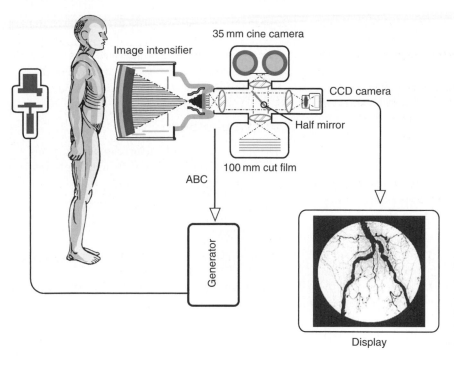

Figure 10.4 *Image intensifier output shared by a 100 mm cut-film camera, a cine-camera and a video camera. The input can be switched between two fields of view.*

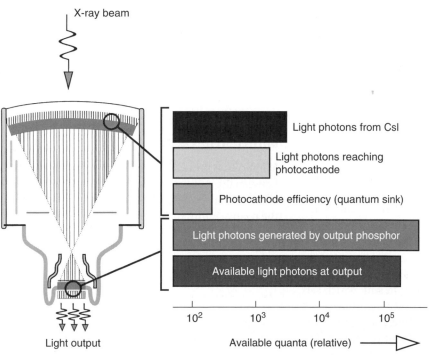

Figure 10.5 *Gains and losses from the input of the image intensifier to the output. Calculations are given in Box 10.1 quantum sink.*

The metal window has an absorption loss of about 5 to 8% and following this the X-ray absorption by the CsI phosphor is about 50 to 60%. The calculation in Box 10.1 explains the bar graph presented in Fig. 10.5. For an image intensifier having a 23 cm diameter field of view and 2.5 cm output screen the incident dose is $0.2\ \mu Gy\ s^{-1}$ which would represent a $5 \times 10^5\ cm^{-2}\ s^{-1}$ photon flux.

Box 10.1 The flux gain of an image intensifier

Using the reference values for exposure stated at the beginning of this section, and assuming a useful X-ray flux of 3×10^5 (after window and absorption loss) the following calculation can be made.

Light conversion

The input phosphor CsI:Na has 50% conversion efficiency to light. X-ray effective energy 60 keV and the mean photon energy of the light produced is 3 eV so

$$\frac{(3 \times 10^5) \times (60 \times 10^3) \times 0.5}{3} = 3.0 \times 10^9$$

There are approximately 7000 light quanta produced for each X-ray photon.

Photocathode electrons

Only a fraction ($\approx 3\%$) of the above light photons produces useful photoelectrons. So the above light flux would give approximately 10^8 photoelectrons; these are accelerated by the high voltage onto the output phosphor, each absorbed X-ray photon producing about 300 electrons.

Output phosphor

The kinetic energy of the accelerated electrons is converted into visible light at the output phosphor. Depending on the output phosphor type approximately 0.063 light photons are produced for each electron of energy 1 eV. For an electron stream having an effective energy of 30 kV this would give

$$10^8 \times (30 \times 10^3) \times 0.063 = 2 \times 10^{11} \text{ photons}$$

This produces approximately 2000 light photons per photoelectron.

Flux gain

The total light produced at the output screen by the electrons is $10^8 \times 2000 = 2 \times 10^{11}$. The available X-ray flux produces 3×10^9 light photons at the input so the flux gain is $2 \times 10^{11}/3 \times 10^9 = 66$. These are the gains and losses plotted in Fig. 10.5.

10.2.1 Image intensifier gain

The gains and losses through the image intensifier conversion processes are plotted in Fig. 10.5.

The lowest efficiency in the chain is the X-ray absorption by the input phosphor, which depends on three major factors: the phosphor's composition (K-edge energy), phosphor thickness and X-ray to light conversion efficiency; this is the area of most statistical uncertainty termed the **quantum sink** which sets a limit to image quality. All subsequent stages will only amplify the fractional difference (contrast) between any two points on the input phosphor. The intensification factor is a measure of the electronic gain or increase in the light intensity at the output compared with the input phosphor. There are two parameters for measuring intensification factor:

- Image minification
- Flux or electronic gain

MINIFICATION GAIN

Minification gain is derived simply from the area ratio between the input and output screens of the intensifier which produces an increase in gain in proportion to the relative radius of the input and output phosphors. The image is brighter when minified since the number of photons will be squeezed onto a smaller area, giving a minification gain in brightness, so:

$$\frac{\pi r_{in}^2}{\pi r_{out}^2} \qquad (10.1)$$

The output phosphor diameter is typically 2.5 cm. Since area also varies with the square of the diameter ($\pi r^2 \times 4\pi/4d^2$) a 40 cm diameter image intensifier will give a minification gain of $40^2/2.5^2 = 256$. The minification gain varies with input field size and has typical values between 50 and 250.

Radiation exposure increases with decrease in field size (zooming) since the minification gain is smaller. The increase in exposure rate is obtained by simply squaring the diameters i.e. zooming from 36 to 17 cm produces a 362/172 or 4-fold increase in dose maintaining the same noise figure.

FLUX GAIN

As the high voltage electrons are accelerated from the photocathode onto the output phosphor they gain kinetic energy. The amount of light produced at the output phosphor depends on the kinetic energy deposited by the electrons on the phosphor. The number of light quanta emitted by the output screen for every light quantum emitted by the input phosphor is the lumen, electronic or flux gain:

$$\frac{\text{light photons from output phosphor}}{\text{light photons at photocathode}} \quad (10.2)$$

This depends on the operating potential of the image intensifier; typically 25 to 30 kV. Box 10.1 calculates flux gain by comparing the input light to output light ratio.

The differing luminescent spectra from input and output screen make this a somewhat dubious measurement. The luminance (candela m^2) is increased also by the minification gain by up to 200 so a **total gain** (luminance, brightness or intensification gain) of 10 000 is available; this increases to 15 000 for large field (40 cm) intensifiers.

A more useful measure of image intensifier performance is given by the conversion factor, which directly compares the light output with X-ray exposure.

10.2.2 Conversion factor

This is a measure of the efficiency of image intensifier converting ionizing radiation (X-rays) measured in $\mu Gy\, s^{-1}$ to light output whose luminance is measured in candela (cd) as cd m^{-2}. So the conversion factor is:

$$\frac{\text{output phosphor luminance}}{\text{input phosphor dose}} \quad (10.3)$$

The output phosphor luminance is measured with a photometer; the incident radiation with a calibrated dosimeter. The X-ray beam quality must be defined and is usually taken as 2 mm Al pre-filtration giving 7 mm HVL. If a $0.5\,\mu Gy\, s^{-1}$ input phosphor dose

Table 10.1 *Conversion factor multipliers.*

Given	Required		
	mR^{-1} s	μGy^{-1} s	μC kg^{-1} s
mR^{-1} s	1.0	0.115	3.9
μGy^{-1} s	8.7	1.0	34.0
μC kg^{-1} s	0.256	0.03	1.0

gives 400 cd m^{-2} output luminance the CF would be 200. Typical values of conversion factor range from 100 to 1000 cd m^{-2} per μGy s^{-1} depending on intensifier input area.

The conversion factor varies with the area of the input field, since although the radiation dose per unit area does not change minification gain will alter, so the CF value for the same dose rate increases with intensifier input area since the intensification factor (light output) increases.

If the amount of light seen at the output is kept constant then as conversion performance decreases (as the image intensifier gets older) more radiation will be required at the input.

UNITS FOR THE CONVERSION FACTOR

The conversion factor for an image intensifier can be expressed in:

- millirads (cd m^{-2} mR^{-1} s^{-1})
- micrograys (cd m^{-2} μGy^{-1} s^{-1})
- microcoulombs (cd m^{-2} μC kg^{-1} s^{-1})

The approximate multipliers for these are given in Table 10.1.

10.2.3 Image noise

In the fluoroscopic image, noise may be due to quantum fluctuations or electronic noise introduced from various parts of the circuitry (either high voltage noise in the image intensifier or low voltage noise from the semiconductors). **Quantum noise** is associated with statistical fluctuations in the number of photons per unit area (mm^2) that contribute to image formation. The image chain is designed to be high in contrast and very sensitive to radiation. For this reason, substantial quantum mottle is to be expected. Box 10.2 shows a typical specification for a modern image intensifier and the associated noise values.

Electronic noise is associated with the imaging system electronics, which includes image intensifier

Box 10.2 Specification for a modern image intensifier

Overall resolving power: 2.5 Lp mm^{-1} giving five resolvable elements per mm (50 resolvable elements per cm).

Integration time of image chain: 0.2s, including the eye.

Fluence at face: 0.2 μGy s^{-1} input dose is about 5×10^5 X-ray photons per second.

Overall absorption/conversion efficiency: 40%, so useful photons equals 2×10^5.

Image frame rate: 5 fps (0.2 s per frame) giving $2 \times 10^5/5 = 40\,000$ photons cm^{-2} per image. From the resolving power, for each 50 resolvable elements, photon density is $40\,000/50 = 800$ photons.

The **quantum noise** associated with each resolvable element is therefore $\sqrt{800}$ giving a quantum noise figure of 3.5%.

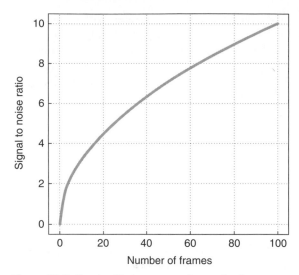

Figure 10.6 *Graph of frame summation and noise reduction.*

Increasing the iris aperture would have the converse effect.

DETECTION QUANTUM EFFICIENCY

The image intensifier image is inherently noisy owing to the low X-ray photon density used during fluoroscopy investigations (screening). A typical noise figure can be calculated for an incident exposure of 0.2 μGy s^{-1} photon density to estimate the quantum noise figure for a real-time fluoroscopy images, calculated in Box.10.2.

In order to obtain diagnostic quality images from an image intensifier with minimum noise level a certain density of X-ray photons is required. The detection quantum efficiency (DQE) relates the intensifier's input screen absorption efficiency and its X-ray-to-light conversion efficiency as an SNR figure. This then describes the signal-to-noise ratio (input SNR) at the input phosphor, for total absorption, compared to the output SNR of the image:

$$DQE = \left(\frac{\text{output SNR}}{\text{input SNR}} \right)^2 \qquad (10.4)$$

An ideal system would convert 100% of the photons into useful information but in practice losses occur at both the input and output window of the image intensifier, as already shown. The DQE measurement therefore takes into account:

- The percentage of X-ray photons penetrating the input window

with video or charge-coupled devices. This noise may be introduced by noise in the image intensifier high voltage supply, noisy amplifiers in the camera electronics, noise associated with a charge-coupled device, noise in the analog-to-digital converter.

Noise in dynamic fluoroscopic imaging is reduced by displaying individual noisy images in rapid succession. The human visual system has an integration time of between 100 and 200 ms. When displaying images in rapid succession, acquired at (say) 30 fps, the eye integrates the individual frames. Since noise is a random process, integrating images over several frames reduces the noise content by the square root of the number of frames used in the integration (Fig. 10.6).

IRIS CONTROL

Iris control is a light aperture positioned between the image intensifier and video camera. Its action is similar to those found in ordinary 35 mm cameras. A small aperture decreases the efficiency of light capture by the video camera so a greater X-radiation density is required at the image intensifier face, this will:

- Increase photon density
- Decrease quantum noise so improving SNR
- Increase patient dose

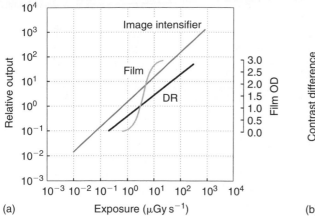

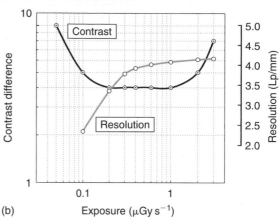

Figure 10.7 *(a) The dynamic range of an image intensifier covers several orders of magnitude. The lower limit is given by the dark current noise of the photocathode; the upper limit is due to the X-ray exposure on the conductivity between photocathode and output phosphor. (b) Low contrast visibility (plateau region) is optimum between 0.15 and 1.0 μGy s^{-1} and resolution is approaching maximum.*

- The percentage of X-ray photons absorbed by the input screen
- The percentage of absorbed quanta forming the image

Typical DQE values from modern equipment vary between 50 and 70%. It is a critical measure since the difference between a 40% DQE and a 50% DQE would give a relative contrast improvement of approximately 25% with a 20% lower radiation dose. In order to obtain maximum DQE:

- The input metal window must give maximum transmission.
- The input phosphor must offer maximum absorption to X-rays.
- There must be maximum light conversion.
- There must be an increase in detector size.
- The highest SNR for imaging chain should be obtained.

The electronic noise in a video camera determines the dynamic range of the image intensifier/video image chain; a common SNR value is 1000:1 with current systems approaching 2000:1.

The DQE is commonly measured using a ^{241}Am source, which gives a gamma ray with 60 keV energy; this corresponds to a filtered X-ray beam with a peak energy of 120 kV$_p$. The output signal is measured using a photometer with a time constant (integration time) which closely matches the eye. There is a great deal of variation in methods chosen for measuring

the DQE and manufacturers' figures should only be taken as a very rough guide.

10.2.4 Dynamic range

The linear transfer curve in Fig. 10.7a shows the dynamic range of an image intensifier as output luminance for an input dose rate; this range covers several orders of magnitude. The limiting factors are:

- The **lower limit** is due to the image intensifier dark current which is inherent electronic noise in the system equivalent to a dose of 0.001 μGy s^{-1}.
- The **higher limit** is imposed by the high X-ray photon flux which induces separate currents within the photocathode which reduces electron velocity and produces a decreased light output.

10.2.5 Resolution

The spatial resolution is often conveniently measured in terms of line pairs per millimeter (Lp mm^{-1}) by using a line pair test pattern consisting of an etched tungsten or tantalum grating. This is a measure of fine object detail in the output image. Overall resolution of the image intensifier improves with increased dose rate at the image intensifier face but low contrast visibility is the limiting factor which again restricts the dose rate to within 0.15 to

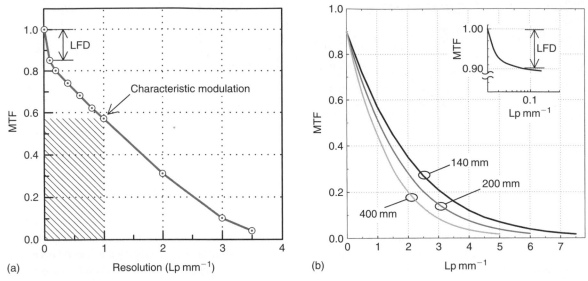

Figure 10.8 (*a*) *MTF of an image intensifier (linear plot) showing the low frequency drop influencing the entire MTF curve. Characteristic modulation is the MTF value for 1 Lp mm⁻¹ which is 0.57 in this case. (**b**) MTF curves (log–linear scale) for three sizes of input field showing an increased resolution with decreasing field (zoom) size.*

$0.2\,\mu\text{Gy s}^{-1}$ as shown by the resolution curve in Fig. 10.7b where 3.5 to 4.0 Lp mm⁻¹ is currently the best performance value.

LOW FREQUENCY DROP

A typical MTF for an image intensifier is shown in Fig. 10.8a using linear axes in order to emphasize the low frequency fall-off, common to all image intensifiers. The MTF response quickly drops from an initial value of 1.0 to about 0.8; the percentage drop is called the low frequency drop (LFD) and represents a fall of 8 to 10% in resolution value and is responsible for the degradation of all spatial frequencies. There are two main reasons for this rapid fall in resolution:

- X-radiation scatter in the input window and phosphor
- Light diffusion at the output window

The first can be reduced by using a thin metal window (aluminum or titanium) and a CsI:Na crystalline input phosphor. Light diffusion at the output screen can be reduced by using a fiber optic plate as an interface. The contrast improvement for larger objects is significantly improved as the LFD is reduced to about 6 or 8%. The **characteristic modulation** of an image intensifier is measured as the MTF value for 1 Lp mm⁻¹ (typically 0.57); this is sometimes used as a measure of overall resolution.

The spatial resolution is increased by decreasing the input field of view. The MTFs in Fig. 10.8b show a 40 cm image intensifier zoomed to decrease the field size through 20 to 14 cm so improving resolution.

TEMPORAL RESOLUTION

Fluoroscopy offers real-time visualization of an object in motion (for example a contrast bolus). The temporal resolution of a system is the ability of an imaging system to localize this object in time from frame to frame and follow its movement. **Image lag** is due to the slow response of the vacuum tube video camera. The image formed on the target of the camera tube is not completely extracted between fields or frames, since complete decay of the signal on the camera target takes between one to eight frames, depending on the camera design and setup. Thus, each image contains a small fraction of several preceding images. Lag is not seen in semiconductor CCD cameras since they operate differently.

Temporal resolution is important in digital subtraction angiography and cardiac imaging, where there are fast moving events so lag is kept to a minimum. Noise can be addressed by increasing radiation dose rate or by using post-processing techniques.

Table 10.2 *The typical performance figures for an image intensifier having three zoom values 29, 22, and 16 cm respectively.*

Variable	Operating mode			Units
	Normal	Zoom 1	Zoom 2	
Entrance field size	29	22	16	cm
DQE at 60 keV	65			%
Conversion factor	240	120	65	cd m^{-2}/mR s^{-1}
				cd m^{-2}/μGy s^{-1}
Limiting resolution center:	4.4	5.0	5.6	Lp mm^{-1}
93% radius:	3.8	4.6	5.2	
Contrast ratio				
Large area: Small detail	22:1	25:1	30:1	
	13:1	15:1	17:1	

10.2.6 Contrast ratio

The minimum detectable difference between two low contrast objects depends on the dose rate to the surface of the image intensifier. The optimum level is therefore set by the manufacturer and automatic dose control devices aim to keep this reference level so that high quality images are displayed. The 'bath-tub' graph shown in Fig. 10.7b demonstrates that there is an optimal dose rate below which quantum noise degrades low contrast visibility and above which saturation effects influence display quality. The dose rate for modern image intensifiers is typically kept within the 0.15 and 0.2 μGy s^{-1} band; this limit allows an optimum patient dose : image quality ratio.

The ability to register low contrast differences also depends on the SNR. Image noise can be introduced by a variety of factors:

- X-ray scattering at the input window
- X-ray scattering at the input phosphor
- Light scattering within the phosphor itself
- Visible light not absorbed by the photocathode
- Back-scattering of light from the output phosphor toward the photocathode
- Scattering of light at the output window (reduced by fiber optic plate)

The overall effect of these scattering events is to reduce image contrast by causing **veiling glare**. This can be measured as a **contrast ratio** C_v by measuring output light intensity at the display before and after

placing a lead disk in front of the image intensifier face so:

$$C_v = \frac{L_c}{L_d} \qquad (10.5)$$

where L_c is the light intensity at center of image and L_d the light intensity at the same point when a lead disk blocks 10% of the central input area. For a perfect image intensifier L_d would be zero and C_v would be infinite but due to scattering the contrast ratio can vary from 17:1 to 40:1 depending on the condition of the unit. The overall operating specifications for a current image intensifier are listed in Table 10.2.

10.3 DISPLAY

Both soft copy (video) and hard copy (film) are available as output displays for the image intensifier. Figure 10.4 shows three displays. Most recent models of fluoroscopic systems rely solely on a CCD camera output. From this output soft-copy, hard-copy and movie (real-time) displays can be derived (see Chapter 13 on digital fluoroscopy).

10.3.1 Output coupling

Some designs of output screen, for dedicated video camera output have a fiber optic plate which acts as an interface between output screen and video camera tube, this design is shown in Fig. 10.3 and significantly reduces light dispersion at the camera face but it restricts output to a single video camera.

Image intensifiers which share output devices (cine-camera, 100 mm cut-film camera and video camera) use a system of lenses and a split mirror to share the light signal from the output screen. This arrangement is shown in Fig. 10.4 where the output screen is shared between a cine-camera, a 100 mm cut-film camera and video tube.

In most fluoroscopic systems the output from the image intensifier passes through a two lens system serving a film recording device and video camera. The first and second lens transmit the image as a parallel beam to the video camera. A rotating split mirror intersects the parallel beam directing light to either a cut film- or cine-camera for a permanent record. The lens system reduces the light output from the image intensifier and the light intensity is reduced for each imaging device added to the output. In practice only one film camera would be used and this would receive about 70% of the available light.

A dedicated video output for digital systems (digital fluorography) uses a direct fiber optic link between the image intensifier and camera, this would capture 100% of the available light and film records would be taken as video or digital images.

IMAGE LAG OR PERSISTENCE

Theoretically, the electron beam of the vacuum-tube video camera neutralizes the charge on the photoconductive layer during subsequent raster scans and therefore the image data at that location is removed. In practice, neutralization is not complete, which results in persistent remnant image data called afterimage or image lag.

Only 60 to 70% is neutralized in the vidicon and 90 to 95% in the plumbicon (an improved vidicon design). Since the vidicon exhibits a considerable amount of image lag or persistence it will not be suitable for certain applications, such as cardio-vascular work, where rapid movements are being recorded. Plumbicon cameras exhibit very little lag but produce images that are more mottled or noisy than those produced by the vidicon since the relatively high lag in the vidicon smoothes or integrates the statistical variation of light in the image. Both designs of vacuum-tube video cameras have now been

Table 10.3 *Comparing properties of vacuum tube video cameras with semiconductor CCD camera.*

	Vidicon	Plumicon	CCD
Target	Sb2S3	PbO	Si
Sensitivity (μA lumen^{-1})	Varies	400	700
Resolution (relative)	0.55	0.65	0.4
Lag (relative)	10	1	0.1
Dark current (nA)	20	<1	5
Life (h)	4500	4500	>500 000

replaced by semiconductor CCD cameras which have superior sensitivity, a very quick response and minimum lag. Properties of different camera types are listed in Table 10.3. The CCD resolution can also challenge the resolution capability of the vidicon.

CHARGE-COUPLED DEVICE

This is a solid-state imaging sensor commonly found in domestic 'cam-recorders'. The device needs no electron gun, deflection system or evacuated tube seen in video camera tubes. Its simple design is shown in Fig. 10.9a where a semiconductor photosensitive surface (8 × 6 mm being typical) divided into many thousands of separate islands of photodiodes arranged in rows and columns. Electrons are captured in the charge-coupled layer of the semiconductor, the electron number is in proportion to light intensity.

Readout of this stored information is different from other camera technology. An electron beam is not used, but each line of information (stored electrons) is shifted electronically and read out as a video waveform. The camera operates on a voltage of about 12 V, compared with 200 to 300 V for a video tube resolution of 2000 × 2000 pixels. A lens system focuses the image onto the semi-conductor surface.

Spatial resolution approaches that of a vacuum-tube camera but since the output is more amenable to digitization higher quality charge-coupled device (CCD) cameras, being developed, are rapidly replacing the tube cameras (Fig. 10.9b).

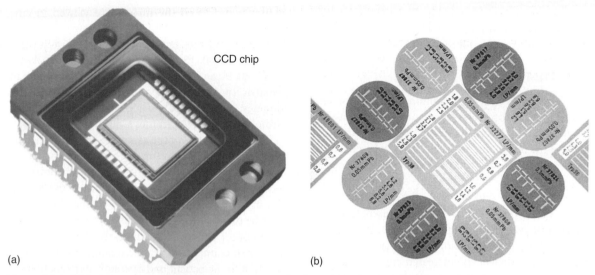

(a)   (b)

Figure 10.9 *(a) A charge-coupled device used as a camera for fluoroscopy (courtesy Toshiba Inc.). (b) A test image showing good spatial resolution across the field of view and lack of picture distortion.*

10.3.2 Recording

This is used to capture the video image for subsequent display or hard-copy film recording. Multiple film copies using a film formatter can be readily achieved. Rapid video recording is obtained by using a solid-state image memory. It provides limited storage (four to five frames) but offers instant playback and reduces a patient's radiation dose.

VIDEO TAPE RECORDER

Although the economics of a video recorder are very favorable (maximum number of images on a video tape cassette), the quality of the images commonly recorded is much poorer than those obtained by cine-fluorography since the images are obtained from a relatively low resolution television system. High definition video recorders matching HD-video standards are becoming available. Major disadvantages are:

- The access times to individual images stored on magnetic tape may be long.
- Direct or random access is not available.
- Contact between the heads and the tape causes wear and leads to image degradation.
- A video tape deteriorates in storage and images become noisier.

VIDEO DISK

An alternative video image storage device which has a limited storage capacity but allows instant playback of any stored image uses a video magnetic disk. Images can be selected after a patient investigation for film recording before the disk is erased and re-used.

DIGITAL RECORDING

The output from the video camera is digitized and the image is stored as a matrix (512×512, 1024×1024 or larger matrices). Many such digital images can be stored during a patient study and then selected for film hard copy on a laser film formatter. Dynamic frames can be collected at up to 30 fps (see Chapter 13).

10.3.3 Hard-copy film recording

Real-time events can be viewed on the video monitor but it is sometimes important to obtain permanent records during patient investigations. There are five common methods for obtaining permanent film images:

- Spot film cassette
- Rapid sequence 100 or 105 mm cut film
- Serial film changer (film cassette)
- Cine-fluoroscopy
- Digital recording

The video camera monitoring an image intensifier input can also be used for providing a video or digital image for storage and retrieval.

SPOT FILM CASSETTE

Spot film cassette is the traditional method of film recording. Fluoroscopy is interrupted and the cassette moved sideways from its protective shelter to be in front of the image intensifier face. The tube current is then increased from 1 to 3 mA used for fluoroscopy to 300–400 mA for film exposure. The area for film recording can be selected thus allowing for multiple exposures on the one film–cassette combination. The major disadvantage of this technique is the time required for the cassette to move into place and for the X-ray tube to deliver the increased current (filament heating). The overall delay time is about 0.75 s and the image cannot be viewed on the video monitor while the cassette is in place. Modern systems allow up to two exposures per second for a range of format sizes.

The spatial resolution is the highest of the hard-copy devices, about 5 to 6 Lp mm^{-1}, which is limited by the size of the focal spot. The radiation dose to the patient is the highest of any of the hard-copy devices per image obtained.

RAPID SEQUENCE CUT FILM CAMERA (100 AND 105 MM)

These devices can acquire permanent images on small format, 100 mm cut film or 105 mm roll film, at a rate of up to 10 images per second. The camera views the light output of the image intensifier deflected from the semi-transparent mirror between the tandem lens system (see Fig. 10.4). When the mirror is in place about 85% of the light is directed onto the cut-film camera.

The main advantage of this recording system is the reduction in patient and staff radiation dose, about one third of that from a spot film cassette. However, the spatial resolution of the 100 mm camera is inferior to the film cassette. An advantage, however, is the reduction of unsharpness (caused by organ movement) by the short exposure times. Cut film typically requires 1.5 μGy per frame. Frame rates are usually 1 to 6 fps and the film resolution 3 to 4.5 Lp mm^{-1} depending on image intensifier field size.

CINE-FLUOROGRAPHY

Cine fluorography records the moving image, in real time, on 35 mm cinemato-graphic film. After the reel of film is processed the images are viewed in cine mode.

A variety of framing rates are available in Europe: 12.5, 25, 50, 100, 150 frames s^{-1} and in the USA: 15, 30, 45, 60, 90 and 120 frames s^{-1}. Rapid heart rate in pediatric cardiology can be followed at 120 to 150 frames s^{-1} (90 to 120 fps USA) and typically adult cardiology at 50 to 60 frames s^{-1} (30 to 60 fps).

The drive control of the camera is part of the generator and must be able to run at a selected frame rate in a reproducible way. In addition, the synchronization between the shutter-open interval (when the 35 mm film in the camera is stationary) and the X-ray pulse must be maintained. This avoids any radiation during the transport phase of the film as this kinetic blurring would reduce image quality, increasing at the same time radiation to the patient and operator. Examinations of the heart (cardiology) are performed using cine techniques. Cine-fluorography normally employs a double imaging system involving both anterior and lateral planes of the heart where pulsed radiation exposures are synchronized with the film transport mechanism.

An X-ray tube with a small grid-controlled focus is used for cine operation. Automatic cine systems employ a photomultiplier or semiconductor photodetector as a sensor to achieve specific shorter pulse widths rather than use pre-set values. The radiation for each individual cine frame is switched off by the automatic exposure control system.

Geometric blurring is reduced by automatically applying the smallest focal spot within the tube loading and voltage range for best contrast; this change of focal spot size also depends on the object transparency.

10.3.4 Overall performance

The general specification for a large field image intensifier having three zoom settings is summarized in Table 10.2. Both conversion factor and image pincushion distortion **increase** with **increasing field size**. Resolution, contrast ratio both improve with **decrease** in field size and relative patient dose also increases.

Image intensifiers have undergone major improvements owing to the stringent requirements for digital fluorography. A typical signal-to-noise ratio exceeds 1000:1 and low frequency drop would be less than 8% due to aluminum or titanium input windows having a transmission factor of >95% at 60 keV.

A 100 mm film cassette for hard copy is shown in Fig. 10.4 but various hard-copy devices are used.

Automatic exposure and display brightness controls are incorporated into all fluoroscopy systems. These alter the generator kV and mA to give a constant input dose rate to the image intensifier.

The overall image resolution, contrast and noise is the product of the image intensifier, video camera and display type. Of this image chain the image intensifier is the major weakness due mostly to the quantum sink effect described earlier so significant improvements in image quality will depend on image intensifier improvements.

The image intensifier is capable of about 6 Lp mm^{-1} for a 17 cm (6.5 inches) diameter field of view. Resolution decreases with increasing input diameter as shown in Table 10.4. A 36 cm (14 inches) image intensifier is chosen for imaging the full body width. It has a DQE of 52% and a low frequency drop of 6%; a conversion efficiency (G_x) of 150 cd m^{-2} mR^{-1} s^{-1}. The final resolution of the fluoroscopy display is the product of all the components of the system.

Improved input face materials (thin metal window and CsI:Na phosphors) have produced significant improvements in resolution. A 20 cm image intensifier has a resolution of 5 Lp mm^{-1} when using cut film, almost matching spot film, and the cut film fluoroscopy investigation has a much lower radiation dose. High definition video displays (1049/1249 lines) approach the resolution of modern image intensifiers and this is not a limiting factor particularly with the current 2046 and 2498 line video displays.

The resolution of the image-intensifier and video display combined can be estimated from the resolvable video line-pairs:

$$R_s = \frac{\text{image intensifier size}}{V} \quad (10.6)$$

where V is the vertical resolution. This is used for calculating the system resolution already given in Table 10.4.

SENSITIVITY

Sensitivity is the ratio of the camera signal strength to the input illumination and is analogous to the film-screen characteristic curve. The gamma for plumbicons is 1.0 and for vidicons 0.7 so the image contrast is preserved at the output of a plumbicon but slightly reduced for a vidicon. The sensitivity, signal strength for the same illumination, is higher in

Table 10.4 *Image intensifier specifications.*

Field diameter	40 cm (16″)	32 cm (12.5″)	20 cm (8″)	15 cm (6″)
Resolution (Lp mm^{-1})	4.0	4.2	5.5	6.0
Contrast ratio	20:1	25:1	30:1	30:1
Dose (relative)	0.25	0.5	0.75	1.0
Pincushion (%)	9	4.5	1.4	1.0
CF (cd m^{-2} mR^{-1} s^{-1})	166	100	60	50

plumbicons than in vidicons. The dark current that flows when no illumination is present is equivalent to film fog and ideally should be zero. The dark current in plumbicons is about 25 times less than that of vidicons. CCD gamma value is also 1.0 and the dark current is very low (see Table 10.3).

10.4 X-RAY TUBE AND GENERATOR

The rating (loadability) of the X-ray tube and the power output of the generator exceed that of conventional X-ray units. The basic electronic fluoroscopy imaging chain is shown in Fig. 10.10. It includes:

- X-ray tube
- High frequency generator
- Image intensifier
- A video camera
- A hard copy film camera
- A video display for real-time viewing

Most fluoroscopy systems are now controlled by some form of microprocessor which accepts feedback from the outputs of the image intensifier and display in order to maintain a constant image quality (brightness/contrast/noise) for an optimum patient dose. The X-ray tube is grid controlled to give a pulsed output synchronized with the display.

10.4.1 The X-ray tube

Table 10.5 lists the specifications for a typical X-ray tube suitable for fluoroscopy. X-ray tubes have maximum thermal capacity and heat dissipation. These permit high patient throughput and are usually synchronized with imaging systems (e.g. cine-camera) using pulse mode.

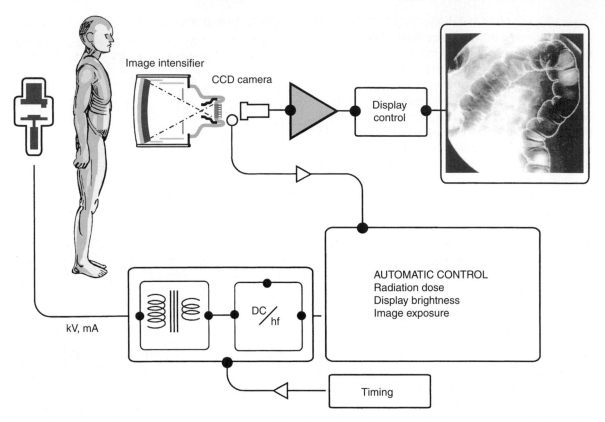

Figure 10.10 *General design of a fluoroscopic system with an image intensifier and feedback mechanisms to the X-ray tube and generator. The fluoroscopy imaging chain shows the image intensifier feeding a video/CCD camera.*

Table 10.5 *X-ray tube specifications.*

	Medium duty	**Heavy duty**
Construction	Glass	Metal/ceramic
Focal spot (mm)	0.6/1.2	0.4/0.8
Target	12°	8°
Heat storage	0.4 MJ (0.6 MHU)	1 MJ (1.3 MHU)
Maximum power	450 W	2000 W

Patient separation from the image intensifier face usually gives a magnification of about 1.25 yielding a resolution of 6.25 Lp mm^{-1} for a focal spot of 0.8 mm and 4 Lp mm^{-1} for a 1.2 mm focal spot. The focal spot size, however, is not a limiting factor for image resolution since the image intensifier has an upper limit of about 4 Lp mm^{-1} but if magnification views of ×2.5 are chosen large focal spot sizes will significantly influence image unsharpness. Fluoroscopic X-ray tubes typically have dual focal spot sizes 0.3 and 1.0 mm which allow magnification views with minimum unsharpness and optimum thermal rating.

The influence of focal spot size on resolution is critical, as the curve in Fig. 10.11 demonstrates. The influence of focal spot size on image resolution R follows a general formula:

$$R = \frac{m}{F(m-1)} \tag{10.7}$$

where m is the image magnification and F the focal spot size of the X-ray tube.

10.4.2 Generators

High frequency power supplies are used almost exclusively with power ranges from 15 to 80 kW depending on application (small mobile or large fixed installation). The larger generator should permit continuous operation at 2000 W and allow an acquisition rate of up to 8 frames per second (fps). Since the K edge of iodine is 33 keV an effective X-ray energy

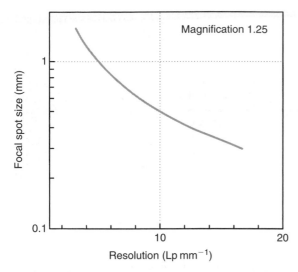

Figure 10.11 *The change of potential resolution with X-ray tube focal spot size.*

of ×2 or 70 keV is chosen which translates as a peak value of 100 kV.

The high frequency generator combines the advantages of a constant-potential generator with less cost (about 30% less). Additional features include:

- Reduced patient dose due to low tube voltage ripple (2 to 10%)
- Space savings of 60 to 80% obtained relative to conventional generators

Tube voltage must be independent of changes in tube current and line regulation and should have a maximum 5% tolerance for X-ray tube voltage, tube current, and exposure time.

Contrast and sharpness are partly influenced by the X-ray system. Movement unsharpness especially is influenced by exposure time and the pulse rate of the generator. The X-ray tube voltage (kV_p) determines the penetrating power of radiation and therefore is responsible for the contrast.

High frequency generators produce many X-ray tube voltage pulses per second, depending on the firing frequency of the inverter–high tension transformer system. The operating frequency is between 5 kHz and 20 kHz.

10.4.3 Pulsed beam fluoroscopy

If the grid-pulsed X-ray tubes are used with high frequency or constant-potential generators to produce a precise pulsed output in synchrony with the fluoroscopy video system then temporal resolution is improved with much reduced patient dose. In pulsed fluoroscopy a square wave pulse is generated immediately before the beginning of each readout cycle. The duration of the radiation pulse must be short in order for the pulse to begin and end between the end of one readout cycle and the beginning of the next.

The ideal configuration for pulsed fluoroscopy is to use a grid-controlled X-ray tube to minimize the rise and fall time of the X-ray pulse (Fig. 10.12). Many high frequency generators use 'saw tooth' or 'square' wave shape generators to simulate a pulsed waveform. This technique is less than ideal because of the inherent (cable) capacitance of the secondary circuit producing pulse distortion. Pulse shapes generated in this way will have longer rise and decay times during which low energy radiation will be produced. Most of this radiation will be absorbed so increasing patient radiation dose.

If the patient is exposed to fewer pulses per second dose rate is reduced in direct proportion to the pulse rate. For frame rates between 5 and 15 frames per second, the dose savings will depend on acceptable noise levels. The X-ray beam is pulsed by using a grid controlled X-ray tube. This cuts out inductive/capacitive delays introduced by the high voltage cable as would be given by electronically switching the high frequency generator so providing very sharp cut-off pulses.

10.4.4 Collimation: the dominant region

Chapter 4 has already shown the different independent circuits of high frequency generators, with feedback from AEC–ABC systems for a selection of a dose reference values.

The measured dose rate ($\mu Gy\ s^{-1}$) at the image intensifier input screen is proportional to the signal produced by the photomultiplier or semiconductor sensor, which samples the optical light intensity of the image intensifier output screen. **Selective dominant measurement** (SDM) systems allow selective sampling of an area of the image intensifier output screen. The SDM measuring field is part of the object that contains the relevant information regarding the lesion. The SDM system controls all fluoroscopy modes through the automatic brightness control (ABC)

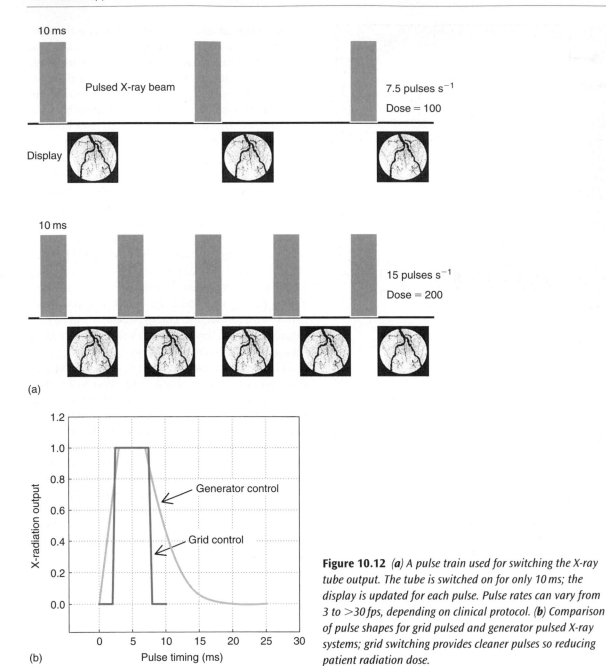

(a)

(b)

Figure 10.12 *(a) A pulse train used for switching the X-ray tube output. The tube is switched on for only 10 ms; the display is updated for each pulse. Pulse rates can vary from 3 to >30 fps, depending on clinical protocol. (b) Comparison of pulse shapes for grid pulsed and generator pulsed X-ray systems; grid switching provides cleaner pulses so reducing patient radiation dose.*

system. Figure 10.13 shows selective measurement of the dominant regions, illustrating the sampling of different portions of the output screen for the different medical applications in fluoroscopy.

If the object is moving within the region of interest then this can lead to large changes in brightness levels. In order to minimize this effect the feedback controls can:

- Monitor the peak video value
- Monitor the minimum value
- Use the mean value of these extremes

Monitoring the peak value does prevent the display from being overdriven, but other parts of the

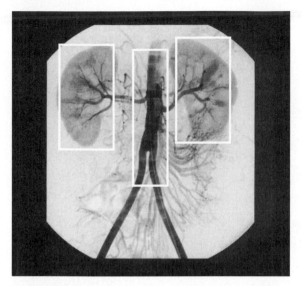

Figure 10.13 *An example where three dominant regions of interest are available; any one of which can be selected for optimum display. The anatomy of interest is the dominant factor controlling image quality.*

image can become too dark and for this reason the minimum value should also play a part. Control taken from a photodetector (photomultiplier) sampling the image intensifier light output can only give a mean value. A better method selects regions of the image (usually splitting the display into three rectangles). The particular display region which covers the anatomy of interest is operator selected and this is then the dominant region which supplies luminance information to the ABC circuit.

10.5 FEEDBACK CONTROLS

The absorption of X-rays depends on the transparency of the object and for different thicknesses of patient the image intensifier output will vary greatly in brightness producing a changing image quality. In order to stabilize the image signal two methods are used:

- Automatic brightness (or dose) control maintains a constant dose rate at the intensifier face.
- Automatic gain control (AGC) maintains a constant video display brightness.

Both types of regulation are used in modern fluoroscopy equipment.

The image intensifier–video image chain is calibrated at the time of manufacture so that a certain dose at the image intensifier face produces optimum image quality at the output. The dose rate which provides optimum image brightness is pre-set by the manufacturer and is typically 0.15 to 0.2 μGy s^{-1}.

10.5.1 Automatic brightness control

Many systems have automatic brightness control that is designed to reduce exposure by allowing more rapid increases in operating kilovoltage as patient attenuation increases. These units may allow a lower patient dose rate for the same perceived noise but may also result in loss of image contrast due to higher kV_p.

The automatic brightness control (ABC) maintains a constant average dose rate at the input window of the image intensifier so giving a constant displayed image brightness independent of X-ray absorption by the patient. Manufacturers use various techniques for measuring this input dose, two of which are:

- The image intensifier light output is monitored by a small photomultiplier or photodiode.
- For a dedicated video camera where the output screen and camera face are connected by a fiber optic plate, the video signal from a central (dominant) area of the image is monitored.

The first method is preferred since it provides a direct measure of image intensifier performance prior to the video chain.

Slight signal loss is inevitable since the optical coupling is modified and is not as efficient as the fiber optic plate. Signal sensors which provide feedback control are shown in Fig. 10.14a:

- A photodetector which monitors image intensifier output controlling kV and mA
- The display video signal whose amplitude alters video amplifier gain

The photodetector system monitoring the image intensifier output (pd in the diagram) also adjusts the luminance levels for film exposure when using 100 mm cut film or cine-camera. The automatic brightness control (Fig. 10.14 a) ensures consistent dose rate at the image intensifier face which maintains image quality at the display monitor.

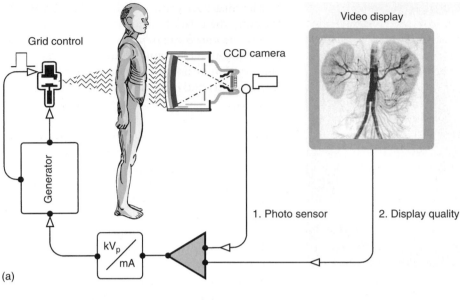

(a)

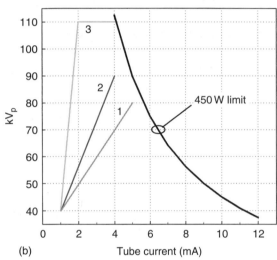

(b)

Figure 10.14 (**a**) *Automatic brightness (dose) control using signals from [1] a photodetector (pd) and [2] the display video signal controlling the X-ray generator to provide a consistent image quality at the display by controlling kV_p and mA supplied to the tube.* (**b**) *An automatic brightness control program which alters kV and mA for increasing thicknesses of patient (slopes 1, 2, 3), so that the same input dose rate is maintained at the intensifier face; the 450 w isowatt curve shows the power limit of the X-ray tube which must not be exceeded. The plotted values are described in the text.*

Feedback control of the tube current is a simple operation but the response may be slow since it takes time for the filament to heat up; this type of exposure control is not suitable for cine applications. Current control of the X-ray tube can lead to difficulties when imaging very thin patients, since these patients are relatively radiotransparent leading to high transmission values at the image intensifier. If feedback is obtained using current control only, the current reduction may be too great and lead to noisy images.

Automatic brightness control is therefore achieved by adjusting both current and kilovoltage levels. The radiation dose at the image intensifier input can be maintained in one of three ways:

- A change in kV_p at fixed mA
- A change in mA at fixed kV_p
- Both kV_p and mA changed

Current control usually dominates, but a kilovoltage over-ride exists when preset values of current might be reached which would exceed rating levels. Figure 10.14b plots kilovoltage against tube current control and shows the maximum permitted level (480 W in this case) which forms the 'isowatt' limit for the particular X-ray tube.

In some X-ray tube designs this can approach 2000 W. A function similar to the ones shown plotted here is used by the fluoroscopy system to calculate the kV_p, mA, and dose rate so maintaining a constant object transparency. The linear functions plotted in Fig. 10.14 b differ according to the emphasis placed on mA or kV; slope (1) predominantly alters mA while (2) alters mA and kV with equal measure.

In addition the video signal itself can be maintained by applying an AGC; both types of regulation are used in modern fluoroscopy equipment as shown in Fig. 10.14a. Choosing a 'worst case' condition of an extra-large patient acting as an effective X-ray absorber the ABC first adjusts the tube current in order to achieve the set input dose figure for the image intensifier (typically 0.2 μGy s^{-1}). If a current limit is reached the kV is then increased keeping the overall power within the rating of the X-ray tube.

When investigating thick body parts the ABC will increase mA and then kV in order to maintain video signal strength (display brightness). This may not be sufficient for loss of image brightness and if exposure limits are installed the machine will change iris aperture or increase video amplifier gain (automatic gain control AGC); both these adjustments will increase image noise. In special cases high level control (HLC) increases mA still further in order to overcome limitations but this results in a much increased patient dose, exceeding the upper limit of 100 mGy min^{-1} (10 R min^{-1}) at the patient surface. In most fluoroscopic machines the ABC uses a reference central area of the image intensifier; this is the dominant area so the anatomical area of interest should always be central in the field of view. Fluoroscopic equipment with automatic brightness control commonly gives a range of exposure rates for particular studies.

ISOWATT/ANTI-ISOWATT OPERATION

The value of tube voltage and tube current relate directly to the transparency of the examined object because the dose rate at the input screen of the image intensifier is adjusted to a fixed value (typically 0.175 μGy s^{-1}) at the time of installation. This information is used in various automatic control systems to automatically preset technique factors when recording images.

Operating at maximum X-ray tube power (isowatt fluoroscopy using the 450 W curve in Fig. 10.14b) cannot be used for imaging since tube ratings would

be exceeded (see specifications in Table 10.5 for the medium duty tube).

Anti-isowatt fluoroscopy (curves 1 and 2 in Fig. 10.14b) offers a good compromise between contrast and dose for all objects. The brightness of the image intensifier output screen is measured and used by the automatic brightness control system and compared with reference values to maintain image quality. The brightness is kept at a constant value by the reference to these values controlling tube voltage and tube current during any changes in the transparency of the patient anatomy (i.e. contrast agent injection); the image contrast and brightness are therefore maintained constant.

Minimal radiation exposure (curve 3 in Fig. 10.14b) is used mostly in pediatric radiology, where a certain loss of contrast may be acceptable. Application of this curve means operation at the highest possible tube voltage and low tube current.

10.5.2 Automatic exposure control

When radiography (spot film) is being performed by placing a film cassette in front of the image intensifier, a thin walled ionization chamber located in front of the film cassette controls exposure cut-off by comparing to a reference signal. Fluoroscopy uses a low input dose rate of about 0.15 μGy s^{-1} but during cut-film or cine this dose must be increased to about 0.9 μGy per frame for correct film exposure. Cine-film exposure depends on frame rate which can vary between 30 and 150 frames per second. Increasing frame rate increases radiation dose proportionally since each cine-film frame requires the same exposure level per frame.

Both cine and 100 mm/105 mm photospot cameras require higher light intensities from the image intensifier when recording an image and the exposure signal for these cameras is obtained from the photodetector feedback.

KEYWORDS

automatic brightness control (ABC): adjusts generator output to give constant dose rate at image intensifier face for different patient thicknesses
automatic exposure control: adjusts image intensifier light output for film recording

automatic gain control: adjusts video signal for constant display brightness

barrel distortion: display distortion (also pincushion distortion)

bi-planar: a system using two C-arm fluoroscopy units which have independent positioning. Commonly used in cardiac studies

C-arm: a fluoroscopy design found both in small mobile and large fixed units. The image intensifier is fixed in-line with the X-ray tube on a C structure which is sometimes cantilevered giving oblique views

C-arm: cantilevered connected image intensifier and X-ray tube

charge-coupled device (CCD): semiconductor position sensitive detector (camera)

cine-film: 35 mm panchromatic film

contrast ratio: a low contrast measure. Output light intensity before and after a 10% central region is shielded. (see veiling glare)

conversion factor: ratio of output phosphor luminance (cd m^{-2}) to input dose (μGy s^{-1}); typical values 100–1000 cd m^{-2} μGy s^{-1}

cut-film: 100 mm or 105 mm square film stock

dark current: background current during no input conditions

dual energy subtraction: a method for removing hard and soft tissue contributing to a subtracted image. X-ray energies of 60 and 110 kV$_p$ are commonly employed

field size: area seen by image intensifier input

filtering (spatial): simple filters are smoothing or edge enhancement

filtering (temporal): frame averaging or recursive filtering takes the average value from a small series (typically four) which reduces image noise

flare: light dispersion at the input phosphor surface

flux gain: gain in light intensity between input and output phosphors (electronic gain)

focusing electrodes: high voltage electrodes accelerating electrons

hybrid subtraction: this combines the advantages of both dual energy subtraction and temporal filtering to remove interfering tissue (bone) and vessel movement

image lag: temporal response time

intensification factor: product of minification gain and electronic gain

look-up table: a series of stored values in memory which is used for mathematical transformations (log or nonlinear image processing)

low frequency drop: drop in MTF value which influences entire resolution range

mask: an early image containing tissue detail which is subtracted from later images

minification gain: ratio of input to output screen area

photocathode: placed immediately behind the input phosphor converting light to electrons

pincushion distortion: display distortion

progressive scanning: a non-interlaced video display giving higher definition and less flicker

quantum efficiency: efficiency of converting photons to electrons or vice versa

quantum sink: point loss of signal data

road mapping: subtraction of a contrast filled reference image continuously from the display to reveal catheter placement

veiling glare: ratio of light intensity at center of image with and without lead disk

vignette: loss of peripheral display detail

windowing: displaying only part (usually 256 levels) of the complete pixel depth (usually 4096 levels)

zooming: changing input field size

11

Computers in radiology

11.1 COMPUTER ARCHITECTURE

The concept of computer design starts with Charles Babbage (1792–1871; British mathematician) who in 1822 described an analytical engine to the Royal Astronomical Society. Countess Augusta Lovelace (daughter of Lord Byron) was his assistant and could be identified as the first computer programmer. Important foundation work was started by George Boole (1815–1864; British/Irish mathematician) who developed an analysis of logic in 1847 and Boolean algebra later became the cornerstone of modern computer design. Herman Hollerith (1860–1929; American inventor) meanwhile devised a method in 1880 for automating the process of data handling into an electromechanical counter using a series of cards with punched holes. A similar method was already being used by the weaving industry for controlling their machines. In 1911 Hollerith merged with three other companies to form the Computing Tabulating Recording Company, later to become part of IBM.

Alan Turing (1912–54; British mathematician) published an article in 1936 on 'computable numbers' which gave a precise mathematical concept of computers and he was instrumental in the construction of an automatic computing engine (ACE) in 1948.

Meanwhile, in 1938, an independent development in Berlin by Konrad Zuse (1910–95; German engineer) resulted in a mechanical computing machine the Z1 which was later developed in 1941 into the first automatic digital programmable calculator (Z3) using 2600 electromechanical relays. He later constructed a Z4 model weighing more than one ton.

John von Neumann (1903–57; Hungarian/ American mathematician) studied the art of numerical computation and designed some of the earlier electronic computers. His theoretical treatise on computer architecture governed their design until quite recently.

The parallel development of semiconductor microelectronics: the transistor by Bardeen, Brattain, and Shockley in 1947 (American physicists) and the first integrated circuits by Noyce and Kilby in 1957 (American physicist and engineer) gave the much needed reliability which heralded the practical everyday computer. Noyce also co-founded Intel the microprocessor manufacturer. Modern computers now encroach on all aspects of business, entertainment, education, science, and medicine. Diagnostic radiology relies on them for:

- CT, MRI, ultrasound, nuclear medicine machines as well as microprocessor controlled X-ray generators
- Radiology information systems (RISs), as a computer network for digital image storage and transmission, handling text as well as image data
- Quality control systems where measurements are taken, stored and compared to reference values. A report is then generated

- Nuclear medicine and radiopharmacy inventory and monitoring
- General office word processing, spreadsheet, database, and graphics

Before outline descriptions of these computer systems can be given a basic knowledge of computer science is useful starting with their arithmetic fundamentals.

11.1.1 Computer code

BINARY

The computer uses the binary system as the numerical base for all its internal working. All input signals from radiology equipment or otherwise must first be converted into binary format.

Since the base 2 number system is awkward to describe two common formats are used for describing it: octal, using a modulo of 8 and hexadecimal using a modulo of 16. Table 11.1 compares decimal, binary, octal, and hexadecimal numbering and demonstrates the convenience of octal and hexadecimal when tackling computer programming or problems involving binary notation.

The fundamental unit is the **bit** (short for binary integer) which can either be on or off: this is binary or 2 state logic 0 or 1. Figure 11.1a shows this basic building block and the way it is used to construct larger units. Bits can be put together in groups of 8 to form **bytes** which hold a maximum decimal count of 256 the 8 bits giving 2^8 or 256 decimal possible variations. Bytes can be further grouped into words, 2 bytes forming a 16 bit **word** giving 2^{16}, $\approx 65\,000$ decimal which was the basic word size used in earlier computers and 4 bytes forming a 32 bit word, 2^{32}, $\approx 4.3 \times 10^9$ decimal, which has now become the standard word length.

Larger word sizes of 64 bits are also available in very fast computer systems. These words form the computer memory. Bulk storage devices such as disks have sizes measured in megabytes (MB).

11.1.2 Data transfer and storage

Data transfer can be achieved by either **parallel** or **serial** methods, both are shown in Fig. 11.1b. Parallel connection is much faster than serial but sometimes the device can only handle data at a slow rate, a modem serial connection is an example. Some printers and film formatters are serial devices where slow

Table 11.1 *Four numbering systems.*

Decimal	Binary	Octal	Hexadecimal
00	00000	0000	0000
01	00001	0001	0001
02	00010	0002	0002
03	00011	0003	0003
04	00100	0004	0004
05	00101	0005	0005
06	00110	0006	0006
07	00111	0007	0007
08	01000	0010	0008
09	01001	0011	0009
10	01010	0012	000A
11	01011	0013	000B
12	01100	0014	000C
13	01101	0015	000D
14	01110	0016	000E
15	01111	0017	000F
16	10000	0020	0010

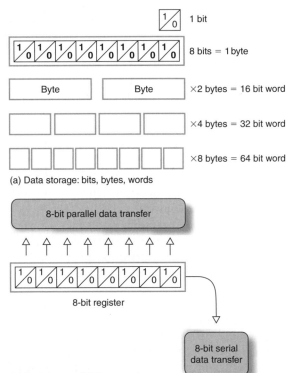

(a) Data storage: bits, bytes, words

(b) Serial or parallel data transfer

Figure 11.1 *(a) The single bit forming an 8-bit byte which is then used to form a 16-bit or 2-byte word. Other word lengths are 32-bit and 64-bit which use 4 and 8 bytes, respectively. (b) A single byte shift register which can move data in serial or parallel fashion.*

mechanical speed cannot match the fast data transfer. Fast devices such as memory or VDU displays are always parallel.

The terms kilo- and mega- do not strictly work out to 1000 and 1 million in binary arithmetic:

$2^{10} = 1024$ byte $= 1$ kilobyte (kB)
$2^{20} = 1048$ kilobytes $= 1$ megabyte (MB)
$2^{30} = 1073$ megabytes $= 1$ gigabyte (GB)

Accurate determination of storage requirements converting bits to bytes uses these values. An image matrix having x and y dimensions 512×512 and 10 bits deep (z axis) would have a total of 2621440 bits:

$$\frac{2\,621\,440}{8 \times 1024} = 320\,\text{kB}$$

Using a similar conversion factor, a high resolution image of $1024 \times 1024 \times 10$ bits is equivalent to 1.25 MB and a computed radiography image plate of $2176 \times 2640 \times 12$ bits would require 8.2 MB of disk storage.

ASCII (AMERICAN STANDARD CODE FOR INFORMATION EXCHANGE)

This is a second computer coding system using binary numbers in groups of 8 digits (bytes). These represent display characters and are commonly met when representing alphanumeric characters. The byte values range from 00000000 to 01111111 which will define 128 separate characters, including upper and lower case alphanumeric. For example 'A' is represented by 01000001 (65 decimal, 101 octal) and 'B' by 01000010 (66 decimal, 102 octal), etc.

11.2 CENTRAL PROCESSING UNIT

A block diagram of a basic computing system, based on a common PC, is shown in Fig. 11.2. The central processing unit (CPU) is a microprocessor semiconductor chip (Pentium series, AMD Athlon etc.). The external devices (disks etc.) connected to a CPU make up a practical computer. Some of these devices only accept information as output devices such as the video display unit (VDU), various printers and film formatters. Others are exclusively input devices such as the keyboard and boot-up ROM. Most of the other peripherals are both input and output devices.

The local bus is a pathway directly linking peripheral components such as the VDU and hard disk. An expansion bus allows a wider range of peripherals (including other computers) to be connected. Hard disk interfaces have a bus standard that allows efficient data transfer.

The integrated drive electronics (IDE) is a part of the computer motherboard. An expanded version of this is the small computer system interface (SCSI, pronounced 'scuzzi'), which accepts a far wider range of devices including disks and printers.

The CPU is the main organizing center of the computer and handles program instructions. Within it are electronic circuits:

- The arithmetic unit which carries out arithmetic operations on binary numbers
- Instruction decoders which examine program instructions
- Logic gates which are the pathway for these programmed instructions

The CPU also has registers that temporarily store words as the CPU is carrying out the various operations. The entire CPU is under a master clock control which provides synchronizing pulses and dictates to some extent the speed at which the CPU can run. Most radiology computer CPUs have the common microprocessor families manufactured by IBM/Intel, Macintosh or Sun.

11.2.1 Computer processor families

A microprocessor chip is shown in Fig.11.3 as part of a computer motherboard which includes other integrated circuits such as memory and control circuitry. The motherboard represents the complete working computer to which peripheral devices (e.g. disk storage units) are connected.

DESIGN SPECIFICATIONS

Within many microprocessor chips there are additional components that let the microprocessor handle complex mathematical calculations and graphical functions more quickly. The Pentium chip, for example, has a special characteristic called 'superscalar technology' which gives this chip set more than one pipeline to execute instructions making it much quicker than those that use just one.

Older design chips used complex instruction set computing (CISC) which gave a slower performance

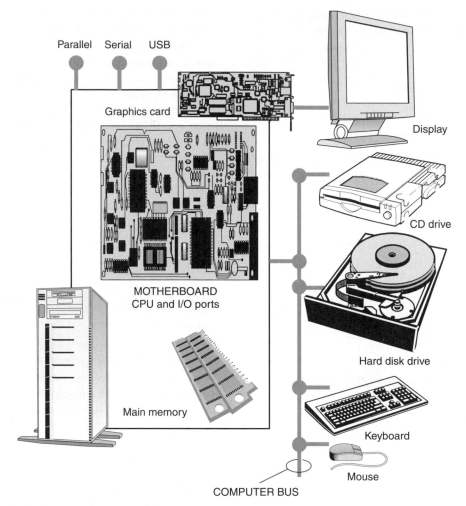

Figure 11.2 *The basic personal computer (PC) showing the motherboard (large central printed circuit board) containing the CPU, main memory and display/graphics board. A main bus-line from the motherboard connects the peripheral devices: mouse, keyboard, hard disk, CD drive, and display. Other parallel, serial, and USB ports are connected to the motherboard.*

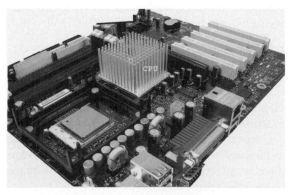

Figure 11.3 *The CPU microprocessor with large heat sink (CPU) attached in its holder on a motherboard.*

than the reduced instruction set computing (RISC) found in PowerPC and Alpha microprocessors. RISC is based on the concept that most computers use only a few simple instructions most of the time thus RISC chips execute those fewer instructions faster in a single clock cycle. Table 11.2 identifies the prefixes for the very large numbers involved in computer specifications and memory size.

CLOCK SPEEDS

Although there are numerous types and standards for microprocessors they all have one measurement in common: the system clock speed measured in

Table 11.2 *The SI prefixes suitable for measuring addressing capabilities of 32 and 64 bit processors.*

Prefix	Value	Bit size
giga-	10^9	32 (4.29×10^9)
tera-	10^{12}	
peta-	10^{15}	
exa-	10^{18}	64 (18×10^{18})
zeta-	10^{21}	
yotta-	10^{24}	

Table 11.3 *The increased complexity and speed of central processing units from 1978 to the present day.*

Processor	Introduced	Transistors
*Pentium	1993	3.1×10^6
Pentium Pro	1995	5.5×10^6
Pentium II	1997	7.5×10^6
Pentium III	1999	8.2×10^6
Pentium 4	2000	42×10^6
*Itanium 2 (64 bit)	2003	410×10^6
*PowerPC G5 (64 bit)	2004	58×10^6
*AMD Athlon 64 (64 bit)	2004	105×10^6

*Pentium, Itanium, PowerPC G5 and AMD Athlon are all registered trade marks.

MHz or millions of clock cycles per second. Clock speed helps to distinguish chip types although they should not be used for judging processing speed since processors may have similar clock speeds but due to internal design differences the processing power can be markedly different. To a certain extent the same would apply to the total number of transistors. In 1965 Intel co-founder Gordon Moore predicted that transistor density on integrated circuits would double about every 2 years; this is popularly known as 'Moore's Law' . Table 11.3 gives an indication of computer processor development showing the increases in transistor density as the computer microchip has been developed by Intel Pentium®/Itanium®, Apple®, and AMD®.

Computer speed is often quoted as millions of instructions per second or MIPS and millions of floating point operations (mega-flops or MFLOPS). A speed of one MIP is equivalent to an integer calculation performed on a $1024 \times 1024 \times 8$ bit matrix

(1 M-byte). Typical speeds given by current computers are 13×10^3 to 128×10^3 MIPS.

A MFLOP would involve a floating point operation on the above matrix; an example would be a count density normalization. A recently constructed 'super-computer' called The Earth Simulator housed in Yokohama, Japan used for meteorology calculations has a reported speed of 36 Teraflops or 36×10^{12} floating point calculations per second!

With increasing transistor density comes increasing power consumption and consequent heating problems. This is a major concern for designers of microprocessors. Figure 11.3 shows a microprocessor chip complete with its very large heat sink; sometimes an individual cooling fan is attached.

HYPERTHREADING

Intel's hyperthreading (HT) technology effectively fools the operating system into thinking that the single processor is actually two processors. It uses pipelines and transistors that are already on the processor, and only adds 5% more to the size of the chip, to hold additional storage areas and state control systems required for storing the existing state of both logical processors. The performance offered by a hyperthreading processor does not match that offered by a true dual-processor system, as both logical processors share a single high-speed cache and external connection.

Hyperthreading PCs can perform up to 35% better than normal processors. since several applications can be run at the same time. For optimum performance the operating system needs to support the distribution of threads across more than one processor; something that is only currently covered by Windows XP. The second condition is that the applications and processes being run need to support hyperthreading too. There are currently few applications that use threading properly.

64 BIT PROCESSORS

The big advantage with a 64 bit processor is obviously its ability to deal with 64 bit numbers. Data can also be fetched in 64 bit chunks and the mathematics performed on numbers twice as long as in a 32 bit CPU. A prime benefit is greater accuracy with less effort when performing large floating point calculations, and its ability to address large amounts of memory. Companies such as HP, IBM, Sun and others have long employed 64 bit reduced instruction set computing processors to drive their Unix-based enterprise servers. Most recent microprocessors employ this architecture (see Table 11.3).

Data stored in random access memory (RAM) is commonly addressed by using two numbers – a base address and an offset. With current 32 bit processors and current operating systems the addressable memory is limited to 4 GB (see Table 11.2).

The 64 bit processor increases this figure by several orders of magnitude, comfortably handling tera-, peta- and exa-bytes rather than just gigabytes of RAM. **Server** applications are the principal beneficiaries of this increased memory handling ability, enabling whole websites and huge databases to be located entirely in memory. That brings with it significant performance advantages compared to fetching data from disk in the case of 32 bit machines, since solid-state RAM is a lot more reliable and access is much faster than disk based virtual memory.

Operating system and application code can be made much bigger, with no need to continually swap memory contents to and from disk (paging), again helping to boost performance. Fewer processors are needed to do the same work and more users can be accommodated by the same number of servers. More complicated applications can also be developed, making the 64 bit CPU an important upgrade, at least in server applications.

On the desktop the advantages of 64 bit are not so clearly defined, although there are some obvious beneficiaries. The ability to handle very large image files entirely in RAM is a real plus point when it comes to image manipulation and compression in radiology.

11.2.2 Memory

The microprocessor has three types of memory:

- Read and write (RAM)
- Read-only memory (ROM)
- Cache memory

READ AND WRITE MEMORY

The computer memory uses semiconductor capacitors and transistors for storing information as bits. The most common type of memory is the RAM (random access memory) or DRAM (dynamic RAM) which uses electric charges held by etched capacitors on a silicon chip. This memory is **volatile**; it only holds information when the power is on. The electric charge representing the stored information drains away so these chips must be constantly refreshed in order to prevent data loss. This makes this type of memory slower than static RAM (SRAM) which uses thousands of transistors to store information. Although SRAM is still volatile it does not need refreshing so is many times faster than RAM although it is more expensive and less compact. If power is removed from either kind of RAM chip all data is lost.

The RAM is the main computer memory and stores programs and data. This can be up to several gigabytes in size, using either 32 or 64 bit words according to CPU type. Program instructions or data in the form of images are stored here, so a large memory is essential; for radiology systems the working memory is typically between 500 MB to several gigabytes. This memory will hold typically several hundred 512×512 images with a gray-scale depth of 10 bits. Large memories have definite advantages in computing speed if large image matrices are being handled, since time consuming disk transfers are reduced.

CACHE MEMORY

Although RAM composes the largest amount of memory in a computer other forms of memory exist. CPU chips have built-in memory space called cache memory. Several types of cache memory exist but their common purpose is to serve as transitional storage between conventional RAM and storage devices such as disk. The cache acts as an intermediate store allowing the CPU to complete some other task; this greatly increases computational speed. Most video display adapter cards which drive video monitors also have dedicated cache memory for image display.

READ-ONLY MEMORY

A specific read-only memory (ROM) contains a permanent pre-programmed instruction set that users cannot alter. These instructions form part of the boot-up sequence when the computer is first switched on by loading input/output instructions into RAM.

VIRTUAL MEMORY

This is commonly supplied by the hard disk as swap files. When the RAM becomes full some data can be written to disk which frees up RAM for more immediate work. RAM and the hard disk then swap data back and forth.

Virtual drive or a RAM disk can be supplied by sections of RAM being treated as a disk. This speeds up the CPU by supplying frequently used programs, which would be stored on the hard disk, from the RAM disk which has a much faster access and data transfer time.

11.3 BULK STORAGE

In most situations in which digital images are acquired in radiological examinations the diagnosis will not be made immediately. Some means must be available to store the examinations' images, perhaps on a semi-permanent basis, for viewing and for making hard-copy images of, later.

Also the digital imaging system must be capable of performing many digital examinations and so information from one examination must be set aside safely while data from the next examination is being acquired. There are many devices used to store images in a digital format:

* Magnetic disks
* Magnetic tape
* Optical disks

The important features to be considered when choosing and specifying a digital auxiliary storage device are:

* **Storage capacity**, the number of bytes that can be stored
* **Transfer time**, the rate (M-bits s^{-1}) at which the information can be moved from main memory to storage device and vice versa
* **Access time**, the time required to retrieve a stored piece of information

Typical values for these characteristics are shown in Table 11.4. Other factors which must be taken into account are the relative cost of storage per image, ease of operation and avoidance of any errors which might occur during image transfer.

There are four main options for storing the high number of images produced during digital imaging procedures. Fast access, short-term storage is always the realm of semiconductor solid state memory and this is becoming less expensive so large G-byte sized memories are common. Semiconductor memory is,

Table 11.4 *Storage devices compared to RAM.*

Storage	Capacity	Access time	Data transfer
Hard disk	30 to 400 GB	10 to 20 ms	2 to 4 Mbits s^{-1}
Optical	400 to 650 MB	150 ms	Very slow
DAT	4 GB	Slowest	Slowest
Flash memory	128 MB to 1 GB	100 ns	36/12 Mbits s^{-1} read/write
RAM (main CPU memory)	256 MB to 4 GB	15 to 100 ns	250 to 300 Mbits s^{-1}

however, **volatile** (it loses stored information when the power supply is removed). Long-term storage which retains its information without a permanent power supply has a much slower access but can hold several hundred gigabytes per disk; this includes magnetic and optical disks as well as magnetic storage tape.

MASS STORAGE

Refers to various techniques and devices for storing large amounts of data. The earliest storage devices were punched paper cards, which were used as early as 1804 to control silk-weaving looms. Modern mass storage devices include all types of disk drives and tape drives. Some of these are listed in Table 11.4 with typical capacities found in radiology and their access time and data transfer speeds. Mass storage is distinct from memory, which refers to temporary storage areas within the computer. Unlike main memory, mass storage devices retain data even when the computer is turned off. The main types of mass storage are:

* Hard disks : very fast and with more capacity than floppy disks, but also more expensive. Some hard disk systems are portable (removable cartridges), but most are not.
* Optical disks: unlike floppy and hard disks, which use electromagnetism to encode data, optical disk systems use a laser to read and write data. Optical disks have quite large storage capacity (4.7 GB). There are several different technologies (CD, DVD, MO) but they have slower read/write cycles when compared with hard disks.

- Tapes: Relatively inexpensive and can have very large storage capacities, but they do not permit random access of data.
- Flash storage: this is a type of semiconductor memory which retains information when removed from its power source. They are becoming valuable large capacity portable stores.

Mass storage is measured in kilobytes (1024 bytes), megabytes (1024 kB), gigabytes (1024 MB) and terabytes (1024 GB).

11.3.1 Magnetic disk

The stored data are recorded magnetically on the disk surface and organized in tracks and sectors as shown in Fig. 11.4a.

FLOPPY DISKS

These are removable 3½ inch diameter disks. The disk material is coated magnetic plastic and is vulnerable to damage. The standard disk density is 1.4 MB. They are rapidly being phased out in favor of the various forms of compact disk (CD) and flash memory.

HARD DISKS

Sometimes known as a Winchester disk, this consists of one or more magnetic disks arranged one on top of the other and rotating at high speed. These bulk storage devices are fixed and not removable. The disk is aluminum coated with magnetic material. The Winchester design is hermetically sealed against environmental contamination. An example of this design is shown in Fig. 11.4b, showing a multi-platter disk and read/write heads that float on the disk surface.

The sizes of early hard disks ranged between 5 and 20 GB but most recent models used for image storage are typically between 400 and 800 GB. They are the main medium for short- and medium-term image storage for radiology. Hard disks offer the cheapest storage medium for archiving information.

Essentially the surface of the disk is treated as an array of data points, 1 or 0. The position of each point is decided by the disk format so the disks need to be formatted before they can be used. Accessing the data in any reasonable time requires the disk to spin very fast. Hard disks spin at between 5400 and 10 000 rpm yielding very fast data storage and retrieval.

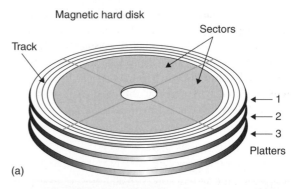

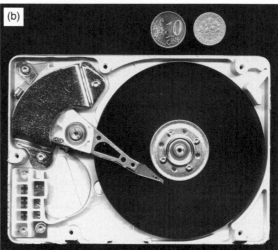

Figure 11.4 *(a) The magnetic hard disk is organized as tracks and sectors which are addressable. (b) A Winchester disk used for storing up to 80 GB of information; the storage size dependent on the number of disk surfaces (platters).*

The performance of a hard disk is crucial to the speed of a computer system. Slow data retrieval will hinder a fast processor performance. The disk average **access time** is the time taken by the drive to locate the right track on which data are stored and the specific place on the track where the data starts. This is quoted in milliseconds and ranges from 65 to 80 ms for slow disks to 10 to 12 ms for the large fast disks. The **transfer rate** is the speed of data transfer and is measured in MB s^{-1}. In order to obtain an accurate view of a hard disk performance both access time and transfer rate should be considered. A high access rate with a slow transfer rate produces a slow drive. A less important measure is the **seek time** which defines the amount of time it takes the hard drive's read/write head to find the data location point.

The main purpose of a hard disk in radiology is to store images. High image transfers of up to 25 images per second are typical for some systems. Magnetic disks with capacities up to about 400 G-byte are available. Such a store would be capable of holding many tens of thousands of 512 × 512 images. The access time is typically about 10 ms.

11.3.2 Magnetic tape

Magnetic tape systems are available for archival purposes which have capacities up to about 4 GB and transfer rates of typically 500 to 800 kB s^{-1} and so have slow data retrieval times. However, it is a relatively cheap storage medium and its portability has made it a popular medium of image data transfer. There are two types of technology used for tape streamers: helical scan recording and linear (or longitudinal) recording. The linear type offers a better performance over the helical but has lower capacities.

HELICAL SCAN

This includes the 4 mm and 8 mm DAT (digital audio) tape. Helical scan recording uses the same principle as video tape recorders and is inherently slower than the linear type. For this reason it is usually found as a back-up medium. The read/write heads are attached to a helical scanning drum and data are recorded in a stripe pattern. The tape moves at less than 1 inch per second. A typical DAT tape can store 4 GB of data.

LINEAR

This includes QIC (pronounced 'quick') tapes. QIC-WIDE tapes offering higher capacities cost appreciably more than the equivalent DAT tape. When data is recorded onto linear tape the tape heads are stationary and the tape moves past at about 100 to 125 inches per second. The data is recorded in straight lines. Extra heads can be added to improve data transfer. The 800 kB s^{-1} can be increased to 1.6 MB s^{-1}. A linear tape stores typically 2 to 4 GB of data.

11.3.3 Digital optical disk

Optical drives include WORM (write once/read many), magneto-optical (MO) and re-writeable optical. These devices are well suited as an archival

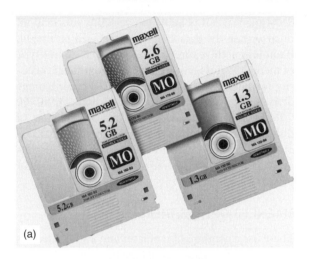

(a)

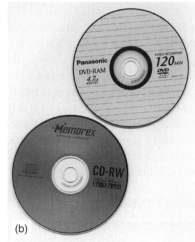

(b)

Figure 11.5 *A collection of large volume storage media showing (**a**) magnetic optic (MO) disks having capacities of 1.3 to 5.2 GB along with (**b**) a 700 MB CD-RW and a 4.7 GB DVD-RAM.*

medium because of their very large storage capacities, typically in the gigabyte range, and slow transfer rate (mega-bits per second (Mb s^{-1})) which is much slower than that of digital magnetic disk. A collection of magnetic and optical storage media is shown in Fig. 11.5.

The information is physically stored on the disk surface by burning a tiny indentation, using a laser. Some optical disks can only be written to once, but read from many times, hence their name WORM. This is very different to the digital magnetic disks which can written to many times, i.e. data stored on the disk can be erased and overwritten by new data.

So, while it is not possible to overwrite information, once written the data cannot be replaced or altered. Radiology archives are particularly keen on this type of media for storage since it provides sufficient security for patient data and cannot be altered. Storage densities approach 2 GB which can hold up to 450 CT images of $512 \times 512 \times 16$ bits deep. Banks of disks can be held in 'juke boxes' where many of these optical disks can be kept on-line holding thousands of images representing weeks and perhaps months of patient image data.

MAGNETO-OPTICAL DISKS

These use a combination of laser and a small electro-magnet to store data. To change the magnetic information on part of the disk a tiny area on the magnetic surface is heated by the laser. This brings the magnetic layer to its Curie point when new magnetic information can then be written. Once cool the magnetic state is fixed. The process is fast but the extra heating step takes time and consequently slows the writing speed.

Data access is as fast as the optical disk and relies on the polarization of laser light by the magnetic polarity of the data area. The main drawback of magneto-optic disks is the extra time to write information.

THE COMPACT DISK

The compact disk (CD) format is extremely simple, instead of sectors and clusters used on a magnetic hard drive the CD holds its information as a single $0.5\,\mu m$ wide spiral. The data appear as a long string of small depressions ('pits') 0.83 to $3.56\,\mu m$ in length, with variable spaces between them ('lands'). The edge of each pit represents only 1 bit of data. The total length of the data spiral is about 5 km.

The spiral data are recorded on a polycarbonate surface covered by a thin layer of metal to reflect laser light (aluminum, tantalum, gold or silver). A second thinner layer of polycarbonate seals the disk. Data are read by using a semiconductor laser focused by a complex lens system onto the data spiral and reflected by the metal layer.

As the laser moves over each **land**, a strong reflected signal is received by a photodetector. When the laser is over a **pit** the light is slightly defocused, so the reflected signal is smaller. Each signal transition (pit to land, or land to pit) corresponds to a binary 1, while a period with no change corresponds to a zero.

The CD-read only (**CD-R**) format replaces the standard pits and lands with a single layer of photo-sensitive dye, covered by a metal and plastic layer. A new CD-R disk starts with a clear dye layer, but this darkens when heated. The CD records when the laser focuses on points along the data track, creating dark spots where the pits would normally be. The dye recording only records once but the data can be read many times (WORM). Although a cheap method for storing image data the dye fades over time so CD-R disks have a limited life span of about 5 to 10 years depending on disk storage conditions.

RE-WRITEABLE OPTICAL DISKS

The limitations of a CD-R disk are overcome by a re-writable optical disk (CD-RW). This contains a metallic film consisting of an alloy of silver, indium, antimony, and tellurium, initially in a clear crystalline form. The recording laser heats and then cools this rapidly so it liquifies (becoming darker). Heated for a longer period and this metallic layer becomes crystalline again – the recorded data are erased. These 'phase change' materials are not fully stable so there is usually a fixed read/write limit of about 1000 times. However, their record can be archived more successfully than the CD-R. Re-writeable or erasable optical disks provide the same high capacities as those given by WORM or CD-ROM. The average access time for a 4¾ inch (12 cm) erasable optical drive is about 40 to 60 ms; about three times slower than a magnetic disk.

DIGITAL VERSATILE DISK

This was initially called digital video disk but eventually became known as the digital versatile disk (DVD). The format type DVD-R (DVD recordable) is similar in concept to the CD-R and is a write-once medium. It first appeared in 1997 having a capacity of 3.95 GB. This was later increased to 4.7 GB on a single-layer, single-sided DVD-R disk.

Since the DVD format supports double-sided recording and playback up to 9.4 GB can be stored on a double-sided DVD-R disk. Data can be written to a DVD at 11.08 M-bit s^{-1}, which is roughly nine times the transfer rate of the CD-R. DVD-R, like CD-R, uses a constant linear velocity (CLV) rotation technique to maximize the storage density on the disk surface. This results in a variable number of revolutions per minute (RPM) as disk writing/reading progresses from one end to the other. Recording begins at the inner radius and ends at the outer. At '×1' speeds, rotation of the disk varies from 1623 to 632 rpm on a 3.95 GB disk and 1475 to 575 rpm on a 4.7 GB disk, depending on the record/playback head's position over the surface. On a 3.95 GB disk the track pitch, or the distance from the center of one part of the spiral information 'track' to an adjacent part of the track, is 0.8 μm; one half that of CD-R. The 4.7 GB disk uses an even smaller track pitch −0.74 μm.

In order to achieve a six- to seven-fold increase in storage density over CD-R the wavelength of the recording laser and the numerical aperture of the lens that focuses on the DVD must be improved. A CD-R uses an infrared laser with a wavelength of 780 nm; a DVD-R uses a red laser with a wavelength of 635 nm. This allows the DVD-R disk to record marks as small as 0.40 μm compared to 0.834 μm size with CD-R.

The DVD-R uses a similar dye recording process as CD-R. If both sides are needed for recording, then two recordable sides can be bonded together. In this case each side must be read directly by turning the disc over, as dual layer technology is not currently supported.

Its large capacity and durability (this medium has a typical life expectancy of better than 100 years) make the DVD-R a good choice for long-term image archive. Since DVD disks are dimensionally identical to the CD family of disks, they have the advantage of being compatible with existing CD-based recording devices.

The type **DVD+RW** has a better compatibility between machines than DVD-R designs. 'Lossless linking' is a technique developed specifically for DVD+RW which ensures writing can be started and stopped at an accurately defined position. Together with the option of no defect management, this feature allows DVD+RW discs to be written in a way that maximizes compatibility with existing DVD players and drives. DVD-RW and DVD+RW storage is the same at 4.7 GB with data transfer rates of 3.32 Mbps. A new dual-layer DVD recordable technology virtually doubles data storage capacity on DVD+R recordable disks from 4.7 GB to 8.5 GB, while retaining compatibility.

DVD-RAM disks employ phase-change technology with some MO features mixed in rather than the pure optical technology of CD. A 'land groove' format allows signals to be recorded on both the grooves formed on the disk and in the lands between the grooves. The specification for DVD-RAM Version 2.0 has a capacity of 4.7 GB per side. The principal difference between DVD-RAM and DVD-R is one of compatibility. Single-sided DVD-RAM disks come with or without cartridges. Manufacturers claim that DVD-RAM media can be overwritten up to 100 000 times and will maintain data integrity for at least 30 years.

11.3.4 Flash memory

Flash memory is commonly met as small storage devices holding a control code such as in the basic input/output control system (BIOS) in a personal computer. When the BIOS needs to be changed (rewritten), the BIOS code can be written in block (rather than byte) sizes, making it easy to update. Flash memory is not used as a replacement for random access memory (RAM) because RAM needs to be addressable at the byte (not the block) level. Flash memory gets its name because the microchip is organized so that a section of memory cells are erased in a single action or 'flash'. Flash memory uses in-circuit wiring to apply the electric field either to the entire chip or to predetermined sections known as blocks. This erases the targeted area of the chip, which can then be rewritten. The erasure is caused by tunneling in which electrons pierce through a thin dielectric material to remove an electronic charge from a floating gate associated with each memory cell. Flash memory is used in digital cellular phones, digital cameras, LAN switches and removable memory data storage devices. Its great advantage is that flash memory does not need power to sustain the stored data, unlike RAM. Both flash memory devices as well as PCMCIA Type I and Type II memory cards adhere to standards developed by the Personal Computer Memory Card International Association (PCMCIA). Because of these standards, it is easy to interchange flash memory products in a variety of devices. Date transfer rates when attached to USB Version 2.0 are: read at 36 Mb s^{-1} and write at 12 Mb s^{-1}. A selection of removable storage devices using flash memory is shown in Fig. 11.6.

11.4 DATA INPUT/OUTPUT

The central processing unit communicates with the outside world by exchanging information very much as do human beings. There are input 'sensory' signals in the form of image data or keyboard instructions and output 'motor' signals driving disks and printers.

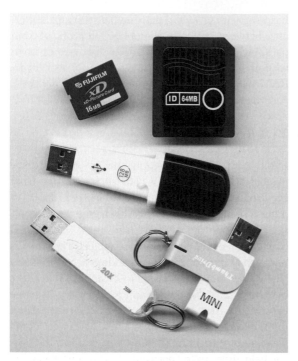

Figure 11.6 *A selection of removable storage devices using flash memory. Their capacity ranges from 16 MB (top left) to 1 GB (bottom right). The bottom three devices use USB connection.*

Each input and output connection must first go through an interface with the computer which is a simple logic device packaging the digital information in coded words or blocks recognizable by either the computer or device. Some devices need confirmation or 'handshakes' after each data transfer so that synchronization can be maintained.

11.4.1 Interfaces

An interface is the connection between hardware either within the computer (disk interface, display interface etc.) or between the computer system and an application device (gamma camera etc.). Interfaces are of two types: serial and parallel depending on the transfer of data; parallel interfaces are obviously much faster than serial interfaces but some data lends itself more readily to serial transmission such as optical data transmission. There are common standards that define interface performance:

- SCSI: small computer systems interface ('scuzzi') is a general purpose high-speed multi-tasking

interface used to connect a computer peripheral device such as printers and disk drives.
- EISA: extended industry standard architecture competitor of IBM's microchannel architecture (MCA) which is a PC design.
- IDE: integrated drive electronics refers to the hard disk drive interface.

PORTS

These can be either serial (RS232) which connects the mouse, keyboard, modem, or parallel, usually used by printers and imagers. The mouse is the most common form of pointing device using a serial port along with the keyboard. The computer keyboard has special keys which are not found on a typewriter keyboard. Modifier keys are used in combination with other keys to change commands, the most useful key being the control key or 'Ctrl'. Other keys are the function keys F1 through to F12 which represent **macro functions** (small programs) or specific commands that launch an application that would otherwise require a set of commands, sequences or multiple keystrokes.

DISPLAYS

These can show gray-scale or color images. The video interface or video card allows the monitor to decipher digital-to-analog converter (DAC) instructions and defines display resolution. Gray-scale monitors are able to display a wide range of grays. The common monitor has 8 bit pixel depth so can display 256 gray levels but high brightness monitors are capable of handling up to 2000 gray levels. These are most valuable for diagnostic radiology displays. Color displays exist as 24 and 32 bit monitors. The 24 bit monitor can display 2^{24} colors or $16\,77\,216$ and gives a true color representation; a 32 bit monitor displays the same number, the extra bits are used for display manipulation which is used for photo-retouching or video production. (Also see Chapter 12, 'The Digital Image'.)

UNIVERSAL SERIAL BUS

This is an external bus standard. The universal serial bus (USB) version 1.1 supports data transfer rates of $12\,\text{M-bits s}^{-1}$ ($1.5\,\text{MB s}^{-1}$). A single USB port can be used for connecting up to 127 peripheral devices from a USB hub. These could be mice, modems, keyboards, printers, storage devices or scanners. A USB also supports hot plugging so the device can be disconnected while the computer is still operational; a request is made before unplugging otherwise data may be lost from any storage device. USB 2.0 is a fully compatible extension of USB 1.1. It uses the same cables and connectors and supports data rates up to 480 Mbps (40 times faster than USB 1.1). This makes USB Version 2.0 ideal for external storage devices, scanners, and CD-RWs. It is expected to completely replace serial and parallel ports.

11.4.2 Communications

The common computer communication uses cables to connect peripheral equipment such as displays, printers, and keyboards. The communication with other equipment, including other computers, is more complex since the speed of communication is most important. This is measured in bits per second or **baud**. The baud rate is roughly equivalent to characters per second: 1200 baud ≡ 120 characters per second. Common baud rates for data transmission are 1200, 2400, 4800, and 9600.

MODEMS

These allow computers to communicate over telephone lines, using a dial-up facility. Their maximum transmission speed is 56 kb s^{-1}, which is far too slow for anything other than e-mails.

BROADBAND TECHNOLOGIES

Broadband services can be delivered over an ordinary telephone line or private network, via a cable connection or across wireless networks. The **digital subscriber line** (DSL), originally designed for delivering video content over 'ordinary' phone lines, is now adapted to deliver Internet data at high speed. The main benefit is that it uses existing phone twisted pair cables and can be used for telephone calls at the same time as being connected to the Internet. A broadband connection typically has a data speed of 512 k-bits s^{-1}. Faster broadband services are also available, such as a 1000 k-bits s^{-1} (1 megabit s^{-1}).

Satellite connection is a special form of wireless communication, using a satellite dish as the aerial. Its main disadvantage is that there is a signal delay between the satellite and the ground station.

Using the Internet usually involves a small request for information (an upload) from the user, followed by a large provision of information (a download) from the Internet (e.g. obtaining image data or checking for new e-mail). For this reason, most access technologies provide higher download than upload bandwidth. This would be an **asymmetric** service (ADSL). Asymmetric services are adequate for most small business or clinic requirements.

Some more advanced applications (i.e. two-way video conferencing) require the same bandwidth in both directions. In these circumstances, **symmetric** services such as leased lines or SDSL are required. When specifying a broadband connection, it is important to distinguish between these two forms and determine the best option. **Latency** is the delay that occurs along the transmission path. This is a factor with satellite connections because the data must travel over large distances. Therefore satellite systems are not suitable for businesses that require real-time delivery of information/data. **Contention** between users occurs because most broadband access services share a single connection path between many customers. For example, the contention ratio may vary from 1:1 (i.e. you are guaranteed that you are the only person using the 512 k-bits s^{-1} service) to 40:1 (i.e. up to 40 users may be sharing the same 512 k-bits s^{-1} service at one time). When usage is light, contention does not pose a problem. However, the quality of the connection can deteriorate if many customers use the connection at the same time. For example, if all 40 users are using a 512 k-bits s^{-1} broadband service at the same time, the access speed is reduced to about 13 k-bits s^{-1}. In reality, this rarely occurs but at peak usage times connection can seem slower because of network congestion. Most of the time broadband delivers up to 75 to 90% of the top speed available at the location. Contention is an issue with services such as ADSL, satellite, and wireless broadband access. Since guaranteed fast broadband access is often more critical to a clinic or hospital, consideration should be given to buying a broadband service with a low contention ratio.

11.5 SOFTWARE

The computer is quite dumb unless it is given some form of instruction for the task in hand. All the previous sections have concerned themselves with the mechanisms or 'hardware' that go together to make a working computer but this will only 'come alive' and do useful work when the appropriate 'software' is loaded into memory. The software consists of programmed instructions carefully written in a logical sequence. Programs can be quite simple (macro-functions mentioned in Section 11.4.1) using a simple English instruction set; these are not very efficient with computing power so can be rather slow. Longer more complex programs which must be very fast and efficient use special coded instructions.

11.5.1 Languages

Both the computer instructions or program and image data are stored in memory and also on disk, in binary format. A computer program consists of a series of binary numbers which when processed identify a unique coded instruction e.g. add, subtract, fetch data, etc.

Early programs consisted of strings of these numbers and consequently programs were very difficult to write. Programs now exist in various languages which simplify program composition. Assembly language is the most primitive but enables precise control of the computer and the way it handles data. Assembly languages are extremely efficient and offer the greatest speed of computation. They are mostly used for fast data handling.

More complex program languages, i.e. C or C++, Pascal, and FORTRAN, are more understandable having short English-like instruction sets. Both types of programs must be translated into the binary coded instructions. This is achieved by using a compiler. The easiest language is BASIC which is a high-level language that is usually compiled as the program is run. It is therefore much slower than the low- and medium-level languages but this is not a limitation if the data itself is keyboard limited. Versions include QuickBasic and Visual Basic.

11.5.2 Operating systems

This is a master control program that manages the internal functions of a computer and essentially makes it work as a computer, moving data in and out of the RAM and finding room for new data by freeing up or swapping memory or copying it onto disk.

MULTI-TASKING

Multi-tasking describes the ability of the operating system to run more than one application in memory simultaneously. Since CPUs and operating systems are extremely fast and memory management is very efficient, the computer can seem to be handling more than one operation at once, using pauses in one application to implement instructions in another program.

One type of multi-tasking is **time-sharing** where the processor works with several users on a cyclical basis. Users do not notice this unless there are many users requiring fast response. Some operating systems allow multi-tasking either on a local scale where different jobs are carried out simultaneously (keyboard input, saving to disk, and printing) or between machines on a **network**. Common operating systems that have been designed for single or multi-user personal computers are:

- MS-Windows
- UNIX
- Apple Macintosh System
- Linux

MICROSOFT WINDOWS

This is a windowing environment or graphical user interface (GUI) similar to Macintosh. MS-Windows is an operating system that utilizes MS-DOS but introduces multi-tasking and memory management. The latter increases the apparent size of RAM by allowing expanded memory, extended memory or virtual memory situated on disk.

Both MS-Windows 95 and MS-Windows NT have no DOS background and run 32 bit applications. Freed from this restriction it allows the full 32 bit code capability of 32 bit processors such as the 486 and Pentium and treats memory as one long segment rather than splitting it up into sections as previously. Each 32 bit program runs in its own protected memory space.

UNIX

This is used on a large variety of computers from PCs to large mainframes. It is designed to support multi-user and multi-tasking. It is a common operating system for radiology. It still has its limitations since it is not very user friendly having more than 200 commands and somewhat restricted error messages. UNIX is able to link computers of different families together (i.e. PCs and mainframes).

APPLE OSX OPERATIONAL PROGRAM

This is a UNIX-based core operating system with protected memory and advanced memory management to increase system stability. Pre-emptive multi-tasking boosts system performance and responsiveness and multiprocessing takes advantage of dual processor systems.

LINUX

A freely distributable open source operating system that runs on a number of hardware platforms. The Linux kernel was developed mainly by Linus Torvalds. Because it is free, and because it runs on many platforms, including PCs and Macintoshes, Linux has become an extremely popular alternative to proprietary operating systems.

11.5.3 Application software

These are the common programs that make the PC an invaluable tool for clinic, laboratory, and office. They include:

- Word processing
- Spreadsheets
- Databases
- Graphics
- Technical drawing
- Computer aided design and drafting (CAD and CADD)
- Desktop publishing

All applications are specific to the computer operating system but most software publishers have versions of their applications that will run on MS-DOS, Windows, OS/2 or UNIX. Macintosh applications are mostly unique to that computer type (Claris).

DATABASE

This is a collection of information organized in such a way that a computer program can quickly select desired pieces of data. The common database is organized by fields, records, and files. A field is a single piece of information; a record is one complete set of fields; and a file is a collection of records. As a simple example, a radiology patient list is a file. It contains a list of separate patient records, each of which consists of three fields: name, address, and hospital number.

An alternative concept in database design is known as **hypertext**. In a hypertext database, any object, whether it be a piece of text, a picture or a film, can be linked to any other object. Hypertext databases are particularly useful for organizing large amounts of disparate information (diagnosis from an image, clinical report, and laboratory information) but they are not designed for numerical analysis. A **structured query language** (SQL) is used for requesting information from a database. It supports distributed databases (databases that are spread out over several computer systems) which enables several users on a local area network to access the same database simultaneously.

SCIENTIFIC APPLICATIONS

Software is available for more specialist applications. Radiology applications would be:

- Laboratory/radiopharmacy management
- Spectrum analyzers
- Equipment quality control
- Image communication and management
- Patient management

11.6 NETWORKING

This is a way of linking several PCs and larger mainframe computers so that they can swap data and share resources such as printers and hard disks. Network servers commonly form the nucleus of a networked computer system where many separate PC or Apple Mac workstations use a common database and program set. In theory any computer on the network can be a **server** but in practice this is a specialized unit consisting of a fast microprocessor with a few gigabytes of RAM and a very large hard disk (also many gigabytes).

11.6.1 Cabling

Connections between computers can use a variety of methods from a set of **twisted pair** wires (commonly used with telephones), handling a restricted data flow, to **co-axial** cables which will handle much faster data rates. **Fiber optic** cables are becoming the connections of choice, however, since these can handle extremely fast data rates and are not prone to electrical interference. Cableless or **wireless** inter-connections using infrared or GHz radio frequencies are available for local area networks.

- **Twisted pair** connections connect low speed peripherals handling 300 to 9600 baud (bits per second). The cable may be unshielded (unshielded twisted pair UTP) or shielded to reduce electro-magnetic interference (EM). Shielded twisted pairs can handle up to 16 M-baud in Token Ring networks.
- **Coaxial cable** dramatically reduces EM interfer-ence and provides a high bandwidth of up to 250 M-baud. The transmission speed does not decrease at such a fast rate as the twisted pair.
- **Fiber optic cable** gives a very large bandwidth of up to 2 G-baud and greatest immunity to EM interference. This is fast becoming the standard communication medium.
- **Wireless connections** or radio-LAN is simply radio communications on an allocated frequency.

TWISTED-PAIR WIRE

This method was formerly associated with the con-nection of low-speed peripheral equipment operat-ing at 300 to 9600 bits s^{-1}. However, it is currently still being used for Ethernet networks. Unshielded twisted-pair wire is inexpensive and is easy to install but it produces and absorbs a large amount of **elec-tromagnetic interference**, which can result in noisy transmission with high error rates. Shielded twisted-pair wire can handle higher data rates over longer distances since it has a better immunity to electro-magnetic interference.

Shielded twisted-pair wire is commonly used for **token-ring networks** (see below) where it attains data rates of 16 M-bits s^{-1}. Data bandwidth decreases with distance.

COAXIAL CABLE

Coaxial cable reduces electromagnetic interference by surrounding a single conducting wire with a solid dielec-tric material (polythene) with a copper sheath. The center conductor may be either solid or stranded, and the outer sleeve may be either solid or braided. Coaxial cable has a high immunity to electromagnetic interfer-ence and a large bandwidth of up to 250 M-bits s^{-1}. In a similar way with twisted-pair cabling, the bandwidth of coaxial cable decreases with distance, although not as drastically. Examples of coaxial cable are the **thick-net** Ethernet, using a large diameter special-purpose cable, and **thin-net** Ethernet using general purpose coaxial cable, which causes greater attenuation and lower noise resistance.

FIBER-OPTIC CABLE

Fiber-optic cable provides a huge increase in bandwidth (>2 G-bits s^{-1}), although some transceivers limit this bandwidth to around 250 M-bits s^{-1}. It also provides the greatest immunity to electromagnetic interference. Although fiber-optic cable itself is relatively cheap the installation costs and connections are high.

Fiber-optic cable is becoming the standard means for connecting local area networks. Data transmission relies on the presence or absence of light of a specified wavelength to convey binary information; this is called intensity modulation. An optical fiber will have a typ-ical attenuation of 20 dB, so that a fiber system trans-mitting light with a wavelength of 850 nm would have a limit of about 10 km. There is an insertion loss of 1 to 2 dB for every termination or connection.

WIRELESS LINKS (WI-FI)

Radio (RF) and infrared line-of-sight transmission is used in a variety of communication methods. They include cellular, microwave, and satellite techniques. Frequencies have been allocated between 2 and 5 GHz. Transmission is coded for security and it can quickly link computers in the same building. It has distance limitations. The 802.11 family of standards refers to specifications developed by the IEEE for wireless LAN technology, describing the interface between a wireless client and a base station or between two wireless clients. Data transmission rates of up to 54 M-bits s^{-1} are currently available.

11.6.2 Network architecture

This is the design of a communication system which includes the hardware, software access methods, and protocols used for controlling data flow between a group of users. It defines the method of control, i.e. whether computers can act independently or are con-trolled by other computers monitoring the network. Network architecture can be separated into:

- Local area network
- Wide area network

Computers connected together in a network allow data exchange and communication using either a local area network (LAN) or a wide area network (WAN). The most basic form of computer connection uses cables and the data are sent as information **packets** which travel at various speeds depending on transmission technique. The speed of transmission is measured in **bauds** or **bits per second**. The **baud rate** is approximately equal to characters per second; 1200 baud is 120 characters per second. Transmission speed is limited to the highest baud rate that connected devices have in common. Networks can connect just two or three computers to common output devices (i.e. printers) but may include many more (50 to 100 computers). WANs use telephone or fiber-optic lines to link computers at a distance.

LOCAL AREA NETWORK

This is a method for connecting a group of computers, usually near to one another so it is called a local area network (LAN). LANs enable resources to be shared within a department. The computers and peripherals (laser film formatters, large disk storage, printers etc.) are connected by a simple cable or optical fiber link. Points or nodes on the network (usually the separate computers used as workstations) provide connections which can transmit, receive or repeat a message. Networking is commonly met in radiology in management systems or when similar digital imaging machines are linked: CT, MRI, and DSA to diagnostic workstations. A local area network can form the basis of a picture archiving and communications system (PACS) that communicates with other departments, clinical centers, and hospitals so that patient diagnostic images can be dispatched more effectively. Networking radiology equipment provides several benefits:

- Images can be accessed via a common disk store (server) and reported from a single point.
- Single film output devices can be used for department hardcopy.
- Protocols dictate uniformity of format in the department.

There is usually a fast machine controlling a large disk store transmitting or **down-loading** information and programs as well as sending it back or **up-loading**. The central archive storage medium of the LAN (file server) is a fast computer and holds all the department's image and program data; this supplies other machines in the network (workstations).

Most LANs are confined to a single building or hospital or connected to a group of hospitals. Each **node** (individual computer) in a LAN executes its own independent program and has access to data and devices anywhere on the LAN. This means that many users can share expensive devices, such as laser printers, as well as a common **database**. There are many LAN designs, **Ethernet** being the most common for PCs. Most Apple Macintosh networks are based on an AppleTalk® network system, which is built into Macintosh computers. Other LAN designs are the WLAN (or LAWN), which is a wireless local area network using a high frequency radio link rather than wires to communicate between nodes.

LANs area capable of very fast data transmission but distances are limited, and there is also a limit to the number of computers that can be attached to a single LAN, consequently two or more LANs are commonly connected through **routers**.

WIDE AREA NETWORK

A wide area network (WAN) is a computer network that spans a relatively large geographical area. A LAN can be connected to other LANs over any distance via telephone lines and radio waves. A system of LANs connected in this way forms a wide area network (WAN). Computers connected to a WAN are often connected through public networks, such as the telephone system. They can also be connected through leased lines or satellites. The largest WAN is the Internet.

PROTOCOLS

These are the rules and encoding specifications for sending data. The protocols also determine whether the network uses a **peer-to-peer** or **client-server** architecture (see later).

11.6.3 Network topology

This describes the geometric arrangement of devices on the network, either in a linear arrangement or as a ring of workstations or input/output devices. The topology of any practical distributed network will be a hybrid of these basic topologies. There are four principal topologies used in LANs:

- **Bus topology**: All devices are connected to a central cable, called the bus or backbone. Bus networks are relatively inexpensive and easy to install for small networks. Ethernet systems use a bus topology.

- **Ring topology**: All devices are connected to one another in the shape of a closed loop, so that each device is connected directly to two other devices, one on either side of it. Ring topologies are relatively expensive and difficult to install, but they offer high bandwidth and can span large distances.
- **Star topology**: All devices are connected to a central hub. Star networks are relatively easy to install and manage, but bottlenecks can occur because all data must pass through the hub.
- **Tree topology**: A tree topology combines characteristics of linear bus and star topologies. It consists of groups of star-configured workstations connected to a linear bus backbone cable.

These topologies can be mixed; for example, a bus-star network consists of a high-bandwidth bus, called the backbone, which connects a collection of slower-bandwidth star segments.

TREE OR BUS TOPOLOGY

The extension of the computer bus is only suitable for very limited distances. Bus topology is a method of extending this communication using nodes to connect various computer systems or input output devices. Bus topology is a special case of tree topology which has a single trunk shown in Fig. 11.7a.

Using this design the bus can be extended by up to 300m (1000 ft) without a repeater, which is a data amplifier used for extending the length of a network. Each branch of a tree network can act at full bandwidth since many messages can be sent along the bus at the same time. It is possible for messages to collide with each other and therefore need to be re-transmitted. Tree topology is a decentralized LAN used by Ethernet and AppleTalk where a single connecting line or bus is shared by a number of nodes including shared peripherals and file server. AppleTalk, used by Macintosh, is a low bandwidth network design suitable for small network systems. The advantage of a tree topology is that failure of a node does not disrupt the network.

Bus topology is a multi-point trunk in which all nodes share a common physical channel. Communication takes place through multiply accessible broadcasts, with each node having a unique address. Electromagnetic signals propagate in both directions on the bus. A terminator at each end of the bus terminates these signals. Since the signals propagate in both directions, it is necessary for nodes to arbitrate for access to the bus. Bus arbitration can be handled

through contention or token protocols. The nodes on the bus do not repeat data packets, single-node failures will generally not affect network operation; there is no overhead or delay involved with the retransmission of data packets. This topology is easily expandable, since additional nodes simply tap into the bus through a connector. Examples of bus topology are the ubiquitous Ethernet.

Tree topology consists of a central trunk with bifurcations creating branches, with the trunk and each branch being a multi-point circuit. Bus topology is simply a special case of tree topology with a multi-point trunk and no branches, so the description of bus topology also applies to tree topology. Tree topology has a head end or hub (root) connecting with several independent network buses (branches). Each branch can operate at the full bandwidth of the bus. This also explains how individual Ethernet networks are **bridged** together to form networks with greater usable bandwidth.

RING TOPOLOGY

Ring topology networks use point-to-point connections between nodes, forming a closed loop or ring (Fig. 11.7b). The transmitted data circulate from node to node around the ring in one direction, each node serving as an active **repeater** to the next until the data packet arrives at the addressed node. Each repeater is connected to a host computer. If the data packets traveling on the ring are addressed to the connected node, the repeater copies the data to the computer. Ring topologies require a control **protocol** which determines the sequence in which devices transmit data and provides contention arbitration between nodes. The ring is an efficient communication topology because connection of future nodes requires connection to only two neighboring nodes. Disadvantages are the need for active repeaters at every node (which requires greater complexity than does bus topology); lengthening of communication paths as the ring expands; and, unless elaborate repeaters are used, termination of network function if an active component fails or if the ring configuration is disrupted.

TOKEN RING TOPOLOGY

This is typified by point to point connections forming a closed loop shown in Fig. 11.7b. Each node acts as an active repeater to the next so ring networks can extend a greater distance than bus networks.

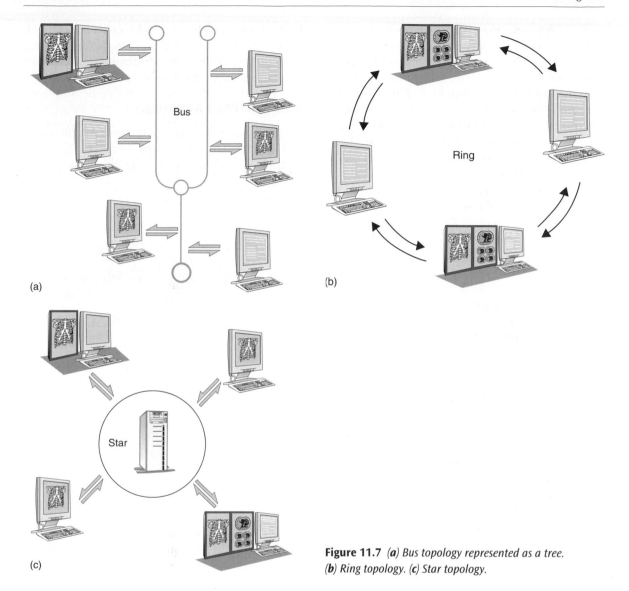

Figure 11.7 *(a) Bus topology represented as a tree.*
(b) Ring topology. (c) Star topology.

Computers and other equipment on a token ring communicate by means of a piece of software called a token which is passed between the devices. The token is a 'pass' that gives priority to the machine that possesses it at any time. The token is passed from machine to machine. A machine can only send a message (image or data) on the network if it has the token. The drawback is that only one computer can use the network at any one time slowing down the system. Other disadvantages of the ring system include the need for active repeaters at each node and the lengthening of the communication path as the ring expands. Failure of a node can disrupt the network. Fiber optic distributed data interfaces (FDDI)

use ring topology where two independent rings exist; data circulates in one ring only, the second being held in reserve for fault recovery purposes. The IBM token-ring specification has been standardized by the IEEE as the IEEE 802.5 standard.

STAR TOPOLOGY

In this design all nodes are connected to a single central exchange or hub, typically through serial connections. The primary function of the hub is that of a network switching element, which routes network communication among the various peripheral nodes (Fig. 11.7c). Wiring costs are high since each workstation connects to the central router but timing can be controlled more easily, preventing messages from colliding.

Multiply interconnected star topologies exist in which two or more hubs are connected to form an extended network. The topology of this extended network is called a meshed star. The star topology has several advantages. It allows for point-to-point communications between the hub and peripheral nodes, requiring no complex network control procedures, since the hub is the supreme network arbiter. Also, it involves simpler connections between the peripheral nodes and the hub, since most of the protocol processing and routing functionality is built into the hub itself. The main disadvantage is that the hub can be a single point of failure. If the hub fails, the entire network will be disabled. Thus, high reliability and redundancy measures are required for the hub, which can make the hub equipment expensive. The UltraNet design network is an example of the star topology. **Gateways** and **bridges** allow separate networks to be connected so that local traffic within a network does not add to the overall traffic of the combined network. When users need to communicate with others in different zones they send information through the gateway.

ETHERNET

Ethernet is a local area network (LAN) architecture developed by the Xerox Corporation in cooperation with DEC and Intel in 1976. Ethernet uses a bus or star topology and supports data transfer rates of 10 Mbps. The Ethernet specification served as the basis for the IEEE 802.3 standard, which specifies the physical and lower software layers. Ethernet is the most widely used LAN technology (Token Ring is second). Ethernet broadcasts packets to as many as 1024 nodes on a network segment via twisted pair, coaxial or fibre optic cabling. Shielded twisted pair is used in 10BASE-T Ethernet LAN. To extend the 10BASE-T Ethernet network throughout a department, floor or building, links are established between multi-port repeater units.

Ethernet tends to be faster and more efficient than many other network designs and is capable of handling a great deal of information data and allows workstations to send data virtually simultaneously. It uses the CSMA/CD access method (carrier sense multiple access/collision detection); when a device wants to gain access to the network, it checks to see if the network is free. If not, it waits a random amount of time before retrying. If the network is free and two devices attempt access at exactly the same time, they

both assume standby to avoid a collision and each then waits a random amount of time before retrying. The general classification of Ethernet encompasses data transmission rates from $10 \, \text{Mb s}^{-1}$ to $100 \, \text{Mb s}^{-1}$.

FAST ETHERNET NETWORKS

Table 11.5 lists the current Ethernet specifications and Table 11.6 gives the typical transfer times for a standard resolution digital chest radiograph; the broadband ADSL speed is given for comparison. Currently, Ethernet is by far the most widely deployed LAN access method; various estimates rank Ethernet at 85.4%, followed by Token Ring at a distant second with 10.6%. ARCNET, FDDI, and other methods make up the remaining 4%.

A **switched Ethernet** is an Ethernet network running through a high-speed switch. Changing to a

Table 11.5 *The five specifications for Ethernet.*

10Base5 – 10 Mbps	Thick coaxial cable attached to network nodes via transceivers that tap into the cable. This was the first Ethernet design. Also called thick Ethernet, ThickWire and ThickNet.
10Base2 – 10 Mbps	Thin coaxial cable attached to network nodes via BNC connectors. It is also called thin Ethernet, ThinWire and ThinNet.
10BaseT – 10 Mbps	Telephone wire. All stations use twisted pair to connect in a star configuration to a central hub, also known as a multipart repeater. Widely used due to the low cost and flexibility of twisted pair wire.
100BaseT – 100 Mbps	Fast Ethernet: 100BaseTX uses two pairs of twisted pair, 100BaseT4 uses four pairs and 100BaseFX uses multimode optical fibers.
Gbit Ethernet – 1000 Mbps	The most recent Ethernet standard.

Table 11.6 *Ethernet bandwidths, and typical transfer times for an uncompressed 10.8 MB digital chest radiograph.*

Network technology	Bandwidth	Chest radiograph (10.8 MB)
ADSL (example)	$512 \, \text{kbits s}^{-1}$	2.8 m
Ethernet	$10 \, \text{Mbits s}^{-1}$	8.6 s
Fast Ethernet	$100 \, \text{Mbits s}^{-1}$	0.86 s
Gigabit Ethernet	$1 \, \text{Gbits s}^{-1}$	0.086 s

switched Ethernet network means replacing the Ethernet hub with a switch. Instead of sharing rates of $10\,\mathrm{Mb\,s^{-1}}$ for Ethernet or $100\,\mathrm{Mb\,s^{-1}}$ for fast Ethernet among all the users on the network segment, the full bandwidth is made available to each sender and receiver pair. If the switch and network interface adapters provide full-duplex operation then the total bandwidth is $20\,\mathrm{Mb\,s^{-1}}$ or $200\,\mathrm{Mb\,s^{-1}}$ between nodes. A major advantage in migrating to switched Ethernet is that the existing interface adapters are still used.

WIRELESS NETWORKS

The wireless LAN avoids cable problems and provides a unique flexibility and portability in configuration. It also allows networking in situations where cable installation is either expensive or impractical. Wireless LANs use either an allocated radio frequency or infrared link to transmit and receive coded binary information. In 1985 the Federal Communications Commission (FCC) in the USA allocated several frequency bands (e.g. 2.0 to 2.4 GHz) to communication systems for digital data transmission.

It uses **spread-spectrum modulation**, which is a form of amplitude modulation (AM) and frequency modulation (FM). It uses not only a carrier frequency but also a second auxiliary signal in the modulation process; this auxiliary signal is the spreading code. The receiver must have information about the spreading code used by the transmitter in order to make sense of the information. This prevents eavesdropping on communications.

An infrared wireless LAN (or photonic LAN) uses the same data transmission technique as used for television remote-control units. Infrared photons can be used to send information from a transmitter on one computer to a receiver on another. A photonic system must provide either direct line-of-sight access or access to a common reflective surface such as a ceiling or window. Interference with photonic LANs can come from excessive ambient light (e.g. sunlight or fluorescent light) or obstructing solid bodies. Photonic LANs operate most effectively in large, open areas.

The IEEE 802 standards are a set of network standards developed by the IEEE. These are listed in Table 11.7. A simple wireless network is shown in Fig. 11.8.

11.6.4 Network component parts

Any network contains certain important component parts. A basic network example is shown in Fig. 11.9. A list of the individual components is given in Table 11.8. These are identified as follows.

HUB

A common connection point for devices in a network. Hubs are commonly used to connect segments of a LAN. A hub contains multiple ports. When a packet arrives at one port, it is copied to the other ports so that all segments of the LAN can see all packets. A passive hub serves simply as a conduit for the data, enabling it to go from one device (or segment) to another. So-called intelligent hubs include additional features that enables an administrator to monitor the traffic passing through the hub and to configure each port in the hub. Intelligent hubs are also called manageable hubs. A third type of hub, called a switching hub, actually reads the destination address of each packet and then forwards the packet to the correct port.

REPEATER

A network device used to regenerate or replicate a signal. Repeaters are used in transmission systems to regenerate analog or digital signals distorted by transmission loss. Analog repeaters frequently can only amplify the signal while digital repeaters can reconstruct a signal to near its original quality. In a data network, a repeater can relay messages between sub networks that use different protocols or cable types. Hubs can operate as repeaters by relaying messages to all connected computers. A repeater cannot do the intelligent routing performed by bridges and routers.

SWITCH

A device that filters and forwards packets between LAN segments. Switches operate at the data link layer (layer 2) and sometimes the network layer (layer 3)

Table 11.7 *Wireless standards.*

Specification	Wireless standard		
	802.11a	802.11b	802.11g
Maximum speed ($\mathrm{Mbits\,s^{-1}}$)	54	11	54
Theoretical range outdoors (m)	30	120	50
Theoretical range indoors (m)	12	60	20
Operating frequency (GHz)	5	2.4	2.4

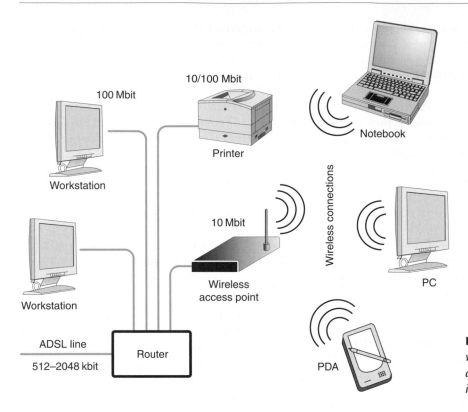

Figure 11.8 *A simple wireless network showing data rates and common input/output devices.*

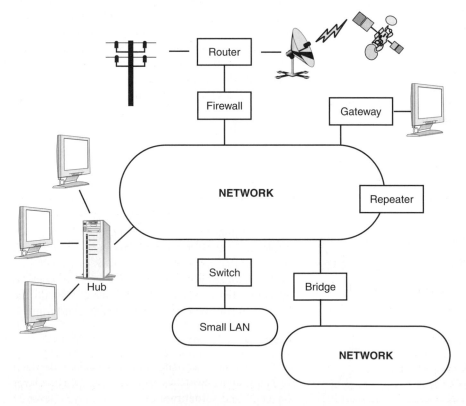

Figure 11.9 *Basic network showing component parts mentioned in the text.*

Table 11.8 *Component parts of a computer network further identified in Fig. 11.9.*

System component	Function
Hub	A common connection point with multiple ports. Passive hub: Simple data steering. Intelligent hub: Able to monitor data. Switching hub: Reads destination address before data steering.
Repeater	Regenerates/amplifies digital and analog signals; non-intelligent. (see Bridges and Routers)
Switch	A device that filters and directs data packets between sections of LAN.
Router	Connected between two networks and usually located at gateways so configuring best route between any two hosts.
Bridge	Connects two LAN segments such as Ethernet and Token Ring.
Gateway	Connects workstation to the network.

of the OSI Reference Model and therefore support any packet protocol. LANs that use switches to join segments are called switched LANs or, in the case of Ethernet networks, switched Ethernet LANs.

BRIDGE

These are devices which connect two LAN segments together, of similar or dissimilar type (Ethernet and Token Ring). Bridges are inserted into a network to improve performance by keeping traffic contained within smaller segments. Bridges are faster than routers. Transparent bridging protocols are where the workstations are unaware of bridges in the network. Ethernet uses this protocol.

ROUTER

A device that forwards data packets along networks. A router is connected to at least two networks, commonly two LANs or WANs or a LAN and its Internet service provider's network. Routers are located at gateways, the places where two or more networks connect. Routers use headers and forwarding tables to determine the best path for forwarding the packets, and they use protocols such as Internet Control Message Protocol (ICMP) to communicate with each other and configure the best route between any two hosts. Very little filtering of data is done through routers.

GATEWAY

A node on a network that serves as an entrance to another network. In enterprises, the gateway is the computer that routes the traffic from a workstation to the outside network that is serving the Web pages. In homes, the gateway is the Internet service provider (ISP) that connects the user to the Internet.

In enterprises, the gateway node often acts as a proxy server and a firewall. The gateway is also associated with both a router, which use headers and forwarding tables to determine where packets are sent, and a switch, which provides the actual path for the packet in and out of the gateway.

FIREWALL

For most users, the primary reason for implementing a firewall is to protect intrusion from unauthorized users. In the default configuration of most firewalls, all traffic originating on the Internet is blocked from entering the network, denying external users access to the confidential clinical network. There will be times when a certain selectivity is required about the type of traffic that enters the network (clinical Web sites and teaching files). With the hospital's own internal Web server, for example, Internet users will want connection. In these cases the firewall will need configuring so that this traffic is recognized. Configuring a firewall mainly sets rules for the interactions between the private network and the Internet.

Firewalls can be implemented by software or hardware methods. As a rule, protection of a hospital or office network will be best achieved with a hardware solution in the form of an Internet router. These relatively inexpensive devices usually include a range of features, such as the ability to share a broadband cable or DSL Internet connection, a firewall component, and an integrated server for allocating IP addresses to systems on your network.

For a single computer accessing the Internet a software firewall is more cost-effective. A wide variety of software-based firewall solutions exists. Windows operating systems include a native firewall which blocks requests originating from the Internet and allows the operator to select and sanction different types of TCP/IP (Transfer Control Protocol/Internet Protocol) requests on the network, and gives control over how the system will respond to common requests. The various types of firewall techniques are:

- Packet filter: Looks at each packet entering or leaving the network and accepts or rejects it based on user-defined rules. Packet filtering is fairly effective and transparent to users, but it is difficult to configure. In addition, it is susceptible to IP spoofing.
- Application gateway: Applies security mechanisms to specific applications, such as file transfer protocol (FTP) and Telnet servers. This is very effective, but can impose a performance degradation.
- Circuit-level gateway: Applies security mechanisms when a TCP or user datagram protocol (UDP) connection is established. Once the connection has been made, packets can flow between the hosts without further checking.
- Proxy server: Intercepts all messages entering and leaving the network. The proxy server effectively hides the true network addresses.

In practice, many firewalls use two or more of these techniques in concert.

One additional but related feature found in many software firewall packages is the ability to restrict access to the Internet by certain programs. For example, an exact specification which authorizes access to an Internet connection, such as Internet Explorer or Outlook Express. This feature is especially useful since it can help ensure that any malicious applications installed on your system (virus, worms or Trojan horse programs) cannot access the Internet, thus rendering them useless.

REDUNDANT ARRAY OF INDEPENDENT (OR INEXPENSIVE) DISKS

A redundant array of independent (or inexpensive) disks (RAID) is a collection of disk drives that employ two or more drives in combination for fault tolerance and performance. RAID disk drives are frequently installed on **servers** (see below).The basic design of a network often contains a central file server that is the central mass storage. The file server is commonly a very fast PC with a large disk store which holds the applications programs and data files or image files for all the workstations in the network. In a peer-to-peer network all the workstations act as file servers. In a more common client–server network a single large PC with a very large disk store is the central file server for all the workstations or clients. Most network servers

run 24 h a day 7 days a week so reliability is essential. A network serving a small number of users (15 to 20) is called a work-group server and typically has 128 M-byte RAM and a 100 G-byte disk as a starting size which can be expanded as necessary.

11.6.5 Servers

A common network design utilizes **client–server architecture** which is a network in which each computer or process on the network is either a client or a server. **Clients** are PCs or workstations which run the specific applications (acquiring image data, accessing patient records, etc.). Clients rely on servers for resources, such as files, devices, and even processing power.

A **server** is a powerful computer specifically configured with large memory and hard disk storage on a network that manages network resources. A current specification would be dual 3.2 GHz CPUs with between 2 and 16 GB of DDR memory and 128 MB of cache memory. It would have a very large disk storage capacity; a typical arrangement is shown in Fig. 11.10 which holds twelve 400 GB hard disks giving a total storage of 4.8 TB. The various components are 'hot-swappable'; that is, the computer boards or connectors can be unplugged and re-arranged or replaced while the computer is on without the operating system crashing.

Servers are often dedicated to perform no other tasks besides their server tasks. A **file server** is a computer and storage device dedicated to storing files that can be accessed by any user on the network. A **print server** is a computer that manages one or more printers, and a **network server** is a computer that manages network traffic. Figure 11.7c shows a file server acting as the central point in a star network. A **database server** is a computer system that processes database queries. On multiprocessing operating

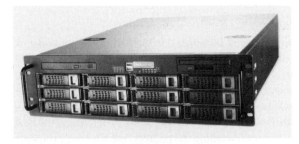

Figure 11.10 *A commercial server which has a bank of twelve hard disks giving a total of 4.8 TB.*

systems a single computer can execute several programs at once. A server in this case could refer to the program that is managing resources rather than the entire computer.

In client–server applications, clients can be distinguished as either **thin client or fat client**. A thin client has little or no computing power and no hard disk; it is designed to be minimal so that the bulk of the data processing occurs on the server. A **fat client** includes a computer with a disk drive. Client–server architectures are sometimes called two-tier architectures.

PEER-TO-PEER ARCHITECTURE

Often referred to simply as peer-to-peer, or abbreviated P2P, this is a type of network in which each workstation has equivalent capabilities and responsibilities. This differs from client–server architectures, in which some computers are dedicated to serving the others. Peer-to-peer networks are generally simpler, but they usually do not offer the same performance under heavy loads.

11.6.6 Internet

This was set up in the early 1970s for the United States military as a computer network able to survive nuclear warfare. Four university computers were linked to form a high speed network and in 1988 the administration of the network passed to the National Science Foundation. Other independent networks around the world found it easier to route their traffic through this common backbone than link directly to each other.

The Internet is a wide area network (WAN) connecting millions of PCs and mainframes by cable and radio links across the world using common communication protocols, the major one being TCP/IP. This allows very different types of computers to communicate with each other. Communication can be via a **modem** which allows digital data to be transmitted along a telephone line. Modem speed should be at least 14 400 baud. Modems are commonly classified by a series letter, V.32 and V.34 being typical. These refer to 14.4 and 28.8 k-baud respectively. An **Internet service provider** (ISP) connects the user to the on-line community. An account is provided on the central computer service provider enabling the user to log onto the server via a modem. The user's PC then acts as a terminal for the central **server**.

Computers on the Internet are divided into **clients** and servers. Clients are the desktop units that access the Net. Servers are the 'workhorses'; many of them are mainframes which use UNIX as their primary operating system. TCP/IP allows users to operate their normal operating systems (Windows, OS/2, etc.) and translates this information into a version that can be understood by the internet UNIX servers. Lines of communication are controlled by routers.

Medical interests on the Internet are handled by various servers around the world having archives containing, for instance, radiology teaching files belonging to various university medical schools; these can be down-loaded by the Internet user. There are now 168 countries linked to the net and in May 1995 responsibility for the Internet's backbone was handed over to private companies.

TRANSMISSION CONTROL PROTOCOL/ INTERNET PROTOCOL

TCP/IP is the suite of communications protocols used to connect hosts on the Internet. TCP/IP uses several protocols, the two main ones being TCP and IP. TCP/IP is built into the UNIX operating system and is used by the Internet, making it the *de facto* standard for transmitting data over networks. Even network operating systems that have their own protocols, such as Netware, also support TCP/IP.

SIMPLE MAIL TRANSFER PROTOCOL

SMTP (pronounced as separate letters) is a protocol for sending e-mail messages between servers. Most e-mail systems that send mail over the Internet use SMTP to send messages from one server to another; the messages can then be retrieved with an e-mail client using either POP (Post Office Protocol) or IMAP (Internet Messaging Access Protocol). IMAP provides a message store that holds incoming mail until users log on and download it. In addition, SMTP is generally used to send messages from a mail client to a mail server. This is why you need to specify both the POP or IMAP server and the SMTP server when you configure your e-mail application.

JAVASCRIPT

This is an object-oriented scripting language based on the concept of prototypes. The language is most well known for its use in websites.

HTML

Short for HyperText Markup Language, the authoring language used to create documents on the World Wide Web. HTML is similar to SGML (Standard Generalized Markup Language), although it is not a strict subset. HTML defines the structure and layout of a Web document by using a variety of tags and attributes. Tags are used mainly to specify hypertext links. These allow Web developers to direct users to other Web pages with only a click of the mouse on either an image or word(s).

ATM

Short for Asynchronous Transfer Mode. A network technology based on transferring data in cells or packets of a fixed size. The cell used with ATM is relatively small compared to units used with older technologies. The small, constant cell size allows ATM equipment to transmit video, audio, and computer data over the same network, and assure that no single type of data hogs the line.

ATM creates a fixed channel, or route, between two points whenever data transfer begins. This differs from TCP/IP, in which messages are divided into packets and each packet can take a different route from source to destination. This difference makes it easier to track and bill data usage across an ATM network, but it makes it less adaptable to sudden surges in network traffic.

HTTP

Short for HyperText Transfer Protocol, the underlying protocol used by the World Wide Web. HTTP defines how messages are formatted and transmitted, and what actions Web servers and browsers should take in response to various commands.

FTP

Short for File Transfer Protocol, the protocol for exchanging files over the Internet. FTP works in the same way as HTTP for transferring Web pages from a server to a user's browser and SMTP for transferring electronic mail across the Internet. Like these technologies FTP uses the Internet's TCP/IP protocols to enable data transfer. FTP is most commonly used to download a file from a server using the Internet or to upload a file to a server (e.g. uploading a Web page file to a server).

WI-FI

Short for Wireless Fidelity and is meant to be used generically when referring of any type of 802.11 network, whether 802.11b, 802.11a, dual-band, etc. Any products tested and approved as Wi-Fi Certified® by the Wi-Fi Alliance are certified as interoperable with each other, even if they are from different manufacturers. A user with a Wi-Fi certified product can use any brand of access point with any other brand of client hardware that also is certified. Typically, however, any Wi-Fi product using the same radio frequency (for example, 2.4 GHz for 802.11b or 11g, 5 GHz for 802.11a) will work with any other, even if not Wi-Fi certified. Formerly, the term 'Wi-Fi' was used only in place of the 2.4 GHz 802.11b standard, in the same way that 'Ethernet' is used in place of IEEE 802.3.

11.7 COMPUTER SYSTEMS IN RADIOLOGY

The diagnostic radiology department is not the sole generator of medical images in a hospital. Cardiology, oncology, and endoscopy suites and even pathology laboratories all add to the image storage and transmission problem. The clinician requires a single workstation with an interface to these other disciplines including the ability to present and manipulate medical image data. The traditional PACS that supports only dedicated 'thick client' workstations that display images alone does not address this integration requirement; the enterprise PACS must. A true enterprise PACS must also provide delivery of these data sets.

11.7.1 Hospital information systems

The hospital information system (HIS) is the main hospital-tracking computer for initial patient acceptance and personal details, order request placement (examination and referral details), and any necessary billing and insurance details. This computer also holds the central administration for the entire hospital complex (salaries and employment details etc.).

In general, two types of RIS-HIS integrations are now offered, one type via a broker and another without a broker. The brokerless technology is preferred, as there is less opportunity for data inconsistencies. When functions are combined (administration or image acquisition and reporting), the line between study management (HIS, RIS) and image management (PACS) responsibility becomes blurred.

It is preferable to have a common platform (single server) that incorporates image management and study management capabilities. This method ensures a seamless flow of data (both patient information and image as well as data available for clinical audit). Full integration is a complex task that requires cooperation from PACS, RIS, and machine manufacturers that maintain a networking standard complying with the latest Digital Imaging and Communications in Medicine (DICOM) requirements.

11.7.2 Radiology information systems

The radiology information system (RIS) is responsible for maintaining patient referral, scheduling, and financial information within the department and collating the interpretations of examination results. The connection between the RIS and the PACS is critical since bottlenecks can easily be created in a busy system. At the patient acceptance desk the work list provides a direct point of entry of patient demographic information into the system. In the various imaging (modality) rooms (projection radiography, CT, MRI etc), the images can only be acquired if they are associated with the relevant patient information, previously collected by the RIS. The RIS should be able to handle the following duties:

- **Diary**: Handles all procedures associated with incoming orders, scheduling, worklists and documentation
- **Diagnostic**: Manages procedures necessary for carrying out a diagnosis (worklists, dictation, voice recognition, transcriptions)
- **Archive**: Administrative procedures for image archiving (digital and film)
- **Statistical reporting**: User definable clinical auditing
- **Inventory**: manages departmental consumables and initiates ordering (radiopharmaceuticals, film stock and disposable items)
- **User setup protocol**: Enables authorized system administrators to define and configure department functions and access
- **Central server database**: Allows patient information to be shared across other departments (linking with HIS)
- **Enterprise connection**: This serves as the interface between the RIS and other information systems

including World Wide Web and hospital ISP for e-mail
- **Firewall**: Protection of RIS integrity

CONNECTION WITH PACS (HL7)

The **radiology information system** is a separate computer system responsible for maintaining patient information, scheduling, and financial information along with diagnostic information and interpretations of examination results. Many RISs are used independently of the radiology PACS; the RIS standardization is based on Health Level 7 (HL7), a standard communication language for medical information developed by the Healthcare Information and Management Systems Society (HIMSS).

Figure 11.11 is the simple plan, which shows the integration of HIS, RIS and PACS networks in a hospital. Two standards dictate system operation: HL7 for the hospital and radiology systems and DICOM for PACS and the imaging equipment (modalities).

To avoid data redundancy and, consequentially, data inconsistencies, most PACS rely on the RIS as

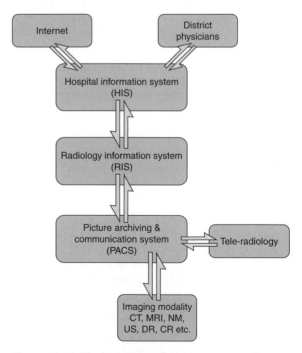

Figure 11.11 *The integration of computer systems in a hospital. In order to reduce intrusion a single contact between other hospitals and the Internet is made via the HIS. Tele-radiology interchange between accepted clinical sites is made via the PACS.*

the primary source of patient information. As a result, the PACS does not work efficiently without a robust connection to the RIS. This connection is often made through a **broker** acting as an intermediary translator where the relevant data are exchanged and translated (from HL7 to DICOM or vice versa). This connection is not ideal, as data inconsistencies can still occur and most image interpretation functions will require seamless functionality of two different systems. Intimately integrated PACS and RISs, a need recognized by many users, are now offered by several suppliers.

11.7.3 Picture archiving and communication systems

DEFINITION

Picture archiving and communication systems (PACS) is a method for acquisition, storage, and transmission of radiology images. Once a clinical study has been acquired from the radiology imaging system such as CT, MRI, image plate (CR or DR), it is first stored on a fast access medium for reporting and then subsequently archived on a large capacity magnetic or optical disk. The PACS connects imaging devices as a network and allows connections to other networks in wider localities so that images can be transported between rooms, departments and even other hospitals (tele-radiology capability). Any PACS installation should have the four basic components:

- High quality workstations for PICTURE (image) viewing allowing diagnosis, reporting, consultation, and clinical review
- ARCHIVING on magnetic or optical media for short- or long-term storage
- A local area network (LAN) or wide area network (WAN) that allows fast and efficient COMMUNICATION for the transmission and retrieval of patient and image data
- SYSTEMS that include interfaces and gateways to the hospital information system (HIS) and radiology information system (RIS) offering one integrated system to the user

In operation an efficient PACS will improve a diagnostic radiology service by providing:

- Good quality images available for treatment planning and consultation in multiple locations simultaneously, transferring these easily to remote locations

- Consistent quality radiographic images reducing or eliminating the need for retakes
- Image manipulation: enhancement techniques for improving quantitative analysis and visualization for diagnosis
- Images that are more accessible for education, quality assurance, risk management, and medical audit purposes
- A lower patient radiation dose by operating a clinical audit of the department's workload together with image enhancement of low dose images

A well designed PACS should eliminate the film record so cutting costs and loss of data. The ability to transmit high quality images rapidly over long distances (satellite link) to other clinicians for consultation is an essential item for outlying hospitals.

Figure 11.12 identifies the basic organization for image acquisition. Each machine (CT, MRI, DR/CR, ultrasound, nuclear medicine etc.) complies with the DICOM standard so has a common protocol. The patient work list for each machine is preloaded from the RIS/PACS servers giving all the necessary information (name, number, study type) for a secure and consistent acquisition. Unnecessary views, incorrect orientation, wrong exposure levels (adult versus children protocols) are (hopefully) eliminated.

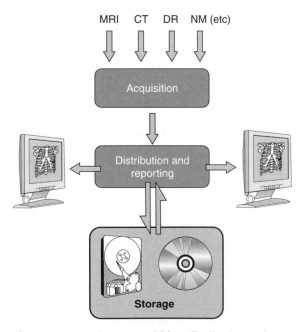

Figure 11.12 *An image acquisition, distribution, and storage pathway fundamental to all PACS designs.*

THE DICOM STANDARD

This is the standard data transmission protocol for clinical data and images set up by the American College of Radiology (ACR) with members of the National Electrical Manufacturer's Association (NEMA) in 1984. The ACR–NEMA Digital Imaging and Communications in Medicine (DICOM) standard has now been adopted by the majority of medical product manufacturers inside and outside radiology. The DICOM standard is a means for obtaining image data and associated information into and out of imaging equipment, whether it be an acquisition, archiving, display or hardcopy device.

In a radiology department operating different makes of equipment specific interfacing is necessary to get the machines to 'talk' to one another (if at all). If each piece of equipment, regardless of manufacturer, has a DICOM interface then interconnection between these machines is straightforward. The DICOM interface uses its own software operating system and executes the DICOM protocol so that the image data are formatted for transmission and provides network connection with other devices. Intrahospital and tele-radiology applications are accommodated into this protocol. The key features of the DICOM standard include:

- An effective framework necessary for claiming conformance to DICOM, requiring product manufacturers to complete a DICOM conformance statement
- Communication of patient and scheduling information thus integrating equipment with hospital and departmental information systems
- A means for querying patient studies and retrieve images as selected by the user
- The management of hard-copy devices connected to the network with basic film layout and remote hardcopy tracking
- The transfer of imaging studies from computer radiography, computed tomography, magnetic resonance, nuclear medicine, and ultrasound
- The interchange of images on storage media such as optical or magnetic disks

The European standards body (Committee European de Normalisation: CET TC 251) has adopted DICOM for the European Standard MEDICOM and the Japanese Industrial Association of Radiation Apparatus (JIRA) has incorporated DICOM into its standards. The direct connection of medical equipment to standard TCP/IP network environments is also specified by DICOM bringing flexible network solutions using a variety of network standards.

WORKFLOW INTEGRATION

The required functionality for a RIS–PACS interface, in addition to providing connections between HL7, DICOM, and other proprietary message protocols, is that it can also buffer HL7 messages. This is necessary because HL7 implementations are often event based, so that all systems have to be continuously in the 'listen mode' in order to ensure that no event is lost. Many radiology systems are not designed for this so data can be lost. Consequently, an intermediary is required which will capture the events and buffer them for later querying. The Integrating the Healthcare Enterprise (IHE) initiative started by the Radiological Society of North America (RSNA) in conjunction with the Hospital Information and Management Systems Society (HIMSS) represents an attempt to achieve a standard for workflow integration through the so-called IHE Initiative.

ACQUISITION

The diagnostic imaging systems input their digital images into the various workstations attached to the PACS network, these are then stored and distributed by the PACS. These digital imaging systems include all the common modalities. Projection radiography, traditionally performed with screen-film cassettes, has been replaced by either CR or DR digital units. Digital mammography using either full field or partial field imaging can also replace film-screen devices. Table 11.9 gives an idea of the RAM memory occupied

Table 11.9 *Size of various digital matrices.*

Imaging system	Matrix size	Size (MB)
Computed radiography	2048 × 2500 (10)*	6.4
Direct radiography	2688 × 2688 (12)	10.8
Computed tomography	512 × 512 (16)	0.5
Digital subtraction angiography	1024 × 1024 (10)	1.3
Nuclear medicine	128 × 128 (12)	0.025
Ultrasound	640 × 480 (8)	0.3
Mammography	4096 × 3277 (12)	20.0
Cardiology	512 × 512 (10)	0.32

*Values in parentheses are pixel depth.

by various image matrices. The entire study, comprising several image matrices, commonly resides in memory during the acquisition cycle. It is therefore essential to specify RAM memory sizes in the gigabyte region, otherwise valuable computer time can be taken transferring images to a virtual memory space on the hard disk.

DISTRIBUTION AND REPORTING

The PACS network provides communication between users and output devices. To avoid patient data repetition of entry (and therefore the possibility of data inconsistencies), most PACS take this information from the RIS which is then the primary source of patient information. The PACS depends on a reliable connection to the RIS in order to work efficiently. This connection is often made through a **broker**, which is an independent mostly hardwired unit where the relevant data are exchanged and translated

(from HL7 to DICOM or vice versa). This connection can produce problems as data inconsistencies can occur. It also can be a source for future incompatibility between RIS and PACS data handling. The aim is to provide a **brokerless** connection.

THE NETWORK

This connects all the components of a PACS and is the highway that provides the data connection. Some common network technologies have been described in Section 11.6.2. Commonly associated with the PACS network are intermediate ancillary computers which transfer images to the PACS or information to and from the RIS. These ancillary computers should be minimized since conflicts in data handling do occur between several computers working on the same network (multi-tasking).

An outline design for a basic PACS for radiology is shown in Fig. 11.13.

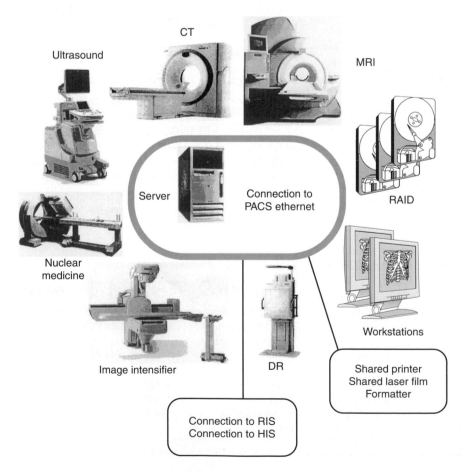

Figure 11.13 An outline design for a basic PACS for radiology. Gateways connect the PACS fileserver to the radiology (RIS) and hospital (HIS) information system. A tele-radiology microwave link is also possible.

ARCHIVE STORAGE

The PACS **server** is responsible for controlling access to information, and images and data flow. The server is typically a rack mounted dual computer system with multiple hard disks (see Section 11.6.5). The archival system is an important component of a PACS and is responsible for short- and long-term image storage. It also duplicates image data as backup in the event of system malfunction and disaster recovery. Since magnetic disk stores offer the largest and cheapest method of storing image data these often perform both tasks of short-term and long-term archiving. The advantage with this fast large storage capacity is that clinical data are always on-line, even for images going back several years.

ARCHIVAL SYSTEMS

These are often made up from multiple storage devices suitable for short-term (and rapid access), long-term (often slower access), and duplicate (often

off-site for disaster recovery) storage of image data. The rapid development and decrease in cost of hard disk storage has blurred the division between short- and long-term archives. Although many PACS installations have been able to eliminate the film record the majority of PACS do supply hard copy printed on dry laser printers.

The capacity of a PACS facility can be measured by the number of images accessed. Storing $1024 \times 1024 \times 10$ bits requires 1.3 MB. Table 11.10 lists bulk storage devices available for PACS systems and their capacity. Optical disks are arranged in a 'juke-box' configuration holding many hundreds of gigabytes but retrieval time can be very slow indeed. Critical design problems now emerge. In order to increase storage capacity and access time some form of **data compression** must be introduced, preferably without image data loss (see later).

Digital archiving enables multiple image storage sites, which allows disaster recovery. A redundant array of independent disks (RAID) is a design for archiving which uses cheaper disk storage rather than a single large optical disk. Speed of access and reliability are improved. Table 11.11 lists the most common diagnostic clinical studies, image matrix sizes, and total storage needed for each complete study. Table 11.12 gives a size estimate for the total archive space needed for a medium sized radiology department seeing 100 000 examinations per year.

Levels of access are available from immediate (most recent cases) to less immediate (cases older than a certain time period, e.g. weeks, months). The standard computer hard drive or magnetic disk, also known as a direct-access storage device, is the fastest medium from which to retrieve data. Presently available devices have

Table 11.10 *Archival image storage, access timing, capacity, and cost.*

Technology	Timing *	Capacity
Magnetic disk	1 to 50 ms	100 MB to 10 GB
Optical disk	30 s to minutes	1 GB to 10 GB (TB devices)
Tape (DAT)	Minutes	10 to 100 GB (TB devices)
Digital video disk	Seconds	1 GB to 10 GB (TB devices)
RAID	10 to 300 ms	10 to 100 GB (TB devices)

* Time for retrieval of a 10 MB file (typical chest radiograph in Table 11.6).

Table 11.11 *PACS storage needed for clinical examinations.*

Imaging system	Matrix size and pixel depth	MBytes per image	Images per study	Total storage (MBytes)
Computed radiography	2048 × 2500 (10)	6.4	2	12.8
Direct radiography	2688 × 2688 (12)	10.8	2	21.6
Computed tomography	512 × 512 (16)	0.5	100	50
Digital subtraction angiography	1024 × 1024 (10)	1.3	50	65
Nuclear medicine	128 × 128 (12)	0.025	20	0.5
Ultrasound	640 × 480 (8)	0.3	30	9
Mammography (low resolution)	2300 × 1900 (12)	6.5	4	26
Mammography (high resolution)	4096 × 3277 (12)	20	4	80
Cardiology	512 × 512 (10)	0.3	500	150

Table 11.12 *Estimated hard disk storage for 100 000 examinations per year.*

Image	Exam storage (Mbytes)
Projection (computed radiography, direct radiography)	560 273
Computed tomography	453 516
Magnetic resonance imaging	29 004
Digital fluorography	11 338
Digital subtraction angiography	66 797
Ultrasound	56 625
Mammography	102 422
Cardiac	66 797
Nuclear medicine	102 422
TOTAL	1.38 TB

a capacity of 100 to 800 GB and a rapidly decreasing cost. Continued decreases in cost indicate that magnetic disks will satisfy long-term storage for the near future.

Since magnetic disk technology has become very reliable and still offers the cheapest method for storing large numbers of images 'on-line' then the 1.4 terabyte (TB) capacity indicated in Table 11.12 is not a limitation. Some form of reliable back-up is essential, however, in order to protect from catastrophic breakdown.

Optical disks, magneto-optical disks, and digital video disks (DVDs) are often integrated for automated access having the added advantage that they can be removed and so offer solutions for long-term storage. Tape is also a removable archive storage medium. It has very high capacity, tens to hundreds of gigabytes or many terabytes per tape library, and low cost, but it is a slower medium than optical disks, in terms of random retrieval times, because of its serial data storage. It is best used for disaster back-up or long-term permanent storage.

COMPARISON OF IMAGE STORAGE SYSTEMS

No single storage medium possesses the requirements of a large storage capacity and high image transfer rate combined with short access times. As a result of this most digital imaging systems comprise a combination of different storage devices. They contain a fast semiconductor memory capable of storing digitized images in real time. However, because of the relatively high cost per bit of semiconductor memory this type of storage is limited. The semiconductor memory is used again for the next exposure so if the data already stored is to be retained it must be transferred to the auxiliary memory: magnetic disk. The magnetic disk serves as intermediate storage and will retain its data if the power is lost. However, older studies can be erased after a period of time or when the disk runs out of memory space.

If the images are to be archived then, again, the magnetic hard disk is the most suitable medium. The hard disk has the lowest specific storage costs and does enjoy very fast data transfer times. If a number of archived studies are requested then any data stored on optical disk should first be transferred to magnetic disk. From the disk it would be placed in solid state semiconductor memory for viewing purposes. During a viewing or reporting session the data stored in the semiconductor memory would constantly be updated and replaced as a new patient study as requested from the hard disk.

WORKSTATIONS AND DISPLAYS

The soft-copy display workstation or system, the last element of the imaging chain, is perhaps the most visible 'face' of a PACS. The soft-copy displays provide a dynamic and changeable presentation of the image data to the clinician. A soft-copy display workstation has two major components: software and hardware. At the software level, the graphical user interfaces (GUIs) implemented by the manufacturer enable various functionalities necessary for viewing an image such as image query and retrieval, image display, and various image manipulation functions such as window levelling and zooming. At the hardware level, two technologies are currently used for soft-copy display of medical images: the cathode ray tube (CRT) and the liquid crystal display (LCD). The soft-copy display station is a critical component of a PACS that can affect its acceptability and efficiency. Various display technology options and qualities are discussed later. **Workstations** are connected to the network. The **soft-copy display** workstation provides instant presentation of image data to the clinician, radiographer or technologist. The display can be flat panel or cathode ray tube (see Section 12.8, Electronic displays) and can be either thin or fat client (see Section 11.6.5).

SECURITY

The same network, server, and workstations provide image distribution to 'designated remote' areas of the enterprise (the intensive care unit, operating room, emergency room, etc.). This approach can also be used with other means to extend the network beyond its physical reach (i.e. shared or dedicated WAN extensions including satellite connections).

The thin client Web-based approach is an increasingly popular strategy for enterprise-wide image distribution. This approach avoids the problems with distributing large image data sets (and the very demanding infrastructure requirements of a traditional PACS network and workstations) by distributing compressed images. The security settings of the system should be verified to ensure firewall protection and patient confidentiality. In the USA these should be in accordance with state and federal (e.g. the Health Insurance Portability and Accountability Act (HIPAA)) requirements.

PACS TIMING

The timing performance of the system should be tested. The user should establish timing benchmarks for common processes. The timing tests might include common tasks such as image and study transfer times from the acquisition system to display and to archive, RIS report retrieval, single image retrieval (from the cache and the short-term and long-term archives), patient folder retrieval (from the short-term and long-term archives), switching from one study to another, marking a study as 'dictated', log-out and log-in functions, system reboots, and Web-display retrievals (from the server and from the archive).

11.7.4 Image compression

Image data from large matrices occupies a great deal of room in the computer memory and disk store. A radiographic image contains a great deal of redundant information. If this is removed before storage then simple image compression can be achieved without information loss. Other more complex forms of image data compression alter the pixel depth from 8 to 3 or 4 bits.

DIFFERENCE VALUE

Instead of storing the total value for each pixel the difference value from its neighbor is stored reducing the image storage requirements considerably. The absolute value for the pixel is kept at each line of the matrix.

The image matrix depth can be reduced (8 bits) if the pixel density is represented not by a total density value but by a comparative figure obtained by reference to its neighbor. Small relative numbers can then be used to form an image. Following an image profile line by line the next pixel need only be incremented or decremented when comparing it to its neighbor. An example is shown in Fig. 11.14 and the list of stored difference values is given in Table 11.13 showing the significant decrease in stored number values. For this profile a 5 bit (32 decimal) matrix would be needed to store the original signal values whereas, as Table 11.13 shows, only 3 bit storage is needed for the difference values, representing a 40% space saving or 20% if a sign bit is kept. This method of encoding retains all the original image information.

Pixels in image areas which contain little detail have neighboring pixels with the same value, these can be compressed by storing these values along with the number of pixel locations having this value as a **run length**. Storage areas can be significantly diminished since radiographs contain a significant proportion of

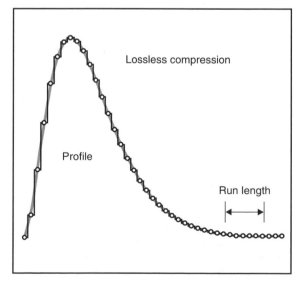

Figure 11.14 *Image compression using a difference value technique on a single line of image data.*

Table 11.13 *Difference value compression.*

Image value	Stored difference value
8.7	6
14.9	6
20.1	6
23.6	3.5
25.6	2.0
26.2	0.6
25.7	−0.5
24.4	−1.3

black or white pixel values. Figure 11.14 shows image compression using a difference value technique.

PIXEL AVERAGING

Images can also be compressed by replacing small pixel regions with single pixels which are the average of all values in the region. Storage can be reduced by 75% using a 2:1 pixel averaging method or 88% using a 3:1 method. There is a slight loss of image detail which may be unacceptable. Digital subtraction angiography (DSA) only concerns vessel architecture so a computer algorithm can trace the vascular tree and generate a map of data which only belong to the vascular components. **Data mapping** requires only a fraction of the original storage. There are two major techniques for compressing and decompressing images; they either retain all the original image data or drop some of this information that is deemed diagnostically uncritical (lossy decompression).

NO DATA LOSS

These algorithms include **run-length encoding** and are based on the observation that image areas which contain little detail have neighboring pixels with the same value so these locations can be stored as a pixel value and pixel range (a 'run length'). Storage requirements can be considerably reduced since large areas of radiographs consist of black background. The radiograph can be further cropped by using electronic shutters so only areas of diagnostic importance are saved.

LOSSY COMPRESSION

Pixel averaging techniques selectively reduce image information by replacing numbers of pixels with single pixels which are the average of all values in the region. Storage requirements can be significantly reduced by

using 2:1 or 3:1 pixel averaging although image quality is degraded (information loss) which may result in loss of diagnostic information. Other lossy methods can be employed to retain only those features of importance in an image. For instance cardiac or DSA images where vessel detail only is required can retain image information about the vascular tree, rejecting background detail which may be of no diagnostic importance. This vessel map requires only a fraction of storage space. **Fractal compression** offers the greatest efficiency for image storage but the time taken for compressing each image imposes a serious limitation.

Image communication systems for medical images have bandwidth and image size constraints that result in time-consuming transmission of uncompressed raw image data. Thus, image compression is a key factor for improving transmission speed and storage, but there is a risk of data loss.

LOSSLESS COMPRESSION

This is preferred since the image data can be recovered completely. Lossless compression is not very effective in many cases, and can even result in an image file that is larger than the original. Image compression involving a small amount of data loss, termed **lossy compression**, provides a means of reducing storage load and transmission bandwidth. JPEG (Joint Photographic Expert Group) and the recently developed JPEG2000 are accepted as reliable and fast compression procedures. The radiology standard DICOM3 (Digital Imaging and Communications in Medicine, Version 3.0) provides rules for compression using lossless methods. The context where the use of lossy compression of medical images is clinically acceptable is beyond the scope of the DICOM Standard (National Electrical Manufacturers Association, 1996). DICOM provides a mechanism for supporting the use of run-length encoding (RLE) compression, which is a lossless compression scheme.

WAVELET-BASED IMAGE COMPRESSION

Fourier transform techniques are conventionally used for analysis of signals and images. The usefulness of the Fourier transform is its ability to analyze a signal in the time domain for its frequency content. However, Fourier analysis has its problems in that the sines and cosines which are used are periodic and extend to infinity in both directions. Real signals and images contain transient components that are highly localized in time and space. These components do not resemble any of the Fourier basis functions and thus are not represented faithfully. The windowed or short-time Fourier transform overcomes some of these problems but the time–frequency resolution is fixed over the entire time–frequency plane. To overcome these limitations attempts have been made using transforms with functions of limited duration. These basis functions are localized in position as well as frequency and are termed **wavelets**. The undoubted value of wavelet analysis has led to considerable research in applications such as signal and image compression, removing noise, feature extraction, and texture analysis as well as in communication improvements.

Wavelet-based image compression has good compression results in both rate and distortion sense. Some modern wavelet-based compression methods such as compression with reversible embedded wavelet (CREW) and set partitioning in hierarchical trees (SPIHT) have been suggested to the JPEG2000 image compression standard as possible candidates.

11.7.5 Remote access: tele-radiology

The transmission of images over a WAN involves telephone or radio communication links between hospitals or clinics; the term tele-radiology describes this branch of a PACS design.

Conventional voice telephone links are unsuitable for long distance image transmission due to data speed limitations so dedicated digital links have been developed; dedicated microwave frequencies have also been allocated.

A tele-radiology system consists of two or more sites connected as a wide area network. Video teleconferencing facilities may also be incorporated into such a system using a small CCD camera situated on the display station so that face-to-face contact can be established for security purposes. The essential points to be considered with a tele-radiology system are:

- Image transmission speed
- Individual workstation display quality
- Communication links
- Number of patient studies to be transmitted
- Security

Box 11.1 Image transmission times

Using a 9600 baud telephone line

Transmitting a CT image of $512 \times 512 \times 12$ bits, and image size 2.09×10^6 bits.

Transmission time is

$$2.09 \times \frac{10^6}{9600} = 3.6\,\text{min}$$

Using a co-axial or wireless link giving 10 Mbit s^{-1}

Transmission time is

$$\frac{2.09 \times 10^6}{10 \times 10^6} = 0.3\,\text{s}$$

Transmitting a $2048 \times 2048 \times 12$ bit chest radiograph, the transmission time is

$$\frac{5.0 \times 10^7}{10 \times 10^6} = 5.0\,\text{s}$$

Using a fiber optic cable giving 1 Gbit s^{-1}

Transmission time is

$$\frac{5.0 \times 10^7}{10 \times 10^9} = 0.05\,\text{s}$$

A CT image typically contains in excess of 1 million bytes. These require immediate storage for display and diagnosis (processor semiconductor memory) and then intermediate storage (magnetic disk). Box 11.1 calculates the transmission times for this image and indicates the practical advantage of very high speed transmission. The practical transmission (downloading) of this data from intermediate or permanent storage to other localities (clinics or hospitals) depends on the speed of data transmission; 2 or 3 s may be tolerable for each image. More than 10 s would not be acceptable, unless it was accomplished prior to requirements (downloading during lunch breaks or outside work time), anticipating reporting requirements.

KEYWORDS

ASCII: American Standard Code for Information Exchange. Each character of text is represented in byte mode. Capital A is 65 decimal; B is 66 and so on

assembly language: a type of computer language which is complex but enables the most efficient way of programming the computer, particularly for speed

back up: copying data from one storage medium to another, e.g. from hard disk to floppy disk. Protection against data destruction

BASIC: Beginners All purpose Symbolic Instruction Code. A very user friendly programming language (unlike assembler). Versions are GW Basic, Quick Basic, Visual Basic

BIOS: (basic input/output system). A set of programs encoded on a ROM chip. It enables the computer to perform basic input/output instructions during boot-up

binary: numbers written in base 2, the fundamental counting system used by computers (see bit and byte)

bit: each bit in a computer memory can represent 1 or 0

boot: the process a computer goes through when it starts up. BIOS loads the operating system from the disk (hard or floppy)

BUS: a multi-wire connection that carries data between different parts of the computer or between computers

byte: a unit of storage capacity made up from 8 bits. This will hold any number from 0 to 256. The byte is the composite building block common to all computers. Several bytes make up a word. Memory and disk sizes are usually quoted in bytes: kilobytes (1000 bytes), megabytes (1 million bytes), gigabytes (10^9 bytes)

C: A fast and widely used programming language

cache: an area of memory used to store a copy of information recently read from or written to a hard disk. This greatly speeds up program operation. Cache sizes can vary; the bigger the better

CD-ROM: compact disk read-only memory. Used as a storage medium for programs and data. Very high capacity (2 GB) can store images but is quite slow to read them out

client: a workstation or personal computer in a client–server network

client–server architecture: a network having a client(s) as a personal computer, or workstations as the requesting machines and the server supplying programs, files, and the patient database (information and images)

CPU: central processing unit. The central micro-processor chip, e.g. i486, Pentium

database: a program that stores information so that it can be easily retrieved by searching and sorting facilities

database server: the computer responsible for storing patient information

default: when a program requests an answer and gives you the most common answer which is accepted as a default when the enter or return key is pressed

expanded/extended memory: methods of adding extra memory beyond the basic 640 kbytes. Expanded memory can be fitted to all PCs. Extended memory can be added and simply extends the existing main memory from 1 Mbyte up to 8 or sometimes 16 or 64 MB

file: a section of information stored on disk and given a name

file server: a very high speed computer in a network that stores programs and data files shared by users. It acts like a remote disk drive

floppy disk: a small disk, either 5¼ or 3½ inches, which can be removed and used on other machines

hard disk: a fixed disk drive and rigid disk used as the main bulk storage device on a computer; usual sizes are 200, 500 and 2000 MB (1 to 2 GB)

interface: hardware or programs that sit between two or more pieces of hardware and act as an intermediate data exchange mechanism or translator for dissimilar machine types

macro: a stored sequence of instructions (usually keystrokes) that can be implemented by pressing just one key

math co-processor: a companion chip to the CPU that carries out arithmetic functions. Program speeds increase by up to 6 times when using image processing or graphics

modem: modulator/demodulator. A piece of hardware that connects the computer to a telephone line for communication

multi-tasking: running more than one program or doing more than one job simultaneously on the same computer or connected group of computers

network: several computers linked together with their output devices shared (printers, film formatters etc.)

operating system: a program that is automatically loaded into the machine at start-up (boot-up), and performs all the basic or housekeeping instructions i.e. disk transfer of program material, erasing or relocating data etc.

parallel port: input/output connection connecting the PC with usually display devices (printer or film formatter). The fastest method of data output

pixel: picture element, represented by dots on the display screen. Images can be from 512×512 to over 2048×2048 pixels

redundant array of independent disks (RAID): two or more magnetic disk drives connected to provide increased performance and error recovery. Originally called 'inexpensive disks' but since all magnetic disk drives have become inexpensive this term has been changed to 'independent'

RAM: random access memory, where data can be written to and read from. Stored data is lost when power is removed (computer switched off)

ROM: read-only memory. Contains the start-up programs of the computer. This data is obviously not lost when the computer is switched off

serial port: connection between input/output devices where data queues up 'in line'. This is much slower than the parallel port but is more universal between computer types (RS232 interface line)

server: a computer in a network shared by multiple users. This term defines both hardware and software

thick (fat) client: a client workstation in a client–server environment that performs all processing with little interaction with the server

thin client: (1) thin processing client in a client–server environment that performs very little data processing. (2) Thin storage, the client downloads the program from the server and performs some processing but does not store anything locally. All programs and image data are on the server

12

The digital image

12.1 SIGNAL INPUT

Essential devices connected to radiology computers are the keyboard, a pointing device such as a mouse, disk drives (floppy or hard disk), and a source of signal data from machines such as ultrasound, gamma camera, CT or MRI as well as digital or video image data from radiographic equipment: DSA and image plate.

12.1.1 Analog to digital conversion

The input data is first converted to binary format using an analog-to-digital converter (ADC); the principle is shown graphically in Fig. 12.1 where the varying voltage levels are converted to their binary equivalent numbers. Conversion accuracy depends on the number of bits used which influences the step size.

An ADC with $2N$ steps can more accurately handle the analog voltage but takes a longer time for its conversion than an N step converter.

Most signals from radiology equipment start as varying analog voltages seen in Chapter 8 as film density changes or video signals. These varying signal voltages must be represented as a digital value before being accepted by the computer for signal processing and displayed as a digital image. This is represented as a stepped graph in Fig. 12.1 where a varying voltage is sampled and the voltage level converted into a

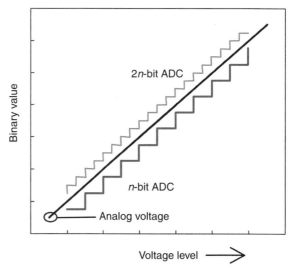

Figure 12.1 *The conversion of analog voltage signals (x-axis) into digitized values (y-axis), showing step digitization using a low and high bit number ADC.*

binary number which represents voltage amplitude or height.

12.1.2 Data sampling

If the analog signal is represented by a moving voltage waveform then how often should it be sampled? If sampling is too slow it will fail to pick out rapid fluctuations and too many samples would require excessive data points and create storage problems.

ALIASING

The example in Fig. 12.2 shows the same signal (A) being sampled prior to AD conversion. The number of samples taken faithfully represents the sinusoidal waveform but is the signal being over-sampled? Since the fastest fluctuation of the waveform corresponds to the highest frequencies this information will be lost if the sampling is reduced. It is important to digitize or sample the signal at a rate which faithfully reproduces the original detail (resolution or signal frequency).

If the original signal (A) is considered as a simple frequency f then this can be digitized accurately if the sampling frequency is at least $2f$. This is represented by waveform B in the diagram. The critical sampling frequency of $2f$ is the **Nyquist frequency** (H. Nyquist, 1889–1976; US mathematician); sampling rates below this frequency would lose high frequency information (example C in Fig. 12.2) causing aliasing artifacts in the image. This can be seen in the common

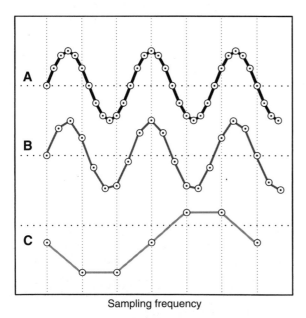

Sampling frequency

Figure 12.2 *The sinusoidal waveform (A) is being over sampled. The waveform (B) is sampled at the Nyquist frequency which achieves accurate signal digitization. Fewer sampling points (C) misrepresent the original data which now has a lower frequency; this signal has undergone aliasing.*

'wagon wheel effect' in western movies, where the film transport rate is slower than the revolutions of the spoked wheel, which then seems to be rotating backwards.

SHANNON SAMPLING THEOREM

This states: 'An analog signal containing components up to a maximum frequency f (in hertz) may be completely represented by regularly spaced samples of $2f$ or twice the signal frequency'.

The sampling rate T is

$$T = \frac{1}{2f}$$

The minimum sampling frequency $2f$ is the Nyquist frequency.

For example, an audio waveform with frequency components of 20 kHz must be sampled at least at 40 kHz intervals. A frequency of 1 MHz should be sampled at 2 MHz. The sampling interval would be $1/2f$ or $1/2 (2 \times 10^{-6})$ which is a sampling period of 5×10^{-6} s. This sampling frequency implies that we can recover the complete analog signal avoiding spectral overlap or **aliasing**. In practice a slightly higher rate is chosen to capture all the fast frequencies. Aliasing is a serious artifact in high resolution digital images (CT) where fine detail is smoothed out (bony structure) because high frequency information has been lost through data sampling error.

QUANTIZATION ERROR

Since analog signals are constantly varying the action of sampling and converting to a binary value introduces errors. Digitization accuracy depends on the bit number n of the ADC. The maximum quantization error q_{max} when digitizing an analog signal with an amplitude range of A and increment size N where $N = 2n$ is

$$q_{max} = \frac{A}{N}$$

For a range of 10 V and a 3-bit ADC the q_{max} value is 1.25 V.

The average error q_{av} is half this at 0.625 V, so

$$q_{av} = \frac{A}{2^{n+1}}$$

The average digitization error for a range of bit sizes is listed in Table. 12.1. Quantization error in a digital image is illustrated in Fig. 12.3 where a single digitized step value can represent a range of analog voltages. A video signal of 1 V with a noise of 1 mV (dynamic range or SNR of 1000:1) will require at least a 10 bit conversion since the least significant bit would represent 1 mV.

The original signal from the video camera (attached to an image intensifier) is a varying analog voltage, i.e. a moving video voltage level, that describes the light intensity on the camera face which in turn is directly related to the X-ray intensity at the image intensifier input face. The video voltage is transformed into a digital signal using an ADC as previously described. The ADC must have a linear response over the full dynamic range of the image intensifier otherwise **differential nonlinearity** will cause stretching or compression of values during conversion leading to image distortion. The binary output from the ADC forms the digital image matrix.

12.2 THE IMAGE MATRIX

While they are being acquired digital images are held in a block of semiconductor memory either in the main central processor memory or in a special image computer called an **array processor**. The array processor is a dedicated computer with some functions 'hardwired' to give extra speed. These functions would include data steering into the image memory independent of software program control.

A variety of matrix sizes are used in radiology depending on the degree of resolution required. Common matrix sizes are 512×512, 1024×1024 and 2048×2048 although smaller matrices are used in ultrasound and nuclear medicine.

12.2.1 Forming the image matrix

Separate elements of the matrix are **pixels** and carry intensity information represented on the video display as a gray scale. The analog signal in this case is a video scan line, from a fluoroscopy system image intensifier, which is digitized prior to storage in the image matrix. Figure 12.4 shows how a single scan line is sampled and digitized and each binary value stored in an x- and y-matrix to form the digitized image. The video waveform is measured in decimal millivolt levels (64, 82 etc.) and then converted into a binary value, for instance 92 would be 00111010 and 100 would be 00100110 etc. These values represent signal intensity (gray scale) and are stored in the individual addresses of the image matrix. The signal first undergoes some filtration to remove noise which would interfere with the subsequent analog to digital process in the ADC; each voltage level is represented by a digital binary value as shown by the pulse sequences in Fig. 12.4. The stream of binary digits is accepted and stored by the computer processing unit (CPU) as the digital image.

The positional information (x and y) is obtained from the video raster timing and scan speed. Pixel positions within the matrix are governed by spatial information (position along the scan line) and timing (end-of-line and sync. pulses) of the scanning beam; the video time-base of the camera or display

Table 12.1 *Digitization error.*

Bits	Range	q_{av} (%)
4	16	3.125
8	256	0.2
10	1024	0.05
12	2048	0.012

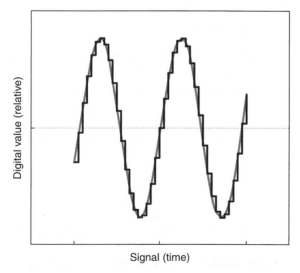

Figure 12.3 *The stepped conversion by the ADC produces varying heights which translate as varying degrees of accuracy in digitization. This is the quantization error.*

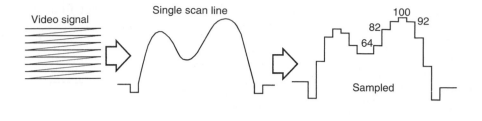

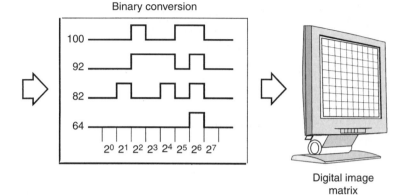

Digital image matrix

Figure 12.4 *The digitization of a video scan line showing the continuous waveform broken down into discrete values at regular intervals. In this example the intermediate decimal figures are converted to binary format.*

supplies these signals from stable clock pulses. The video voltage level, which is proportional to image-intensifier light intensity, is digitized giving the gray-scale information which is stored in each pixel.

Digitizing a video frame acquired in 1/30 s for a 512 × 512 matrix requires that 512^2 samples are digitized in:

$$\frac{0.0333}{512^2} = 127 \times 10^{-9}\ \text{s}$$

or 127 ns or 8 MHz. This sampling frequency would limit the bandwidth to 4 MHz for faithful digitization (1/2 Nyquist rate). Specific signal handling for imaging devices used in nuclear medicine, ultrasound, CT, and MRI are described in their relevant chapters.

12.2.2 Matrix size

Image matrices used for capturing radiology picture data range from a very low definition 32 × 32 pixels to extremely high definition 2048 × 2048. Some image plate digital images exceed even this high figure. Table 12.2 lists typical applications seen in radiology.

As already discussed in Chapter 11 the image matrix is stored in computer memory as a 2-dimensional array (x- and y-axes); each pixel address is from 8 bits to 16 bits deep which is displayed as a gray scale describing signal intensity (nuclear medicine, DSA,

Table 12.2 *Matrix sizes common in radiology.*

Recording medium	Matrix size	Pixels	Pixels mm^{-1}
Film (14″ × 17″)	3500 × 4000	14 M	10
Image plate	2048 × 2048	4 M	4
Video			
625 line TV	512 × 512	262 k	1
1249 line TV	1024 × 1024	1 M	2

MRI), attenuation (CT). Figure 12.5a shows alternative methods for framing the circular field of view offered by many radiology machines (e.g. fluoroscopy, CT, gamma camera, etc.). **Exact framing** encloses the total area within the matrix but is wasteful of matrix area; the alternative is **over framing** where the whole matrix is within the field of view. This closely represents the collimated field of view or the area of patient being examined and gives a larger working image than the exact framing method.

Figure 12.5b shows the decrease in count density for a fixed total count (1 million); as the image matrix increases in size from 64 × 64 to 256 × 256, the individual pixel count N decreases by a factor of 4 from 64^2, 128^2 to 256^2. Since noise content is related to $\sqrt{N}$ the noise component increases with matrix size (for the same total count). Resolution may be improved

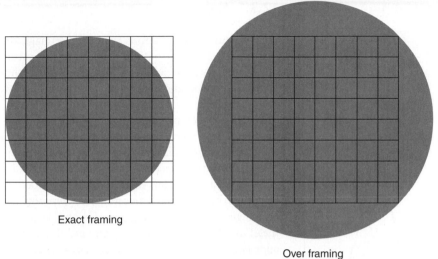

Exact framing

Over framing

(a)

For 1 million counts

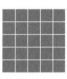

	64 × 64	128 × 128	256 × 256
Matrix size	64 × 64	128 × 128	256 × 256
Pixel size (mm)	6	3	1.5
Pixel count	244	61	15
% noise	1.6	12.7	25.8

(b)

Figure 12.5 (*a*) *A nuclear medicine gamma camera field within a rectangular image matrix showing exact and over framing.* (*b*) *The individual pixel values* N *for three matrix sizes 64 × 64, 128 × 128 and 256 × 256. Image noise is related to EQ.*

with larger matrix sizes but low contrast definition will be lost due to increasing noise.

12.2.3 Image storage

Image memories are specified by:

- Storage capacity
- Transfer rate
- Access time

Storage can be located in the computer RAM memory which has very fast transfer rates and data access time but has limited storage capacity or disk storage (Winchester disk) which has a transfer rate of $1\,MB\,s^{-1}$ corresponding to an image transfer rate of 4 fps at 512^2 as shown in Table 12.3; disk retrieval or access is about 10 ms. Optical or magneto-optical disks are suitable for long-term (archival) image storage since their access times are much longer.

Table 12.3 *Data storage for two image sizes.*

	$512^2 \times 8$	$1024^2 \times 10$
Total memory	256 kByte	1.25 MByte
Transfer rate		
4 fps	$1\,MByte\,s^{-1}$	$5\,MByte\,s^{-1}$
15 fps		$18\,MByte\,s^{-1}$
60 fps	$15\,MByte\,s^{-1}$	
Storage		
5 s duration	75 MByte	90 MByte

12.2.4 Image display

DIGITAL TO ANALOG CONVERSION

Data output from the computer most commonly appears as images on a color or black and white monitor, other output devices would be film formatters

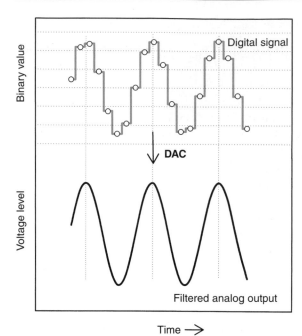

Figure 12.6 *A simple DAC example showing conversion of digital values to voltage levels and filtering the step waveform to get a smooth analog signal for display.*

and printers. Digital data for display is converted to voltage levels by a digital-to-analog converter (DAC), the converse of the analog-to-digital converter.

The action of a DAC is shown in Fig. 12.6 where each digital value (represented by a different height column) gives a 'staircase' waveform which is then filtered giving a smooth output waveform which is mixed with video sync pulses to give a complete video scan line for the display.

12.3 DIGITAL IMAGE QUALITY

Quality of digital images depends primarily on the image matrix size. Smaller matrices have poor resolution but better noise characteristic and therefore better low contrast discrimination. As the matrix size is increased resolution improves but the count or photon density in each pixel must be increased in order to maintain a certain minimum noise level. This factor is crucial to digital image quality so the size of the image matrix should be chosen with care and should not be unnecessarily large.

12.3.1 Noise

Since the number of photons available for image formation is related to patient dose image quantum noise increases as patient dose is decreased (all other parameters being unchanged, i.e. detector efficiency, matrix size).

The interaction between a position sensitive detector (gamma camera, image intensifier etc.) with a uniform flux of radiation (gamma or X-ray) obeys the random processes covered by statistical laws, i.e. Poisson and Gaussian distributions described in Chapter 1. Thus if such a detector was represented by an image matrix each matrix pixel would contain a mean number x counts with a standard deviation of approximately $\sqrt{x}$. The statistical error or noise can be expressed as $x/\sqrt{x}$. For a pixel count of 100 the estimated noise figure would be 10% and the standard error 0.1. For a pixel count of 10 000 the values would be 100 and 0.01 respectively. Box 12.1 gives other examples involving low contrast detection demonstrating that noise content influences the level of low contrast differences that can be visualized in a digital image.

Digital image matrices can contain multiple noise sources including:

- **The detector**. This is responsible for quantum noise or the interaction of the photon flux with the phosphor. The number of quanta making up the image determines the image noise content; this is seen in low radiation dose investigations using image intensifiers, image plates, and low count density scintigraphs.
- **Digitization accuracy**. Conversion of the analog event into a binary coded precision gives error to the image (Fig. 12.3).
- **Magnification**. Decreasing the field of view can decrease photon density and so increase noise.
- **Image subtraction**. Digital subtraction of one image from the other leaves behind the sum of the noise content of both images (e.g. digital subtraction angiography or DSA).

12.3.2 Resolution and contrast

Image resolution for a digital matrix cannot be better than the dimension of an individual pixel. The real dimensions of a pixel as mm^2 or cm^2 depends on the size of the field of view.

Box 12.1 Low contrast and noise

Fluoroscopy

3×10^5 protons give an approximate skin dose of 10 mGy. The quantum noise is $\sqrt{3 \times 10^5} = 547 = 0.18\%$, so low contrast differences of 1% will be visible even at reduced patient radiation dose.

Nuclear medicine

An image having a total count of 10^6 on a 128×128 matrix has an individual pixel density of

$$\frac{10^6}{128^2} = 61$$

so the quantum noise per pixel is $\sqrt{61} = 7.8$ or 12%. Increasing the total counts to 2 million reduces this to 9%.

Tomographic imaging

SPECT (see Chapter 16) requires an accurate uniformity measurement with a variation of only 1%. A 30 million flood field collected by a 64×64 matrix would give 7324 counts per pixel and a quantum noise figure of approximately 1%. A 128×128 matrix would require four times the number of counts.

Table 12.4 *Pixel sizes for radiology matrices.*

System	Matrix size	Pixel size (mm^2)
Nuclear medicine		
38 cm camera	256×256	1.5
Computed tomography		
28 cm (head)	512×512	0.55
45 cm (body)	512×512	0.87
DSA		
20 cm II	512×512	0.4
	1024×1024	0.2
Image plate		
8″ × 10″	1760×2140	0.01
Laser imager		
14″ × 17″	4260×5182	0.008

From Chapter 8, image resolution is measured in line pairs per mm (Lp mm^{-1}); if two lines are x mm apart then $1/x$ mm represents x mm^{-1}. If two lines separated by 0.5 mm can just be resolved then the image resolution is 2 Lp mm^{-1}. The resolution of a digital image, in line pairs per mm, depends on pixel size p and can be calculated as $\frac{1}{2}p$.

Pixel size is determined by the field of view (for instance film size or image intensifier size) and matrix size m so that pixel size is FOV/m. A 43×43 cm film ($14″ \times 14″$) digitized on a 1024 matrix would have a pixel size of 0.4 mm giving a resolution of 1.25 Lp mm^{-1}; hardly acceptable considering the original film data may have yielded 3 mm^{-1}. Table 12.4 lists some common digital images used in radiology and the area occupied by the individual pixels.

The resolution of a digital matrix usually matches the machine resolution. Information cannot be gained by using a 1024×1024 matrix having resolution of 1.25 Lp mm^{-1} if the machine is only capable of 0.5 Lp mm^{-1} resolution.

This point is clearly seen in nuclear medicine where digital images of 256×256 represent the maximum resolvable detail that the gamma camera is capable of. Employing larger image matrix sizes degrades image quality by introducing more noise into each pixel. For a fixed total count density each pixel n would reduce in magnitude so increasing noise as $\sqrt{n}$.

Line-pair value A resolution of 1 Lp mm^{-1} would require 2 pixels mm^{-1} and 5 L p mm^{-1} would require 10 pixels mm^{-1}. An image intensifier having an input face of 250 mm would give a resolution of 1 mm on a 512×512 matrix. Mammography using a field size of $7″ \times 9\frac{1}{2}″$ (18×24 cm) would need a matrix of 2048×2048 to resolve detail approaching 0.1 mm.

Matrix size is sometimes increased for display purposes. Some CT machines reconstruct their images using a 512×512 matrix but display them as a 1024×1024 matrix by **interpolation**. This does not increase system resolution, merely improves the cosmetic appearance of the image and will be described later.

CONTRAST

This is dependent on count density in a digital image matrix. It was shown in Section 12.3.1 that noise plays an important role if small density differences are to be seen. Contrast is therefore a question of signal to noise which is demonstrated in Box 12.1. The low contrast visibility depends on noise fluctuations.

12.4 DIGITAL IMAGE PROCESSING

The great advantage of digital image matrices is the ability to manipulate the raw image data using computer techniques. Real improvement and feature enhancement can be achieved that contributes significantly to diagnosis.

12.4.1 Spatial filtering

Contrast occurs at different scales in an image; fine structure occurs on a small scale while slow changes in gray level occur over a large scale. Spatial filtering techniques can be used to emphasize features of different sizes. Sharp edges, fine detail, and image noise or mottle all occur over a small scale. Spatial filtering techniques can be used to enhance these edges and fine structure and reduce the effects of noise. There are two types of digital spatial filter: a **low pass**, smoothing filter used to reduce noise and a **high pass** edge or contrast enhancing filter.

The general application of a small filter mask or kernel to an image matrix is shown in Fig. 12.7. Using the labels from this diagram the mathematical expression for the 3×3 filter (9-point) can be described, either as:

$$P_8 = (A \times P_1) + (B \times P_2) + (C \times P_3) \\ + (D \times P_7) + (E \times P_8) + (F \times P_9) \\ + (G \times P_{13}) + (H \times P_{14}) + (I \times P_{15})$$

or

$$P_8 = \sum_{x,y}^{3} k(x, y) \times f(x, y)$$

or

$$g(x, y) = \sum^{3} \sum^{3} k(x, y) \times f(x, y)$$

or

$$g(x, y) = k(x, y) \times f(x, y)$$

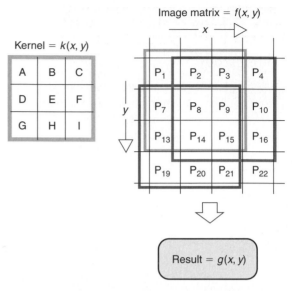

Figure 12.7 *Action of matrix filtering using a small mask (kernel) which is moved over the image matrix. The center pixel in the image matrix is modified for each mask position.*

These same equations describe placing the kernel $k(x, y)$ over the image matrix $f(x, y)$ and storing the product of the entire matrix multiplication $\otimes$ as the output filtered matrix $g(x, y)$.

LOW PASS FILTER (SMOOTHING)

Low pass filters are used to reduce noise or mottle. The process is often called image smoothing, i.e. removing the apparent 'graininess' due to image noise. Figure 12.7 shows that for each pixel in an image the gray level value is added to the sum of the gray levels in the eight surrounding pixels.

The example in Fig. 12.8a shows a single profile through a section of an image having a uniform pattern interrupted by a noise spike. The average of each pixel is obtained by addition of the gray levels of the adjacent pixels.

This new averaged or smoothed data is shown after filtering with this smoothing kernel. The effect of the noise spike has been reduced with a loss, however, in spatial resolution or detail. The original pixel gray level is replaced by the average of these nine pixels. This process is repeated for all the pixels in the image. Figure 12.8b shows the frequency shape for this low pass filter; all values above the threshold are heavily

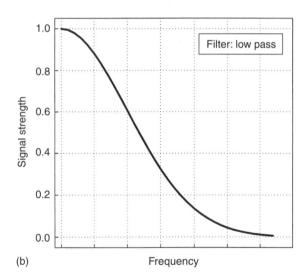

Smoothing filter

−1	−1	−1
−1	−2	−1
−1	−1	−1

Matrix with noise

After filtering

Noise

Profiles

(a)

(b)

Signal strength

Frequency

Filter: low pass

Figure 12.8 (a) Smoothing a section of a digital image using a 9-point kernel to remove a noisy pixel (last in the third row); the profile for this row is shown below the matrix. After filtering the sharp edge (between the 1's and 0's) is smoother but the noise component has vanished. (b) The shape of a low pass filter which will reject higher frequencies.

attenuated. The smoothing action given by this filter when applied to a noisy image is shown in Fig. 12.9.

HIGH PASS FILTER (EDGE DETECTION)

These are used to enhance of an edge or contrast in an image. An edge is defined as a change in gray level and contrast is defined as a change in optical density in an image. Figure 12.10a shows a pattern of numbers representing a step change in an image matrix and the kernel used to modify the values in the matrix. This 3×3 filter now has negative values. Each of the original values is multiplied by the central kernel value, 8, while the two neighbors are multiplied by the outer^{-1} kernel

values. The original data is replaced by the sum of these three operations, giving the filtered matrix. The effect of this operation is to emphasize the location of edge structures in an image. Figure 12.10b gives the shape of the high pass filter which has the effect of heavily attenuating those values below the threshold slope. The angle of this slope can be varied by the kernel values.

The image data in a matrix can be enhanced by using low pass or high pass filters. Since noise contains a great deal of high frequencies it can be greatly reduced by passing the data through a low pass filter removing scattered noise peaks in an image or reducing them in height. If edges are an important feature in the radiograph then an edge enhancement can be

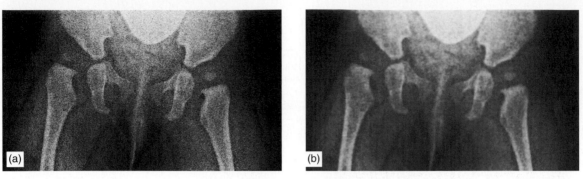

Figure 12.9 *A noisy image (a) having undergone a simple smoothing routine (b).*

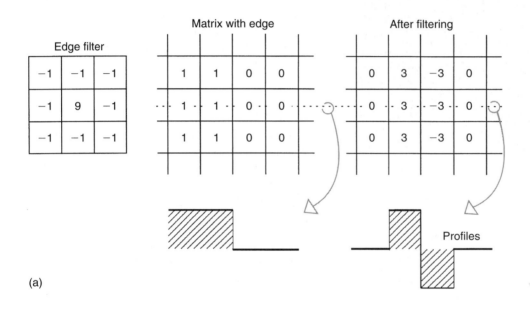

(a)

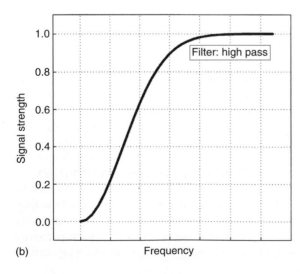

(b)

Figure 12.10 *(a) Edge enhancement produces an exaggerated differential profile. (b) The shape of a high pass filter which will reject low frequencies while accentuating high frequencies.*

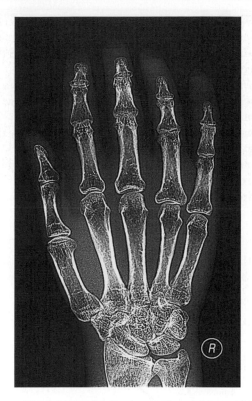

Figure 12.11 *Image detail enhanced by applying a high pass filter to a hand radiograph.*

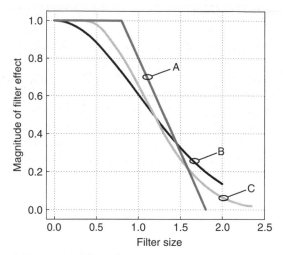

Figure 12.12 *A linear filter (A) and two types of Butterworth filter (B and C). The x-axis is a measure of the filter matrix size.*

applied. This can be seen in Fig. 12.11. Digital filters can be used to enhance detail in an image and help to reduce noise but they are computationally expensive. For example, each pixel in a 1024 × 1024 image (about a million pixels) requires nine multiplication and one addition.

SPECIFIC FILTERS

Two commonly used filter types are Hanning and Butterworth. The filter amplitude at any particular frequency depends on the cut-off frequency F and the 'roll-off' value Q decides the filter's shape. If F or Q is high then the filter is high-pass: accentuating edges in the image. Low values of F and Q give a smoothing action. These filters can be designed so that even though a general smoothing is carried out the tail of the filter characteristic passes sufficient high frequency information to preserve edge detail.

Figure 12.12 shows three filter shapes: (A) a simple linear ramp and two varieties of Butterworth filter (B and C).

UNSHARP MASKING

Many techniques are available for edge detection and enhancement and certain manufacturers (Kodak) have produced adaptive unsharp masking (AUSM) for effectively and rapidly edge enhancing their computed radiography image plates. Unsharp masking follows a common principle which is the formation of the initial mask by over-smoothing the clinical image. This is then subtracted from the initial image and then resulting matrix added to the original image. This action reduces noise and emphasizes any detail that may be present.

The AUSM is thus not a linear process. The general equation describing it would be

$$O(j,k) = I_i(j,k) + \beta[I_i(j,k) - I_b(j,k)]$$

where $I_i(j,k)$ is the input image, $I_b(j,k)$ is the unsharp mask formed by blurring or over-smoothing the initial image and β is a boost function which depends on the application. $O(j,k)$ is the output image.

12.4.2 Temporal or recursive filtering

Noise reduction is particularly important in radiological imaging where patient radiation protection requires that the minimum amount of radiation is used for the imaging procedure. As a result the noise component in an image can be significant, e.g. fluoroscopy or in nuclear medicine examinations. When dealing with a sequence of similar digital images such as a dynamic acquisition, noise reduction can be obtained by averaging a number of images in the sequence. The signal-to-noise ratio obtained by averaging any number of images, N, will be improved by a factor $\sqrt{N}$ as plotted in Fig. 12.13. When several images are added together any image signal (feature) remains relatively constant, but the noise due to its random nature is uncorrelated and the fluctuating values will tend to average or cancel out. This is described more fully in Chapter 13. It has already been seen that image noise decreases as the pixel count increases. Increasing the pixel count can be achieved by increasing either radiation dose or time per study in the case of nuclear medicine and MRI; an alternative procedure is to add successive images.

12.4.3 Look-up tables

Signal pre-processing is achieved by both analog and digital means where non-linear outputs are desirable. The analog method relies on fixed circuits whereas digital methods use a 'look-up table' (LUT) which holds stored values of the desired nonlinear conversion (i.e. logarithmic numbers). An LUT is stored in ROM or RAM depending on whether the signal conditioning is fixed or variable. A display look-up table (Fig. 12.14) relates the brightness produced on the screen to the number stored in memory.

Usually a linear look-up table is used (curves A and B) which produces a steep or shallow linear change in monitor brightness for a given linear change in the input digital data. However, it is possible to vary the shape of the look-up table so as to enhance dark or bright sections of the image (curve C). Table 12.5 gives an example where a linear input can be converted into a clipped-linear function or a logarithmic function.

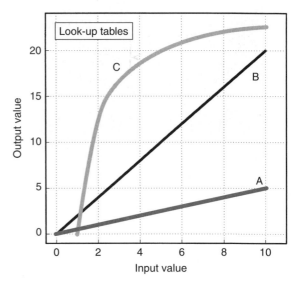

Figure 12.14 *Three LUT examples linear (A and B) and non-linear (C) that can be used for input signal modification. The input values are represented by the x-axis while the output values derived from the stored LUT are given by the y-axis.*

Table 12.5 *Values for a look-up table (LUT) that gives a clipped or logarithmic output.*

Table entry	LUT value	
	Clipped linear	**Logarithmic**
20	20	3
40	40	7
60	60	20
80	80	55
100	80	148
120	80	–

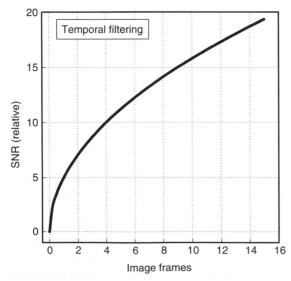

Figure 12.13 *Temporal filtering reduces image noise as a square root function of the image frames that are summed. In practice five images are usually averaged.*

TRANSLATION TABLES

A common application for look-up tables involves the alteration of display characteristics. When a video signal is acquired and digitized it is converted to a sequence of numbers. Each number represents the amount of radiation detected in different parts of the field of view. The image may be displayed on a viewing monitor in its raw state but some form of data processing is usually required. Figure 12.15a shows an input video signal that can be shaped in order to correct for detector response nonlinearity before conversion to an analog display signal.

The common linear gray scale can be transcribed into other formats including color scales, both linear and nonlinear. This is achieved by digitally changing the original linear gray scale into three nonlinear signals (by using look-up tables) and feeding these into the red, green, and blue amplifiers of the color display. Figure 12.15b shows the generation of a red, orange, yellow, white thermal scale from the original linear gray scale.

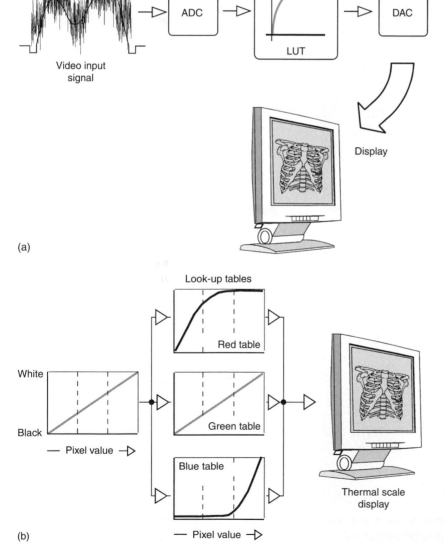

Figure 12.15 (*a*) The position of a look-up-table after the ADC in an imaging system (digitized video signal) which alters the detector characteristic before display. (*b*) Three LUTs used for driving the red–blue–green guns of a color display to give a thermal color scale (red, orange, yellow, white).

The gray-scale pixel values are sampled by the RGB amplifiers. The green LUT has values linearly following the gray-scale value. The red LUT saturates rapidly with the gray scale so is only evidently changing at low values. The blue LUT only responds to high pixel values giving white saturation.

12.4.4 Histogram equalization

If the total image gray scale is represented as a histogram by plotting image densities against frequency of occurrence as shown in Fig. 12.16 it can be seen that a considerable number of pixels are either entirely white or entirely black and contribute nothing to the image content. If these pixels are removed from the displayed image then the pixels holding gray-scale information in the middle of the histogram can be displayed utilizing the full gray scale range. This enhances the contrast differences. The image in Fig. 12.16 shows an example where extreme pixel values are ignored leaving the entire gray scale to represent the pixel values which contain useful diagnostic information.

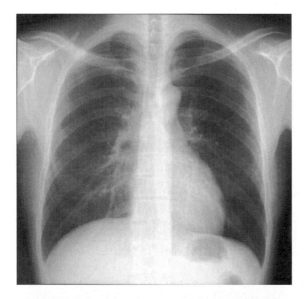

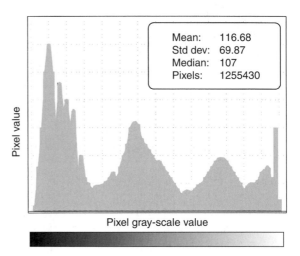

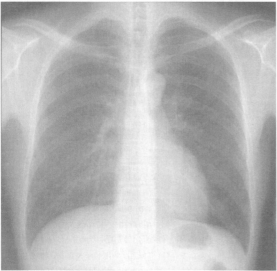

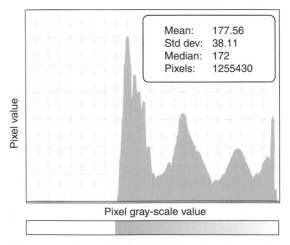

Figure 12.16 *Histogram equalization of an image showing the full gray scale (top radiograph) and a restricted gray scale applied to a selected group of pixel values (bottom radiograph).*

12.4.5 Windowing

Histogram equalization and LUTs are effective methods for improving the image contrast. The contrast resolution of modern digital imaging systems is 10 to 12 bits, i.e. the range of contrast covers 2048 and 4096 gray levels, respectively. However, the eye is only capable of distinguishing about 35 gray levels, a fraction of the information provided. Windowing a section of the stored data allows a selected anatomy to be viewed with improved contrast. This is a common method for improving low-contrast visibility in CT.

Windowing can be used to display only a small range of contrast in which low contrast variations will be enhanced. Figure 12.17 shows windowing of a large digital scale 0 to 4095. Most display systems have a resolution of 8 bits, i.e. only a maximum of 256 gray levels can be displayed simultaneously.

A window permits a small section of these stored values to be displayed using the full 8 bits or a reduced bit number if greater contrast between structures is required.

By varying the position and width of the window it is possible to display a section of the total range on a black to white scale.

The center and width of the window may be chosen independently. It is therefore possible to represent any gray level range of the digitized signal with maximum contrast resolution on the viewing monitor. The maximum window possible is all 4096 gray levels displayed simultaneously as black to white. The minimum range occurs when one level is set to black and the next level up is set to white. Thus the maximum contrast between adjacent levels is obtained.

12.4.6 Interpolation

A degree of image improvement can be obtained by pixel doubling or interpolation, which is commonly found in CT displays where 512×512 images are interpolated as 1024×1024. The distribution of pixel densities shown in Fig. 12.18 shows a coarse bell shaped profile. If the number of pixels of this data set is increased by inserting pixels which have an average value of their neighbors then a much smoother image results as seen in the example by the curve outline. The appearance of the image improves but the resolution remains the same.

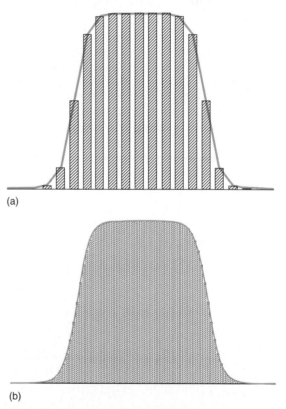

(a)

(b)

Figure 12.18 *Interpolation showing how the real data in a coarse matrix (n × n) can be interpolated to give a larger matrix (2n × 2n). This is commonly performed with medium resolution images (CT or MRI) where 512 × 512 matrices are interpolated and displayed as 1024 × 1024 matrices.*

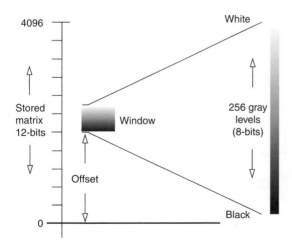

Figure 12.17 *Windowing a selected group of values stored in image memory for display using 256 gray levels. The full range of stored values covers 0 to 4096. Window width W and off-set O are indicated.*

12.5 DIGITAL IMAGE DETECTORS: COMPUTED RADIOGRAPHY

Digital imaging systems, such as computed tomography, ultrasound, and nuclear medicine, gained widespread acceptance in the 1970s. In the 1980s, magnetic resonance imaging, computed radiography (CR), and digital subtraction angiography furthered the trend toward digital imaging. Even with these advances routine projection radiography, using film-screen cassettes, continues to supply images for an estimated 65% of diagnostic examinations (Fig. 12.19).

Projection film-screen radiography is being replaced by three practical digital radiography cassette systems:

- Computed radiography (CR), which uses a photostimulable phosphor for capturing the X-ray image
- Charge-coupled detector (CCD), which uses a CCD camera to read the image produced by a phosphor detector
- Direct radiography (DR), which uses a combination of X-ray detector and electronic readout

All three digital systems are capable of replacing film-screen images in a variety of diagnostic applications.

The ideal digital imaging system should conform to the requirements listed in Table 12.6 but unfortunately all the present digital imaging systems fall short of these requirements either technically or by reason of their cost.

In 1983 researchers at Fuji laboratories developed an erasable X-ray imaging device based on the X-ray excitation of a phosphor layer and subsequent reading the stored image data with an infrared laser (photostimulable luminescence). Results showed that the imaging plate was more sensitive than conventional X-ray film with intensifying screens.

Luminescence is a phenomenon which has been exploited widely in radiation detection and medical imaging. The interaction of ionizing radiation with luminescent materials elevates electrons from the valence to the conduction band by ionization. Electrons

Table 12.6 *Ideal digital radiography system.*

Physical design	• Compatible size with film cassettes • Immediate readout • Robust • Cost effective
Image capture	• High quantum efficiency • Low dose
Image quality	• Spatial and contrast resolution as good as film • Wide dynamic range • DICOM compatible

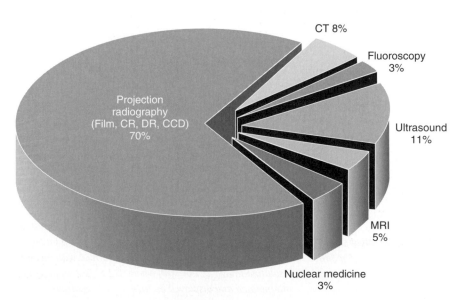

Figure 12.19 *Pie diagram showing proportion of imaging procedures by percent.*

CT 8%

Fluoroscopy 3%

Ultrasound 11%

MRI 5%

Nuclear medicine 3%

Projection radiography (Film, CR, DR, CCD) 70%

trapped at impurity centers at some intermediate energy may be released promptly (fluorescence), after a delay as a consequence of their own thermal energy (phosphorescence), by application of heat (thermoluminescence) or by exposure to visible or infrared radiation (photostimulable luminescence).

Computed radiography uses a sensitive phosphor plate to record the patient's image in place of the traditional film-screen. The image plate looks very similar to the traditional phosphor screen, however it functions very differently. In the photostimulable phosphor plate (also known as an imaging plate, storage phosphor plate or computed radiography (CR)) the phosphors demonstrate phosphorescence or photoluminescence so they are able to store X-ray energy and later, when stimulated by (laser) light, free the energy as emitted light. The simplified diagram in Fig. 12.20 shows the essential features of a computed radiography imaging system comprising the exposed image plate which is then read or developed by a laser scanning device (reader). The output from this is fed to an image array processor where the digital gray-scale image is formed. A certain degree of

image processing can be performed at this stage (edge enhancement). The resulting image can then be displayed as hard (film) or soft copy (video display). The digital image can then be stored on an optical or magnetic disk for future reference.

12.5.1 The photostimulable image plate

The image plate consists of a radiographic screen containing a special class of phosphors which when exposed to X-rays, stores the latent image as a distribution of electron charges, the energy of which may later be freed as light by stimulation with a scanning laser beam. This has been seen before as thermoluminescence in Chapter 6. Figure 12.21a shows the electron transport from the valency band to the conduction band, then returning to be trapped in the forbidden zone. Figure 12.21b shows the action of selective heating with a fine infrared laser beam (laser readout) where the trapped electron (carrying X-ray exposure/image information) is ejected from the forbidden zone back into the valency band. This electron

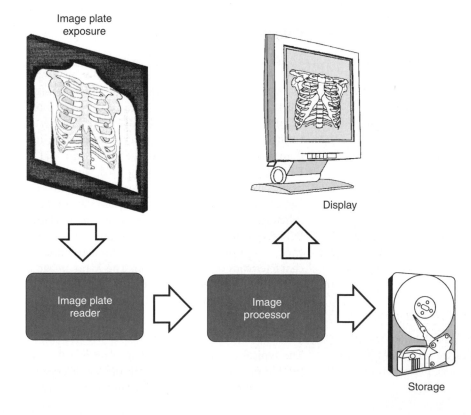

Figure 12.20 *A simplified block diagram of a computed radiography system.*

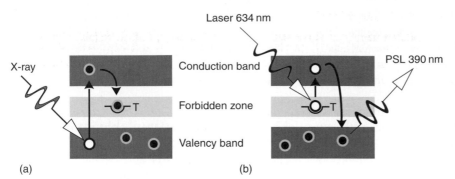

(a)   (b)

Figure 12.21 *Phosphor exposure to X-rays (**a**) elevating a valency electron to the conduction band and subsequently being trapped in the forbidden zone. (**b**) Heating the phosphor with an infrared laser beam ejects this electron with the emission of light.*

movement causes light emission which is collected by a photosensitive detector as image data.

In a digital radiography application, the image plate is positioned in a light-tight cassette or enclosure, exposed and then read by a raster scanning the plate with a laser to release the luminescence. The light signal is detected by a photomultiplier tube, and the output electrical signal is digitized to form an image matrix. The final result is a digital projection radiograph.

This gives a two stage device where the image plate is first exposed to X-rays and then the electronic image is produced by scanning with a laser. This has the advantage of being fully compatible with existing X-ray equipment designed for film-screen imaging; it has the disadvantage of requiring readout and processing steps that take about the same time as conventional film to obtain a diagnostically useful image. In summary:

1 The image plate is placed inside a cassette and exposed to the standard X-ray beam.
2 A latent image is formed which is read by a laser scanning device.
3 The laser stimulates the image plate so that the stored energy, carrying the image details, is emitted as ultraviolet light; this is the photostimulable luminescence (PSL).
4 A photomultiplier is used to collect this light emission and present it as an electrical signal. The electrical signal is digitized and forms the image, ready for processing and recording.
5 The image plate is then erased by exposure to strong light.
6 The imaging process can then be repeated.

Recent CR systems can process 65 to 70 cassettes an hour, accepting mixed cassette sizes, and the time from cassette exposure to image presentation can be less than 90 s.

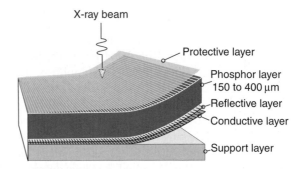

Figure 12.22 *The sandwich construction of the image plate showing the phosphor layer placed on an antistatic conductive metal film.*

PHOSPHOR COMPOSITION

The photostimulable phosphors in the imaging plate have a property termed phosphorescence or photo-luminescence (see Chapter 6) which in this context means they are able to store X-ray energy and later, when stimulated by (laser) light, free the energy as emitted light. A class of europium-activated barium fluorohalide compounds, of general form BaFX: Eu are suitable and have been reported, where X may be the halides Cl, Br or I. The phosphors used in radiography are mixtures of three different barium fluorohalides doped with europium as an activator; $BaFI:Eu^{2+}$, $BaFCl:Eu^{2+}$, and $BaFBr:Eu^{2+}$; the atomic energy levels of the europium activator determine the characteristics of light emission. The X-ray image is recorded on a plate coated with crystals of an appropriate composition phosphor.

CONSTRUCTION

The typical commercial imaging plate is a 0.5 mm flexible plastic plate coated with phosphor crystals, such as $BaFBr:Eu^{2+}$, in a plastic binder. Figure 12.22

Table 12.7 *CR specifications. Processing time 110s.*

Cassette size	Matrix size	Pixel size (μm)	Reading specification (pixels/mm)	
			Standard	High density
35 × 43 cm (14 × 17″)	2048 × 2500	200 × 200	5	10
35 × 35 cm (14 × 14″)	2048 × 2048	200 × 200	5	10
24 × 30 cm (10 × 12″)	2048 × 2500	150 × 150	6.7	10
18 × 24 cm (8 × 10″)	1792 × 2392	100 × 100	10	10

shows the basic construction for a high resolution imaging plate with a phosphor thickness of 150 μm. Routine image plates can have a phosphor thickness up to 0.4 mm thick.

A variety of plates for general radiology, mammography, tomography, and subtraction applications have been developed. Spatial frequencies of 2 and 3 Lp mm^{-1} have been reported for standard and high-resolution work; special applications (mammography) approach 10 Lp mm^{-1}. Table 12.7 lists commonly available CR cassettes. This range has the advantage of being fully compatible with existing X-ray equipment designed for film-screen imaging.

12.5.2 X-ray interaction (image recording)

PREPARING THE IMAGE PLATE FOR X-RAY EXPOSURE

To prepare the imaging plate for an X-ray exposure, the plate is exposed to intense light to erase any previous image. For X-ray imaging, the plate is placed in a cassette and is used just like a film screen cassette with standard radiographic equipment. When exposed to X-rays, the europium atoms in the phosphor crystalline lattice are ionized (converted from 2+ to 3+), liberating a valence electron:

$$EU^{2+} \rightarrow \text{X-ray irradiation} \rightarrow Eu^{3+} + e^-$$

These electrons are raised to a higher energy state in the conduction band where they can move throughout the crystal lattice. The presence of impurities (e.g. bromine) introduces energy levels in the **forbidden zone** called F-centers.

Once in the conduction band, the electrons travel freely until they are trapped in the F-center in a metastable state with an energy level slightly below that of the conduction band, but higher than that of

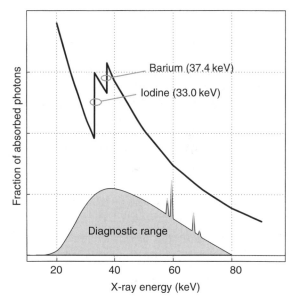

Figure 12.23 *The relative photon absorption for a BaFBr:Eu^{2+} image plate phosphor showing K edges for iodine and barium together with a typical diagnostic X-ray spectrum.*

the valence band. The number of trapped electrons is proportional to the amount of X-rays absorbed locally. The trapped electrons constitute the **latent image**. Due to thermal motion, the electrons will slowly be liberated from the traps, and the latent image should therefore be read without too much delay. At room temperature, the image should, however, be readable up to 8 h after exposure.

X-RAY ABSORPTION

Figure 12.23 shows the X-ray absorption spectra for imaging plates of differing thickness. The sharp upswings near 33 keV and 37 keV show the K-edge characteristics of iodine and barium, respectively.

X-RAY SCATTERING

The incident X-rays are absorbed by the phosphors of the imaging plate, but a portion of these X-rays is first scattered and finally absorbed by phosphors at places different from the initial positions of incidence. Consequently, the image is blurred. The proportion of this scattering is of the order of several percent, and the resulting effect upon the overall CR response characteristics is comparatively slight.

12.5.3 Image readout

Reading the exposed image plate is performed by scanning the surface with a small (50 to 200 μm) point of light from a helium–neon laser. The laser light **stimulates** the trapped electrons moving them up to the conduction band where they make their exit returning to the lower energy valence band. This movement involves the transformation of europium from the 3+ to the 2+ state involving liberation of energy, and the emission of light. For the readout:

$$Eu^{3+} + e^- \rightarrow \text{(influenced by IR laser 633 nm)}$$
$$\rightarrow Eu^{2+} + hf(\text{PSL at 390 nm})$$

Triggering the **emission** of this shorter-wavelength (blue) light is called **photostimulated luminescence (PSL)**.

The energy levels in the crystal are critical to the effective operation of the detector (Fig. 12.21). The energy difference between the traps and the conduction band ET must be small enough so that stimulation with laser light is possible, yet sufficiently large to prevent random thermal release of the electron from the trap. There are very small losses due to some excited electrons missing the traps and returning immediately to the valency band.

The wavelength of the emitted light must be efficiently detected by a photomultiplier and have good wavelength separation between stimulated and emitted light quanta so avoiding contamination of the measured signal (PSL). The PSL intensity is proportional to the original X-ray exposure.

STIMULATION SPECTRA

Figure 12.24a shows the light wavelengths necessary to stimulate two common image plate phosphors. The stored energy is proportional to the original X-radiation and is released by stimulating the lattice with radiation of a much lower energy band; the bandwidth of the stimulation radiation is shown to be quite broad, ranging from 500 to 750 nm which releases the electrons from their traps.

The optimum wavelength for stimulating these phosphors is seen to be 600 nm, in the infrared

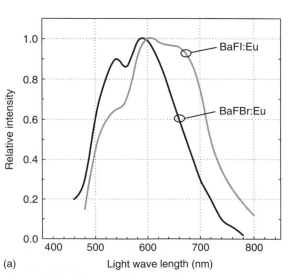
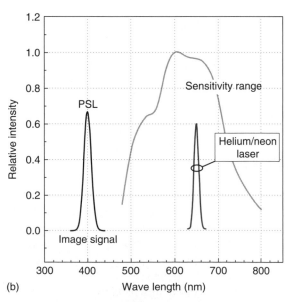

Figure 12.24 (a) The broad range of wavelengths necessary to stimulate emission from the image plate phosphor. (b) The stimulation and emission spectra for a typical image plate. The relative intensity of emitted light in the 400 nm band is directly proportional to the X-ray exposure at the plate over approximately five decades.

region. The stimulation spectrum is a close match to the helium–neon laser emission spectrum. The ready availability of helium–neon lasers which emit light with wavelength 633 nm means that the phosphor should have high emission sensitivity when stimulated. Figure 12.24b shows the laser wavelength He/Ne superimposed on the stimulated spectrum together with the PSL wavelength.

PHOTOSTIMULATED LUMINESCENCE

The wavelength of emitted (output) radiation should be in the range 100 to 500 nm where photomultiplier tubes have high quantum efficiency. The emission spectrum peaks in the wavelength region of 400 nm, which is close to the peak spectral sensitivity of the emission detector (photomultiplier) wavelength.

The response time of the photostimulated luminescence (PSL) is fast (0.8 μs) so it is possible to read many megabytes of image data within a few seconds using a scanning laser beam. The PSL has a wavelength of 390 nm (ultraviolet) and the laser wavelength is 632.8 nm (infrared). The PSL with a wavelength of 390 nm (UV) has a FWHM of 150 mm giving a possible 10 pixels mm^{-1}, the laser scanning pitch is 5 to 10 pixel mm^{-1}. If the PSL decay is 0.8 μs then a 5000 × 4000 pixel matrix will take: $(2 \times 10^7) \times (0.8 \times 10^{-6}) = 16$ s. Each reading is digitized to 10 bits and the image plate has an 80% photon capture efficiency.

READOUT MECHANISM

Reading the plate after exposure is accomplished by scanning a laser beam in a raster over the plate and measuring the light emitted with a photomultiplier tube via a linear light guide. The difference between the stimulation and emission wavelengths is critical for efficient detection of the emitted light. By using a filter that absorbs red light but is transparent to green light, the emitted light is selectively detected by a photomultiplier.

The component parts required for reading an exposed image plate are shown in Fig. 12.25 where the He–Ne laser beam scans the image plate by means of a rotating mirror. The laser beam scans the imaging plate in a transverse direction while the plate is moved past the scanning beam.

The emitted light is collected using a light guide and is fed to a photomultiplier tube where the light is converted to an electrical signal which is amplified to an electric output signal. This signal is converted by ADC and the image is stored in a computer as a digital matrix.

The shorter wavelength PSL is collected by a photomultiplier tube (PMT) and fiber-optic light guide. The PMT signals are logarithmically amplified, then

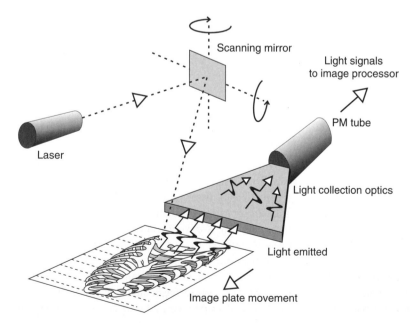

Figure 12.25 *Image plate readout procedure using an infrared He–Ne laser beam scanning the plate using a rotating mirror. The PSL is picked up by a photomultiplier tube and its signal fed into a digital imager.*

passed through analog conversion and filter circuits, and transmitted to an analog-to-digital converter. The digitized signal is stored in an image matrix, each pixel having a gray-scale value determined by the amount of light emitted from the corresponding spot on the imaging plate, which can be used to give a film image or be part of a digital image display system. The screen is then completely erased with an intense light source before reuse.

The final result is a digital projection radiograph. Since the diameter of the laser beam can be made very small, the spatial resolution is strongly influenced by this. The image may be processed in a variety of ways depending upon the clinical application and the final image may be recorded on photographic film by digital-to-analog conversion followed by the modulation of a He–Ne laser beam in a film formatter which scans the film.

Computed radiography response characteristics are largely determined by the broadening of the laser light spot in the image plate reader. This broadening depends upon the response characteristics of the laser (scatter characteristics of laser light within the phosphor layer) and the laser beam diameter.

PRE-READING

In practice, depending on the laser intensity, the readout of a stimulable phosphor plate yields only a fraction of the stored signal. This is a disadvantage with respect to sensitivity and readout noise, but it can be helpful by allowing the plate to be 'pre-read', i.e. read out with only a small pan of the stored signal, to allow automatic optimization of the sensitivity of the electronic circuitry for the main readout. When reading the image from the plate the computer builds a density histogram of the picture so that optimum gray scale can be allocated to the available countdensity (histogram equalization).

ERASURE

To prepare the imaging plate for an X-ray exposure, the plate is exposed to intense light to erase any previous image. Ease of erasure of the residual image increases the fading characteristics of an image plate. This is due to the fact that the same PSL centers are related to both fading and erasure characteristics. Efficient image erasure can be achieved by improving the image erasure unit within the image reader. This improved method of erasure consists of a two-stage

process, i.e., first irradiation with light including an ultraviolet component and then with light containing no ultraviolet.

12.5.4 Image quality

Current commercial image plate systems offer matrix sizes of 1760×2140 for standard resolution (ST) and 2000×2510 pixels for high resolution (HR). These are digitized to 10 bits. The effective resolution is 2.5 Lp mm^{-1} for 35×43 cm ST plates and approximately 5 Lp mm^{-1} for 18×24 cm HR plates. Chest X-ray systems commonly employ a 3584×4096 by 12 bit deep matrix having 5 to 10 pixels mm^{-1} resolution. When reading the image from the plate the computer builds a density histogram of the picture so that optimum gray scale can be allocated to the available count density (histogram equalization).

The image may be processed in a variety of ways depending upon the clinical application and the final image may be recorded on photographic film by digital-to-analog conversion followed by the modulation of a He–Ne laser beam which scans the film.

Using low and high kV images, a subtraction image may also be synthesized in which bone or tissue can be cancelled (see later). Similarly, subtraction angiography is possible. A variety of plates for general radiology, mammography, tomography, and subtraction applications have been developed. Current commercial image plate systems offer matrix sizes of 1760×2140 for standard resolution (ST) and 2000×2510 pixels for high resolution (HR). These are digitized to 10 bits. The effective resolution is 2.5 Lp mm^{-1} for 35×43 cm standard plates and approximately 5 Lp mm^{-1} for 18×24 cm high resolution plates. Chest X-ray systems commonly employ a 3584×4096 by 12 bit deep matrix having 5 to 10 pixels mm^{-1} resolution.

DYNAMIC RANGE AND SENSITIVITY

The imaging plate has a much wider dynamic range than film-screen systems (see Chapter 7). Unlike film-screen it has a linear characteristic curve, giving it a much wider exposure latitude than film-screen image systems. With X-ray film and intensifying screens, speed is defined by the exact combination of film with screen but image plates have no such speed limitations, since each type can be used over a wide range of exposures. Speed performance of the imaging plate is rated at between 20 and 2000. The imaging

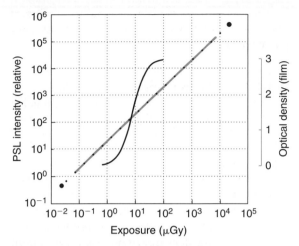

Figure 12.26 *Image plate dynamic range compared to film.*

plate thus allows exposures ranging from low dosage (high sensitivity) to high dosage (low sensitivity), specifically adapted to the anatomical area in question and the exposure method employed.

Figure 12.26 plots exposure versus response (dynamic range) and shows the increase in sensitivity and the extended response of the imaging plate for very low radiation dose. The practical dynamic range is 1:10000 compared to film-screen of 1:1000. The response of the luminescence is linear from 8 X-ray photons per pixel to 4×10^4 photons per pixel: a range of 1.0 to 5×10^3.

DOSE RESPONSE

Because of certain 'pre-scan operations' which are performed prior to the actual readout of the imaging plate, an automatic gain control is achieved; overexposed images are recorded with equal 'brightness' as underexposed images. There is a small patient radiation dose saving, although the required amount of X-radiation to the plate is roughly the same as film-screen systems for the same image noise. The wide exposure latitude and 'automatic gain control' allow dose reduction but at the cost of increased noise. The uniform density despite over- and underexposure is one of the great benefits of the system as compared to conventional film-screen systems; almost no retakes due to incorrect exposures are necessary.

Additional benefits are those common to all digital techniques, including post-processing such as changing window level and width, exact measurement of distances, angles, and areas, zooming, panning, and not the least, digital archiving and communication.

RESOLUTION AND CONTRAST

A variety of plates for general radiology, mammography, tomography, and subtraction applications have been developed. Spatial frequencies of 2 and $3\,\mathrm{Lp\,mm}^{-1}$ have been reported at 40% MTF for standard and high-resolution screens, respectively. Recent image plates can achieve $7\,\mathrm{Lp\,mm}^{-1}$ and certain specialized mammography plates can approach $10\,\mathrm{Lp\,mm}^{-1}$.

With the aid of image processing the computed radiography image plate system is capable of accentuating response at any desired spatial frequency. This provides appropriately enhanced diagnostic images for any body region and exposure method. Without image processing, the sharpness is determined by the pixel size and the type of imaging plate used (standard or high resolution). The 12 bit (4096) pixel depth gives a much wider contrast response than film. Unlike analog film, the CR image can be windowed to accentuate small contrast differences. Film can only return a contrast range of between 5 and 6 bits (32 to 64 gray levels).

GRANULARITY AND NOISE

Since the imaging plate has a wide exposure latitude, it is necessary to specify acceptable granularity levels for the type of exposure being considered. In high speed (low dosage) exposures, the granularity is determined chiefly by the quantum mottle of X-ray energy; in low speed (high dosage) exposures, it is determined by the structural mottle of the imaging plate. As exposure levels increase, the resultant image carries larger amounts of diagnostic information (signal) so the signal-to-noise ratio increases. Figure 12.27 shows the granularity curves (RMS) as a function of exposure. The noise affecting image quality in an imaging plate consists of:

- X-ray quantum noise
- Light photon noise
- Fixed noise

The noise characteristics of the system are determined primarily by the imaging plate, being quantum limited up to approximately $100\,\mu\mathrm{Gy}$. At higher doses, **quantum mottle** becomes dominated by the **structure mottle**.

X-RAY QUANTUM NOISE

X-ray quantum noise, a Poisson distributed spatial fluctuation of X-ray quanta, arises in the process of absorption by the imaging plate; the associated noise power is inversely proportional to the X-ray dose absorbed by the detector (IP).

If the incident X-ray dose is constant, then the associated noise is determined by the absorption characteristics of the imaging plate, and the major issue consists in ascertaining the extent to which the effective thickness of the imaging plate can be increased so as to increase X-ray absorption while still maintaining the image plate response characteristics. X-ray quantum noise can be reduced by decreasing the thickness of the protective layer on the phosphor surface. This protective layer is indispensable in order to prevent physical and chemical changes in the phosphor layer, but should preferably be absent from the viewpoint of image quality. This is because the stimulation beam is scattered within the protective layer, thereby causing deterioration of the response characteristics (sharpness).

LIGHT PHOTON NOISE

Light photon noise (fluctuation of photoelectrons at the photomultiplier) arises in the process of photoelectric transformation of the PSL light; the associated noise power is inversely proportional to number of photoelectrons. The noise power is also inversely proportional to:

- The incident X-ray dose
- The X-ray absorption of the imaging plate
- The light condensing efficiency of the light guide which collects the PSL light
- Photoelectric conversion efficiency of the photomultiplier

Therefore, an important design requirement with respect to the imaging plate consists in improving the absorption characteristics while also increasing the brightness of emission by the photostimulabe phosphor. The reading device must possess a high-output laser beam (in order to raise the level of light emission) as well as a highly efficient light condensing system and a light detector of high photoelectric conversion efficiency.

FIXED NOISE

Possible sources of fixed noise include image plate structural noise, laser noise, analog circuit noise, quantization noise in the AD conversion process, etc. Image plate structural noise arises from non-uniform spatial distribution of the phosphor within the phosphor layer of the imaging plate, this gives a non-uniform PSL at the phosphor surface. The size distribution of the phosphor particles (i.e. the statistical dispersion of the grain size) is the dominant factor with respect to fixed noise and overall reduction of the fixed noise level can be obtained by decreasing phosphor grain size.

MOIRÉ PATTERNS WITH STATIONARY GRIDS

Antiscatter grids are commonly employed in projection radiography; the grid lines superimposed on the image can cause Moiré fringe noise. Film images have virtually no problems with Moiré interference, however, when stationary grids are placed in parallel with the image plate laser scan pattern serious interference patterns can be generated. Moiré reduction can be achieved by a filtering process that removes components having a specific frequency. A 40 line cm^{-1} grid has a frequency of 4 cycles per mm so the Moiré fringe pattern can be significantly reduced by passing the image signal through a filter tuned to this frequency.

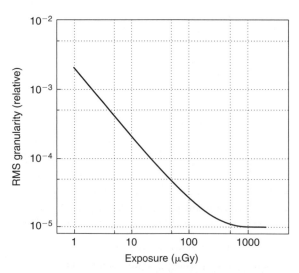

Figure 12.27 *Image plate granularity measured as a relative root mean squared noise value. Granularity falls rapidly with radiation dose.*

DETECTIVE QUANTUM EFFICIENCY

The signal-to-noise ratio is a straightforward method for measuring image quality. The detective quantum efficiency (DQE) uses the transmitted and received signal-to-noise ratios of an imaging device as an index for the comprehensive evaluation of sensitivity and image quality (resolution, contrast and graininess). The DQE is a factor that indicates the efficiency with which detected image information is transmitted and then displayed as an image. It is defined as the value obtained by dividing the square of the input signal-to-noise SNR_{in} by the square of the final image signal-to-noise ratio SNR_{out} where Q is the number of input X-ray quanta and ν is the spatial frequency, so:

$$DQE_{\nu,Q} = \frac{SNR_{out}^2}{SNR_{in}^2} \qquad (12.1)$$

The ideal DQE for the X-ray image sensor is 1 (that is, 100%). The DQE index thus provides comprehensive evaluation of sensitivity and image quality. The DQE is radiation dose dependent as its value should always be quoted along with the dose level used in its measurement. For diagnostic imaging exposure levels (10 to 30 µGy) the image plate shows a slightly better DQE value than film screen for low spatial frequencies (Fig. 12.28). For spatial frequencies above 2 Lp mm^{-1}

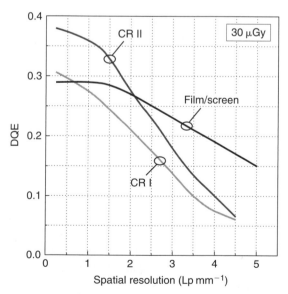

Figure 12.28 *Detective quantum efficiency (DQE) for a mammography film-screen combination compared to a standard large area image plate (CR.I) and an image plate used for mammography (CR.II).*

the DQE value falls rapidly due mainly to fixed noise sources. Patient dose is also influenced by the DQE of an imaging system since image quality is largely determined by SNR_{out} and patient dose related to SNR_{in}.

12.5.5 Image processing

Computed radiology images can be acquired over four decades of exposure (1:10 000; see Fig. 12.26) so some form of image processing must be performed to optimize the radiograph for output display. A manufacturer will supply a set of computer algorithms that can be applied to the digital image for laser film (hard copy) or monitor display (soft copy). In general, the digital image processing applied to CR consists of an analysis phase, followed by contrast enhancement, frequency processing, or both. In general, the primary image processing consists of an image analytical phase, followed by contrast enhancement and frequency processing.

IMAGE ANALYSIS

The **image analysis phase** performs a histogram analysis of the pixel gray-scale values in the digital image and the appropriate look-up table for the anatomy is selected for the display; this protocol is chosen by the operator. The image recognition stage (sometimes called exposure data recognizer or segmentation) precisely identifies the collimated region of exposure and a histogram analysis of the pixel gray values is made to assess the actual exposure to the plate. Proper recognition of the exposed region of interest is extremely important as it affects future processing applied to the image data. For example, if the bright white areas of the image caused by collimation at the time of exposure are not detected properly, the very high gray values will be taken into account during histogram analysis and will increase the 'window' of values to be accommodated by a given display device (soft copy or hard copy); contrast in the image will thus be decreased. This algorithm feature tends to improve image appearance by removing the bright white background in images of small body parts or of pediatric patients.

CONTRAST ENHANCEMENT

Conventional contrast enhancement, sometimes called gradation processing or tone scaling is performed

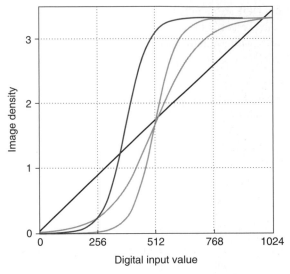

Figure 12.29 *Gradation processing creating sigma responses which emulate a film-screen response and so enhance contrast levels.*

after the analytical phase. This chooses the best characteristic curve (usually a nonlinear transformation of X-ray exposure to image density) for application to the image data. This is equivalent to altering the film gamma of the sigma characteristic curve (Fig. 12.29).

SPATIAL FREQUENCY PROCESSING

Edge enhancement algorithms adjust the frequency response characteristics of computed radiography systems and typically apply a nonlinear **unsharp masking** filter, which suppresses noise by image smoothing. Unsharp masking is an averaging or summation filter that blurs the image which is then subtracted from the original image data; this has the effect of noise suppression. Using this method it is possible to emphasize specific spatial frequencies by changing the mask size and weighting parameters. Low-frequency image information can be amplified by using a relatively large mask, conversely high-frequency or edge information can be enhanced by using a small mask size.

DUAL-ENERGY SUBTRACTION TECHNIQUE

In this method, X-ray energies are separated by the insertion of a copper filter between two image plates which are then given a single exposure (Fig. 12.30a,b). The low-energy image is recorded on the front image

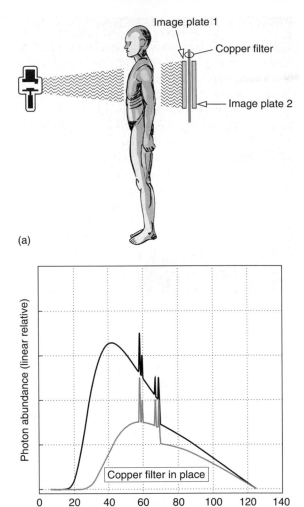

Figure 12.30 *(a) The positioning of the copper filter between the image plates 1 and 2. (b) The X-ray spectra obtained before and after the copper filtration supplying a spectrum with predominantly low energy photons and the second with predominantly high energy photons.*

plate and a high-energy image is recorded on the back. Owing to the difference in energy the absorption ratio of X-rays through bone and soft tissue will differ for the two images. By subtracting these two images using weighted factors, bone or soft tissue detail can be selectively displayed (Fig. 12.31).

12.5.6 Image display

The X-ray images recorded on the imaging plate are scanned by a narrow He–Ne laser beam and the

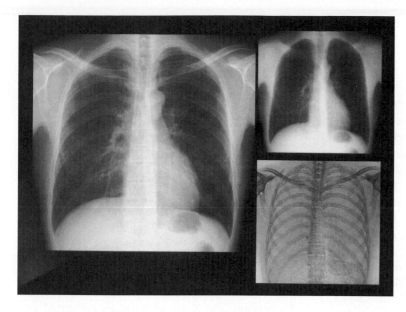

Figure 12.31 *An example of dual energy subtraction showing lung fields and rib cages obtained from the composite image (courtesy Fuji Medical).*

issuing light collected by a photomultiplier whose signal output is digitized to either 10 or 12 bit accuracy and stored in the memory of an image processor (dedicated computer). The image processor enhances the information (smoothing, edge enhancement etc.) before display, which can either be a high resolution video display or hard-copy film.

THE VIDEO DISPLAY

This should give a minimum resolution of 1024 lines but 2048 or more would be more appropriate for revealing information in higher definition imaging plates.

FILM HARD COPY

A second semiconductor or helium–neon laser is used for transferring the image information from the array processor memory onto film. The array processor feeds the image information from its memory into a digital-to-analog converter; this analog signal then modulates the intensity of the laser while scanning the film. The film is a single emulsion with a peak sensitivity at 633 nm to match the laser output. Two images can be printed onto a single sheet of film; one can be unaltered image data, the other can be edge enhanced.

COMPARISON WITH FILM-SCREEN

Compared to other integrating image detectors (film and video cameras) the dynamic range of the imaging plate system is much wider; approximately $1:10^5$. The noise level is equivalent to 3 X-ray photons per pixel which compares to the film fog-level of 1000 X-ray photons per equivalent area. The plate yields reproducible results over many repeated uses. Particular radiology advantages:

- Broad dynamic range showing low contrast differences
- Digital manipulation of the image (edge enhancement)
- Electronic storage and retrieval of image(PACs)
- Patient dose reduction

The limitations of film recording, compared to image plate are:

- Expense
- Poor contrast ≈5% difference visible
- Absorbs only 30 to 50% of available X-ray photons
- Not easily transferable to digital storage

12.6 DIGITAL IMAGE DETECTORS: CHARGE-COUPLED DEVICES

Charge-coupled devices (CCDs) are now used as the image-acquisition component of cameras in video and digital photography. CCD digital radiography systems use these devices together with minification optics to image the light emitted by a scintillator, most often a conventional intensifying screen designed for film-screen radiography. CCD-based systems are available from a wide variety of manufacturers.

12.6.1 Image capture

Originally invented by Bell Laboratories in 1969, CCDs were quickly adapted for use as electronic camera devices when their sensitivity to visible light was recognized. They are used in a wide variety of indirect-conversion X-ray imaging devices for radiology, including large-area radiographic imaging systems and commonly as robust image-intensifier camera systems in fluoroscopy, having replaced the more delicate vidicon/plumbicon tubes.

The basic CCD consists of a series of metal oxide–semiconductor capacitors that are fabricated very close together on a semiconductor surface. The CCD is a silicon wafer that has been etched to produce a matrix of photosensitive elements insulated from each other (Fig. 12.32). Each pixel element on the CCD is typically $9\,\mu m^2$. Matrix sizes of 1024×1024 are commonly available with larger matrices for specific applications. A CCD chip with dimensions $2.5 \times 2.5\,cm$ can have 1024×1024 or 2048×2048 pixel elements on its surface; even larger CCD chips of $8 \times 8\,cm$ have been produced.

Each element in the CCD can be made to act as a signal storage capacitor by applying a suitable biasing

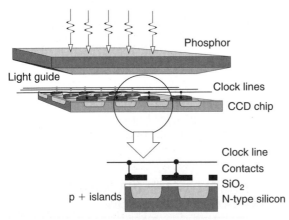

Figure 12.32 *The basic design for a charge-coupled device used in radiography. The three part construction includes X-ray phosphor, a light guide which directs the X-ray to light interactions onto the CCD surface. A cross section of the CCD shows the data/clock lines which move information via the contacts across the chip.*

voltage. Exposing the CCD to light generates a signal proportional to light intensity. Signal readout does not require an electron scanning beam unlike the vidicon/plumbicon camera tube. The clock lines select each row of pixel detectors in turn, then shift the contents from each detector to its neighbor causing the line to read out sequentially into a shift register and amplifier which produces an analog voltage. This process is virtually instantaneous. The voltage signal is converted to a digital value by an analog-to-digital converter and the digitized signal used for constructing the digital image matrix. Bit depths can be 8, 10 or 12.

Using the CCD for radiography requires a phosphor layer, acting as an X-ray converter. The CCD chip is fitted either with a luminescent screen or attached to the output screen of the image intensifier. In both cases a fiber optic light guide is necessary to match the imaging area of the phosphor with the CCD dimensions. The X-ray photons are converted into visible light photons which are detected by the CCD and form the digital image. The CCD has the following benefits over conventional vidicon/plumbicon camera tubes:

- There is no scanning electron beam to cause drifting.
- The fixed geometry of the CCD camera is uniform and distortion free (pincushion/barrel distortion).
- The CCD has a wide dynamic range (12 bits or 4096 gray levels).
- It has a low electronic noise.

12.6.2 Small field units

For small field-of-view applications such as dental radiography (typically a $25 \times 50\,mm$ detector size), an intensifying screen is used as the X-ray converter. The light emitted from the screen is collected by the CCD chip. For applications in which the field of view is only slightly larger than the area of the CCD chip, as in digital biopsy systems for mammography, a fiber-optic taper is placed between the intensifying screen and the CCD. This serves as an efficient lens that focuses the light produced in the screen onto the surface of the CCD chip. Typical fiber-optic tapers used in digital biopsy have front surfaces that measure $50 \times 50\,mm$ (abutted to the screen) and output surfaces that are $25 \times 25\,mm$ (abutted to the CCD). In these systems light is lost in the fiber-optic taper but most reaches the CCD chip.

DENTAL RADIOGRAPHY

CCD detectors the same size as dental film achieve a resolution of approximately 10 Lp mm^{-1}. The radiation dose for each exposure is only 10 to 20% of that for medium speed dental films. Reductions of approximately 50% are obtained when compared to faster films.

IMAGE INTENSIFIERS

These are fitted with CCD cameras, giving direct digital fluorography. However, recent image intensifiers have spatial resolutions of 4 to 5 Lp mm^{-1} which is not matched by the performance of the present family of CCD cameras.

MAMMOGRAPHY

Direct digital detectors, based on charge-coupled devices (CCD) coupled to phosphor screens are now used as an alternative to film-screen systems for use in small field mammography, particularly for stereotactic localizations in biopsy units (Fig. 12.33). Specifications for such a detector are given in Table 12.8. Systems for small field imaging (typically 5 × 5 cm to 8 × 5 cm) use a single CCD coupled to the intensifying screen either directly, through a minifying lens system, or via a fibre optic bundle.

A concern often shown with respect to digital mammography is the loss of spatial resolution compared with film-screen systems.

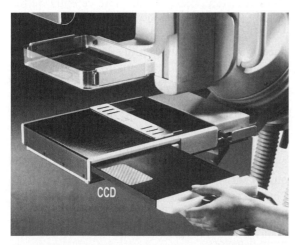

Figure 12.33 *A small field CCD unit forming part of a removable sensor in a mammography X-ray machine (courtesy Siemens).*

In small field mammography, CCD detectors have been used with pixel sizes as small as 24 μm (nominally equivalent to 20 Lp mm^{-1}); this approaches film-screen resolution.

12.6.3 Large field units

In large field of view radiography devices which use CCDs the light emitted from the large screen is focused onto the surface of the CCD chip but loses a very large fraction of the light photons. The amount of light lost is proportional to the demagnification factor required to couple the input area to the output area. Even with near perfect optical coupling, the light loss is significant and a **secondary quantum sink** is created, which is simply a signal bottleneck that can substantially increase image noise (quantum mottle) and degrades image quality. The number of light photons that reach the CCD can be on orders of magnitude less than those emitted by the scintillator. Although an image can be produced if a sufficient number of X-ray photons are used, any X-ray system with a large secondary quantum sink will be inefficient and result in relatively high patient radiation doses.

Lenses and fiber-optic tapers both generally introduce geometric distortions, light scatter, and reduced spatial resolution, and imperfections in the optical fiber bundles can introduce structure distortions and artifacts into the image.

MAMMOGRAPHY

Larger full field systems require an array of CCDs and the image is 'stitched' together. This results in stitching artifacts or loss of information where the segments

Table 12.8 *Typical small field biopsy unit.*

Image area	49 × 85 mm
Image matrix	1024 × 1792 or 2048 × 3584
Phosphor	Gadolinium oxysulfide
Pixel size	48 μm standard
	24 μm high resolution
Contrast	12 bits (4096 levels)
Resolution	10 Lp mm^{-1} standard
	13 Lp mm^{-1} high resolution
DQE	
1 Lp mm^{-1}	45%
2 Lp mm^{-1}	35%

Table 12.9 *The specifications for a full field mammography unit using a scanning beam and moving CCD array.*

CCD size	10 × 220 mm slot
Scintillator	CsI
Image area	220 × 300 mm
Image matrix	4096 × 5624
Pixel size	54 μm standard
	27 μm high resolution
Contrast	12 bits (4096 levels)
Resolution	9.25 Lp mm^{-1} standard
	18.5 Lp mm^{-1} high resolution
DQE	
1 Lp mm^{-1}	50 to 55%
2 Lp mm^{-1}	40%

of the image join. An alternative approach employs a scanning beam technique in conjunction with a moving linear CCD array. One of the current full field systems (Table 12.9) based on a CCD array has a pixel size of 40 μm with a theoretical limiting resolution of approximately 12 Lp mm^{-1}.

12.7 DIRECT RADIOGRAPHY (LARGE AREA)

The hypothetical 'ideal' direct radiography (DR) system would produce images of higher quality than conventional systems. It would have high spatial resolution, contrast resolution, and dose efficiency. The detector itself would be robust, solid state, and much like existing film-screen systems in size, weight, and ease of use, while completely eliminating cassette handling. Because the entire system is digital, it would interface well with the hospital information systems and conveniently output images to printers, archives, and workstations.

Large-area, flat panel, solid state detectors with integrated, thin-film transistor readout mechanisms comply with most requirements of an 'ideal' DR system. Present models give fast access to digital images wherever radiography with stationary X-ray equipment is performed, and can provide image quality that exceeds that of both film-screen and computed radiography (CR). However, CR has a financial advantage and will continue to play an important role in many applications where economic factors predominate.

Differences exist among the available DR detector materials, both in terms of how they capture the X-ray image and in the resulting image quality. Large area flat-panel digital radiographic X-ray detectors can be divided into two classes:

- **Direct conversion detectors**: in which X-ray energy is converted directly into electric charge
- **Indirect conversion detectors**: where an intermediate phosphor is used. The two most common phosphor-scintillators are cesium iodide (CsI:Na) and gadolinium oxysulfide (Gd$_2$O$_2$S).

Both direct and indirect conversion detectors have readout within a few seconds.

EARLY MODELS

Most imaging devices in radiology depend on the process of luminescence. For instance: an intensifying screen in film imaging, an image intensifier with a phosphor scintillator behind its face plate or the image phosphor plate.

Electrostatic imaging, using selenium as the detector, does not rely on luminescence. Amorphous selenium is used as an X-ray detector by first applying an electric charge to its surface (amorphous selenium has a very high resistivity). When exposed to light or X-rays, the selenium plate acts as a **photoconductor**, generating electron–electron hole pairs which results in local surface discharging in areas exposed to X-rays, leaving behind a latent 'discharge' image. Selenium is widely used in photocopiers and has been used in xero-radiography X-ray systems, although xero-radiography was unreliable and eventually replaced by fast screen-film systems and more recently by full field direct radiography devices.

Selenium detector technology has been reintroduced for chest imaging (Philips Thoravision) where the X-ray image was captured by a drum shaped detector and then read directly by a linear array of electrometer probes placed very close to the plate surface. The probes covered the drum vertically, and as the drum rotated past the detector array, the electrometer probes read the image by 'sensing' the differences in charge on the plate surface. The image quality was good for both resolution and contrast. The selenium was about 500 μm thick deposited on a metal surface. The mode of action for the Thoravision unit follows a path common to all selenium detectors:

1   Plate preparation by applying a uniform electrical charge (1500 V) on its surface.

2 Charged surface exposed to X-rays when free electrons generated from the ionizing events locally discharge the plate surface, imparting the image pattern (i.e. chest radiograph).

3 The charge pattern on the surface scanned with a small electrode assembly at about 100 μm from the plate surface. The Thoravision scan time is approximately 10 s.

After readout the plate is recharged ready for the next exposure. The electrical image signals are collected and form an image matrix of typically 2000 × 2000 pixels giving a 2 Lp mm^{-1} resolution 14 bits deep. This selenium image has a good dynamic range and since the image is carried by surface charges it does not suffer from the same disadvantage of light diffusion as luminescent phosphors.

12.7.1 Large area TFT arrays

Advances in photolithography and electronic microfabrication techniques have enabled the development of large-area detectors with integrated readout mechanisms based on thin film transistor (TFT) arrays. This has been made possible by the progress in the manufacture of flat computer display screens which use the same TFT technology. Flat electronic detectors using TFTs provide direct digital registration of X-ray images without the intermediate stage of optical or mechanical scanning.

Large area TFT arrays are used as the active electronic switching elements in practically all flat panel digital radiography systems. In both direct- and indirect-conversion detectors, the image pattern produced during X-ray exposure is stored by the TFT detector matrix as an electric charge (obtained directly from either an electrostatic or indirectly via a photoconductive signal). After the exposure, the TFT-switching electronics directs the stored signals on these charge plates to amplifiers and analog-to-digital converters so producing a raw digital image. This allows immediate readout which is an important feature of all flat panel electronic detectors.

TFT arrays are deposited onto a glass substrate in multiple layers, beginning with read-out electronics at the lowest level, followed by charge-collector arrays at higher levels (Fig. 12.34). Then, depending on the type of detector being constructed, X-ray-sensitive elements, light-sensitive elements, or both are deposited to form the top layer of this complex electronic

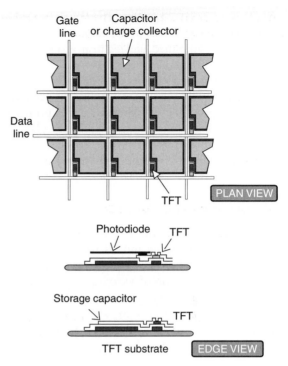

Figure 12.34 *A section of a TFT array showing the small TFT adjacent to a much larger storage capacitor. Data and gate lines enable the image information to be fed out. The selected edge view shows the TFT signals supplied by either a charge electrode or photodiode feeding a storage capacitor.*

structure. The entire assembly is then encased in a protective enclosure with external cabling for computer connections. As with all electronic devices, the more layers that are needed, the greater the complexity of the fabrication process. This generally lowers yield and reliability.

Unlike CCD-based detectors, image signal collection and read-out electronics in flat panel TFT based detectors are immediately adjacent to the layer in which the X-rays interact; either a photoconductive X-ray detector in the case of 'direct' conversion or scintillator plus photodiode detector in the case of 'indirect' converters. These X-ray detectors do not require any form of intermediate stage of optical light-guides, lenses optical coupling, image demagnification or mechanical scanning which allows for a compact design and provides immediate access to the digital images without distortion.

The signals from the individual sensors are read out in sequence. All sensors in the first row are activated simultaneously via a gate line. The signals are led in parallel via the data lines in the column direction to preamplifiers, amplified, and led to an analog–digital converter. When the first row has been completely digitized, the second row is activated. This process continues until the whole X-ray image has been read out. As the process is electronic it can, in principle, achieve very high transfer rates, so this type of detector can acquire dynamic image sequences. This immediate readout is an important feature of all flat panel detectors.

MONOLITHIC PANELS VERSUS TILED ARRAYS

Because fabrication of full-size TFT-detector panels is technically challenging and can have relatively low yields, many manufacturers reduce costs by constructing detectors that consist of two or more smaller panels in a **tiled** configuration. In these detectors, digital image processing is used to 'stitch together' the image sections to eliminate the appearance of the tile junctions.

APERTURE

Detectors for digital radiography are composed of discrete elements, generally of constant size and spacing. Figure 12.35 shows the construction of two flat detector types. The dimension of the active portion of each detector element defines an **aperture** or **pixel pitch**. The aperture determines the spatial frequency response of the detector. The detector element in Fig. 12.35a is 173^2; the active pixel element is 140^2 so the pixel area represents $140^2/173^2$ or 65% of the available area. This is the **fill factor** which has an ideal value of 100% signifying that the entire area of the TFT array is used in pixel formation. However, the area taken by data

lines, transistor and connecting network restricts the area available for the charge collector. The example in Fig. 12.35b shows that even when the detector element has decreased to 140^2 with a pixel area of 100^2 the fill factor (51%) is decreased further since the ancillary components represent a greater proportion of the detector element. Figure 12.36 plots the variation of fill factor with pixel size. Usually as the pixel pitch becomes smaller the fill factor degrades leading to image losses.

BAD PIXELS AND ROWS

Fabricating perfect thin-film transistor arrays is extremely difficult and therefore expensive, so practical

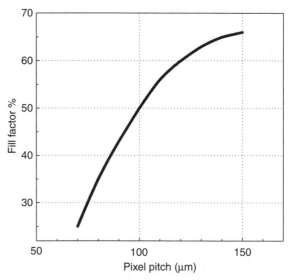

Figure 12.36 *A plot of fill factor versus pixel pitch. The area taken by the TFT and connecting matrix does not alter greatly when pixel sizes are reduced so the fill factor decreases.*

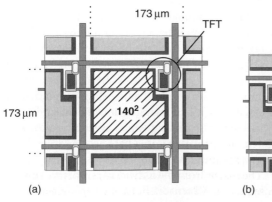

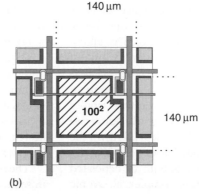

(a)   (b)

Figure 12.35 *A section of the TFT array identifying actual pixel area and pixel pitch or active pixel area (hatched). The fill factor is calculated in the text.*

limits with regard to the number of defects allowed in these devices must be established by each manufacturer. Defects may show as individual bad pixels or entire bad pixel columns or rows. As fabricating methods improve, TFT matrix quality and size will also improve. This is most commonly demonstrated in computer flat panel TFT displays which use the identical fabrication technique.

DETECTOR ELEMENT AND MATRIX SIZE

The physical dimensions of the X-ray detector have an obvious influence on the radiographic examinations performed. It is critical that the detector be sufficiently large to capture the desired anatomic views. Electronic detectors for standing radiographic examinations, for example, would ideally have an active detector that is at least 35 × 43 cm (14 × 17″) in size and allow both vertical (35 × 43 cm) and horizontal (43 × 35 cm) imaging orientations. Rectangular formats also correspond to workstations, monitors, and X-ray printers which normally provide output of the same aspect ratio.

The maximum spatial resolution of an image is defined by detector-element size (pixel pitch) and spacing. For example, spatial frequencies above $2.5 \, \mathrm{Lp \, mm^{-1}}$ would be limited by a system with a $200 \, \mu m$ detector-element size. The limiting frequency for a $139 \, \mu m$ pixel DR system is $3.6 \, \mathrm{Lp \, mm^{-1}}$, encompassing all the spatial frequency of interest for general radiographic imaging. Chest radiography $200 \, \mu m$ pixel spacing $2.5 \, \mathrm{Lp \, mm^{-1}}$ is adequate for most diagnostic tasks.

The calculations in Box 12.2 give examples of current DR pixel sizes and their expected resolution. Figure 12.37a plots the relationship between pixel size and image resolution measured in $\mathrm{Lp \, mm^{-1}}$. The formula used is derived from that seen previously in Section 12.3.2.

Box 12.2 Pixel size and spatial resolution

If the pixel size is in μm (p) and the resolution cut-off in $\mathrm{Lp \, mm^{-1}}$, then by using the formula

$$\mathrm{Lp \, mm^{-1}} = \frac{1000}{2p}$$

a pixel size of $100 \, \mu m$ will give

$$\frac{1000}{2 \times 100} = 5 \, \mathrm{Lp \, mm^{-1}}$$

Similarly $139 \, \mu m$ will give $3.59 \, \mathrm{Lp \, mm^{-1}}$, and $70 \, \mu m$ will give $7.1 \, \mathrm{Lp \, mm^{-1}}$.

Figure 12.37a plots size of pixel with spatial resolution limit.

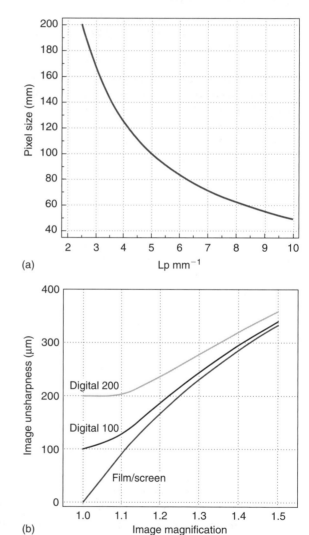

(a)

(b)

Figure 12.37 (a) The relationship between pixel size and spatial resolution, as calculated from the formula in Box 12.2 measured as line pairs per mm (Lp mm⁻¹). (b) The image unsharpness plotted for a DR detector having 100 and 200μm pixel dimensions. Image magnification (x-axis) is across a 22 cm cross section using a 70 cm SID.

DETECTOR UNSHARPNESS

Four factors determine overall **image receptor unsharpness**:

- Focal spot size
- Imaging geometry (SID and OID)
- Patient movement
- Detector unsharpness

The first two factors influence the geometric unsharpness and have been dealt with in the analog image (Chapter 8). If the exposure time is short movement unsharpness will be small and can be neglected.

However, for a digital image and its pixilated construction (matrix) other factors influence the image unsharpness (laser readout scan pitch, pixel dimensions); these together contribute towards the **detector unsharpness**. These contributions can be combined in quadrature to give an overall unsharpness U. Image magnification M is included which represents object distance from the imaging surface:

$$U = \frac{1}{M}\sqrt{(M-1)^2 f^2 + F^2} \qquad (12.2)$$

where f is the focal spot size and F the receptor unsharpness. For magnification $M = 1$ where the object is on the surface of the imaging detector/cassette the formula can be simplified to:

$$U = \sqrt{f^2 + F^2} \qquad (12.3)$$

Overall unsharpness is not increased significantly if a sufficiently small focal spot is used.

In Fig. 12.37b, eqn 12.2 has been used to compare film-screen (with theoretical detector unsharpness of zero) with two digital detectors, plotting 100 and 200μm pixel sizes.

Mammography requires smaller pixel sizes, probably in the range of 50 to 100 μm per pixel; most recent offer 70 μm or 7 Lp mm^{-1}. Although some detectors can offer substantially higher pixel pitch, it should be remembered that any advantages that may be gained by using larger image matrices also have drawbacks in practical implementation, including:

- Lower fill factor
- Image noise levels
- Increased data volume
- Increased archiving requirements
- The requirement for image size reduction for displaying on video monitors

Differences exist among the available detectors, both in terms of how they capture the X-ray image and in the resulting image quality. These can be appreciated by distinguishing two distinct flat panel digital radiography technologies currently available:

- **Direct conversion detectors**, in which X-ray energy is converted directly into electric charge using a photoconductive detector (selenium).
- **Indirect conversion detectors**, in which X-ray energy is first converted to light by an X-ray scintillator. The two most common scintillators are cesium iodide (used in X-ray image intensifiers) and gadolinium oxysulfide (used in conventional X-ray intensifying screens).

Both direct and indirect conversion detectors have instantaneous readout.

DETECTOR MATERIALS

The common phosphor materials used for indirect conversion DR panels are terbium doped gadolinium oxysulfide (Gd_2O_2S: Tb^{3+}) and thallium doped cesium iodide CsI:Tl. The physical properties of these together with selenium and the common phosphor used in CR image plates (BaFBrX) are compared in Table 12.10.

The linear attenuation coefficients for detector materials used in flat panel direct radiography are compared in Fig. 12.38. Gadolinium shows higher absorption over the diagnostic imaging range (50 to 100 kV) and selenium shows the lowest absorption.

Table 12.10 *Physical properties of common detector materials.*

Parameter	Direct/indirect DR system		
	a-Se	**CsI:(Na)**	**Gd_2O_2S:(Tb^{3+})**
Equivalent Z	34	55	64
Density (kg m^{-3})	4500	4510	7440
Sensitivity*	50	19	13
Signal**	0.6	0.87	0.92
Practical detector thickness (μm)	500 to 1000	500 to 600	500 to 600
K edge (keV)	12.6	33	50.2
Absorption at 60 keV (%)	52	80	90

*Sensitivity = electron–hole pair.
**Signal = comparative fluorescent yield.

12.7.2 Flat panel detectors: direct conversion

Direct-conversion flat panel digital detectors use the X-ray photoconductor material, **amorphous selenium** (a-Se), to directly convert X-ray quanta into an electric charge pattern. This is the simplest method, since it requires no intensifying screens, intermediate steps or additional processes. Amorphous selenium is well developed technologically; it has been used for decades in photocopiers, photocells, and exposure meters for photographic use, as well as in solar cells. Because selenium is used in its amorphous form, large area selenium plates can be made by vapor deposition, a highly reproducible and cost-effective technology.

Amorphous selenium has acceptable X-ray-detection properties and extremely high intrinsic spatial resolution. A typical design uses a 1000 μm thick layer of amorphous selenium deposited on a 2560×3072 lithographically fabricated array of thin film transistors (TFT array described above). Selenium is a photoconductor that, when exposed to radiation, alters its electrical conductivity proportional to the intensity of the radiation. In a first step, prior to the X-ray exposure, a homogeneous electrical charge (a 5 kV **bias voltage**) is applied to the surface of the selenium through an electrode layer. In the second step the selenium is exposed to the X-ray beam and these photons are absorbed in the selenium layer, liberating electrons. These electrons pass to the surface of the selenium layer where they neutralize part of the applied charge. This discharge is proportional to the radiation intensity and results in a latent charge image. Electric charges are drawn along the electric field lines directly to the charge-storage-capacitor electrodes connected to TFT. In the third step this pattern of charges is electrically scanned, and converted into a digital signal stored as a charge by each TFT. Detector elements are effectively separated by electric-field shaping within the selenium layer. Therefore, the entire selenium surface is available for X-ray charge conversion. Charge-collection electrode design results in effective **fill factors** approaching 100% (see later). Data is captured at 14 bit depth and digitized to 12 bits per pixel detector element.

The selenium detector is very susceptible to humidity and temperature variations so requires extensive protection from the environment. Typical specifications for a commercially produced DR flat panel direct detector using a-Se are listed in Table 12.11 and the basic construction outlined in Fig. 12.39. More recent developments have produced full-field mammography systems using a-Se direct conversion detectors with a pixel pitch of 70 μm and spatial resolutions of 7.0 Lp mm^{-1}.

12.7.3 Flat panel detectors: indirect conversion

Indirect flat-panel digital radiography detectors use doped phosphor scintillators commonly used in

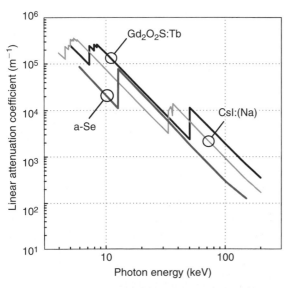

Figure 12.38 *Linear attenuation coefficient for direct detector selenium and indirect detectors cesium iodide and gadolinium oxysulfide.*

Table 12.11 *DR panel direct (amorphous selenium).*

Component	Specification
Active area	35×43 cm
Detector	a-Se over TFT
Element array	2560×3072
Active element	129×129 μm
Element pitch	139×139 μm
Fill factor	86 to 100%
Spatial resolution	3.6 Lp mm^{-1}
Pixel depth	14 bit
DQE @ 60 keV	60%
Dynamic range	1:10000
Display time	7 s

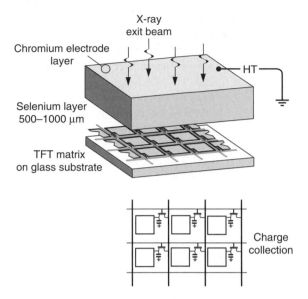

Figure 12.39 *The essential components of an a-Se direct conversion flat panel detector. The TFT layer on its glass substrate reads the pixel information from the selenium X-ray detector. This has a high voltage power supply attached, which supplies a bias voltage via the top electrode layer before exposure.*

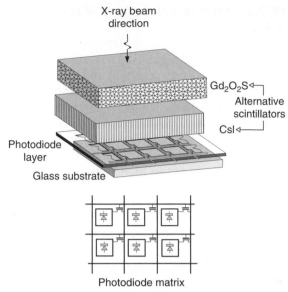

Figure 12.40 *Two indirect scintillation detector designs using gadolinium oxysulfide (unstructured) and cesium iodide (structured) with photodiode + TFT signal collection.*

film/screen and image intensifiers (gadolinium oxysulfide and cesium iodide). These phosphors are used as the image converter layer producing light when exposed to X-ray photons.

Indirect-conversion systems, in common with direct-conversion systems, use large TFT arrays. In addition a photosensitive p-i-n silicon photodiode layer (<1 μm thick) is placed as a top layer forming a photodiode/TFT sandwich. On top of this is the phosphor scintillator layer approximately 500 μm thick. The photodiode/phosphor layers replace the single X-ray photoconductor layer (a-Se) that is used in direct conversion devices.

When X-rays strike the scintillator, visible light is emitted proportional to the incident X-ray flux. Visible light photons are then converted into an electric signal by the photodiode array, which is transferred to be stored as a charge on the TFT capacitor. The signal is read out by activation of scanning control lines for each row of the device, in an identical manner to the direct conversion DR. The principle of operation of an indirect detector is shown schematically in Fig. 12.40.

The phosphor materials used for indirect-conversion fall into two categories:

- **Unstructured**: commonly, terbium doped gadolinium oxysulfide produced as a uniform layer of crystals held in a binder
- **Structured**: thallium doped cesium iodide, a material borrowed from image intensifier technology

UNSTRUCTURED SCINTILLATORS

Terbium doped gadolinium oxysulfide (Gd_2O_2S:Tb), similar to the familiar intensifying screen material in film radiology, is used as the X-ray/visible light converter. All indirect conversion DR systems which use phosphor materials (both unstructured and structured) lose some of the light energy by scattering. Scattering causes the light to spread laterally over distances equal to or greater than the thickness of the scintillator so light photons generated from a single X-ray photon interaction can spread to a number of adjacent pixel sites, so reducing spatial resolution. Table 12.12 lists a typical specification and Fig. 12.41 shows commercially available fixed and portable cassettes using an indirect scintillator flat panel detector.

STRUCTURED SCINTILLATORS

In order to reduce the problem of light scattering some manufacturers use structured scintillators developed

Table 12.12 *Indirect conversion: Gd_2O_2S:Tb unstructured scintillator.*

Component	Specification
Active area	22.5 ×28.7 cm (8.8″ ×11.3″)
Detector	Gd_2O_2S:Tb + photodiode over TFT
Thickness	500 μm
Element array	2256 × 2878
Pixel pitch	100 μm
Element pitch	140 μm
Fill factor	52%
Spatial resolution	5 Lp mm^{-1}
Pixel depth	12 bit
Display time	3 s

from image intensifier technology. This phosphor consists of doped cesium iodide crystals grown directly onto the detector. The structure consists of discrete and parallel monoclinic 'needles' of CsI:Tl, 5 to 10 μm wide and up to 600 μm long. The crystals are highly hygroscopic (readily absorbing water vapor) and quickly degrade if not completely sealed. The monoclinic crystalline structure behaves in a similar manner to fiber-optic channels, steering light to the photodiode detector. Since light spreading is greatly reduced thicker layers of phosphor material can be used, increasing the number of X-ray photon interactions and thus the quantum efficiency. Table 12.13 lists a typical specification for this model.

12.7.4 Comparisons: detector performance

X-ray image quality depends on maintaining a high signal-to-noise ratio throughout the entire imaging chain. Evaluation and selection of a digital radiographic system should involve a thorough analysis of the complete imaging system, including the X-ray detector itself and the environment in which the system will be used. Beyond this, DR systems must provide connectivity to DICOM and HIS/RIS systems as well as to the image processing needed to produce high-quality display-ready images.

QUANTUM EFFICIENCY

In order to contribute to image formation X-ray photons must first interact with the detector material. The probability of photon interaction or quantum

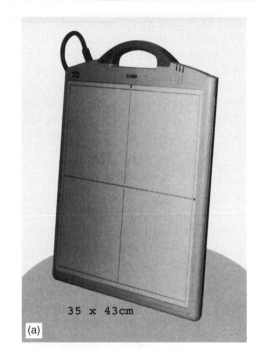

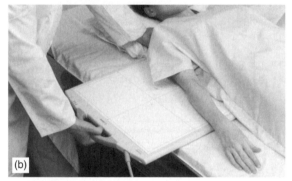

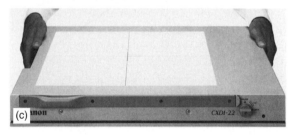

Figure 12.41 *Indirect conversion portable (a and b) and fixed cassettes (c) (courtesy Canon plc.).*

efficiency (η) for a photon energy E is given by:

$$\eta = 1 - \exp[-\mu(E)t] \tag{12.4}$$

where $\mu(E)$ is the linear attenuation coefficient of the detector material, at the chosen energy E, having a thickness t. In practice X-ray beams used in radiology are polyenergetic, so the quantum efficiency is expressed as an 'effective' value covering the spectrum of X-rays incident on the detector.

The quantum efficiency of the detector material can be increased by increasing detector thickness or by using materials having a higher μ. Using eqn 12.4, Fig. 12.42 plots the quantum efficiencies of three detector materials (Se, CsI and Gd_2O_2S,) for a photon energy range from 40 to 100 keV and detector thickness of 500 μm. Quantum efficiency is generally highest at low energies, decreasing with increasing energy. Quantum efficiency increases markedly above any K edge. Gadolinium shows a consistently high quantum efficiency over the total range 40 to 100 kV while selenium shows a marked drop off in efficiency for the higher photon energies.

DYNAMIC RANGE

In practice, the required dynamic range into two components:

- The ratio between the X-ray attenuation of the most radiolucent and most radio-opaque paths through the patient to be included on the same image
- The precision of X-ray signal to be measured in the part of the image representing the most radio-opaque anatomy. If, for example, there was a factor of 50 in attenuation across the image field and it was desired to have 1% precision in measuring the signal in the most attenuating region, then the dynamic range requirement would be 5000.

The dynamic range requirements for certain applications may exceed the capabilities of available detectors. Figure 12.43 shows the linear dynamic range given by digital radiography, compared to the sigma response of film-screen. A theoretical range of 5 orders of magnitude is given by both digital detector systems as against the film-screen of 1 to 2 orders of magnitude. In practice the dynamic range for a digital detector is restricted since a photon deficient, low exposure value (below 0.2 μGy) gives a noisy image. High doses are also possible without image degradation although patient high exposure levels are to be discouraged.

Table 12.13 *Indirect conversion: CsI:Tl structured scintillator.*

Component	Specification
Active area	43 × 43 cm (17″ × 17″)
Detector	CsI:Tl + photodiode over TFT
Thickness	550 to 600 μm
Element array	2688 × 2688 pixels
Pixel pitch	143 μm
Element pitch	173 μm
Fill factor	68%
Spatial resolution	3.5 Lp mm^{-1}
Pixel depth	12 bit
Display time	10 s

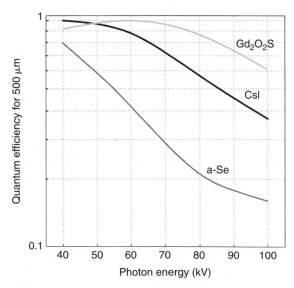

Figure 12.42 *The quantum efficiency for gadolinium oxysulfide, cesium iodide and selenium. Detector thickness is 500 μm in all cases.*

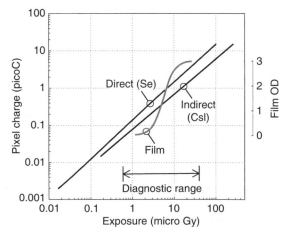

Figure 12.43 *Dynamic range graph for direct DR (a-selenium), indirect DR (CsI) and film. The diagnostic photon energy range is marked.*

FILL FACTOR DIFFERENCES

Before exposure the selenium detector plate is prepared by applying an electric field using a bias electrode on the top surface of the selenium. As X-rays are absorbed in the detector electrons and holes are released within the selenium material which locally discharge the surface electric field (see Fig. 6.15). Electric charges within the selenium are drawn directly to the charge collecting electrodes (Fig. 12.44). The entire selenium surface is available for X-ray charge conversion and, importantly, with properly designed charge collection electrodes, effective fill factors approaching 100% are achievable. Figure 12.44 illustrates the better fill factor obtainable with a direct selenium detector in spite of the TFT pixel size limitation. This is not the case for indirect scintillation detectors.

UNIFORMITY

It is important that the radiographic imaging system provide uniformity, i.e. the sensitivity be constant over the entire area of the image giving a 'fixed pattern noise'. In an analog imaging system, great pains must be taken in the design and manufacture of detectors to ensure that they provide uniform response. In a digital system, the task is much easier, because, at least over a considerable range, differences in response from element to element can be corrected.

SENSITIVITY

The final output from virtually all X-ray detectors is an electrical signal, so that sensitivity can be defined in terms of the charge produced by the detector (before any external amplification) per incident X-ray quantum of a specified energy. The sensitivity of any imaging system depends on photon absorption (Fig. 12.38) and on the primary conversion efficiency (the efficiency of converting the energy of the interacting X-ray to a more easily measurable form such as optical quanta or electric charge). Conversion efficiency can be expressed in terms of the energy

necessary to release a light photon in a phosphor, an electron–hole pair in a photoconductor (or semiconductor) or an electron–ion pair in a gaseous detector. Sensitivity values (hole–pair formation) for some typical detector materials have already been given in Table 12.10.

12.7.5 Comparisons: image quality

Digital radiography projection images originally used storage phosphor imaging plates (see photostimulable phosphor plate). A major disadvantage with such plates is that the handling process involves similar work operation as for common film-screen systems so patient throughput is not improved. The need for 'on-line' imaging offered by direct radiography systems has been a significant advance since, in such systems, the image is read out from the image receptor in seconds without moving it from the exposure position.

IMAGE SPATIAL RESOLUTION

This varies substantially, depending on physical detector characteristics. As already mentioned, limiting spatial resolution is determined by the pixel spacing in the detector. The frequency that characterizes this limiting resolution is known as the Nyquist frequency. It is simply the inverse of twice the pixel spacing.

The MTF of the direct-detector system remains high up to the Nyquist frequency. The small observed drop in MTF for the direct conversion detector results only from the physical size of the pixel. Higher Nyquist frequency and MTF allow visualization of finer diagnostic details.

Geometrical factors, such as focal spot size and magnification between the anatomical structure of interest and the plane of the image receptor, photon scattering, and patient movement are extrinsic sources of image unsharpness. Factors that influence the intrinsic spatial resolution of the detector arise from its effective aperture size, spatial sampling interval between measurements and any lateral scattering

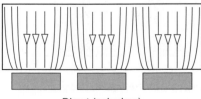

Direct (selenium)

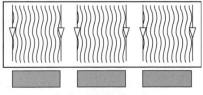

Indirect (scintillator)

Figure 12.44 *Fill patterns for direct and indirect detector designs.*

effects of the X-ray or light photons within the detector or readout.

MODULATION TRANSFER FUNCTION

This describes the fraction of each frequency component that will be preserved in the captured image. The MTF of all current technologies except the direct-conversion detector falls off substantially at higher spatial frequencies (Fig. 12.45). Owing to the set pixel dimensions of all direct digital TFT systems the MTF is cut off abruptly at a line pair value determined by the pixel dimension. However, the MTF of the direct-detector system remains high up to this Nyquist frequency.

Digital radiography systems currently suffer from an inferior spatial resolution compared to film. However, the digital systems have far better low contrast resolution than film.

ANTISCATTER GRID

Any digital imaging system that includes an antiscatter grid has the potential for interaction between the grid lines (i.e. lead septa) and the rows of pixels that constitute the digital image. For example, grid line artifacts often manifest in a 'corduroy pattern' of lines on the image owing to image aliasing: however, some high-strip-count grids do not leave apparent grid lines on digital images. Artifacts that can be produced by grid interaction are not always obvious and can degrade image quality, so caution and proper selection of the grid are advised.

NOISE

X-ray image quality depends on achieving a high signal-to-noise ratio throughout the entire imaging chain which would include:

- Good quantum efficiency of the phosphor
- Optimum signal transfer/collection by the charge capacitor
- Noise free readout of the stored signal

Direct radiography systems convert X-ray image information into electronic charges held by the TFT capacitor. Because indirect-conversion systems rely on light, substantial scatter occurs before the energy is converted to charge; this reduces signal-to-noise ratio.

THE QUANTUM SINK

Figure 12.46 illustrates signal losses and signal gains through the various energy conversion stages of a flat panel electronic detector system.

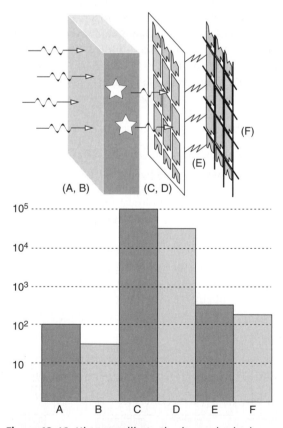

Figure 12.46 *Histogram illustrating loss and gains in a direct radiography detector.*

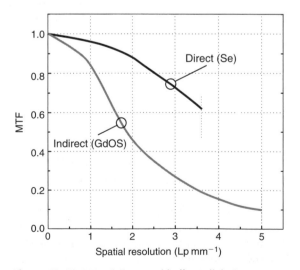

Figure 12.45 *MTF of direct and indirect digital systems.*

Assuming a certain photon flux incident on the detector surface (Column A where $N = 100$). A fraction of these are absorbed and interact given by the quantum detection efficiency with the detector (Column B where $N \approx 40$). The mean number of photons interacting at this stage represents the **primary quantum sink** of the flat panel detector. Photon fluctuation defines the SNR of the imaging system; the SNR increasing as $\sqrt{N}$ of the interacting photon number. This is the primary SNR of the imaging system defining the SNR of the imaging system as a whole. So the system is **X-ray quantum limited**. The total SNR will become further reduced as the signal passes through the imaging system from light production, signal transformation and image signal output.

Further losses occur at subsequent stages and are reduced if the detector provides adequate quantum gain. Columns C and D illustrate light photon creation in the photodiode and the escape of light photons from the phosphor. Here, light absorption, scattering and reflection processes are important.

Further losses occur in the coupling of the light to the photodetector which converts light to electronic charge (Column E) and in the spectral sensitivity and optical quantum efficiency of the photodetector (Column F). The statistical fluctuation of the light or charge at this point becomes an additional important noise source.

If the conversion gain of the phosphor is not sufficiently high to overcome these losses and the number of light quanta or electronic charges at a subsequent stage falls below that at the primary quantum sink, then a **secondary quantum sink** is formed.

In this case the statistical fluctuation of the light or charge at this point becomes an additional important noise source. Even when an actual secondary sink does not exist, a low value of light or charge will cause increased noise.

This becomes especially important when a spatial-frequency-dependent analysis of SNR is carried out and, as discussed earlier, its effect is to cause reduction of the detective quantum efficiency with increasing spatial frequency.

DETECTIVE QUANTUM EFFICIENCY

The detector modulation transfer function, when expressed as a function of spatial frequency, is not a useful measure of overall system performance. Digital images can be processed to alter apparent image sharpness: however, excessive processing can lead to an increased image noise. Detective quantum efficiency (DQE) is the best and most widely accepted overall measure of detector image-quality performance and is a useful quantity for characterizing the overall signal and noise performance of imaging detectors.

Detective quantum efficiency combines spatial resolution (i.e. modulation transfer function) and image noise (i.e. noise power spectrum) to provide a measure of the signal-to-noise ratio of the various frequency components of the image. The DQE of real detectors does not have a single value, but varies depending on kV_p and exposure (μGy or mR). The information available in the image is limited by the number of X-ray quanta incident on the imaging detector, which in turn is related to patient dose.

Higher detective quantum efficiency values suggest greater image quality, although the results should be evaluated at all frequencies to estimate the ability of the image to depict both small and large image structures. DQE describes the efficiency in transferring the signal-to-noise ratio contained in the incident X-ray pattern to the signal-to-noise ratio of the detector output (see eqn 12.1).

An ideal imaging system accurately records every incident X-ray quantum and is characterized by a DQE of 1.0 for all frequencies. Real imaging systems, however, always have a DQE of less than 1.0 because of inefficiencies in detecting the incident X-ray quanta and internal sources of noise. Since noise is predominantly high frequency, it often causes the DQE to decrease with increasing spatial frequency.

Because of the light scatter inherent in indirect detectors, there is a trade-off between X-ray absorption and MTF. Increasing the thickness of the scintillator of an indirect detector may increase the low-frequency DQE, but the high-frequency DQE will be reduced by the lower MTF that results from increased light-scatter. Since DR systems using selenium are not limited by light scatter, detector thickness and so X-ray absorption can be increased without a great loss of MTF.

DQE for a film-screen detector typically has a value on the order of 0.2 at a spatial frequency of 0 cycles mm^{-1} and this may fall to 0.05 at a few cycles mm^{-1}. The maximum reported DQE for film-screen and computed radiography are typically 0.15 to 0.25. By comparison, the maximum DQE of a DR system, measured under similar conditions, is nearer 0.5 (Fig. 12.47).

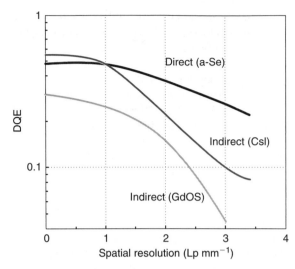

Figure 12.47 *DQE as a function of spatial frequency for three detector systems a-Se, gadolium oxysulfide and cesium iodide diagnostic exposure levels at 70 kV$_p$.*

Table 12.14 *Comparison of DQEs in various detectors at 1 and 2 Lp mm^{-1}.*

DQE value Lp mm^{-1}	Selenium (%)	CsI (%)	GdOS (%)	BaFBr (CR) (%)
1	50	45 to 50	25	25 to 35
2	40	20	15	20 to 26

The selenium detector is more susceptible to humidity and temperature variations than the storage phosphor detector and therefore requires extensive protection from the environment.

TEMPORAL RESOLUTION (IMAGE ACQUISITION TIME)

For serial or static radiographic imaging, the precision of a pixel value (bit depth or the number of gray levels) is related to the readout time; the larger bit depths requiring a longer readout time, generally resulting in more precise image values.

Since image readout involves charge collection from each TFT pixel element, an incomplete charge transfer can lead to inaccurate pixel values later if a subsequent exposure is used without taking the residual charge into account; the result is an electronic memory artifact.

Rapid serial image acquisition, as in the case of 20 to 30 frames per second fluoroscopy, can lead to image artifacts owing to X-ray induced residual charge trapping. For these reasons, not all direct radiography designs are practical for use where high exposure levels or high-speed image acquisition is required.

FACTORS INFLUENCING DETECTIVE QUANTUM EFFICIENCY

These include less than complete X-ray absorption, factors which reduce the amplitude of the signal profile (as measured by MTF), and additional sources of noise. Indirect technologies suffer other sources of added noise that are practically absent in direct detectors. The brightness and lateral spread of the light event produced by an absorbed X-ray depends on the depth of interaction in the scintillator (similar to film intensifying screens). This important source of variability adds noise to the image and substantially reduces the DQE, particularly at high frequencies. In a direct-conversion system the number of electrons produced and their lateral spread (virtually none) are both independent of the depth at which an X-ray interacts.

The major advantage of the selenium detector is its high detective quantum efficiency which is significantly higher than that of other image detectors, both digital and conventional (see Table 12.14). Like photostimulable storage phosphors, selenium detectors possess a very wide dynamic range; unlike storage phosphors, as mentioned before, selenium detectors do not require stimulation for image readout, which eliminates a source of image noise and improves image quality. The spatial resolution is comparable to that of storage phosphor systems; however, the absence of light scattering in the detector provides an improved sharpness impression.

12.7.6 Digital image post-processing

There are numerous examples of digital radiology's capability for image processing. Image contrast characteristics are no longer dependent on exposure conditions as in the case of film-screen imaging (contrast resolution), but they can now be influenced and optimized by post exposure image enhancement. Image processing algorithms can also improve the optical appearance of detail structures up to the nominal detector spatial resolution by using spatial filtering, either edge enhancement or smoothing or a combination of both; image smoothing reduces image noise before applying edge enhancement.

Contrast of lung structure and the mediastinum together with soft tissue information can be enhanced by 'histogram equalization'. This prevents less important gray-scale value information from being included in the determination of displayed image contrast and influencing the display quality of diagnostically important areas so improving the contrast resolution in the area of interest.

Different gradation curves taken from look-up tables are available for primary contrast processing. The flat panel X-ray detector with its wide range of exposures and large-contrast resolution requires sensible image processing in order to extract the full diagnostic information. Image processing of the digital image performs basic tasks such as:

- Dynamic range management
- Contrast and gray-scale management
- Consistent image quality which is device-independent (hard copy/soft copy)

Local processing using soft-copy review can alter contrast and brightness (using window width and window level) which provides enhanced visibility of important structures. Finally, electronic archiving, combined with networking capabilities allows a cost-effective storage of images that can then be duplicated anywhere and at any time without loss of quality.

DYNAMIC RANGE VARIATION

Variation of dynamic range compresses the input dynamic range into the available dynamic range of the output device. A mammography system has a very large input dynamic range (12 bits or nearly three times that of film). On output, a typical monitor can display only 256 shades of gray (8 bits) while a typical printer can only achieve a maximal optical density of 3.5. Breast thickness compensation algorithms give dynamic range compression. It allows the visualization of the entire breast from the chest wall through to the skin line.

CONTRAST ENHANCEMENT

Contrast management selects the local and general contrast. Large-scale contrast variations, with confusing diagnostic content, can be compressed while small-scale variations (nodules, vessels) can be enhanced. Edge enhancement algorithms (detail contrast) aid detection of object boundaries. Contrast and edge enhancement are usually associated with

unacceptable increased image noise. However, the very high DQE of the flat panel detectors (high signal-to-noise ratio) overcomes this drawback.

GRAY-SCALE EXPANSION

Gray-scale expansion or contraction maps the input digital levels to match the output luminance levels on either the monitor or hard copy. A particular film speed can be simulated by the application of a nonlinear transform (from a look-up table) which mimics a film characteristic curve (optical density versus exposure). A secondary transform can be applied to remove the nonlinear (and non-optimal) characteristic curve of the output device. For this to be effective the output device must be pre-calibrated; quality control for display devices plays an important role.

12.8 ELECTRONIC DISPLAYS (SOFT-COPY DISPLAY)

With the increasing importance of digital imaging and the general acceptance of comprehensive picture archiving and communication systems in hospitals and clinics the electronic or 'soft-copy' display has been improved to give an image quality better than that delivered by early control console or primary viewing monitors. The cathode ray tube (vacuum tube) monitor has been the dominant display device but now is being rapidly replaced by clinical quality flat panel TFT displays.

12.8.1 Cathode ray tube video monitor

MONOCHROME B/W DISPLAYS

In monochrome CRT displays, the visible image is formed one line at a time as the single narrow electron beam is moved in rectilinear scan fashion across the face of the phosphor screen (Fig. 12.48). Because of the need to deflect the beam through relatively large angles, electromagnetic deflection is normally employed. The horizontal deflection coils in the yoke assembly produce a vertically oriented magnetic field which sweeps the beam from left to right as each line is scanned. A ramp or sawtooth-like current waveform is applied to these coils. The vertical deflection coils move the beam downward as each frame is constructed, then reposition the beam for the start of

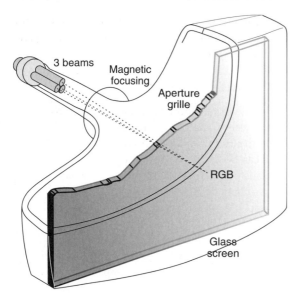

Figure 12.48 *CRT design and scanning method.*

Table 12.15 *Luminance units.*

Steradian (dimensionless)	sr
	surface of sphere = 4π sr hence 1 sr = $1/4\pi$
Luminance	cd m^{-2} (nit)
Lambert	1 cd sr^{-1} cm^{-2} = 10^4 cd sr^{-1} m^{-2} or 10^4 lumen m^{-2}
Foot lambert	1 lumen ft^{-2} approximately 3.426 cd m^{-2}
Typical viewbox	2000 cd m^{-2} or 0.2 cd cm^{-2}

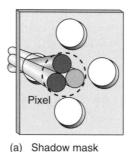 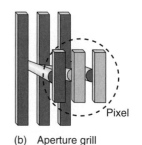

(a) Shadow mask   (b) Aperture grill

Figure 12.49 *(a) Shadow mask and (b) aperture grille design.*

the next frame. The frame rate (e.g., 70, 80, 100 Hz) determines the frequency of the vertical deflection control voltage.

LUMINANCE

Luminance describes the rate at which visible light is emitted from a surface (light box) or display device (CRT or flat panel display). The SI unit for **luminance** describing the energy of visible light is the lumen-second and the unit for luminance is 1 lumen per steradian per m^2; this is the candela per m^2 or sometimes referred to as a 'nit'. In contrast **illuminance** describes the rate at which visible light strikes a surface and the unit is the lumen per m^2 or lux, a unit identical to luminance except there is no solid angle dimension. Table 12.15 lists some equivalent non-SI luminance units. Monochrome display devices capable of producing maximum luminance of up to 500 cd m^{-2} are currently available, with 300 cd m^{-2} a typical value. These levels are to be compared to the luminance level of typical radiographic film illuminators, 1000 to 2000 cd m^{-2}, or mammography illuminators, 3000 cd m^{-2}. Use of a larger beam current will lead to greater display luminance, but this will tend to enlarge the beam spot size and thus reduce image resolution. Larger beam current and image luminance also reduce the useful life of the display device by hastening the normal fall-off

of phosphor efficiency and cathode depletion with time.

COLOR DISPLAYS

Phosphor materials used in screens determine the color displayed on the CRT, and will also influence the luminance capability of a display device since some phosphors are more efficient than others in converting electron beam energy into visible light.

The operation and design of color CRT display devices is similar to that for monochrome but contain three electron guns instead of one. Each beam illuminates one of three screen phosphor elements producing red, green, and blue (fluoroescent) light. Each beam is modulated by its own electronic signal, and the relative strength of the three beams determines the perceived color of the pixel being produced. The electron beam is never perfectly focused, so either a **shadow mask** or **aperture grill** is placed in front of and parallel to the phosphor screen (Fig. 12.49).

SHADOW MASK DESIGN

The first method used a shadow mask which is simply a sheet of metal with minute holes, each one coinciding with the position of a group of three red, blue, and green phosphor dots called a triad. The mask contains a matrix of round apertures in front of the pixels which directs the electron beam, making it sharper and preventing color blurring between triads (Fig. 12.49a). For a color display having a **shadow mask** capable of displaying 800 pixels per line, the mask will have 800 openings from left to right through which the three beams must pass. These openings are positioned precisely in front of the display pixels so that the beam will be collimated on to the appropriate phosphor spot. The shadow mask has a serious disadvantage, however: it blocks a significant percentage of the electron beam reaching the phosphor screen, so the image intensity is poor.

APERTURE GRILLE

Sony introduced the Trinitron design which was the first example of an aperture grille tube, using a mask formed by extremely fine wires, strung vertically behind the display screen. Rather than groups of circular phosphor dots in triads, aperture grille tubes have continuous vertical stripes of red, blue, and green phosphor. Each pixel is made of three vertical bars, one for each primary color (Fig. 12.49b).

The vertical-only masking is sufficient to give the required masking effect and has the bonus that more of the focused electron beam penetrates through to the phosphor. The aperture grille tubes can have a much darker tint of glass and still get a brighter picture than would be possible with a shadow-mask display. The result is far better contrast and a more vivid display.

The aperture grille wires are susceptible to vibration so to stop this damper wires are strung horizontally across the grille, making contact with the vertical wires and damping out any mechanical vibrations. There are usually two of these wires, at one third and two thirds of the way up the screen. Because they are in the path of the oncoming electrons, they cast a shadow on the screen that is usually just visible as two faint black lines. Since the advent of Trinitron, other manufacturers have developed their own versions of aperture grille technology.

Although a mask or grill is important to the operation of the color CRT, its presence contributes to increased veiling glare due to electrons which scatter off the mask and eventually strike the screen in unintended areas. This effect becomes more pronounced as the number of pixels per line is increased, which tends to limit the maximum pixel matrix sizes for color display devices. It is also more pronounced in shadow masks than in aperture grills. The mask-initiated veiling glare in color CRTs is one of the major quality issues in using color CRTs for viewing monochromatic medical images.

FLAT SCREEN GEOMETRY

A color monitor's three electron beams originate from a single fixed point and have to be swept from side to side by the deflection yoke. This means the edges of the screen are further away from the gun than the center, which creates three problems when it comes to keeping the image sharp right into the corners:

• Beam focus
• Beam shape
• Colour convergence

In practice, the electron beam coming from a gun is not perfectly straight so it tends to spread out; it therefore needs to be focused into a spot on the phosphor mask.

In early color tubes, when the focusing plates in the gun were fixed, the need to maintain focus dictated that screens had to be curved to maintain a constant distance from the gun to the screen. Screen curvature produced image distortion. Additional problems were seen at the extreme edges where the shape of the beam would appear elliptical as it cut through the shadow mask and met the phosphor, reducing resolution; and second, the three individual beams controlling red, blue, and green dots had to be focused together so that they converged at the same point.

These three factors made it almost impossible to find monitors whose focus, sharpness and color convergence are as good at the edges as they are in the middle of the screen.

The aperture grille tube was one of the first technologies to start flattening out monitors, allowing the screen to be flat in the vertical direction. In order to produce a flat screen in the horizontal direction dynamic beam shaping and focusing was introduced.

Dynamic focusing techniques use electromagnetic coils in a similar way to the deflection yoke to constantly influence the focal point of the beam, as well as its shape, as it gets scanned across the screen allowing completely flat-screen CRT monitors.

12.8.2 Resolutions and refresh rates

The analog nature of the electron beam in CRTs means that they can be steered and pointed anywhere on the screen, displaying any resolution up to the limit of their amplifier electronics.

VERTICAL SCAN FREQUENCY

The electron beam illuminates the pixels on a video monitor screen (cathode ray tube) scanning the picture left to right, top to bottom, in the same way as a page of text is read. The phosphor coating that the electron beam illuminates only glows for a limited period of time; to remain visible it must be refreshed consistently by the electron beam.

The number of times this happens is the **refresh rate** or the **vertical scan frequency**, the value given in hertz. If this rate is set too low, the phosphor's illumination level fades between refreshes and a visible flicker effect is obvious which degrades the image and produces viewing fatigue. A figure of about 70 Hz is the recommended minimum but sometimes 85 Hz or even 90 Hz is necessary if long viewing times are envisaged. The maximum refresh rate is determined by the design limits of the **video graphics card** and the monitor itself.

HORIZONTAL SCAN FREQUENCY

The horizontal scan frequency is the number of times per second that the electron beam scans a horizontal line, from the left of the picture to the right measured in kHz. This is decided by the number of pixels per scan line. There is a relationship between this and the maximum vertical resolution the monitor can handle. Another related attribute is known as the **bandwidth**.

On every scan line the beam has to switch to a different value for every pixel. At 1800×1440 it has to change 1800 times on every line. For a refresh rate of 85 Hz the bandwidth is then $1800 \times 1440 \times 85 = 220$ MHz. This is the pixel modulation or the number of pixels drawn per second. Pushing a monitor past its maximum bandwidth will give distortion and detail loss.

The above figures are underestimated because within the horizontal and vertical refresh times provision must be made for flyback – the time taken to return the electron beam to the start position (top left of the screen), so the true maximum number of addressed pixels will be less than the bandwidth.

A correction factor of about 1.2 to 1.35 should be used in the calculation of required bandwidth to obtain a given resolution and refresh rate, so: 220×1.35 gives a required bandwidth approaching 300 MHz.

GRAPHICS CARD AND DRIVE ELECTRONICS

When setting resolutions and refresh rates the graphics card needs to be of high enough quality to drive the monitor at an appropriate resolution. This is largely a function of the card's RAM-DAC, the part that converts the digital frame buffer into an analog video signal, which drives the CRT beam. Generally speaking the RAM-DAC frequency decides the graphic card's maximum resolution and refresh rate.

The **video amplifier** converts the extremely low power signal from the graphics card into a driving signal powerful enough to sweep the electron beam across the display. The horizontal scan frequency determines the bandwidth of this amplifier; a diagnostic quality monitor requires a 500 MHz bandwidth.

12.8.3 Flat panel liquid crystal display

Flat panel liquid crystal displays work on the twisted-nematic principle. Nematic crystals have long molecules all aligned in the same direction but otherwise randomly arranged. A twisted-nematic liquid crystal flat panel display consists of several layers; usually five:

- The liquid crystal layer itself sandwiched between two substrates, which have been aligned 90° to each other, so that the direction of the liquid crystals is twisted by 90° when no voltage is applied
- At the top and bottom of this sandwich are polarizing filters, also arranged at 90° to each other

The liquid crystal elements of each pixel are arranged so that in their normal state (with no voltage applied) the light coming through the passive filter is polarized and thus blocked. The crystals are normally transparent but can alter the orientation of polarized light passing through them. When a voltage is applied across the liquid crystal elements they twist by up to 90° in proportion to the voltage, changing their polarization and letting more light through from the **backlight** source. These two stages are illustrated in Fig. 12.50. This **transmissive** property of liquid crystals suits them for controlling the intensity of picture elements (pixels) in the flat display. Varying the voltage varies the amount of twist in the liquid crystal, allowing

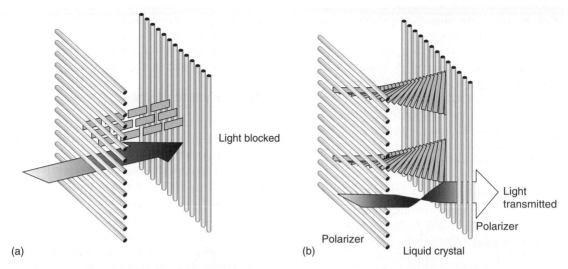

Figure 12.50 *Liquid crystal modulation of the transmitted light for a flat panel display showing (**a**) no voltage applied so light is blocked. (**b**) Applied voltage twists liquid crystal allowing light to pass.*

shades of gray. In order to introduce color each pixel needs three closely grouped liquid crystal elements, each fitted with a red, green or blue filter, in the same way as the phosphor regions of a CRT.

Construction of a flat panel color display is shown in Fig. 12.51. The first layer in the sandwich has the **backlight**, which provides the actual display illumination. Next comes the series (a) and (b) described above: a polarizing filter, a glass panel, the liquid crystal cell, a second glass panel and a second polarizing filter.

The separate liquid crystal elements need to be addressed. So each of the nearly 2.3 million red, green, and blue elements in a standard 1024×768 display needs to be able to be activated individually; this is achieved by using a thin film transistor array (previously described in Section 12.7.1). The twist of each separate liquid crystal element or pixel is controlled by a separate thin film transistor which has been etched onto a glass substrate. Each transistor can hold the voltage applied to its associated pixel until the next time the screen is refreshed. So TFT screens can use very fast-twist liquid crystal and image flicker is avoided.

The active transistor matrix provides a method of electronically addressing or controlling the pixel array. In order to display an image on the screen, one row of pixels receives an appropriate voltage; the display driver, under program control, generates a voltage to columns holding active elements. Where an activated row and column intersect, a TFT turns on an element

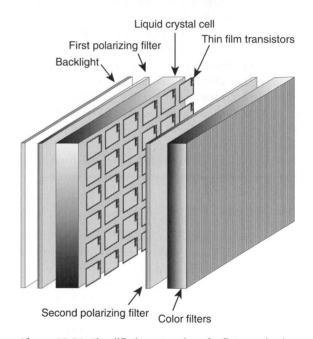

Figure 12.51 *Simplified construction of a flat-panel color display showing the layer of controlling thin film transistors between the polarizing filters.*

electrode generating an electrical field that controls the orientation of the liquid crystals. The transistors control the degree of twist and hence the intensity of the red, green and blue elements of each pixel forming the image on the display. This process repeats sequentially for each of the 1280 rows in a display; a 1280×1024 resolution display requires nearly 4 million thin film transistors for controlling this operation and the total time for image formation is about 20 ms.

A high definition clinical display with a pixel matrix of 2560×2048 will have 16 million transistors. The LCD flat panel minimum viewing angle is typically 120° horizontally; it is not uncommon to see some models having viewing angles of 140° or even wider. Since a TFT display is a single large integrated circuit it is difficult to manufacture these large silicon wafers with few enough defects; consequently, the prices are high.

The fixed pixels of a flat panel make it hard to display lower than native resolutions without aliasing distortion, and impossible to display higher. This is a major limitation of flat panels.

12.8.4 CRT versus flat panel: advantages and disadvantages

LCD flat panel displays take up very little space on the work desk. Even if more recent CRT displays are fitted with short-neck picture tubes, they are still much larger and heavier than an LCD panel with equivalent screen area. A CRT monitor typically needs 100 to 150 W in use, while an LCD panel may need only 15 to 20 W. LCD panels are then more acceptable in restricted areas such as control rooms for fluoroscopy, CT, and MRI and in other confined spaces without loading the air-conditioning units.

IMAGE GEOMETRY

This is one aspect of a flat panel LCD that is perfect, since the individual pixels of an LCD panel are fixed within a matrix when the panel is manufactured, and the shape of the image can never drift out of alignment unlike a CRT display.

IMAGE SHARPNESS

LCDs suffer from image distortion. Although they create the impression that they have very good sharpness a close-up inspection will reveal that a black border surrounds each pixel. This is due to the connections on the integrated circuit linking each trio of thin film transistors to the drive electronics (see Fig. 12.35). This is more obvious for a text character which is visibly broken up into its constituent parts. Except for high definition flat panel displays (5 megapixel) clinical displays can be degraded.

The red, green, and blue elements of each pixel are not perfectly aligned in flat panel displays. So **color convergence** of an LCD is never perfect and a CRT display is superior in this respect.

NATIVE RESOLUTION

An LCD panel has a fixed number of pixels. This means that it has a fixed, native resolution above which it is impossible to go. It also means that switching down to lower resolutions produces aliasing distortions as the position of the pixels in the computer's image buffer do not match the actual, physical positions of the panel's pixels. In contrast, a CRT can cope with a much wider range of resolutions. Table 12.16 indicates a maximum resolution for the CRT but intermediate resolutions can be chosen, unlike the liquid crystal display.

VIEWING ANGLE

This is a problem with flat panel displays. However, several manufacturers have produced top quality clinical displays that can be viewed satisfactorily from the side and so satisfy viewing by more than just one person.

CONTRAST

The color contrast of flat panels is limited since each transistor is driven digitally by a 6-bit signal. This only provides 18-bit as opposed to the CRT which can give a 24- or 32-bit color depth. Gray-scale LCD panels with 3 sub-pixels can be modulated to give an 18-bit gray scale.

DISPLAY QUALITY

CRT technology has one inherent advantage over TFT displays: there are always some 'dead' pixels that are always black, due to faults in silicon fabrication.

Table 12.16 *CRT video monitor compared to LCD.*

	CRT	LCD
Scale	Gray	Color
Viewable size (mm)	300×400	302×376
Pixels	2560×2048	2560×2048
Luminance (cd m^{-2})	300	500
Power (W)	250	80
Monitor depth (mm)	600	70

These can be present on a new panel display or appear over time.

ISO 13406-2 was drafted in 1999 and finalized in 2001. This is quoted by most manufacturers and defines the acceptable number of dead pixels. This Standard covers most aspects of TFTs including uniformity of colors, contrast, and brightness as well as reflectivity, flicker, and pixel defects.

Four types of defect are defined:

1 The first is where a whole pixel is continuously lit. This gives a white spot on an otherwise dark screen.
2 The second type is the opposite of the first: a continuously dark pixel giving a dark spot on a bright screen.
3 The third type is more complex, although in our experience more common. It refers to individual subpixels, where a failure in any third of a pixel will give a colored pixel on either a bright or dark screen. As an example, the TFT on which I am writing this has a continuously lit blue sub-pixel. It therefore does not show up on a white screen, but on a dark screen a blue dot is noticeable.
4 The fourth type of defect is referred to as a fault cluster and is the number of Types 1, 2, and 3 defects in a five-by-five pixel area.

There are also four classes to the Standard. Each class prescribes how many of each type of defect are allowable in each million pixels.

1 For Class I screens this is easy; no defects are allowed.
2 For Classes II and III up to 11 defects are allowed per million pixels.
3 Class III is where these defects are clustered.
4 Class IV has Type 4 defects and fails to meet the Standard.

12.8.5 Displays for radiology

Reporting and viewing radiology images requires high performance monitors (either CRT or LCD). Unlike domestic video screens which display 240 lines interlaced to 480 lines (512 lines in Europe), displays employed for diagnostic imaging may address as many as 2000 horizontal lines on the screen in non-interlaced (i.e. progressive) mode, and the image refresh rate may exceed 70 images per second. In commercial television, each line is painted during a period of about 53 μs, and modulation of beam intensity sufficient to represent all needed image details as luminance variations must take place in that time period. In a high line rate medical imaging display, time per scan line can be as low as 5 μs, necessitating much faster modulation of the electron beam current and a much higher bandwidth requirement.

CONTRAST

Contrast is defined in CRT and LCD monitors as the ratio of black to white. The darkest 'black' and the brightest 'white' give the best image quality. The brightest white is given by the monitor with the highest luminance ($cd\ m^{-2}$). The black level is influenced mostly by ambient light conditions. An ACR Standard for digital image data management states that image luminance should be at least $170\ cd\ m^{-2}$. DIN 6868/57 requires contrast ratio of 100:1 for application class A (primary diagnosis of radiography) and 40:1 for application class B (primary diagnosis with all other imaging modalities and review). For reporting digital radiographs a luminance of at least $200\ cd\ m^{-2}$ is necessary. Figure 12.52 shows a commercially available 5 megapixel flat panel display

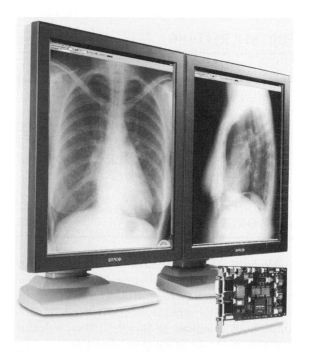

Figure 12.52 *A commercially available flat-panel display giving high resolution and uniformity over a large viewing area. The specially designed display driver board is shown in the foreground (courtesy Barco plc.).*

Table 12.17 *Comparison for standard and medical grade CRT and LCD monitors.*

	1 Megapixel	2 Megapixel	3 Megapixel	5 Megapixel
CRT specification				
Maximum matrix size	⩽1024 × 1280	⩽1200 × 1600	⩽1728 × 2304	⩽2048 × 2560
Active pixel size (mm)	0.28 to 0.3	0.28 to 0.3	0.17 to 0.23	0.15
Amplifier bandwidth (MHz)	160 to 200	160 to 200	250 to 290	>330
Luminance (cd m^{-2})	100	100 to 300	200 to 300	200 to 300
LCD specification				
Native resolution	1280 × 1024	1600 × 1200	2048 × 1536	2560 × 1048
Pixel pitch (mm)	0.2805	0.255	0.207	0.165
Screen area (mm)	359 × 287	408 × 306	424 × 318	422 × 338
Viewing angle (°)	170	170	170	170
Contrast	550:1	1000:1	600:1	600:1
Luminance (cd m^{-2})	400	400	500	500
Power consumption (W)	64	70	79	72
Pixel clock rate (MHz)	85	120	200	330

with a large screen area having a native resolution of 2560 × 1048 and a high luminance. Table 12.17 compares standard (domestic) quality CRT and LCD monitors with the more expensive clinical quality displays.

FURTHER READING

Image Processing for Scientific and Technical Applications, 2nd edition. Bernd Jahne. CRC Press, 2004.

The Image Processing Handbook, 4th edition. John C. Russ. CRC Press, 2002.

Digital Image Processing, 2nd edition. Gonzalez and Woods. Addison-Wesley, 2002.

KEYWORDS

amorphous silicon (a-Si:H): the semiconductor material used for photosensitive detectors in conjunction with the TFT layer. Used as an intermediate light converter for indirect flat-panel detectors

amorphous selenium (a-Se): the photoconductor material used in direct flat-panel detectors

contrast resolution: the smallest exposure change that can be detected. Ultimately, this is limited by the exposure range and the quantization (number of bits per pixel) of the detector

detective quantum efficiency (DQE): a measure of noise performance that is obtained by comparing the image noise of a detector with that expected for an 'ideal' detector having the same signal–response characteristics. The only source of noise in an ideal detector results from the incident X-ray quantum statistics

detector size: the detector size describes the useful imaging area of an imaging device

detector element: a detector element is the smallest resolvable area in a digital imaging device

exposure range: the range of exposures over which a detector can capture an image. Digital radiography and computed radiography are capable of capturing an image over a much larger range of exposures than film-screen. This has been shown to reduce the number of retakes that result from over- or under-exposure

image noise: all images have unwanted fluctuations that are unrelated to the object being imaged. These are collectively described as image noise. In addition to the X-ray quantum noise, which cannot be avoided, imaging systems contribute additional noise to an image. The electronic components of all digital detectors add noise. Indirect-conversion detectors have additional noise sources caused by the conversion of X-ray energy to light and the varying degree to which that light spreads before being absorbed by the light-sensitive photodiode

limiting spatial resolution (LSR): the highest number of line pairs that can be seen in an image or target consisting of a series of periodic bar patterns of increasing spatial frequency. LSR is an unreliable measure of performance because it depends on the contrast of the target, the number and length of the target patterns, as well as the exposure and display conditions. Modulation transfer function is a much more reliable measure

matrix size: the matrix size of a digital detector is the number of detector elements. This is normally expressed in terms of the number of detector elements in two orthogonal directions

modulation transfer function (**MTF**): a measure of the ability of an imaging system to preserve signal contrast as a function of spatial frequency. Every image can be described in terms of the amount of energy in each of its spatial frequency components. MTF describes the fraction of each component that will be preserved in the captured image

Nyquist frequency: the highest spatial frequency that can be represented in a digital image. The Nyquist frequency is determined by the pixel spacing

photodiode: an electronic element which converts light into charge. Indirect-conversion detectors require fabrication of a light-sensitive amorphous silicon photodiode on top of the thin film transistor array

photoconductor: in direct-conversion detectors, the amorphous selenium layer forms a continuous X-ray-sensitive photoconductor which converts X-ray energy directly to charge. This charge can be directly 'read out' by the TFT array, a simple and robust design that does not require complex photodiode fabrication steps needed by indirect-conversion detectors

pixel: A 'picture element', the smallest area of an image which is represented in a digital image. A digital radiography image consists of a matrix of pixels which is typically several thousand pixels in each direction

quantization: while all X-ray detectors respond smoothly and continuously to the incident exposure, digital images require the detector response to be quantized into a fixed number of levels that can be represented digitally. This number is typically 12 to 14 bits or 4096 to 16 384 unique levels for flat panel X-ray detectors

scintillator: A material that absorbs X-ray energy and re-emits part of that energy as visible light. Two modern high-efficiency X-ray scintillators are cesium iodide and gadolinium oxysulfide. Cesium iodide is commonly used in X-ray image intensifiers and is highly hygroscopic, which means it readily absorbs water from the air. Cesium iodide must be hermetically sealed to avoid water absorption or it will degrade rapidly. Gadolinium oxysulfide is commonly used in X-ray intensifying screens to expose film. It is a highly stable material, but has significantly more light spread than a layer of cesium iodide with equal X-ray absorption

signal-to-noise ratio (**SNR**): because noise ultimately limits our ability to see an object (the signal), SNR can be used to describe the detectability of a particular object under well-defined exposure conditions. The SNR in an image is always less than or equal to the SNR of the incident exposure. Detective quantum efficiency (DQE) is a measure of the efficiency with which the SNR of the incident exposure is preserved in an image

thin film transistor (**TFT**): an electronic switch commonly made of amorphous silicon on flat panel detectors. The TFT allows the charge collected at each pixel to be independently transferred to external electronics, where it is amplified and quantized

tiling: a process whereby several flat panel detectors are joined to obtain one larger detector

Digital fluorography

13.1 INTRODUCTION

Initial attempts used for storing fluorographic images used video techniques. The video images from the camera tube were captured on a video disk which was then displayed without further irradiation of the patient. This gave great benefits regarding reduction of patient dose but had limitations regarding image quality, speed of display, and image storage. The development of digital fluorography allowed much faster image acquisition and storage and, more importantly, digital image manipulation. The patient dose reduction was significant. The machines used for digital fluorography commonly use C-arm geometry although under- and over-table designs now use digital acquisition. A digital imaging system offers the following advantages:

- Dose reduction
- Wide dynamic range
- Image storage
- Instant imaging (filmless)
- Dynamic imaging (up to 30 fps)
- Image copying without loss of quality
- Image data transfer (PACS)

13.2 BASIC SYSTEM

The imaging chain of a modern digital fluorography (DF) system is shown in Fig. 13.1. The important component parts are:

- The image intensifier
- Input phosphor
- Photocathode
- Output phosphor
- Coupling optics
- The video camera: Plumbicon, CCD
- The amplifier
- The analog-to-digital converter
- The signal conversion circuit and look-up table

A large field of view (40 cm) image intensifier is commonly used for DSA so that both legs can be imaged during 'bolus chasing' or serial studies. Specifications for a typical image intensifier suitable for digital fluorography have been given in Table 10.4.

13.3 IMAGE MATRIX SIZE

A general formula relating matrix size M and image intensifier field size D with resolution R in Lp mm^{-1} is:

$$R = \frac{Mm}{20D}$$

where m is the image magnification, usually taken as 1.25 due to patient offset from the image intensifier face. This is plotted in Fig. 13.2 for three matrix sizes 512^2, 1024^2 and 2048^2 showing the combined effect of

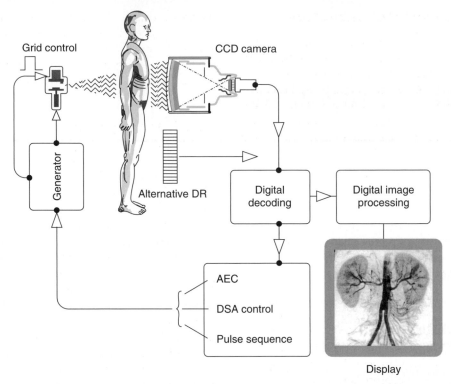

Figure 13.1 *Basic components for a digital fluorography imaging system. The image intensifier output influences exposure settings maintaining a fixed exposure rate at the image intensifier face. Image data are digitized and stored in memory. Look-up tables are used for controlling automatic control and display settings.*

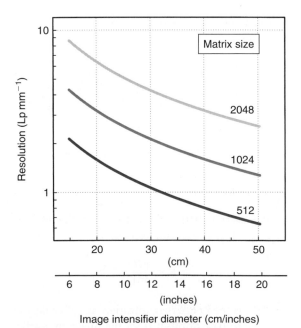

Figure 13.2 *Combined plot of the image resolution given for image intensifier sizes and three matrix sizes.*

image intensifier size and expected resolution given by these three matrix sizes.

Cardiac investigations require the greatest resolution and a rough indication of a system's ability to resolve small vessels r is given by the formula:

$$r = \frac{2D}{M}$$

For a 512^2 matrix which may represent an image intensifier field size of 200 mm, it will resolve 0.78 mm or 1.25 Lp mm^{-1}. A 1024^2 matrix using the same intensifier will resolve 0.4 mm or 2.5 Lp mm^{-1} but for the same noise content the higher resolution 1024^2 matrix will require $\times 4$ the dose of a 512^2 matrix.

The spatial resolution of a digital fluorography system depends on the setting of the image intensifier decreasing from 0.27, 0.19, and 0.14 mm for field sizes 33, 23, and 17 cm, respectively, representing matrix resolutions from 1.8, 2.6, and 3.5 Lp mm^{-1}, respectively. For comparison a film-screen resolution is approximately 5 Lp mm^{-1} at 200 speed.

FOCAL SPOT AND IMAGE RESOLUTION

The digital image matrix rather than the image intensifier limits the spatial resolution, although the limitations are reasonably well matched. At higher magnifications geometrical unsharpness becomes a problem which can be reduced by utilizing smaller focal spot sizes (switching from 1 mm to 0.6 mm). The dependence of image resolution R on the X-ray tube focal spot is described by:

$$R = \frac{m}{F(m-1)}$$

where F is the X-ray tube focal spot size and m the image magnification (typically 1.25 as before).

IMAGE STORAGE

Storage of images in digital fluoroscopy introduced the idea of **last-image hold**, where the last frame acquired in a clinical sequence is retained in memory and displayed on the monitor. Owing to the short exposure time span this image will have a noisy appearance unless some type of processing is used (integration or smoothing).

13.4 IMAGE PRE-PROCESSING

13.4.1 Recursive filtering

This is a common method used to achieve noise suppression without increasing patient dose; several image frames are integrated for display to reduce noise. This process has the effect of degrading temporal resolution however. This filtering technique is usually performed during the time period of frame flyback ('on the fly'). With this technique, several of the most recent frames are averaged into the current image with weighting factors that are inversely proportional to the age of the frame being averaged. The most recent frame is given the highest weighting factor, and the oldest is given the lowest. Frames that are intermediate in age are given proportionally intermediate factors. The amount of noise and lag can be controlled by changing the number of frames to be included in the summation. Lag may be reduced by using filtering techniques that identify moving objects in a series of successive images and precluding their associated pixels from the averaging process. This technique is known

as motion artifact reduction or motion detection. The result is a quiet image in areas where objects are stationary or moving relatively slowly compared with the frame rate. Objects in motion are presented with little or no lag but may have considerable noise.

13.4.2 Look-up tables

Look-up tables (LUTs) play an important role in DSA during acquisition, exposure control and display. An LUT can be stored in ROM or RAM depending on whether the signal is to follow a fixed or variable program. The **transmission** characteristics of the video imaging chain can be altered from its linear response to a nonlinear one (e.g. logarithmic). The **automatic exposure** control determines the optimum exposure required for the chosen acquisition protocol (frame rate and dose etc.). LUTs then set generator voltage, current, and timing (pulse width). The iris diaphragm on the video tube input is also adjusted for optimum display brightness. The video **display** itself is also controlled by an LUT; the table is operator selected to give linear or a variety of nonlinear scales. This is used in conjunction with the windowing facility.

13.4.3 Image data transfer

Transfer rates and storage times are listed in Table 13.1 for two matrix sizes. The large storage requirements should be accommodated by fast RAM memory and then transferred to the hard disk for post-acquisition

Table 13.1 *Image data transfer (in MB s^{-1}) and storage (MB).*

Transfer time (fps) and storage (fps)	Matrix size	
	$512 \times 512 \times 10$	$1024 \times 1024 \times 10$
Transfer time		
7.5	2.4	9.4
30	9.6	37.5
60	19.2	
Storage (5 s duration)		
7.5	12	47
30	48	187
60	96	

processing. Memory size is therefore critical in DF systems.

No single storage medium possesses the requirements of a large storage capacity and high image transfer rate combined with short access times. As a result of this most digital imaging systems comprise a combination of different storage devices. They contain a fast semiconductor memory capable of storing digitized images in real time. However, because of the relatively high cost per bit of semiconductor memory this type of storage is limited. The semiconductor memory is used again for the next exposure so if the data already stored is to be retained it must be transferred to the auxiliary memory which is a magnetic disk. The magnetic disk serves as intermediate storage and will retain its data if the power is lost. However, older studies can be erased after a period of time or when the disk runs out of memory space.

If the images are to be archived then a RAID magnetic disk archive is the most suitable medium. The optical disk has the lowest specific storage costs but does not enjoy very fast data transfer times. If a number of archived studies were requested by the radiologist then this data stored on optical disk would first be transferred to magnetic disk. From the disk it would be placed in solid state semiconductor memory for viewing purposes. During a viewing or reporting session the data stored in the semiconductor memory would constantly be updated and replaced as a new patient study is requested from the digital magnetic memory.

13.4.4 Image quality

IMAGE NOISE

Fluoroscopic noise in the image may be due to quantum or electronic noise. Quantum noise is associated with statistical fluctuations in the number of photons per unit area (mm^2) over the detector. Decreasing exposure in order to reduce patient radiation dose increases quantum noise. Since the image chain using either an image intensifier or a flat field DR detector is designed to be very sensitive to X-ray photons then substantial quantum mottle is to be expected.

Electronic noise is associated with the imaging chain electronics, including image intensifier with their charge-coupled devices (CCD camera). This noise can be introduced by the image intensifier high-voltage supply, the CCD itself or its camera amplifier and the analog-to-digital converter.

Table 13.2 *The improved resolution given by an image intensifier with an increased contrast ratio.*

Contrast ratio	I.I. Diameter (cm)	Resolution (Lp mm^{-1})
20:1	21	5.2
	17	5.8
	13	6.2
30:1	30	5
	23	5.6
	15	6.8
	11	7.5

Noise in dynamic fluoroscopic imaging is reduced by displaying individual noisy images in rapid succession. The human visual system has an integration time of between 100 and 200 ms. When displaying images in rapid succession, acquired at (say) 30 fps, the eye integrates the individual frames. Since noise is a random process, integrating images over several frames reduces the noise content by the square root of the number of frames used in the integration.

RESOLUTION AND CONTRAST

The theoretical attainable resolution given by an image intensifier has been listed in Table 10.2. This is usually not a limiting factor since digitization can cause a major resolution loss. Table 13.2 shows how resolution can be improved by increasing the contrast ratio of an image intensifier.

TEMPORAL RESOLUTION

Since fluoroscopy is capable of seeing an object in real time with motion, such as the progression of a contrast bolus, then image blurring or **lag** between frames must be minimal. The temporal resolution of a system is the ability of an imaging system to localize an object in time from frame to frame and follow its movement. **Image lag** is due to the slow response of the image chain, mainly the video camera. The image formed on the target of the camera tube is not completely extracted between fields or frames, since complete decay of the signal on the camera target takes between one and eight frames, depending on the camera design and setup. Thus, each image contains a small fraction of several preceding images. Lag is not seen in semiconductor CCD cameras since the charge signal is swept at very fast rates. Temporal resolution is important in digital subtraction angiography and cardiac imaging, where there are fast moving events.

13.5 IMAGE DATA POST-PROCESSING

After the initial processing of the acquired image data (amplification and log transformation) and before producing the clinical image the image data is subjected to a series of post-processing measures that are used to improve image quality. These are:

* Windowing
* Spatial filtering
* Temporal or recursive filtering

Edge enhancement, windowing, and magnification are a few of the image post-processing features that can improve the diagnostic quality of the images. Quantitative analysis programs are also available in the form of ejection fraction calculation and wall motion measurements.

WINDOWING

The digitized image is held in a matrix of 512^2, 1024^2 or 2048^2 pixels, where each pixel is represented by 10 or 12 bits. Theoretically, this can give 2048 or 4096 gray levels but since the eye can only appreciate about 35 gray levels only a fraction of the stored information can be displayed at any one time. This post-processing procedure is called windowing and allows small contrast changes to be amplified. Chapter 14 describes how stored values from 0 to 4096 can be displayed as a 256 level gray scale (window width) and placed, by operator control, at different levels of the stored range.

SPATIAL FILTERING

This is a post-processing procedure where raw data images obtained from the image intensifier contain noise due to quantum effects and electronic noise. The effect of this noise can be reduced by subjecting the data to **low pass filtering** or **smoothing**. This was demonstrated in Chapter 12. **High pass filtering** is used for emphasizing edge detail in the picture; this is important for enhancing small vessel detail in contrast angiography. It is commonly called **edge enhancement**.

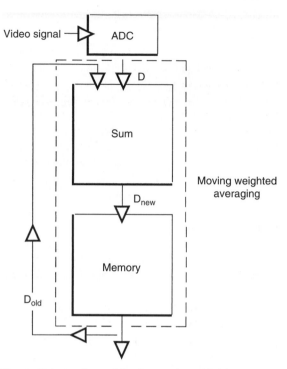

Figure 13.3 *Moving weighted averaging which is incorporated into a digital subtraction angiography system.*

TEMPORAL (RECURSIVE) FILTERING

Image noise reduction using spatial filtering techniques is limited to individual images. Reduction of noise is particularly important in digital fluorography owing to low dose imaging which has a low signal-to-noise ratio.

A very effective method for removing noise is to average several image frames, where stored image D_{old} is incorporated into the acquired image producing a matrix of average values D_{new}; the schematic in Fig. 13.3 shows the data flow. This is a pre-processing procedure when several images are summed (typically four). The useful signal strength increases linearly whereas the noise component, because of its random nature, does not show any correlation between images and its presence is reduced. This is best seen by studying the standard deviation of the image noise. Comparing the individual image noise value σ with the average noise σ_n obtained by summing n images:

$$\sigma_n = \frac{\sigma}{\sqrt{n}} \tag{13.1}$$

Box 13.1 Moving weighted imaging

The averaging technique used in Fig. 13.3 is applied to five samples, 8, 12, 8, 10, 8, and 12, collected at set time intervals and temporally smoothed using the formula:

$$D_{new} = \frac{D_{old}}{K} + \frac{D}{K}$$

When a smoothing factor K of 1 is used then the values do not change. If $K = 1.5$ then at the start:

(a) $D_{new} = 0 - \dfrac{0}{1.5} + \dfrac{8}{1.5} = 5.3$

and

(b) $D_{new} = 5.3 - \dfrac{5.3}{1.5} + \dfrac{12}{1.5} = 9.76$

The temporally smoothed values then become

5.3, 9.76, 8.58, 9.52, 8.5, and 10.8

The contribution from each sample, from 8 through to 12 in this example, decreases proportionally with time, giving the running or moving weighted averaging.

There is an improvement in noise by a factor $\sqrt{n}$, so averaging over four images halves the noise content. A continuous process for temporal smoothing uses a moving weighted average where noise reduction is calculated, not from a fixed number of images but from all the part images. An example of moving weighted averaging is given in Box 13.1.

Temporal filtering exaggerates image lag since it combines video camera lag over the image number summed. For this reason the number of images being summed at any one time is small. **Motion correction** can be used if the difference signal between images is used as a motion detector and the contrast of a moving object is emphasized above the noise component.

13.6 DIGITAL SUBTRACTION ANGIOGRAPHY

In order to distinguish vascular pathology and separate vessel detail from background anatomy a digital image is taken before and after contrast medium injection and the two images subtracted to reveal the isolated vessels. Early attempts suggested that this technique could be a relatively non-invasive venous procedure but since this gave poor image quality arterial injection techniques were adopted. These gave superior image quality in spite of their more invasive character.

13.6.1 Mask image

This is a technique for producing images of the blood vessels isolated from overlying structures. To achieve this, two images of the same region, separated in time, are acquired:

- The first image, called the **mask**, is taken prior to the injection of a contrast agent.
- The second image, called the **contrast** image, is the mask but it now contains the contrast agent.

An image frame of vessels just containing iodine contrast is obtained when the mask image is subtracted from the contrast image. The subtracted image contains any differences which exist between the two images, i.e. the addition of the contrast media and any movement artifact.

13.6.2 The digital subtraction angiography system

The component parts of a digital subtraction angiography (DSA) system are outlined in Fig. 13.4. The starting point in any DSA system is the signal from the detector: either an image intensifier/CCD camera or flat field DR.

The image frames are acquired and kept in the RAM image store. Two memories are used for the subtraction process; one holds the mask image and the other the contrast image. The memory contents are subtracted in a separate arithmetic unit and then undergo windowing before being converted back into a displayed image (using a DAC in the case of an analog video signal). They are then displayed on a high resolution monitor. Multiple images of the investigation are stored on a magnetic hard disk. A very large computer memory (RAM) is essential for image manipulation, its size varying between 512 MB and 1 GB. A fast CPU controls data acquisition and processing.

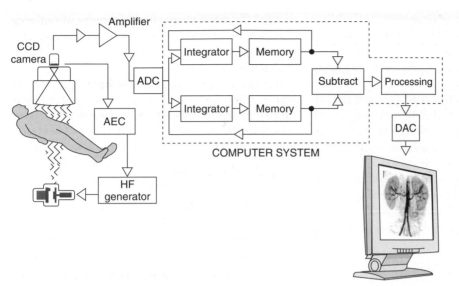

Figure 13.4 *A basic digital subtraction angiography system design showing the log amplification of the video signal and the temporal smoothing feedback in dual memory circuits before subtraction and display. A post-processing module allows the operator to choose image manipulation routines.*

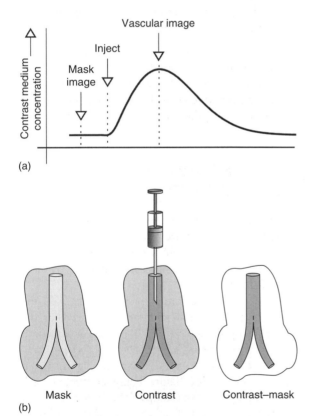

Figure 13.5 *(a) The arterial and venous phases of a digital subtraction angiography study. (b) In the basic DSA technique a mask image (M) is first stored then the relevant vessels are injected with contrast medium and a second image stored (C). Subtracting these images yields the difference image free of surrounding anatomy(D).*

Digital subtraction presents images of vessels in isolation from their background (soft tissue and bone). Two images are acquired from exactly the same anatomical region before and after injection of a contrast medium. The contrast density/time curve of Fig. 13.5a shows the timing which coincides with the peak arrival of the iodine-contrast bolus. Figure 13.5b illustrates the subtraction process. The first pre-contrast image is called the mask M containing background anatomy. The post-contrast image contains the vessels together with the background C. After some data processing (smoothing, edge enhancement etc.), the mask is subtracted from the contrast image to reveal the vessels in the difference image D as $C - M = D$.

The improved SNR that this imaging process yields over plain film contrast imaging and the benefits of image storage and transmission have made DSA the technique of choice for contrast angiography. The noise component of each image (M and C), being random, does not subtract but adds so the noise component increases in the subtracted frame D. This is not serious in the high photon flux images of DSA but can become a problem in low photon/low dose techniques.

13.6.3 Logarithmic subtraction

An essential requirement for DSA is that the contrast signal obtained by subtraction corresponds linearly with the concentration of the contrast medium. Direct subtraction of the two sets of images will not produce an image that is independent of the overlying structures, e.g. the contrast signal would be reduced in regions overlying a bone compared with soft tissue regions.

Logarithmic subtraction is used to insure that an artery of uniform diameter that traverses regions of varying thickness appears in the subtracted image with uniform contrast. The logarithm of the video signals is obtained prior to subtraction. The reason that log amplification is used prior to subtraction can be explained using the simple Beer–Lambert formula for the transmission of monochromatic radiation through matter. Figure 13.6a identifies the various parameters used in the calculation:

- I_0 is the incident radiation fluence
- I_t the transmitted intensity before contrast
- I_c the transmitted intensity after iodine contrast
- x_t and μ_t are the tissue thickness and attenuation coefficient, respectively
- x_v and μ_v the vessel thickness and iodine attenuation, respectively

For the **mask image**, if the intensity of radiation incident on a tissue thickness is x_t then the transmitted intensity is I_t

$$I_t = I_0 e^{-\mu_t x_t} \tag{13.2}$$

If a contrast medium, e.g. iodine, is added to a vessel overlying the tissue then the equation for the transmission after iodine contrast I_c is modified to include the extra vessel thickness x_v of iodine which has an attenuation coefficient μ_v:

$$I_c = I_0 \exp[-(\mu_t x_t + \mu_v x_v)] \tag{13.3}$$

The subtraction image is obtained by subtracting the mask image from the contrast image. Direct subtraction of the transmitted intensities I_s produces a complex expression which is not independent of the overlying structures and which is directly related to the input intensity I_0:

$$\begin{aligned} I_s &= I_c - I_t \\ &= I_0 \exp[-(\mu_t x_t + \mu_v x_v)] - \exp(-\mu_t x_t) \end{aligned}$$

$$\tag{13.4}$$

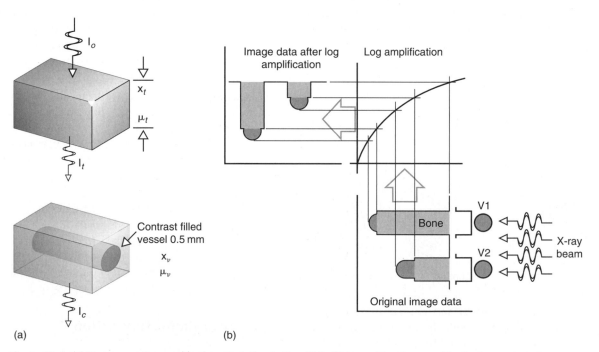

(a) (b)

Figure 13.6 (a) The parameters used in the calculation in Box 13.2. (b) Log subtraction graphically demonstrated showing that after log amplification the contrast filled vessels V1 and V2 lying behind bony tissue (shown as steps) are represented without distortion in the log amplified data. The graphed log values are stored as a look-up table.

However, subtracting the logs of the transmission:

$$
\begin{aligned}
I_s &= \log I_c - \log I_t \\
&= -(\mu_t x_t + \mu_v x_v) - (-\mu_t x_t) \\
&= -\mu_t x_t
\end{aligned}
\tag{13.5}
$$

In comparison to linear subtraction the logarithmic method does not retain stationary anatomical structure which may obscure small signal levels from the opacified vessel. In this way the resulting signal forming the DSA display is not influenced by patient size and produces an output pattern of intensities which depend only on the product of the thickness and attenuation coefficient of the injected contrast medium. Box 13.2 compares the linear and logarithmic methods.

The logarithmic transformation can be implemented either in an analog fashion using logarithmic amplifiers prior to analog to digital conversion, or using an LUT after digitization (Fig. 13.6b). The latter

is the preferred approach as log amplifiers can present stability problems and add noise to the signals. The digital arrangement can be fine tuned to the dynamic range of the input data, although quantization errors can still occur.

In spite of logarithmic amplification tissue variations still give irregular attenuation of vessels in the image field of view. Some form of extra compensation is necessary in the form of either tissue equivalent material or some form of shaped filtration. DSA wedge filters have been developed which can be adjusted to compensate for object thickness differences and, under operator control, these significantly reduce non-uniformities in the image.

13.6.4 Misregistration (movement artifact)

This is a major limiting factor in DF due to small movements in bone–tissue interfaces which can give edges that far exceed that given by the vessels themselves. This is demonstrated in Fig. 13.7 where a profile across a soft-tissue/bone interface is shown with the same profile a short time later plus the vessel contrast signal. The boundary between soft tissue and bone has changed, however.

Box 13.2 Comparing linear and logarithmic subtraction

Use the parameters identified in Fig 13.6a and derivations in eqns 13.2 to 13.5. For a tissue thickness x_t of 5 cm μ_t is 0.018 cm^{-1}. For a vessel diameter x_v of 0.5 cm μ_v is 0.03 cm^{-1}. The incident photon density I_0 is 1.0. The **mask signal** I_t is $I_0 \exp[-(\mu_t x_t)]$. The **contrast signal** I_c is $I_0 \exp[-(\mu_t x_t - \mu_v x_v)]$.

Using **linear subtraction**, for the DSA image

$$
\begin{aligned}
I_{\text{lin}} &= I_c - I_t \\
&= (-\mu_v x_v) I_0 e^{-\mu_t x_t} \\
&= -0.015 e^{-0.09} \\
&= 0.0137
\end{aligned}
$$

For increased tissue thickness (say 8 cm), similarly

$$
\begin{aligned}
I_{\text{lin}} &= -0.015 e^{-0.144} \\
&= 0.0129
\end{aligned}
$$

Using **log subtraction**, for the DSA image

$$
\begin{aligned}
I_{\text{log}} &= \ln I_t - \ln I_c \\
&= -(\mu_t x_t) - (\mu_t x_t - \mu_v x_v) \\
&= \mu_v x_v
\end{aligned}
$$

which is 0.015 regardless of tissue component $\mu_t x_t$.

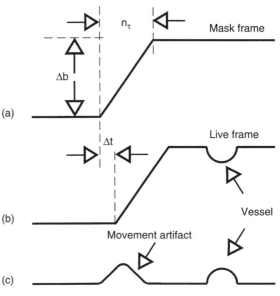

Figure 13.7 *Misregistration across a bone/soft-tissue interface during subtraction angiography. The parameters are identified in the text.*

The magnitude of this misregistration artifact C is given by:

$$C = \frac{\Delta b}{n\tau} \cdot \Delta t$$

where Δb is the brightness change at the bone/tissue boundary, t is the image pixel interval (sampling period in the ADC) and n is the number of pixels in the boundary region. The difference Δt is the magnitude of the misregistration.

Several methods have been devised for dealing with misregistration. Re-masking by retrospective selection of an alternative mask (time-interval difference) often reduces misregistration artifacts and in practice, misregistration in temporal subtraction studies can be either improved or salvaged by remasking.

PIXEL SHIFT

If movement artifacts cannot be corrected by alternative mask selection then the image pixels *in toto* can be shifted vertically or horizontally. This provides better alignment of the two images so improving subtraction.

13.6.5 Digital subtraction angiography programs

The exact procedures used for producing the highest quality subtracted image vary from manufacturer to manufacturer but they all contain the same basic principles described here. The signal-to-noise ratio of the subtracted image decreases during the subtraction process although the unwanted image data are removed and the noise content of each image is summed. Owing to its random nature noise cannot be reduced by image subtraction.

The signal-to-noise ratio of the final DSA image (SNR) depends also on the concentration of contrast medium C (iodine or barium) and the radiation dose D (photon density) so that

$$\text{SNR} = C \times \sqrt{D}$$

Increasing the concentration of contrast material is therefore a more effective improvement than increasing patient dose.

An effective way to improve image SNR is to integrate (add) image frames. Noise reduction depends on the number of similar frames added. If N frames are integrated, each having a noise value of σ then the noise in the summed image is $\sigma/\sqrt{N}$. Image integration reduces both quantum and electronic noise sources whereas increasing dose only affects quantum noise.

SNAP-SHOT IMAGING

This uses digitally enhanced single images utilizing one mask and one contrast image. It is the basic DSA technique and is also called digital spot imaging previously illustrated in Fig. 13.5b with image frames M and C.

REMASKING

If a series of contrast images is taken and a single mask used for constructing the subtracted image then patient movement (voluntary or involuntary) will lead to misregistration errors. These errors can be reduced by selecting images from the acquisition series that can be used for suitable updated masks.

Extending the snap-shot example shown in Fig. 13.5b where the mask M and contrast filled image C gave a difference image D, a series of contrast images taken during bolus transit $C_1, C_2, C_3, \ldots, C_n$ would provide the subtracted images:

$$C_1 - M = D_1, \quad C_2 - M = D_2, \ldots, C_n - M = D_n$$

If during this series there is patient movement during (say) contrast image C_8, which contains peak contrast together with some misregistration errors yielding a sub-optimum subtraction image D_8, then a new mask can be obtained from C_{10} (a frame which matched the shifted anatomy). The desired image would be equivalent to $C_8 - C_6$. If D_8 and D_{10} are subtracted the result would be equivalent to

$$\begin{aligned} D_8 - D_6 &= (C_8 - M) - (C_6 - M) \\ &= C_8 - C_6 \end{aligned}$$

So although the difference images D_6 and D_8 are the stored images an updated remasked difference image can be derived from them since the original mask image M cancels out in the equation yielding the required image which is $C_8 - C_6$.

ROAD MAPPING

Road mapping involves superimposing real-time images onto a previously acquired mask so that intraluminal manipulation of the catheter can be followed.

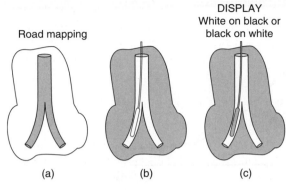

DISPLAY
White on black or black on white

Road mapping

(a)   (b)   (c)

Figure 13.8 *Road mapping used for presenting a real-time image of the catheter position (**a**). A vessel contrast image is taken which is then continuously subtracted (**b**) after catheter insertion to give the real-time image (**c**).*

Table 13.3 *Dual energy subtraction image series.*

Mask and contrast	Bone	Soft tissue	Iodine
Mask			
M_L, low kV mask	High	Medium	NA
M_H, high kV mask	Medium	Medium	NA
Contrast			
C_L, low kV image	High	Medium	High
C_H, high kV image	Medium	Medium	High

Figure 13.8 identifies the basic concept. A static image is used as a reference when advancing a catheter along the vessel being studied. The current fluoroscopic display is compared with the **reference image**, which contains contrast and thereby clearly delineates the position of the catheter within the vessel. The reference image may be from a recent angiographic run or may be produced by acquiring a last-image hold frame of the contrast-filled vessel. In this way the reference image is used as a mask for subtracting from the real-time fluoroscopic display. As the catheter is advanced, it is seen progressing along the vessel lumen.

A refinement on the method for acquiring reference images is peak opacification. During the reference acquisition, a small bolus of contrast material is allowed to flow through the vascular tree instead of the entire vessel being filled with contrast material. The digital system acquires images and saves and displays only the maximum pixel values at each pixel location. The resultant image is then available as a mask for road mapping. The technique results in a reasonably noise-free reference image and requires less contrast material.

DUAL ENERGY AND HYBRID SUBTRACTION

Using two X-ray energies for acquiring image data is a technique that can be used to eliminate either bone or soft tissue detail. The technique depends on the energy dependence of X-ray attenuation through matter. In Chapter 3 it was shown that in the diagnostic range as the energy of the incident radiation increases the linear attenuation coefficient μ decreases. The decrease in μ is much greater for bone than the decrease for soft tissue. To obtain soft tissue cancellation which will produce a bone-enhanced image two radiographs, one with a low kV_p and one with a high kV_p, are acquired of the same anatomical region. When the low energy image is subtracted from the high energy image the soft tissue detail cancels leaving mainly bony detail. Bone cancellation is obtained by subtracting this bony image from the original low energy image. Table 13.3 identifies the high and low energy masks and contrast image series.

Patient motion is the main limitation to vascular imaging using temporal subtraction methods. Artifacts caused by involuntary motion, usually of soft tissue, e.g. due to bowel gas or peristaltic or cardiac movement, are very difficult to suppress. Dual-energy subtraction is relatively insensitive to patient motion as attenuation coefficients of either gas or soft tissue change little between the two energies.

Thus subtraction of the dual-energy images removes effects due to involuntary motion due to bowel gas. However, only one material can be eliminated using dual-energy subtraction. If an iodine contrast is introduced between the low and high energy images, while motion artifacts will be alleviated the image obtained by subtraction will now not only contain the vessels containing iodine contrast but also any overlying bone.

The image acquisition sequence during bolus transit for dual energy subtraction is detailed in Fig. 13.9a. A pictorial sequence in Fig. 13.9b shows a pair of images acquired at both low and high X-ray energies prior to the arrival of the contrast agent in the region of interest. Using energy subtraction these two images are combined to eliminate soft tissue and leave only bone structures as a pre-contrast mask:

$$M_L - M_H \rightarrow \text{bone image } M_B$$

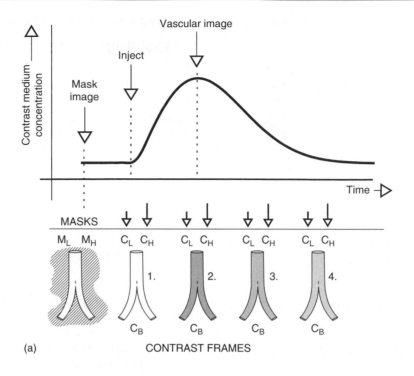

(a)

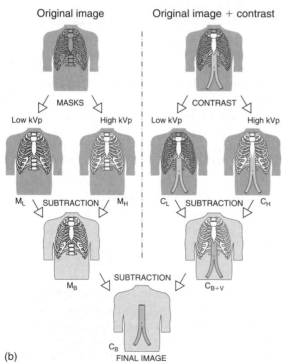

(b)

Figure 13.9 (*a*) The hybrid subtraction sequence representing passage of contrast medium through the vessel and the series of temporal frames C_L and C_H taken at low and high kilovoltages. (*b*) The image series formed during a dual energy subtraction series ending with the final image which contains only the vessel detail free from bone interference.

A series of low and high energy image pairs is then acquired as the contrast bolus flows through the region of interest. Each of these pairs is processed to suppress soft tissue components and to yield a post-contrast image of iodinated vessels plus bone residuals:

$$C_L - C_H \rightarrow \text{bone} + \text{iodine } C_{(B+V)}$$

Finally, a temporal subtraction of the dual-energy mask and post-contrast images removes the bone structures and successfully isolates the iodine-filled vasculature:

$$C_{(B+V)} - M_B \rightarrow \text{iodine image } C_V$$

Hybrid subtraction combines dual-energy techniques and temporal subtraction and successfully cures both overlying bone obscuring vessel detail and movement misregistration problems. The advantage of hybrid subtraction in comparison to temporal subtraction is that it eliminates artifacts caused by soft tissue motion and has the ability to eliminate both soft tissues and bone. However, because of the extra subtraction involved in the hybrid method there is increased noise in the final subtracted image. Hybrid subtraction also involves increased radiation exposure for the patient. However, elimination of motion artifacts may lead to a lower overall dose caused by repeat examinations.

13.7 EQUIPMENT SPECIFICATION FOR DIGITAL FLUOROSCOPY

Major radiography/fluoroscopy (R/F) designs using digital image capture are now based on C-arm geometry. Typical applications cover gastrointestinal, skeletal/orthopedic, vascular, and interventional procedures.

Small **mobile C-arm** machines with an image intensifier and an X-ray tube fixed as an integral unit find a ready application in surgery including orthopedics, bone fracture inspection, foreign body localization, and pacemaker implantation (Fig. 13.10). The image intensifier is linked via a fiber optic plate directly to a CCD device. The video signal provides a measure of light intensity which is related to X-ray exposure input. This forms the ABC feedback maintaining a constant dose rate at the image intensifier face. Table 13.4 lists a typical specification for a small mobile image intensifier unit. The images are stored firstly in memory and subsequently on hard disk. A removable optical disk is sometimes specified for viewing the images on the radiology PACS. Patient

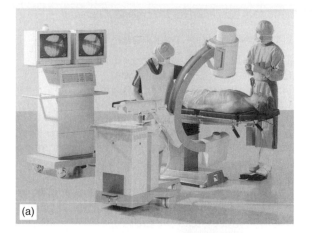

(a)

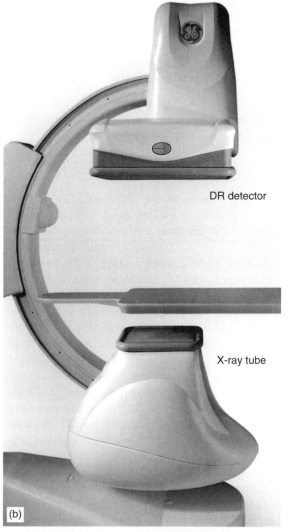

DR detector

X-ray tube

(b)

Figure 13.10 (*a*) *A small mobile C-arm used for small field of view interventional work.* (*b*) *A large flat panel detector on a cantilevered C-arm (courtesy GE Medical Systems).*

Table 13.4 *Specifications for a mobile C-arm unit.*

Component	Specification
X-ray tube	Dual focus stationary anode
Focal spot	0.6/0.8 mm
Image intensifier	15 cm, 560 cd m^{-2}, μC kg s^{-1}
SID	90 cm
Grid	Circular Pb8/40
Display	1024 × 1024 image matrix

radiation exposure can be reduced considerably by using last image hold storage (LIH) in memory. Small mobile C-arm systems are the simplest DF units and are used for:

• Orthopedic intervention
• Foreign body localization
• Cholangiography, cystography, pyelography
• Cardiac pacemaker implantation

The recent introduction of flat field DR detectors has made the mobile C-arm even more robust while maintaining image quality.

LARGE FIELD C-ARM

High output fixed units use cantilevered C-arms holding a large image intensifier and X-ray tube, suitable for vascular intervention studies with or without DSA facilities. Figure 13.10b shows a design incorporating a 22 × 22 cm CsI direct radiography (DR) detector. A typical large C-arm DSA machine would have a heavy duty X-ray tube (metal/ceramic) capable of over 2 kW in continuous operation and having a heat capacity of up to 3 to 5 MHU with dual focal spot of 0.6 and 1.0 mm. This would give an acquisition of up to 30 fps for either a 512 × 512 or 1024 × 1024 × 14 matrix.

The image storage of the system decides its capabilities. In most digital fluorography systems it is common practice to sum more than one image in order to improve the image SNR (recursive filtering). This averaging is accomplished by a data loop where the incoming image is added to the previously stored image. This requires at least 14 to 16 bits per pixel and many image processors have up to three image memories in order to speed this averaging process. Where a sequence of images is acquired they are stored in the main memory which can be 512 MB or larger. After image subtraction the images are stored on disk which is at least 100 GB.

Hybrid subtraction requires two essential components:

Timing: Since the interval between X-ray exposures must be minimized and the pulse widths kept short in order to minimize residual motion artifacts.

Energy consistency: The separation of the two X-ray energies (typically 60 and 110 kV$_p$) is necessary in order to minimize noise in the subtracted hybrid image. The short exposure times and relatively high exposure rates require tube currents of 1000 mA so the X-ray tube must be able to tolerate this high loading.

A suitable X-ray tube would be grid controlled and have a heat storage capacity approaching 2 MJ and a long-term anode loadability figure of 3 kW depending on focal spot size.

CARDIAC DIGITAL SUBTRACTION ANGIOGRAPHY

Digital cardiac angiography can capture non-subtracted images in 512 × 512 × 8 format at 50 fps. Digital cardiac imaging produces considerable image storage problems as shown in Table 11.11 and image frame rates can be reduced to alleviate this problem. The major advantage with digital cardiac imaging is

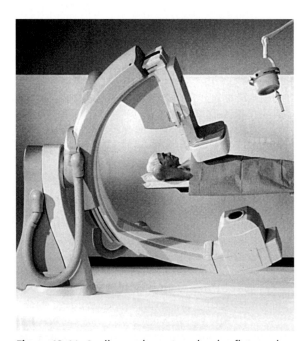

Figure 13.11 *Cardiovascular system showing flat panel detector having a specification listed in Table 13.5 (courtesy of Philips Medical).*

Table 13.5 *Typical specification for a flat detector small field cardiovascular system.*

Component or technique	Specification or use
Detector size (mm)	250, 190, 150 diagonal (square format)
Pixel size	184 × 184 μm
Resolution	2.7 Lp mm^{-1}
Display	1024 × 1024 (14 bits deep)
Frame rate (frames per second)	15 and 30
Image memory	512 MB
Magnetic disk	100 to 400 GB
Image processing	Cardiac subtraction
Clinical analysis	Cardiac ejection fraction

that the images can be retrieved immediately after acquisition (unlike cine angiography). Figure 13.11 shows a cardiovascular system with a flat panel detector having a specification listed in Table 13.5.

PULSED BEAM FLUOROSCOPY

Dose reduction is achieved by rapidly pulsing the X-ray tube using grid control circuits (see Section 10.4.3). In order to deliver a reasonable image noise level and adequate contrast, a large number of photons must be produced within the short time frame of each pulse without substantially increasing the kilovoltage. In conventional fluoroscopy, each frame is formed by integrating the exposure during two 16.7 ms pulses. The X-ray tube typically operates at about 2 mA, which results in 0.07 mAs per frame. To achieve the same noise level with a 10 ms pulse, the pulsed fluoroscopy system needs to operate at 7 mA. For good temporal resolution, the pulse width should be kept much shorter than this, on the order of 3 to 5 ms, requiring a proportional increased mA value per pulse (typically, 10 to 20 mA is not uncommon). This higher value requires an X-ray tube with high loadability; a high anode heat-storage capacity, housing and dissipation rates.

Computed tomography

14.1 INTRODUCTION

One of the major disadvantages associated with conventional planar radiography is its inability to produce sectional information. The image produced on film represents the total attenuation of the X-ray beam as it passes through the patient. It is impossible to distinguish any depth information on the film image. Tomographic techniques have been developed which will separate these superimposed anatomical details and produce slice images which convey depth information.

There are two general classes of tomography in radiographic imaging:

- **Linear,** or conventional tomography, which produces longitudinal sections
- **Computed axial tomography**, which produces sectional or axial slices

14.1.1 Linear tomography

Linear tomography gives longitudinal sectional information by moving the X-ray tube and film in synchrony about a fulcrum or axis. This fulcrum defines the sectional plane of the patient. The images produced are degraded to some extent by blurring caused by interfering absorption on either side of the plane of interest. Linear tomography has suffered a sharp demise with the widespread availability of

computed tomography and so will not be described in this chapter.

14.1.2 Computed tomography

Computed tomography is a digital-imaging process which produces separate axial sectional images (transverse slices) having no intersection interference. Computed axial tomography (CAT or CT) is entirely different from longitudinal tomography and produces radiological images as transaxial sections of the body without any intersectional interference or blurring. The method was first developed in a commercial X-ray machine by Godfrey Hounsfield (UK) in 1973. It was immediately successful as a diagnostic imaging technique since much smaller contrast differences are evident in the CT image, revealing subtle differences between normal and abnormal soft tissue. For example, visible contrast is about 2% on a good radiograph but this is extended to 0.1 to 0.3% for a typical CT image.

14.2 BASIC SEQUENTIAL SCANNER DESIGN

The basic design for a modern transaxial tomographic machine is illustrated in Fig. 14.1a. A rotating X-ray source, collimated as a fan beam, is subtended by a

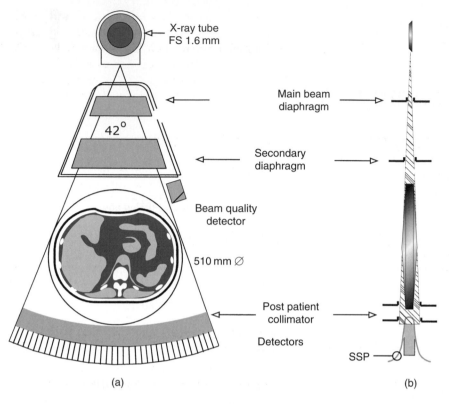

Figure 14.1 (a) Basic computed tomography design showing an X-ray source collimated to a fan beam rotating around a patient abdomen. The X-ray tube and detectors are fixed together as a single rotating unit. (b) The fan beam assembly showing collimator and detector geometry. The slice has a greater thickness in the middle and post patient collimation defines the slice sensitivity profile.

group of up to 800 detectors. The fan arrangement is rotated in a series of **projections** or angles covering the full 360° round the patient. At each projection (up to 1000 is typical for these machines) measurements are made of the beam attenuation. The typical side projection for a fan beam construction, with anode alignment, collimators, and detector array is shown in Fig. 14.1(b). The primary and secondary beam diaphragms (collimators) control the slice thickness. The beam monitor detector measures the beam quality at each projection.

14.2.1 Mechanical

Early CT systems used a mixed rotation and rectilinear scan movement (translation) for their data acquisition, which was very slow: these were the first and second generation machines. **Third generation** machines use fan beam **rotate only** designs and have very fast data acquisition times; approximately 1 to 2 s per slice is common. Image data is obtained by rotating the fan beam around the patient in a series of projections completing a 360° sweep (360 projection ≡ 1° per projection; 720 projections ≡ 0.5° etc.).

Figure 14.2a shows how the rotating fan beam spatially constructs a matrix of data cells over the patient slice during its 360° rotation; these are stored in computer memory as a data matrix or attenuation values. Machine precision in this movement influences the finest resolution of the matrix. The entire fan-beam mechanism (X-ray tube, detectors, and electronics) weighs about 500 kg and must move with a precision better than 0.01 mm.

A small matrix of 5 × 5 elements in Fig. 14.2(b) represents a central area of this data set which contains the individual attenuation coefficients μ. The sum of these is available during data collection as the **ray-sum**. The transaxial image is formed by calculating individual μ values within the matrix using image reconstruction techniques. The final result is a complete digital matrix whose elements represent the individual linear attenuation coefficients for the section or slice in the plane of the X-ray beam. The fundamental mathematics involved was first presented by J. Radon in 1913.

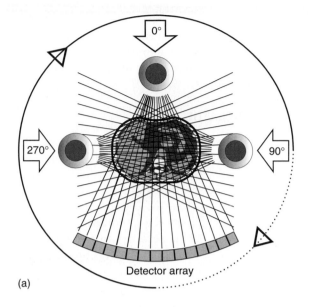

(a)

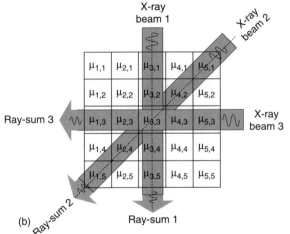

(b)

Figure 14.2 *(a) Image matrix projections for a fan-beam showing construction of matrix cells during fan-beam rotation. (b) A small section of the final matrix showing individual attenuation values combined as a ray-sum.*

An alternative CT design, the so called fourth generation design, had a fixed circle of detectors with the X-ray tube assembly moving inside this detector circle. Very fast scan times were possible but the design suffered from the limited packing density of its detectors and geometrical misalignment problems between the detector ring radius and the X-ray beam origin. It had one advantage over the fan beam design since it could give continuous rotation and therefore faster scan times.

The major drawback of early fan beam designs was that the X-ray tube had to return to its starting (home) position after each rotation; high voltage cable and signal leads connected to the rotating mechanism make this essential. This gave quite considerable interscan delay times. Subsequent spiral/helical scan machines addressed this problem.

SAMPLING FREQUENCY

During each projection the detector signals give information about the total tissue attenuation between the source and detector. High resolution CT requires high density samples. If an insufficient number of projections are taken then streaking is seen. A total of 500 projections are sufficient for a 256×256 matrix with 1 mm resolution whereas 1000 projections require a 512×512 matrix to see 0.5 mm.

14.2.2 X-ray tube and generator

Computed tomography X-ray tubes have a very high standard of performance since they must deliver a stable, intense pulse of X-ray photons for each projection. The X-ray beam is highly filtered by both aluminum and copper to produce a high effective photon energy. X-ray tube specifications are listed in Table 14.1 for two X-ray tubes, one suitable for a low to medium use machine and the other a high throughput or rapid scan machine.

The X-ray intensity or output must not vary over the image acquisition cycle as any variation would be treated as absorption differences in the image; generator stability is typically better than 1%. The linear attenuation coefficient μ is dependent on the kilovoltage so variations in the effective kV energy of the beam will produce variations in the image. In addition it is necessary to maintain the X-ray spectrum to within very narrow limits so that μ does not alter.

Table 14.1 *Computed tomography X-ray tube specifications.*

Design feature	Low–medium	High
Focal spot	1.6 mm	0.8 to 1.2 mm
Anode loading	1 MJ (1.35 MHU)	2.7 MJ (3.5 MHU)
Thermal dissipation	350 kHU	730 kHU
Maximum power	30 kW	40 kW

For large object thicknesses a slice energy of about 30 kW s and a pulse power of 40 kW is necessary in order to generate the necessary minimum number of X-ray photons. The heat capacity of the anode (in excess of 5 MHU) allows a large volume scan consisting of up to 20 to 30 slices.

The **focal spot size** of the X-ray tube determines the minimum point size in the center of the scanned field which is projected onto the detector array. This determines the amount of information distributed over the detector array. As the focal spot increases the point information is spread over a larger number of detectors; this limits resolution. Typical focal spot sizes are between 0.6 and 1.6 mm.

The **anode angles** in CT X-ray tubes are smaller than normal and a common design feature is a completely flat anode surface with an angled cathode/filament assembly. The flat anode ensures more uniform heat transfer and dissipation. The **heel effect** is minimized by setting the cathode–anode axis perpendicular to the detector axis.

Modern machines using a continuously rotating fan beam design can also switch the position of the focal spot (Fig. 14.3). This has the effect of doubling the number of projections during a scan. The direction of the electron beam in the X-ray tube is magnetically

shifted so altering the position of the focal spot on the anode. This small movement effectively halves the detector width for a given number of fan beam projections and doubles the number of ray projections for each sectional image.

X-RAY GENERATOR

High frequency power supplies are used exclusively in CT machines; these provide extremely stable tube current and voltages controlled by a dedicated microprocessor. The X-ray tubes are operated in a fast pulse mode by switching the grids of the X-ray tube. A pulse duration of between 2 and 4 ms and a pulse power of over 40 kW is necessary to give optimum speed of data acquisition and the X-ray tube currents can be up to 800 mA.

BEAM ATTENUATION

Computed tomography operates at about 125 kV$_p$, a little higher in some machines. This is at least 50% higher than conventional radiography and extra beam filtration (2.5 mm aluminum with 0.4 mm copper) ensures that the effective energy is also high (70 to 80 keV). This reduces the effect of 'beam hardening' by the tissues.

Subject contrast of soft-tissue detail from this high effective energy does not depend on photoelectric absorption (in common with most conventional radiography) but the dominant interaction is due to inelastic or Compton scattering which removes X-ray photons from the main beam. Since the fan-beam system has a narrow, highly collimated X-ray source and the detector array is also carefully collimated, the amount of scattered radiation that reaches the detectors is minimized so the image information is carried by the emerging unscattered X-ray beam.

Photoelectric absorption is dependent on atomic number Z and density but Compton scattering depends on tissue electron density (see Chapter 5). Although the electron density per gram of soft tissue is very consistent over a fixed volume of tissue the electrons per unit volume (electrons cm^{-3}) does vary. This gives the tissue differentiation in CT images.

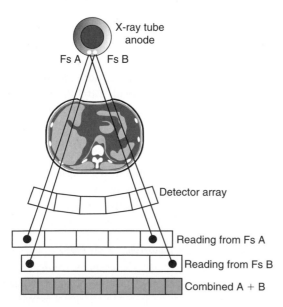

Figure 14.3 *Beam switching by magnetically shifting the X-ray tube electron beam to hit two different areas on the anode. This allows double sampling of the detector which yields two offset readings A and B.*

BEAM HARDENING

As the incident beam passes through the patient lower energy photons are preferentially removed; the effective energy of the X-ray spectrum increases and thus the values of the linear attenuation coefficients decrease. The increase in effective energy causes beam hardening which is influenced by the patient thickness and tissue material; it is worse for bone.

Absorption of a monochromatic X-ray beam with increasing depth of water will give a straight line for I_{in} divided by I_{out} as shown in Fig. 14.4a. However, a typical polychromatic X-ray beam will give a curved response as the lower energies are filtered by the thicker absorption pathway. This nonlinear response is predictable and provides corrections for beam hardening in CT images. The **cupping effect** caused by uncorrected beam hardening is seen in profile across a uniform absorber in Fig. 14.4b. Both tube filtration and correction algorithms reduce beam

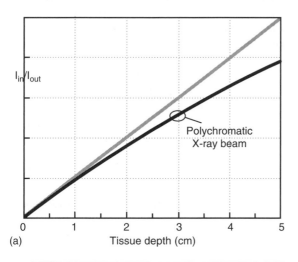

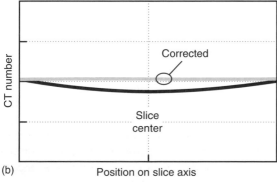

Figure 14.4 *(a) The loss of photon intensity (ratio of input and output beam intensity) from a polychromatic beam with tissue depth. (b) The cupping profile (reduction of CT number value) across the field of view compared to the corrected level profile; maximum error is at the center of the slice.*

hardening artifacts in the final CT image. The corrections work well for soft tissue (water equivalent) but problems can occur in images containing a large amount of bone (head sections). In order to minimize beam hardening it is heavily filtered, using 0.25 to 0.4 mm copper foil; this reduces spectrum width and also X-ray photon intensity. The tube current must be large to compensate for this photon reduction, consequently the heat rating of modern CT tubes must be high as the anode cooling rate limits the number and duration of CT scans. High power output requires oil cooled tubes which often have heat capacities up to 5 MHU.

14.2.3 Collimation and slice thickness

The spatial resolution of a CT system must consider both the resolution in the slice plane together with that perpendicular to it, which is determined by the slice thickness. A high resolution in the slice plane can only be achieved if it is matched by a thin slice, so resolution should be balanced between the slice plane and slice thickness. Owing to the finite length of the detector and the small dimensions of the focal spot, the X-ray beam diverges somewhat in the direction of the slice thickness, so that the latter acquires a slightly wedge shape.

The slice thickness is determined by the collimation shown in Fig. 14.1a and b applied to both the emerging X-ray beam and the entrance to the detectors. The sensitivity profile represents the real slice thickness defined by the full width at half maximum (FWHM) of the sensitivity profile; that is, the distance between the two edges at 50% of the maximum value indicated on the profiles in Fig. 14.5; other methods of measurement are discussed in later sections.

SLICE SENSITIVITY PROFILE

The sensitivity profile is an important factor of a CT machine since it determines the image quality. The steeper the profile slope the less interference from adjacent slices that would cause partial volume effects. The perfect sensitivity profile would be rectangular and for a point source of X-rays this could be achieved by simple collimation; however, for a practical system where the focal spot has a finite size geometrical unsharpness causes penumbra effects and tight collimation at the detector entrance is necessary.

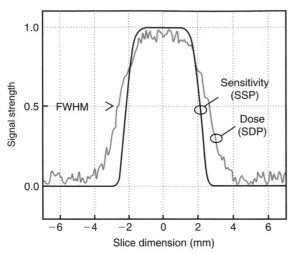

Figure 14.5 *Typical slice sensitivity profile (SSP) and slice dose profile (SDP) for a single slice sequential computed tomography machine. The SDP extends beyond the SSP, adding to the patient dose.*

When opposing beam shapes are superimposed as would be seen in a full 360° data collection series the two diverging beams give a slice section that departs from a true rectangle. The middle of the slice is thicker than the periphery. This is particularly noticeable for thin slices. The general bi-conical shape of a CT slice is indicated in Fig. 14.1b.

SLICE DOSE PROFILE

The slice sensitivity profile (SSP) and the slice dose profile (SDP) have different geometries when measured at the axis, as shown in Fig. 14.5. The larger dose profile contributes to increased surface dose. The xenon gas detectors offer built-in collimation so extra detector collimation is unnecessary and there is good agreement between sensitivity and dose profiles.

14.2.4 Detectors

Three types of detector systems are suitable for CT machines:

- Multiple scintillation detectors with photomultipliers
- Multiple scintillation detectors with photodiodes
- A single multi-chamber inert gas (xenon) detector

Current designs favor gas detectors in spite of their lower quantum efficiency.

GAS PROPORTIONAL DETECTORS

The common detector uses a chamber filled with xenon gas, which is less dependent on stable high voltage supplies, is inherently uniform, and provides in-built collimation as an added bonus. Figure 14.6a gives a design for an integral 768 detector array using pressurized xenon. The xenon gas used to fill the chambers has a high atomic number which increases photoelectric absorption in the detector. Absorption is further increased by keeping the gas under high pressure (up to 20 atm or $20 \times 10^5\,Pa$) and increasing the length of the chambers. Under these circumstances the sensitivity can be about 50% of the scintillation detector. The complete detector array (Fig. 14.6b) is subdivided, using electrode plates, into a large number of chambers (up to 1000). Each one shares the same gas volume minimizing variation in sensitivity between the chambers. The signal strength is not influenced by small supply voltage variations, unlike the crystal/photomultiplier or crystal/photodiode systems. The electrode plates forming the chambers also act as collimators so added collimation is minimal between patient and detector. Each detector anode feeds a dedicated amplifier which is switched to a common A/D converter. The detector electrodes are aligned with the focal spot of the X-ray tube. This is the acceptance angle of the detector decided by the detector collimation and detector aperture size.

Typical detector aperture sizes are between 1 and 2 mm for a detector depth of 100 mm. The fixed detector design of the fourth generation machine has two geometrical centers, that of the gantry–patient and that of the X-ray focal spot. This geometric misalignment between X-ray beam and the center of the detector array gives misaligned beam angles at the detector surface so only shallow depth detectors (photodiodes) can be used to accommodate this differing geometry and the packing density of the detectors (influencing resolution) is restricted. For this reason the fixed detector design has become unpopular in spite of its fast scan times.

SCINTILLATION DETECTORS

Early CT machines used scintillation crystals (thallium doped NaI) and photomultiplier tubes as X-ray detectors. The photomultiplier tubes could not provide the

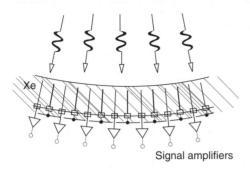

(a) Xenon gas detector schematic

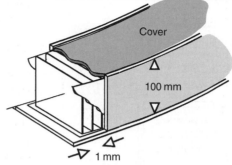

(b) Xenon gas detector design

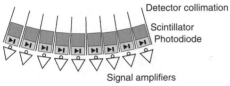

(c) Photodiode detectors

Figure 14.6 *(a) Xenon gas detectors have deep chambers, have a common compressed xenon gas fill and because of their depth provide their own collimation. (b) The complete detector array consists of over 700 separate 1 mm detector elements. (c) Separate solid state (scintillation) detectors combined with their photodiodes require separate collimation to form a detector array.*

packing density that was necessary with fan-beam designs so photodiode detectors were substituted. Cesium iodide superseded sodium iodide as a detector since it gives light photons in the visible range (sodium iodide gives ultraviolet) which can be detected by a simple photodiode which is packed into a very small volume array (example sketched in Fig. 14.6c). Major problems with scintillation detectors are:

- Relatively long afterglow following the detection of an X-ray photon.
- Stable output signals depend on a very stable high-voltage supply.
- Multi-detector uniformity of response is difficult to maintain.

In spite of their high quantum efficiency solid state devices have been replaced by gas detectors which have several advantages.

DETECTOR SIGNALS

These are analog voltage pulses which vary in height according to the level of absorption. They are digitized for processing by a fast analog-to-digital converter (ADC) which is switched to serve the complete detector array. The requirements for an ideal detection system are:

- High efficiency for recording radiation
- Fast response time recording all the detected radiation

- Linear and stable
- Large dynamic range of the detector which is dependent on the accuracy and precision of the ADC

In practice the detector system is a compromise between quantum efficiency which influences patient dose, packing density which influences resolution and response which influences image contrast.

14.2.5 Data acquisition

DATA STORAGE

The CT machine must be capable of acquiring a large number of data samples from its detector array over a very short time to give fast scan times and reduce motion artifacts. Signals from each detector are digitized and transferred to the array processor. For each scan projection a number of mathematical operations are performed on the raw data from the detectors. Separate very fast circuits perform one operation on the signal data and then pass it on to the next circuit using a **pipe-line** process. Image reconstruction is an example of pipe-line processing. Figure 14.7 is a schematic following data acquisition from the detector array through to the array processor. This handles analog to digital conversion then some signal pre-processing before applying filtered back-projection.

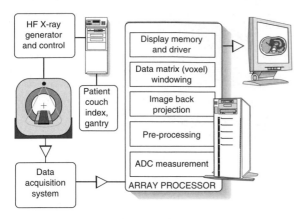

Figure 14.7 *Computed tomography system data collection and control showing pipe-line processing in the array processor to give fast image display.*

While filtering is being performed on one profile, say P, back-projection is occurring with the last profile $P + 1$ and log amplification is occurring with the next profile $P - 1$ etc. The fact that many different processes are occurring simultaneously increases the speed of image reconstruction and presentation. The result is a voxel matrix containing CT or Hounsfield numbers.

The simplified block diagram shown in Fig. 14.7 also gives the main components: the gantry, complete with its X-ray tube and detector array, connected to a computer control system. The image array processor and control console with display are separate. These are linked by a common data bus which transfers information and control signals between a central processor, which holds the acquisition and display programs, and the peripheral systems which collect and process the detector signal data. The array processor reconstructs the section images and displays the final results at the console. Patient positioning is also under computer control, and the overall data flow allows a fully automatic patient handling program to be set up for a particular imaging sequence, i.e. zoomed image sequence of the spine between chosen lumbar vertebrae or a complete set of sectional images following a contrast bolus injection.

COMPUTED TOMOGRAPHY NUMBERS

The absorption coefficient μ depends on the kilovoltage. However, if the tissue absorption coefficient is related to that of water at the same kV a reference

number insensitive to kV change can be obtained. A CT number or **Hounsfield unit** can now be used which is

$$1000 \times \frac{\mu_{\text{tissue}} - \mu_{\text{water}}}{\mu_{\text{water}}} \qquad (14.1)$$

Box 14.1 shows calculations for three different kV values; the CT value remains constant since the water reference also matches the kV value. In practice a range of CT values are produced from -1000 for air, 0 for water and between 2000 and 3000 for bone, some machines producing an even wider range. Figure 14.8 shows values for common tissues. These values are approximately the same between different machines since they are always referenced to water.

DYNAMIC RANGE

The ADC must be capable of responding to a wide variation of attenuation in the patient. This is usually more than 1 000 000 to 1. The dynamic range reflects the ratio of the largest signal (no attenuation) to the smallest signal (maximum attenuation) that can be detected. This allows obese and slim patients to be imaged with the same definition including dense bone and low density soft tissue. Dynamic range is dependent on the accuracy and precision of the ADC of the voltage signal (Box 14.2).

DATA MATRICES

These CT numbers are stored in computer memory and represent a volume slice element or **voxel**. The matrix store must be able to hold a range of voxel values of over 4000. A single voxel is represented in Fig. 14.9a situated in a CT slice. The primary storage matrix for the computed CT numbers must be able to handle values from 0 to 3000 (both positive and negative figures). This requires a memory location of at least 12 bits which is 2^{12} or 4096, plus a 'sign' bit positive or negative. Figure 14.9(b) represents part of a 512×512 voxel memory 16 bits deep. This represents a total storage of 500 kB.

Since the thickness of the tissue is defined by the section width, a collection of transverse images represents a three-dimensional volume of voxel values. Image quality is defined by the dimensions of the sampling ray which determines the attenuation value

Box 14.1 Calculation of computed tomography number

Equation 14.1 is used for the data, and values of μ_{muscle} and μ_{water} at different kV levels are given below.

μ	80 kV	100 kV	150 kV
μ_{muscle}	0.1892	0.1760	0.1550
μ_{water}	0.1835	0.1707	0.1504

At 80 keV: $1000 \times \dfrac{0.1892 - 0.1835}{0.1835} = 31$

At 100 keV: $1000 \times \dfrac{0.1760 - 0.1707}{0.1707} = 31$

At 150 keV: $1000 \times \dfrac{0.1550 - 0.1504}{0.1504} = 31$

Beam hardening

At 100 kV the reference for water is 0.1707 but if the beam effective energy changes to 105 kV in the center of the profile, the μ for tissue changes to 0.1750 then the new CT value is

$$\frac{0.1750 - 0.1707}{0.1707} = 25$$

and not 31, which it should be. This gives the cupping effect seen in Fig. 14.4b.

Box 14.2 Dynamic range of an analog to digital converter

The analog voltage level for a 20 bit binary number is 220 which gives a range of 1:1 000 000. Uncertainty in voltage measurement is therefore $\sqrt{10^6}$ or 1000 which represents 0.1%. At 150 keV the μ value for muscle is 0.155 (0.1% of this value is therefore 0.000155). A positive or negative 0.1% variation in μ gives:

$$\frac{0.155155 - 0.1504}{0.1504} \times 1000 = 32$$

$$\frac{0.154845 - 0.1504}{0.1504} \times 1000 = 30$$

Conclusion

A greater than a 0.1% variation in voltage measurement will influence the calculation of computed tomography number.

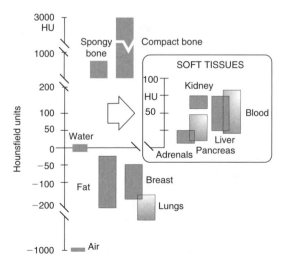

Figure 14.8 *A bar plot of common computed tomography value ranges for tissues and reference materials.*

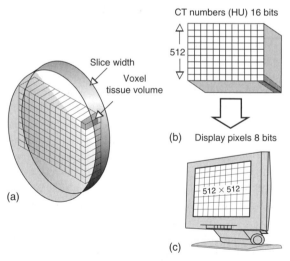

Figure 14.9 *(a) The body slice represented as a digital matrix stored as CT numbers. Each small tissue volume resolved by the matrix is a 'voxel' or volume element. (b) The voxel information is stored in memory by typically a 512 × 512 matrix each voxel occupying a 12 to 16 bit word. (c) The windowed display pixel is stored as a 512 × 512 matrix which can be 4 to 8 bits deep.*

stored in the voxel and its spatial sampling. Uncertainty in the measured voxel attenuation appears as image noise, and the dimensions define the limiting spatial resolution attainable by the scanner.

The entire CT information in a data matrix (as CT numbers) cannot be displayed, since video monitors have limited dynamic range and are usually driven by 8 bit DACs giving 256 gray levels; the entire contents of a raw data matrix, representing CT numbers from $+3000$ for bone to -1000 for lungs would require 4000 gray levels which is not practical for electronic display devices. The display matrix represented in Fig. 14.9c is therefore restricted to only 8 bits deep and a sampling method called windowing has been devised for representing the full 12 bit data on the 8 bit display (described in Chapter 12 and later in this chapter).

14.2.6 Image reconstruction

Absorption signals that have been collected as single-dimensional values must now be displayed as a two-dimensional image. The matrix of absorption coefficients is obtained from the scanning pattern of the fan beam previously shown in Fig. 14.2a and is commonly represented in a 512×512 format. A small portion of such a matrix is shown in Fig. 14.2b where the line source of X-rays (1, 2, 3 etc.) has undergone absorption and the attenuated beam is measured using a detector array opposite the X-ray beam. Only the total absorption figure is known: this is the **ray sum**. The separate matrix values shown in the diagram: $\mu_{(1-1)}$, $\mu_{(1-2)}$ ... $\mu_{(5-5)}$ are found by mathematical reconstruction. The individual values in the matrix can be calculated by using either an **iterative technique** or **back-projection** (or its derivatives). The calculations are performed in a dedicated array processor in order to provide almost instantaneous image display.

INTERATIVE TECHNIQUE

This uses an exact mathematical solution for reconstructing the image slice from the attenuation data. This was the original method for image reconstruction used by Godfrey Hounsfield (1919–2004; British engineer) in the first CT machine. Its disadvantages are that it takes a considerable amount of computer time and is slow. It also suffers from rounding errors

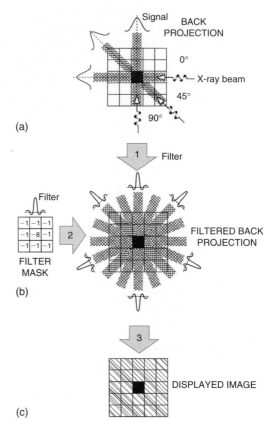

Figure 14.10 (*a*) *Simple back-projection yields a blurred image; the ray-sum signals are collected and the totals back-projected giving a composite signal. After all the projections have been collected and stored the star-burst pattern in* (*b*) *is then filtered using the mask to reveal the true signal displayed in* (*c*). *The calculations are performed in a dedicated array processor in order to provide almost instantaneous image display.*

$(0.95 = 1.0$, etc.) which give imprecise CT values and all the data must be collected before reconstruction can begin.

BACK-PROJECTION

The principle is shown in Fig. 14.10a. A tightly collimated X-ray beam is used and its total absorption provides the ray-sum signal for each matrix row, which is stored in the array processor image memory. This is shown in the diagram (a) for 0°, 45°, and 90° rotated scan positions. Other projections (b)

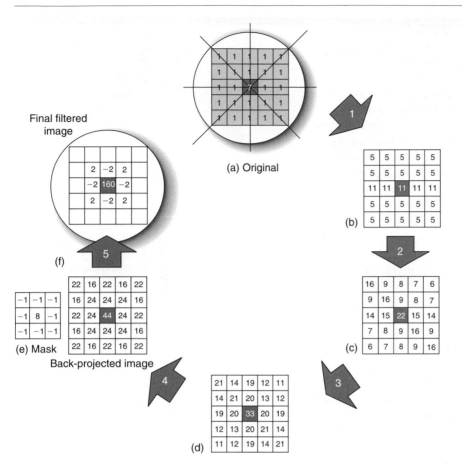

(a) Original

(b)

(c)

(d)

(e) Mask

Back-projected image

(f)

Final filtered
image

Figure 14.11 *A numerical example of filtered back-projection using a simple 5 × 5 matrix. The back-projection proceeds in five stages (stages b to f). At stage e a filter, mask or kernel is applied to retrieve the true point source data.*

provide the complete data set. The central high uptake, from the original, is now distinguishable but it has a star-burst interference pattern. Early attempts at this form of reconstruction used photographic methods and the final images contained star artifacts (there is only one star artifact shown here matching the single high data point in the original image). The artifacts can be removed by just accepting the high values but this is not a satisfactory solution.

FILTERED BACK-PROJECTION

Figure 14.10(b) shows how the star interference may be removed. A **mask** signal with negative going edges (the second stage shown as a small matrix adjacent to Fig. 14.10(b)) acts as a high pass filter removing the remaining back-projected low frequency interference pattern. This results in a clearer displayed

matrix in (c); the original high central value is now clearly seen.

A five-stage numerical example for filtered back-projection is shown in Fig. 14.11 which resembles the previous pictorial example in Fig. 14.10, this having a high central value of 7 surrounded by lower values of 1 (central matrix in Fig. 14.11).

Moving on to the first computation: the horizontal back-projection in (b) stores the total ray sum in each row of (a). In the second stage (c) right diagonal ray sums are then added followed by the vertical (d) and left diagonal ray sums, giving the final image in Fig. 14.11 (e). The next process of **convolution** uses the same mask shown in Fig. 14.10.

CONVOLUTION

The back-projected matrix is subjected to a filter mask, or convolution kernel whose contents are multiplied with the back-projected image. The filter mask consists of a small symmetrical matrix containing a set of numbers. These can have positive or negative values. The filter mask shown in Fig. 14.11(e) is shifted over the back-projected matrix a row at a time multiplying the image pixel by the corresponding filter value e.g. 22 × −1, 16 × −1, etc. until all nine values under the filter have been multiplied giving the filtered back-projection image in (f) with the central area of 160 exaggerated by the edge enhancement filter surrounded by cells of very small numbers (2 and −2). Figure 14.12a shows the filter mask in action for a selected corner of this matrix, 24 being the central value. All the values are summed and the result placed in the central pixel of the image array. The filter mask is then shifted one column and the complete process repeated. The central region of the back-projected matrix is similarly treated giving an enhanced value of 160 (Fig. 14.12b).

In practice the signal data from the CT detector array are first logarithmically amplified to correct for transmission absorption, then beam hardening corrections are made. Each projection then undergoes the convolution process before back-projection (unlike this simple numerical example); the type of convolution filter can be chosen by the user, giving either image smoothing or edge enhancement.

SUMMARY

Algebraic methods are hardly used any more. There are two main reasons for this: firstly, the image calculation is only possible after the acquisition of all scan data, so that there is a longer delay; and secondly, the computing time is considerably longer than with the convolution method. However, since reconstruction methods are finding increasing application in clinical areas such as nuclear medicine and ultrasound diagnostics, where the mathematical conditions for the convolution method are only satisfied inadequately, the flexible and versatile iteration techniques have regained importance.

Since every projection is immediately processed with the convolution method after its measurement there is no delay between the completion of the measurement and the appearance of the image on the screen.

In order to reconstruct a CT image in real time, i.e. while the measurement data is being transferred to the computer, pipe-line processing is used

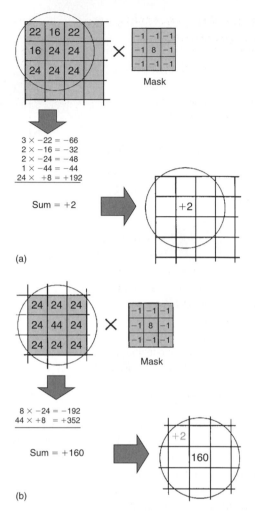

Figure 14.12 *Filtering selected regions of the image shown in Fig. 14.11. The edge of the matrix is shown filtered in (a) yielding a central value of +2. The center region in Fig. 14.11(e) is filtered in (b) using the same mask and gives the high central positive value. This action removes the shadowing artifact associated with back-projection.*

(Fig. 14.7). While the first projection is undergoing analog to digital conversion (ADC) and is being transferred to the computer, the immediately preceding measured projection is already undergoing the necessary preprocessing steps; its predecessor is back-projected and convolved at the same time and its predecessor in turn is already being back-projected. Hardwired special computers are used, which have been especially designed for executing this operation (array processors).

14.2.7 Pre-processing and post-processing

The raw signal data undergoes processing before taking part in image reconstruction and then the reconstructed image itself can be processed to enhance features or remove artifacts.

SIGNAL DATA PROCESSING

A balancing procedure corrects slight sensitivity differences between individual detector channels so that overlying ring artifacts are not seen. This is a common feature of scintillation detector machines. Extended balancing can help to remove streaking caused by sudden density changes (bone to soft tissue). Beam hardening corrections are also applied at this stage. A sampling error is seen in all reconstructive techniques, where the diagonal X-ray beams do not sample complete volume elements. This is corrected by applying chosen weighting factors to each matrix element; the missing sections have a constant area for a fixed beam width and known angle.

IMAGE PROCESSING

Secondary or retrospective reconstruction is performed on an image to enlarge or zoom a smaller portion of the scan view. This causes a real improvement in image resolution, up to the machine's maximum dictated by the physical characteristics of the detectors and collimators. A zoom factor of 1 (real size) may give an image resolution of 1 mm, increasing the zoom to 10 can increase the image resolution to 0.1 mm. Simple magnification of the image does not however involve reconstruction; it merely enlarges the area of interest to fill the display screen.

Mutiplanar reconstruction is also a post-processing technique for combining contiguous axial slices into a three dimensional view. This 3-D data set can then be displayed either as a complete image or as a series of sagittal, coronal, and oblique cuts.

PLANAR PROJECTION VIEW (TOPOGRAM OR SCOUT-VIEW)

These are the names given by different manufacturers to 2-D planar projection views. The scanning system remains in a fixed position with the X-ray tube either above and the detectors underneath the patient or occupying a lateral or posterior aspect.

The patient is then moved through the gantry. The line profiles are then combined to give a longitudinal radiograph. These images are used for determining slice plane position. Slice position is decided and the computer immediately positions the body in the gantry at the chosen point by moving the scan bed. The radiation dose required for these longitudinal views is very low, unlike the CT slice dose itself.

FAST FOURIER TRANSFORMS

This is the preferred method for the reconstruction algorithm for filtered back-projection. The data in each profile are treated as a mixed frequency and the entire image reconstruction then takes place as a series of amplitudes in the frequency domain. (Fourier analysis is explained in Chapter 1.) After filtering, each modified projection is added to the sum of the previous filtered back-projections.

WINDOWING AND IMAGE DISPLAY

Under ideal conditions the eye can distinguish between 50 and 80 gray levels on a good quality computer monitor. Routinely this range is reduced to nearer 35 to 40. Since the full CT data set of 4000 levels cannot be displayed at one time the user must select, or **window**, a range of CT values for display. The CT number range is shown in Fig. 14.13a (-1000 to $+3000$); a window width has been selected with a particular offset, which is the central value.

The range of displayed CT values (as the **window width**) can be displayed at various pixel depths and examples in Fig. 14.13(b) show different window widths (4 to 8 bits) that are used for sampling the available range of CT numbers. The position of the window within the data is the **offset**. If a broad window, from -1000 to $+1000$ is displayed using 256 gray levels, a CT number difference of 8 is represented by one gray level, giving a poor contrast image. Such an image would be useful as an overview only. Small changes in CT number, and therefore greater contrast, can be obtained from narrower windows. If it is too small the image can show a great deal of noise and details in bony structures or fatty tissue could be missed.

The window itself can be moved or offset up or down the scale to include soft tissue or bone detail. CT values outside the window will be shown as white (above the window value) or black (below the window value). For the differentiation of bony or soft tissues

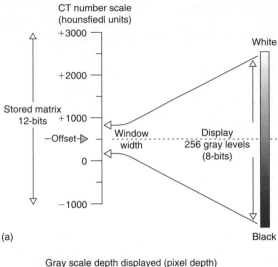

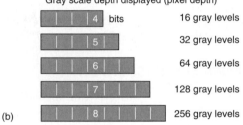

Figure 14.13 *(a) The entire data set stored as CT numbers from +3000 to −1000 occupying 12 bits can only be displayed (b) as separate 4 to 8 bit 'windows' (window width).*

certain window offsets are recommended. For most soft tissue images a window offset of between 35 to 40 and a window width of 200 to 450 covers most detail. For thorax–lung the offset should be −700 and for the inner ear +200. Double windowing is available on some machines where two different density ranges can be displayed together, i.e. negative lung tissue alongside positive detail of the mediastinum. An entire gray scale is available for each of the window widths and, for clarity, a bright contour separates them.

LOOK-UP TABLES

The CT numbers can be displayed on a linear or non-linear scale. Each CT number is referenced to a scale held in the computer display memory as a table of values: this scale is the **look-up table** (LUT). It normally contains a linear set of gray-scale values, so the CT numbers are represented by a linear density scale. However, it can be tailored as a non-uniform table

where tissues of very similar density can be distinguished by allocating steeply changing nonlinear display values. For example a logarithmic scale is often used.

IMAGE FILTERING

The convolution kernel or filter influences the appearance of the image depending on whether a smoothing (low-pass filter) or edge enhancement (high-pass filter) has been chosen. In most CT machines a variety of convolution kernels are available giving standard, light smoothing, extreme smoothing or special high resolution (edge enhancement). Special kernels are also available for reducing beam hardening in head scans.

14.2.8 Image quality

The choice of a machine depends very much on the type of patient case load (e.g. neurology, cardiac) and the patient throughput. For a busy or specialist department a machine capable of a high quality imaging (thin sections, fast scan time etc.) should be considered. Fast scan times (<1 s) will reduce motion artifact (useful in pediatrics). A busy general department would specify a machine with a high power generator and high heat rating X-ray tube giving a large number of sections per unit time. Three-dimensional reconstruction or vascular imaging (bolus transit) may require a spiral acquisition mode (see Sections 14.3 and 14.4).

UNIFORMITY

An important characteristic for assessing image quality is the homogeneity or uniformity over the entire cross section of a homogeneous phantom. Figure 14.14a shows measurements on a water phantom. The degree of homogeneity determines the accuracy of CT number measurement for the same tissue (e.g. liver) at various points across the field of view (FOV). Owing to beam hardening artifacts due to different attenuation through the object the reconstruction algorithm contains correction factors (as a look-up-table) which adjust for these variations. This is important since data measured from different directions of projection (180° opposed ray-sums) would not match. Since beam filtration is already severe in current makes of CT scanner (between 0.25 and

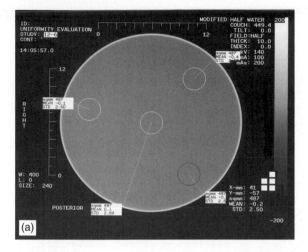

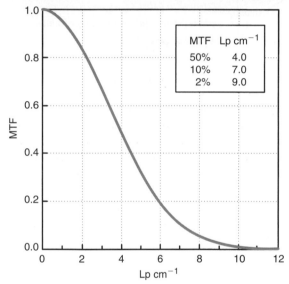

Figure 14.14 (*a*) *A uniformity check giving mean and standard deviation figures for selected areas of a water bath across the field of view.* (*b*) *A modulation transfer function measurement using a point spread function given by a thin wire scanned in the gantry using a general reconstruction protocol.*

0.4 mm copper) the hardening effect is not pronounced so computer correction can be carried out for a wide range of object diameters.

CALIBRATION

An uncalibrated system will have significant influence on overall image quality (resolution, contrast and noise) so calibration of the system components (X-ray tube, detectors, and electronics) must be carried out prior to imaging. The calibration is usually carried out by performing a single scan of a water phantom and inspecting it for inhomogeneity.

RESOLUTION

This is characterized by the ability to distinguish high contrast small objects (high CT number: bony detail) as well as to differentiate close objects (small vessels). Factors influencing resolution are:

- Display matrix and pixel size
- Field of view which can be chosen by zooming

The size of the display pixel can limit image resolution if it is larger than the intrinsic resolution (measured by the MTF). This is true for whole sections where each matrix pixel represents quite coarse resolution. Interpolation from 512×512 to 1024×1024 is purely a cosmetic exercise and does not affect true resolution. Reconstructed pixel size can be derived from:

$$\frac{\text{reconstructed field of view}}{\text{matrix size}} \quad (14.2)$$

Typical values of displayed pixel size are ~0.15 mm for a 512×512 matrix representing a restricted FOV of 7.5 cm (head scan), and 0.3 mm for a 512×512 representing a 15 cm FOV (body scan). Spatial resolution is significantly influenced by the kernel used for reconstruction but data reconstruction beyond a certain zoom factor cannot improve on intrinsic resolution.

Figure 14.14(b) is an MTF example obtained by imaging a 10 μm wire and using standard reconstruction protocols. This, together with the uniformity check, would be part of a routine quality control program. The values given by this curve can be translated into appropriate resolution figures. The 2% value of 8.5 Lp cm^{-1} represents high resolution contrast. A single line or point being the reciprocal of this value: 0.6 mm. Similarly the 50% low contrast resolution value of 4 Lp cm^{-1} translates as 1.3 mm. The 512×512 matrix is therefore sufficient for displaying this detail.

ALIASING

This has already been discussed in Chapter 12. If the discrete sampling frequency of the CT system is too low for the frequency of the object then the high

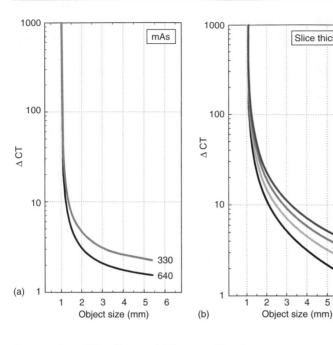

Figure 14.15 *Contrast detail diagrams. The basic contrast detail diagram identifying the resolution limit as the vertical line from 1 mm. (**a**) Increasing radiation dose (330 mAs to 640 mAs) improves image contrast detail. (**b**) Improvement in low contrast detail with thicker slice sections: 1 mm, 2 mm, 4 mm, and 8 mm.*

frequencies will be distorted. The sampling frequency must be at least twice that of the object frequencies to prevent aliasing. This is particularly important in the petrous bone area.

The X-ray beam width and detector dimensions limit the sampling frequency but this is overcome by introducing a ¼ detector shift where the detector array is shifted with respect to the center of the fan beam. This will achieve beam interlacing on opposing projections (0° and 180°, 90° and 270° etc.) and so double the frequency sampling rate.

A smaller department would not require a high rated machine, and costs can be significantly reduced by choosing a low or medium rated design. Reconstruction matrices should be 512 × 512 interpolated to 1024 × 1024 for best display; reconstruction times should be less than 5 s. Magnification views enlarge image detail but do not improve the overall image resolution. However, image resolution can be improved by zooming a section of the matrix and reconstructing this data. This improves image resolution up to the machine's limit. Spatial resolution in zoom mode should be less than 0.5 mm.

CONTRAST

Low contrast detectability is defined as the smallest object size visible at a given percentage contrast level. Image contrast is measured as differences between the object density (in CT numbers) and its background.

Low contrast detectability involves both image noise and spatial information. Image reconstruction kernels influence low contrast detectability and resolution. A standard kernel with some smoothing would give a resolution of just under 1 mm detecting a 5 mm object having a CT value difference (ΔCT) of 0.3%.

$$\Delta\text{CT}(\%) = \left| \frac{\text{CT}_2 - \text{CT}_1}{1000} \right| \times 100 \qquad (14.3)$$

Reconstruction, using a mask or kernal for edge detection, relinquishes contrast information in favor of higher resolution, typically used in the petrous bone region. Object contrast depends on the attenuation property of the tissues and is measured as the difference in attenuation between adjacent structures compared to water:

$$1000 \times \frac{\mu_1 - \mu_2}{\mu_{\text{H}_2\text{O}}} = 1000 \times \frac{\Delta\mu}{\mu_{\text{H}_2\text{O}}} \qquad (14.4)$$

If this attenuation difference in the body is fixed then the contrast in the image ΔCT is only dependent on the size of the structures.

THE CONTRAST DETAIL DIAGRAM

The plot enables both resolution and contrast to be represented on a single graph (Fig. 14.15) and is a convenient method for specifying low contrast detectability.

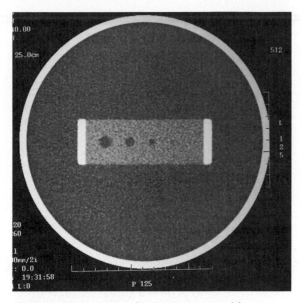

Figure 14.16 *A common low contrast test tool for computed tomography quality control.*

The curve plots detectable diameter as a function of measured contrast. The closer the curve is to the dotted line the better the resolution for low contrast objects. The top of the curve represents high contrast detail (i.e. bone). The CT difference ΔCT is a measure of the contrast. A percentage figure is given on the opposite axis. The region of the curve above the 10% object contrast line indicates the resolution for contrast capability of the system. A difference below 1% describes the noise limits of the system. The 1 to 10% region is the **transition zone** and detectability depends strongly on radiation dose.

A family of curves can be derived for various dose/mAs rates (Fig. 14.15a) or slice thicknesses (Fig. 14.15b). Field of view diameters or reconstruction algorithms can also be compared using contrast detail diagrams. An example of a low contrast test object is shown in Fig. 14.16. Circular plastic objects of 5, 4, 3, 2, and 1 mm are set in a plastic background of different composition yielding a low ΔCT value.

NOISE

Noise, in a CT image, is defined as the standard deviation of CT numbers in a uniform image (usually water bath). For a given CT system noise is inversely proportional to resolution. Generally image noise is proportional to $1/\sqrt{I \times t}$, where $I \times t$ is the

current– time product, mAs. When mAs is doubled the noise decreases by $1/\sqrt{2}$ or 0.707. Dose versus noise is plotted in Fig. 14.17a for two slice thicknesses. Factors affecting noise and low contrast detectability depend on:

- Photon flux reaching the detector: influenced by kV_p, filtration, mAs, and patient size. This latter point is demonstrated in Fig. 14.17(b) showing increasing noise with subject size.
- System noise: mechanical or electrical noise within the CT system.
- Detector efficiency.
- Reconstruction algorithm.
- Age of the X-ray tube.

SLICE THICKNESS

Thin slices are noisier but this is not important for bone detail reconstruction where greater image contrast already exists. Soft-tissue contrast is lost, however, if the sections are too thin. Structures which are at an angle to the slice plane suffer volume artifact which degrades spatial resolution. The visibility of these structures can be improved by using thin slices which separate overlying detail.

14.2.9 Image artifacts

SAMPLING ACCURACY

Mechanical accuracy to high tolerances is essential to prevent loss of resolution. Misalignment by one tenth of a detector area can give aliasing. The number of pixels in the image may be set prior to image acquisition. Usually, the choice is between a matrix size of 256 or 512. The latter may provide higher spatial resolution but with a cost of increased radiation dose if image quality is to be preserved. The larger matrix images contain more pixels and therefore will take longer to store and retrieve and any image manipulation will also require more time.

PARTIAL VOLUME

High attenuating objects projecting partly into a slice will cause a mixed attenuation value. It is assumed that tissue within the voxel is uniform. However, if the slice thickness is large then it might contain a second material, e.g. bone and soft tissue.

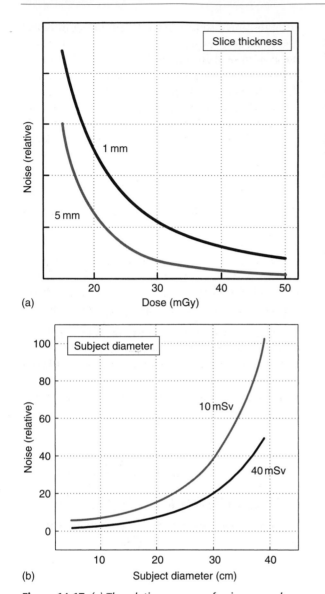

(a)

(b)

Figure 14.17 *(a) The relative measure of noise versus dose for 1 mm and 5 mm slices; the latter give a better contrast. (b) Noise increases quite rapidly with increasing subject diameter (head versus abdomen for instance); increasing radiation dose from 10 to 40 mSv overcomes this.*

Therefore the attenuation coefficient that will be calculated for that voxel will be a weighted average of that for soft tissue and bone based on the relative volumes occupied by both in the voxel. Thinner slice thicknesses reduce this artifact as demonstrated in Fig. 14.18a and b.

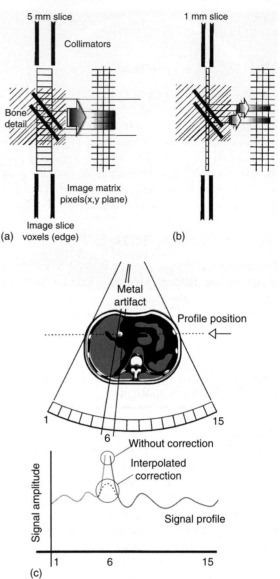

(a)   **(b)**

(c)

Figure 14.18 *(a) Partial volume and slice thickness. The 5 mm slice cannot separate fine bone detail as the voxels include both soft tissue and bone anatomy. The image matrix shows this as a single unsharp object. (b) The thinner slice of 1 mm can separate the closely spaced bone; the image matrix now shows the twin bone detail. (c) Metal artifact reduction by interpolation before and after spike profile due to abnormal high CT values for metal.*

BEAM HARDENING

Filtration of the beam by tissue (bone) removes the lower energy X-ray component. Attenuation then decreases as the effective X-ray energy increases so distorting the CT number values. This has been seen in Fig. 14.4.

DETECTOR NON-UNIFORMITY

A non-uniform response by the array of detectors leads to the production of 'ring' artifacts or a type of halo effect about objects in the image. This usually is not a problem with modern gas detector based equipment. However, when first switching on the equipment in the morning sufficient time must be allocated for the system to reach its operating temperature and for the amounts of gas in each detector to equilibrate.

METAL ARTIFACT INTERFERENCE

This causes star-burst radiating lines from the metal object in the field of view. Corrections to these abnormally high absorption values can be made during reconstruction by placing a threshold on the peak values (Fig. 14.18c).

14.3 SINGLE SLICE HELICAL/SPIRAL COMPUTED TOMOGRAPHY

X-ray computed tomography using sequential or contiguous data collection measures attenuation profiles of a transverse slice from a multitude of angular positions. The X-ray beam is collimated to a fan defining the image plane, incident on a detector as part of a complete fan beam assembly which travels around the patient. Typically, a full 360° are covered to collect a complete set of data. The image is then reconstructed and the patient table moved a small distance through the gantry for the next transverse section. This procedure is repeated slice by slice. Since power and data are transmitted by cable, the tube/detectors are rotated 360° in one direction, stopped, and then rotated 360° in the opposite direction. This is necessary to allow the connecting power and data cables to unwind.

To avoid unsharpness and motion artifacts and maintain high image quality the patient must not move during the data acquisition process. Therefore short scan times are essential. Short examination times (time between slice acquisition) are desirable to limit motion between scans. Patient movement between slices causes loss of anatomic detail and small lesions can be missed if they happen to be located between adjacent slices.

Omission of anatomic levels also causes discontinuities (jagged edges) in three-dimensional (3-D) displays. Scan times are typically limited to 2 or 3 s. These effects are significant drawbacks to separate slice sequential CT. The sequential CT scanner cables which make contact between the X-ray tube and detector banks limit date acquisition to a single 360° slice alternating in a clockwise and counter-clockwise direction.

INTERSCAN DELAY TIME

There are certain limitations to collecting data as sequential axial slices particularly when small lesions are being imaged since these can be missed if they happen to be located between adjacent slices. The sequential slice protocol, although giving complete disk-like sections as shown in Fig. 14.19a, includes delays between slices since the sequential process consists of:

- Fan beam assembly accelerated to scan speed
- X-ray tube pulsed and data collected
- Fan beam assembly halts and returns to its home position
- Table indexed to next longitudinal position while X-ray tube cools

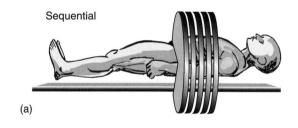

(a)

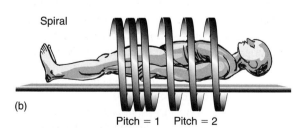

(b)

Pitch = 1   Pitch = 2

Figure 14.19 *(a) Contiguous slice acquisition giving unconnected slices but each one having a complete flat profile. (b) Spiral acquisition where the table moves during continuous acquisition at different pitch settings giving a continuous helical acquisition but the slice shape has a spiral distortion.*

This series of events constitutes the interscan delay time (ISD) and adds a significant time to the clinical study causing problems if the patient must hold their breath or patient movement is present.

Following an iodine contrast bolus through a section of anatomy using a sequential CT produces an incomplete data set due to ISD. Sequential CT examination times are relatively longer due to long rotation times (2 to 5 s in some models) which also influence ISD. Since only a few slices can be acquired larger amounts of contrast medium are required.

In summary a sequential CT machine has several disadvantages:

- Interscan delays are too long.
- Larger amounts of contrast are required.
- Movement slice misregistration can occur.

For these reasons spiral or helical scanning was introduced to include continuous CT data collection where the patient was moved through the gantry while the fan beam was continuously rotating (Fig. 14.19b).

14.3.1 Basic principles of spiral acquisition

Continuously rotating CT machines were developed replacing fixed cables with **slip rings** which transfer the necessary power and signal data. Helical or spiral CT was developed where the patient was moved through the gantry while the fan beam was continuously rotating.

Spiral or helical scanning is achieved by continuously acquiring CT data while the patient is transported through the gantry. The spiral design was first introduced in 1989 and its principle has gained universal acceptance. Recent advances have included multislice helical acquisition. Helical scanning, however, imposes certain limitations on the CT machine:

- A cable-free method for connecting X-ray tube and detectors must be installed.
- X-ray tube power must be substantially increased.
- Image reconstruction algorithms must consider the spiral shape of the resulting section.

Helical or spiral CT allows complete anatomical volumes to be scanned in continuous fashion typically in 20 to 60 s, and then allows reconstruction of the images in a variety of ways from the volume data set.

Several technical developments were necessary to make this capability practical for three-dimensional imaging: slip-ring scanning gantries, high-precision table stepping motors, X-ray tubes with massive thermal loading capacities, and faster computer systems with increased memory. New methods of reconstructing images correcting for the relative motion of the patient and rotating components also had to be developed.

SLIP RING TECHNOLOGY

The first requirement for spiral acquisition for a third generation machine is a continuously rotating fan-beam assembly; fourth generation machines already had continuously rotating X-ray tubes but without the scanner couch increment which was added later.

Since a fan-beam assembly must rotate continuously in helical scanners a method for uninterrupted power supply and data collection must be devised. Slip rings are designed to achieve this (Fig. 14.20). Slip-ring mechanisms employing brushes must be present operating at either low voltages (200 to 300 V), when the generator and X-ray tube must rotate together, or

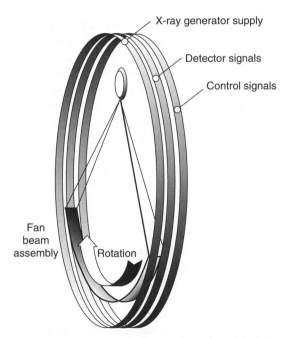

Figure 14.20 *Sketch of slip-ring configuration with sliding contactors to permit continuous rotation of tube and detectors while maintaining electrical contact with stationary components.*

high voltages (up to 140 kV) supplying just the X-ray tube alone. Both low and high voltage techniques have their advantages and disadvantages. Low-voltage (200 to 300 V) connectors require that the high voltage generator for the X-ray tube rotates with the fan beam. These are lightweight high frequency generators forming part of the X-ray tube assembly, the tank unit containing the high frequency transformers and control electronics. This construction adds considerable mass to the already heavy rotational stage, which contains the high power tube housing and related components. Centrifugal forces are therefore an important consideration in helical scanners capable of sub-second rotation speeds.

High voltage designs locate the generator externally away from the fan beam assembly, so reducing weight. CT systems are currently available which use both low tension and high tension slip-ring technology and reliability is equally proven in both instances although the majority of CT designs of X-ray power supplies now use low or intermediate voltage connections across the sliding contactors.

The slip-ring design consists of sets of parallel conductive rings concentric to the gantry axis that connect to the tube, detectors, and control circuits by sliding contactors (small metal or carbon brushes). Continuous data acquisition over long periods of time is possible which eliminates interscan delays caused by the constant stop/start of the tube/detector system.

During rotation the table is moved continuously through the gantry, so complete areas of the head or body can be covered in short time periods; single breath holds are possible in even sick patients. This gives a block or data volume from which single slices are reconstructed. The slip-ring design allows much faster rotation times, in most cases less than 1s.

Data from the detector system can either be transferred optically or by high frequency transmission systems. This is usually achieved photoelectrically by using infrared laser diodes on the edge of the fan beam assembly which aligns with detectors on the fixed gantry.

ROTATION TIME

This is an important parameter and is defined as the time taken for the tube/detector system to rotate 360° around the patient. This can be selected between 0.8, 1.0, 1.5, 2.0, and 3.0 s in modern scanners. If rotation time is decreased, spiral coverage/body length increases

and vice versa. With shorter rotation times, thinner slices, for the same volume, can be acquired in the same amount of time.

Selecting a 100 mm anatomical range using a 10 mm slice, pitch 1 (10 mm feed/rotation), and a rotation time of 1 s, will take a scan time of 10 s. Decreasing the rotation time to 0.8 s will reduce this to 8 s to cover the same range. Shorter rotation times are chosen with thinner slice collimation, since the same range can be covered in the same time but the X-ray tube current may need to be increased to maintain the same mAs and maintain image quality (noise).

14.3.2 X-ray tube and generator

Spiral computed tomography requires higher X-ray power due to large volume continuous data acquisition. One of the limitations of early spiral systems was the heat storage capacity of the X-ray tube and this imposed a maximum acquisition time (typically 30 to 60 s) which resulted in relatively small anatomical volumes being covered in early machines. Higher rated X-ray tubes and smaller gantry distances now enable longer exposure times in spiral acquisition. Multiple spiral acquisitions are possible without incurring lengthy tube cooling delays.

The modern X-ray tube used in CT offers a selection of focal spot sizes from 0.5 to 2.0 mm. Smaller focal spot sizes are preferable for thin section, high resolution slices. Larger focal spots with higher power ratings are necessary for large volume scans requiring low contrast resolution.

X-RAY TUBE RATING

Tubes are now available with anode thermal capacities exceeding 5 million heat units. Table 14.2 gives typical specifications for an X-ray tube and generator necessary to acquire a continuous spiral data set.

Modern helical X-ray tubes are capable of beam currents of 250 to 350 mA for acquisitions of 32 to 100 s. Anode cooling rates must be high since a single helical study with a duration of 40 s at 120 kV_p and 300 mA would dump nearly 2 MHU in the anode.

Designs using liquid metal bearings are now commonplace in order to withstand considerable heating and provide a conductive heat path to supplement radiant heat losses. The addition of a thermal conduction path mainly influences lower temperature cooling and reduces waiting time between helical runs; it does

Table 14.2 *Generator specification for a typical spiral computed tomography.*

Variable	Specification
X-ray tube	
Heat storage	6.3 MHU
Focal spot sizes (mm)	0.7, 0.9, 1.2
Anode angle	7°
Generator	
Power	60 kW
kV ranges	80, 100, 120, 140
mA, maximum	440
Maximum coverage acquisition time	120 s

not improve thermal capacity. There is also some evidence that these newer designs may improve bearing life, one of the major sources of tube failure.

The tube current can be altered during the course of the helical scan sequence, which is useful where body composition or size changes along the patient's body length. A reduction in mean mAs per rotation of 15 to 55% has been recorded for different anatomical regions. These two methods can be combined to give significant radiation dose savings.

During spiral data acquisition noise-free data transmission is essential. Rotating systems use either a separate channel on the slip rings or optical transfer which provide transmission frequencies exceeding 200 Mbits s^{-1}.

FLYING FOCAL SPOT

The number of measurement channels can be doubled by rapid deflection of the X-ray tube focal spot for each projection increasing the image resolution. This is achieved by electromagnetically deflecting the electron beam within the X-ray tube. For each focus position two measured interlaced projections result, since the detector continues to move continuously. The sampling frequency is doubled enhancing the spatial resolution.

TUBE CURRENT MODULATION

The correct tube current selection depends on the individual study. Patient size must also be taken into consideration. In general higher doses and thicker slices are required for low contrast anatomy in order to increase soft tissue differentiation and decrease noise. When the anatomy to be scanned is of a high contrast then thinner slices and lower doses are more desirable as noise is less important for diagnosis of high contrast structures.

Image noise can be improved in helical CT by altering or modulating the X-ray tube milliampere value and so compensate for variations in flux transmission through different body regions. This technique can use a priori information on regional body transmission taken from toposcan or scoutview prescan information of the patient; this sets the milliampere modulation plan. During the helical scan thicker, denser regions of the patient require higher tube current; thinner or less dense regions use a lower tube current. Alternatively, tube current can be modulated during the course of a single tube rotation which is used when the body has cross sections that are not circular (shoulders and pelvis) where the lateral projection through the patient attenuates more than the anterior–posterior projection. Exposure to the patient can be varied by up to 80% in the course of a 0.5 s rotation. As well as dose advantages this has the added advantage of making the image quality more constant for the individual slices in each series.

BEAM FILTRATION

In addition to the inherent filtration of the X-ray tube (typically 3 mm Al), flat or shaped (bow-tie) filters are used. Shaped or 'bow-tie' filters have minimum beam attenuation in the center of the field but more strongly in the periphery. They improve the dynamic range of the detector system and reduce both scattered radiation intensities arising from the periphery and patient dose. The material for these shaped filters has a low atomic number in order to keep the spectral and beam hardening differences between the center and the periphery of the fan beam as small as possible. Teflon (PTFE) is commonly selected as an efficient filter material having high density combined with a relatively low effective atomic number. Copper filters of 0.1 to 0.4 mm thickness are also installed to harden the X-ray spectrum; this additional filtration requires increased X-ray output so that the photon flux is not reduced below certain limits and image noise increased.

FAN-BEAM DESIGN

The demands on mechanical design have risen continuously with the speed of rotation. It is accepted that the X-ray system, detectors and associated electronics demand very high specifications; this is also the case for mechanical design. The centrifugal forces expose the mechanical parts of the scanner to great stress. The fan beam component parts can exceed a mass of 1000 kg. To accelerate this mass to 2 rotations per second, linear drives are installed in the rotary bearing which gives precise uniform motion.

The centrifugal forces which have to expected can be calculated. For an X-ray tube to axis of rotation distance of typically 60 cm and a rotation time of 0.5 s an acceleration of $9.66 \times g$ results. For a typical X-ray tube mass of 100 kg centrifugal forces approaching 10 000 N must be balanced in the assembly. Mechanical registration accuracy approaching 0.1 mm is maintained in order to achieve resolution quality of 1 Lp mm^{-1} or better.

BEAM COLLIMATION

Their design varies between scanner models and manufacturers but generally follows a common pattern. Pre-collimation of the beam is where the width of the X-ray beam is determined by collimators mounted in front of the X-ray tube. A first collimation is provided very close to the X-ray tube focus, reducing the X-ray beam dimension for the given slice width and geometry. This is as close as possible to the patient and helps to limit the dose exposure. This first reduction of the radiation beam is mostly provided by the lead shielding of the X-ray tube itself providing an approximate aperture for the fan beam. A second fixed collimator defines the exact beam dimension. An additional adjustable collimator allows the desired slice width to be selected. The beam path and collimating system of the fan-beam machine with rotating detectors can be seen in Fig. 14.21.

Post-collimation of the X-ray beam is supplied by separate collimators in front of the scintillation detector. They reduce contributions from scattered radiation reaching the detector surface and are constructed as a system of thin lamellae made of strongly absorbing material, typically 100 μm thick tantalum sheets, positioned between the single detector elements and aligned exactly with the shaped geometry of the X-ray beam (comb collimator). This alignment maximizes the signal-carrying primary radiation and minimizes the scatter contribution. The lamellar collimator reduces the proportion of scattered radiation in the measured signal by a factor of approximately 10. However, this detector collimation contributes to **detector dead space** and reduces overall detector geometric efficiency to below 90%.

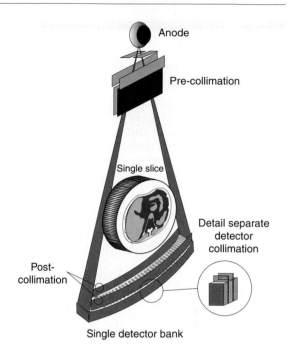

Figure 14.21 *The fan beam design for a single slice spiral computed tomography showing pre- and post-collimation along with separate detector collimation.*

Xenon gas detectors are self-collimating due to the depth of each detector element.

14.3.3 X-ray detectors

DETECTOR EFFICIENCY

The tube load can be reduced for the same noise level if the detector efficiency is improved. CT detector elements used in helical scanners are either solid-state scintillation devices or xenon-gas chambers. Solid-state detectors are typically constructed of a scintillator coupled to a photodiode. Gas ion chambers contain pressurized xenon (20 bar) and show better thermal stability and exhibit less hysteresis than scintillation detectors. Table 14.3 compares gas and solid detectors used in spiral CT.

Faster rotation times require rapid interrogation of the detectors requiring shorter measurement intervals. Under these conditions, xenon detectors have an advantage. There are, however, several new ceramic scintillator materials with faster scintillation decay times that have been introduced. These materials include lutetium orthosilicate (Lu_2O:Ce), gadolinium orthosilicate (Gd_2O:Ce), and yttrium aluminum perovskite ($YAlO_3$:Ce). Current solid-state detectors have

Table 14.3 *Gas and ceramic detectors used in spiral computed tomography.*

Property	Xenon gas	Ceramic scintillators
Efficiency	74% at 120 kV	90% at 120 kV
	71% at 140 kV	85% at 140 kV
Absorption	<50% at 120 kV	95% at 120 kV
Afterglow	0.4% at 100 ms	<0.1% at 100 ms

absorption efficiencies of approximately 99% at $120\,kV_p$. Geometric efficiencies are mainly caused by dead space due to interdetector collimation (see later).

DETECTOR OFFSET

The X-ray tube focal spot can be shifted in order to double detector resolution. Sample spacing in the scan plane can also be improved by quarter ray offset to improve ray sampling within the projection; opposing projections will be offset by one half the detector width (see Section 14.2.2). If the central ray is offset by one fourth of the sampling distance from the center of rotation then this ray will again be shifted by one fourth of the sampling distance in the opposite direction after 180° rotation. High mechanical precision is required for exact registration. The two measurements with the central ray taken in opposite directions are offset relative to each other by half the sampling distance, so the sampling frequency is increased by a factor of 2.

14.3.4 Pitch

Since the patient is moved at a constant rate through the gantry during data acquisition the slice will not be disk shaped but will resemble a coarse screw-thread. The coarseness of the spiral depends on the scan pitch which is controlled by the table feed-rate through the gantry (z-axis) relative to the rotational speed.

The ratio of table increment or displacement per 360° rotation to section thickness is the scan pitch value, which is an important dimensionless quantity with implications for patient dose and image quality. Spiral pitch (p) is calculated as:

$$p = \frac{\text{table travel per rotation}}{\text{slice width}} \quad (14.5)$$

Using the calculation in eqn 14.5 a 10 mm table travel and slice width of 5 mm gives a pitch value of 2. A travel of 5 mm would give a pitch of 1. Intermediate pitch values are also possible. Pitch values of greater than 2 lead to image distortion so in practice the pitch values vary between 1.2 and 1.5. The larger the pitch, the less time it will take to cover a spiral range, and longer ranges can be covered. During a spiral scan length the X-ray tube is on for the entire length of the scan while the table moves continuously through the gantry. If the pitch is greater than 1, this simply means the system is covering a larger axial distance for each 360° rotation. So if the pitch is 2 (for example a 10 mm slice with a 20 mm feed/rotation) then twice the z-axial distance will be covered for one rotation.

TABLE INCREMENT

In spiral CT, the **table increment** per rotation can be selected independently of the selected slice thickness. A larger table increment gives faster acquisition, but leads to a wider **SSP** and consequently lowers resolution. The scan width, specified by the operator, is approximately equal to full width at half maximum of the **SSP** for one reconstructed image from the spiral volume data set.

The table increment is typically between one and two times the size of the selected slice collimation (pitch 1 to 2). The spatial resolution with 5 mm collimation and a table increment of 7 mm (pitch 1.4) lies between that of 5 mm collimation with pitch 1 and 7 mm collimation with pitch 1.

In single-slice spiral CT scanning, a pitch of 1.0 indicates contiguous data collection with no slice gap. A pitch of 2.0 causes a gap equal to one X-ray beam width between adjacent spirals, decreasing patient dose by a factor of 2 but increasing the width of the **section (or slice) sensitivity profile** (SSP) (see Section 14.2.3) and the severity of spiral image artifacts. Pitch values less than 1.0 imply overlapping radiation beams and a corresponding increase in average patient dose.

14.3.5 Image reconstruction and data interpolation

Basic image reconstruction using filtered back-projection is similar to sequential CT and the same algorithms and reconstruction kernels are available. Image quality is a problem in spiral CT scanning since the start and finish points of each slice are different;

image reconstruction requires special consideration. An additional step of data processing slice or section **interpolation** is necessary, however, before image reconstruction can be started.

During continuous rotation of the fan beam and travel by the patient through the gantry the data are continually displaced along the z-axis, and this displacement affects the quality of the resultant axial images and broadening of the **slice sensitivity profile** (SSP), which gives a measure of z-sensitivity. The slice will not be a simple disk shape as shown in sequential CT but will resemble a helix or spiral showing overlap between slices in any 360° section of scan sequence. The degree of overlap depends on the pitch value controlled by the table feed-rate relative to the rotational speed. Resolution in the coordinate perpendicular to the scan plane (in the z-axis) is referred to as the **longitudinal spatial resolution**. The SSP represents the system's response perpendicular to the scan plane in the z-axis (see Section 14.2.3). It gives a measure of slice broadening in the z-axis and compares with the point spread function in the x,y image plane.

In sequential CT, the longitudinal spatial resolution is entirely determined by the slice thickness. In spiral CT, the longitudinal resolution is determined by the table increment per rotation, and by the interpolation algorithm used.

COLLIMATION

The widening of the SSP in spiral CT is reduced by a movable collimator in front of the detector, which is used particularly for defining very thin slices, since these give the greatest deviations from the ideal rectangular form. An idea of the beam collimation is given in Fig. 14.21 where pre- and post-collimation confine the useful X-ray beam to a narrow section, removing the scatter radiation that merely adds to patient radiation dose. As the **slice dose profile** will be wider than the slice sensitivity profile, radiation spreads to an area of patient anatomy not being imaged (a greater area than the section measured by the detector) and contributes to excess patient radiation dose. Manufacturers try to limit this by careful collimation, however, because as X-ray photons are lost the tube output must be increased which places a heavy burden on both the X-ray tube and generator for volume imaging. Although some system designs use post-patient collimation for narrow scan widths to decrease the contribution of scattered radiation along

the z-axis, the nominal slice width is determined primarily by pre-patient collimation, which is the width of the incoming X-ray beam along the z-axis, as well as the spiral interpolation algorithm.

Z-AXIS RESOLUTION

The width of the SSP, measured at half the maximum level (full width at half maximum, FWHM), is the collimated slice thickness. The FWHM suffers from a serious drawback since it gives no information about whether the profile approximates the ideal rectangular shape or deviates significantly from this. Since the shape of the profile is not represented in the **FWHM** value, which is in the specification of the nominal slice width, there is a need for additional measurements. Profile widths at 10% of the maximum value (full width at one tenth of maximum, **FWTM**) and the width of the profile at a height which includes 90% of the area under the profile (full width at tenth maximum, **FWTM**) have been proposed.

In spiral CT, a single data set is obtained which represents the volume covered in the given number of spiral turns, but directly reconstructing any 360° spiral segment would result in image motion artifacts similar to those seen in sequential CT due to patient movement.

In summary, during spiral data acquisition there is continuous rotation of the fan beam while the patient travels through the gantry. Therefore data are continually displaced along the z-axis, and this displacement affects the quality of the resultant axial images, broadening the SSP, as described above. Since this movement also spreads the SDP beyond the SSP margins there is increased patient radiation dose without any contribution to image quality. Careful collimation of the beam can reduce this problem but image quality can also be improved and the SSP sharpened by appropriate selection of pitch and interpolation algorithm.

DATA INTERPOLATION

In sequential CT, SSPs are approximately rectangular with widths equal to the section width (Fig. 14.5), but in spiral acquisition they are extended and more peaked. Since the SSP represents the resolution element along the z-axis this seriously influences resolution when attempting 3-D reconstruction. Since the patient is moved during data acquisition, the information obtained is distorted over the body volume depending on the slice thickness and table increment

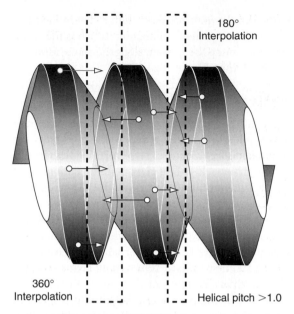

Figure 14.22 *The three-dimensional representation of the spiral data set undergoing 360° and 180° interpolation to remove the spiral section distortion and improve the slice sensitivity profile. For 360° linear interpolation the data are accepted from a wider boundary. The restricted data boundary used for the 180° interpolation allows narrow slice widths.*

per rotation. This data inconsistency causes artifacts but can mostly be compensated by data interpolation. The interpolation methods most commonly employed work from either the full data set (360°) or a half data set (180°). These interpolation principles are illustrated in Fig. 14.22.

The larger pitch settings, where the movement is greater than the slice width, increase the slice distortion and the effective slice width increases and a faster tissue volume is covered with a consequent smaller radiation dose to the patient. In order to overcome this distortion a form of data interpolation is required.

360° INTERPOLATION

To avoid artifacts from the table movement the 360° LI algorithm uses data from a full rotation for the interpolation, they are weighted so that data which are closer to the z-position count more; data which are further away from the z-position to be reconstructed count less. This procedure is indicated in Fig. 14.22 where interpolation is being made between movement z and $z + p$, so correcting for the data offset imposed by the table movement.

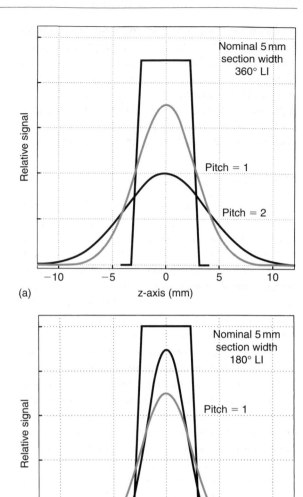

Figure 14.23 *Slice sensitivity profiles in spiral computed tomography result from a convolution of the original profile with the motion function. Profiles are broadened with increasing table feed values for (a) 360° LI and (b) 180° LI.*

As some data are quite distant from the actual slice they cause a widening of the slice profile. So, instead of a 10 mm slice being really 10 mm (as in a sequence scan) a 360° reconstruction with a pitch of 1:1 yields an effective slice about 1.27 times the collimator distance. With a pitch of 2, the slice will be about 2.2 times as wide. The graph in Fig. 14.23a gives an indication of the SSP increase when 360° interpolation is used.

Using two successive 360° rotations on either side of the selected plane involves 720° of projection data and since the patient is displaced twice the distance along the z-axis over the data acquisition, the SSP is considerably broadened. Since the 360° interpolation uses two complete rotations of the fan beam assembly the data acquired with a difference of a complete rotation are then interpolated in the reconstruction.

180° INTERPOLATION

The full 360° LI has now been replaced by a 180° linear interpolation (180° LI) where interpolation from opposing 180° points reduces the spiral range used for reconstruction by distance travelled/2; the SSP now resembles that obtained from a sequential acquisition for the same slice width. The 180° interpolation algorithm uses the data from one rotation which are 180° apart from each other (Fig. 14.22). This is possible since X-ray beam absorption at 0° (the direct ray) is equivalent to the X-ray beam absorption traversing the body at the same level from the opposite side, at 180° (the complementary ray). When processing data in the slice plane for reconstruction then two direct rays separated by 360° are unnecessary. As the distance between the data points is now smaller, the **effective slice width** will be less; with a pitch of 1:1 the effective slice width will be nearly the same as the collimator separation. As the pitch increases, the effective slice thickness increases gradually. Using a pitch of 2:1, the increase will only be a factor of approx. 1.27 wider. This is comparable to a pitch 1:1 with the wider 360° algorithm (graph in Fig. 14.23b). The data are weighted according to their distance from the slice position. From the graph it is clear that with the narrow algorithm even a pitch of 2 can be used without changing the effective slice width significantly. However, artifacts due to data inconsistency remain and image noise increases by about 8% compared to conventional scans. Table 14.4 shows the difference in FWHM and FWTM values obtained after 360° and 180° interpolation.

A major advantage with spiral scanning is the ability to reconstruct a volume data set. It is possible to reconstruct images at varying increments, or slice spacing, within this volume. Since data are continuously acquired, overlapping slices can be reconstructed anywhere within the volume. The advantage of slightly overlapping slices is the increased image quality for post-processing (3-D, multi-projection

Table 14.4 *The variation of full width half maximum (FWHM) and full width tenth maximum (FWTM) with pitch 1 and 2 and 360°/180° interpolation for nominal slice width of 5 mm.*

FWHM or FWTM	Sequential CT	Spiral CT, 360°	Spiral CT, 180°
Pitch = 1			
FWHM (mm)	5.0	6.3	5.0
FWTM (mm)	6.1	11.1	8.0
Pitch = 2			
FWHM (mm)	5.0	10.8	6.5
FWTM (mm)	6.1	19.8	11.3

reconstruction) and preventing any partial-volume effect in axial slices.

If the original volume was acquired using 10 mm collimation and a 100 mm range was covered, then 10 mm slices can be reconstructed at any position within the 100 mm range. If the reconstruction increment is 10 mm, this will give contiguous 10 mm slices every 10 mm. If the increment is 5 mm there will be 10 mm slices every 5 mm resulting in a 50% overlap of the slices. An increment of 1.0 mm will result in a 90% overlap, and so on. So the increment, or slice spacing, can be varied and overlapping slices can be reconstructed without additional dose.

EFFECTIVE SLICE WIDTH

The total effect of the collimation, pitch, and interpolation is described by SSP. The FWHM of this curve is often used as a measure of the effective slice thickness. With the 180° interpolation the FWHM of a pitch 1 acquisition is similar to that of a conventional scan with the same collimation. For larger pitches the FWHM increases linearly up to about 30% at pitch 2. While the SSP of a sequential scan has very steep edges, the SSP of the spiral scan is broader, although sequential and spiral SSP are almost identical at pitch 1, using the same collimation and 180° interpolation.

The increase in effective slice width at higher pitch settings is offset by the increased volume covered. This is particularly important where a thin nominal slice width is required, for example where images are to be used for multi-planar reconstruction (MPR), or 3-D. In practice there is no significant image degradation

Table 14.5 *Broadening of slice sensitivity profile with table speed with 180° interpolation.*

Table speed (mm s^{-1})	Slice sensitivity profile
0	10.0
5	10.1
10	10.2
20	12.8

up to a table pitch of 1.5 (a table feed value 1.5 times greater than the nominal slice thickness). There is a reduced patient radiation dose using an increased pitch value; this is discussed later. The broadening of the SSP with 180° linear interpolation with table increment is indicated in Table 14.5. The slice sensitivity profile (effective slice width) increases significantly only with fast table speeds (20 mm s^{-1}), so increasing slice width and reducing image resolution.

The effective slice width has an important influence on small object detection. The contrast of an object, which is smaller than the slice thickness and located only partly in the scanned slice, is reduced according to the extent to which it is positioned in the particular volume element. This linear partial volume effect is unavoidable, but can be reduced or eliminated altogether by the selection of thinner slices. The shape of the sensitivity profile thus plays an important role for excluding cross-talk between neighboring slices. Figure 14.24 is a film exposure showing the striped pattern of the SSP in a spiral scan where pitch = 1.

GEOMETRIC EFFICIENCY

Geometric efficiency is a measure of the scanner's dose utilization in the z-axis. This is expressed as the ratio of the imaged slice section thickness relative to the z-axis dose profile. For optimum imaging, the geometric efficiency should be 1, but it is often less, especially for narrow beam collimations where post-patient collimation may be necessary to bring the imaged slice thickness closer to the chosen value. The geometric efficiency (G_{eff}) of the detector array can be calculated by comparing the FWHM of the SDP with the SSP:

$$G_{eff} = \frac{\text{FWHM}(z - \text{sensitivity profile})}{\text{FWHM}(\text{dose profile})} \times 100\% \tag{14.6}$$

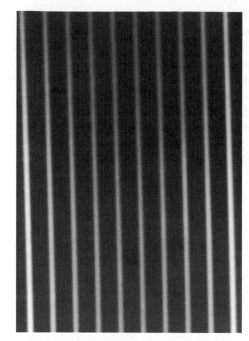

Figure 14.24 *Exposure pattern given by a spiral computed tomography at pitch = 1. This film image shows the gaps between the slice dose profiles for a 5 mm slice width.*

Obviously where the SSP and SDP dimensions are identical, as in the case of sequential CT, the geometric efficiency is 100%. For single-slice spiral CT the geometric efficiency can fall as low as 60%. The geometric efficiency is influenced by the slice thickness so

$$G_{eff} = \frac{z - \text{sensitivity profile}}{\text{slice width}} \tag{14.7}$$

It will be seen that multislice scanners have a poorer geometric efficiency than single-slice.

14.3.6 Image quality

Image quality with spiral CT was always equal in most respects to slice-by-slice CT images. One significant difference was in respect to image noise and slice sensitivity profile. The limitation in terms of available mA values with the early systems resulted in relatively high noise levels and there was a small additional influence due to the interpolation process. The latest CT systems now available no longer have the limitation of reduced mA values for extended spiral acquisitions and hence the noise levels are equal for both modes of operation.

The increase in effective slice width is offset by the increased volume covered. This is particularly important where a thin nominal slice width is required, for example where images are to be used for multi-planar reconstruction (MPR), 3-D or CT angiography. In practice, there is no significant image degradation up to a table pitch of 1.5, i.e. a table feed value 1.5 times greater than the nominal slice thickness.

IMAGE NOISE

CT scanner image quality is generally considered to be X-ray quantum limited under most operating conditions. Image quality with spiral CT was always equal in most respects to slice-by-slice sequential CT images. One significant difference was in the slice sensitivity profile but image noise must be considered.

Every axial image shows the effects of both the axial and the longitudinal resolution on the structures shown. These are the partial volume effect, and spiral artifacts.

The number of photons collected is a function of the incident flux, the patient transmission, the slice width, and the detector quantum efficiency, as well as the number of projections used in reconstruction. Both the effective slice width and image noise in helical scanning are affected by the choice of the algorithm.

With the 360° algorithm, two independent data points one rotation apart from each other are used to generate one data point in the image plane. As a result, the noise is lower compared to the noise in a sequence image. However, the narrow 180° algorithm uses the same data (direct and complementary) twice during interpolation, and so the noise is enhanced compared to sequence imaging.

SPATIAL RESOLUTION IN THE X, Y AXIS (IMAGE PLANE)

Spatial resolution is a measure of how well a detail is delineated in an image. The spatial resolution in the scan plane is referred to as the **axial spatial resolution**. The axial spatial resolution is principally determined by the distances between the X-ray tube, the center of rotation, and the detector, as well as by the width of the focus and the detector elements, and the number of measurements made per rotation. These factors are determined by the construction of the scanner. The resolution in the scan plane can be compared with conventional projection radiography; in CT, however, there is the additional influence of the reconstruction

algorithm. The major geometrical factors influencing the resolution in the scan plane are therefore:

- Focal spot size
- Beam geometry
- Detector element spacing
- Collimation
- Focal spot movement during data acquisition

The factors influencing the spatial resolution in the x,y axes are mostly a fixed characteristic of the machine and there are only limited possibilities to vary these. The most usual variable is the choice of convolution kernel since the focal spot size, detector sampling distance and detector aperture are set according to imaging protocol.

MEASUREMENTS OF SPATIAL RESOLUTION

Subjective measurements commonly use hole or bar patterns set into a plastic base (see Fig. 14.16); these are ideal for basic quality control and should be available for day-to-day tests. Quantitative or objective measurements for investigating the machine's complete resolution capability and inter-machine comparison use indirect methods involving point spread and modulation transfer function (MTF). The MTF is calculated from measurements using a thin metal wire which provides data for obtaining a point source; the MTF test tool should be part of the CT machine test gear supplied by the manufacturer. The point spread function after Fourier transformation gives the MTF. This is the objective measure of the complete spatial resolution measured in line pairs per cm. The effects of detector offset, flying focal spot, and high-resolution comb on spatial resolution can be demonstrated for different scan modes between CT scanners. The spatial resolution obtainable for a given system is calculated for a variety of **reconstruction kernels**. Reconstruction kernels for 'high resolution' are recommended for imaging high contrast objects. Reconstructions with standard or 'smoothing' kernels lose high end resolution but reduce noise and artifacts so improving low-contrast detectability.

THE IMAGE MATRIX DIMENSION

The display resolution depends on the digital image matrix. A matrix of 512 × 512 pixels, with a field of measurement of approximately 50 cm, is the common dimension used in CT calculations, although matrices of 1024×1024 are becoming common with a pixel depth of 12 bits.

The influence of the image matrix on detail perception can be largely excluded when the matrix pixel size is smaller than the diameter of the smallest resolvable detail by a factor of 2 or more (Nyquist frequency).

TEMPORAL RESOLUTION

Since scanning is done more quickly using a spiral acquisition the imaging speed can be less than 1 s per frame, so contrast material can be administered at a faster rate, improving visibility of arteries, veins, and pathologic conditions rich in blood flow. The separation of arterial and venous phases is also possible. Complete organ imaging showing one or more phases of contrast enhancement is achieved by scanning the volume repeatedly during a single contrast cycle. In the latter case the scans are referred to as **multiphasic scans**.

Increased speed allows a complete volume data set to be acquired within one breath hold so avoiding the problem of missed lung regions due to respiration movements.

3-D IMAGING

Since the patient moves through the gantry during data acquisition, true three-dimensional volumes can be acquired that can be viewed in any perspective. These images are free of the misregistration artifacts caused by involuntary motion that would be common in sequential CT. Figure 14.25 shows a 3-D reconstruction from a single spiral data set. The image definition is sufficient for some clinical applications but irregular (jagged) outlines to the bones are evident and prevent fine detail from being shown.

ISOTROPIC RESOLUTION

This refers to identical x-, y-, and z-axis voxel dimensions. Although this is possible with singleslice spiral models it is only really practical in multislice CT scans over reasonably large volumes at sub-millimeter slice thicknesses. Isotropic resolution is necessary when reconstructing 3-D dimensional data sets so that displays are undistorted. The appearance of high power and higher output X-ray tubes and faster rotation times is essential to make isotropic resolution a practical proposition. Isotropic resolution would require a z-axis resolution of at least $5\,\mathrm{Lp\,cm^{-1}}$.

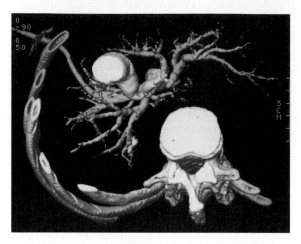

Figure 14.25 *A three-dimensional reconstruction from a single spiral computed tomography data set showing jagged edges to the bone outline caused by slight misplacement of the separate slices.*

Assuming an in-plane resolution (x, y plane) of about 1 mm, current spiral scanners can produce an approximate isotropic sampling aperture. This is discussed in Section 14.4 with multislice CT machines.

COMPUTED TOMOGRAPHY FLUOROSCOPY

This application requires rapid image reconstruction of the object currently in the scan field of view. Movement of the patient couch is under the operator's control. As the images are updated up to 12 times per second, the systems are capable of providing real-time feedback for a range of procedures particularly during interventional procedures.

The ability to follow progress in real time is an advance that was not previously available, but high skin doses to both patient and operator are apparent if CT fluoroscopy systems are used continuously throughout an examination.

14.3.7 Image artifacts

PARTIAL-VOLUME EFFECT

In a CT scan, every part of the patient is represented by a pixel in a reconstructed image. If the slice is relatively thick, each pixel in the CT image will represent a larger quantity of tissue. If this quantity of tissue has different components, i.e. tissue parenchyma and fat or bone and soft tissue, the pixel will be allocated a Hounsfield number somewhere between those of the two types of tissue. Consequently, the outlines of structures in the scan will appear to be vague, while this may not really be the case. The effect is most marked when structures vary in shape or position along the patient's longitudinal axis. Because spiral CT increases the width of the SSP, the partial-volume effect will also increase.

SPIRAL ARTIFACTS

A helical scan gives an effect in the image similar to partial volume averaging where in one direction the partial volume averaging is determined by the collimation and in another direction by the collimation as well as the table increment per rotation. Instead of a perfect circle there is an ellipse-like reconstruction. The artifacts are more apparent when the beam shape has a large top angle, or when large pitches are used. This artifact is seen in spiral scans of the top of the brain. The inclining surface of the skull increases this artifact which can be seen as two crescent shaped bands of increased density along the skull–brain interface which mimics a subdural hematoma. When three or more reconstructions per rotation are made, these bands rotate around the brain in the same direction as the X-ray tube rotates around the patient.

Spiral artifacts are apparent when high contrast objects vary in shape and/or position in an area where low-contrast morphology is important. All artifacts increase with increased pitch.

ROD ARTIFACTS

If a helical scan of a cylinder angulated with respect to the scan plane is made and the table holding the rod is moved during acquisition, then the position of the rod in the scan plane changes. Every projection locates the rod at a different position. Without table movement in a sequential scan, the cylinder would appear as an ellipse. With table movement, the variation in the registered position of the rod, together with the interpolation scheme, gives a distortion of the ellipse extending into the surrounding tissues. These artifacts are especially seen in the liver/rib area.

14.4 MULTISLICE COMPUTED TOMOGRAPHY

Multislice CT scanners (MSCT) which acquired two transaxial slices simultaneously were first introduced in 1992 using two parallel banks of detectors. Another variant was the electron-beam scanner also with a dual set of detectors.

Multi-row detector CT scanning was made available in 1998 using solid detectors and simultaneously imaging four slices in each rotation of the X-ray source. Multislice CT helical scanners are all third-generation (fan beam variation) systems, mostly with low voltage slip rings. Faster rotation sub-second times (0.5 to 0.8 s) reduced examination time significantly, while producing image quality similar to that of single-slice scanners, although multislice helical CT performs differently from single-slice helical scanners with respect to dose, pitch, image artifacts, and its method for image reconstruction.

A great advantage of multisection CT over single-section helical CT is the opportunity for **longer anatomic coverage**. The longer coverage is due to the simultaneous registration of four or more sections during each rotation and the increased gantry rotation speed. The coverage can be up to eight times longer than that of single-section helical CT with the same scanning time. For multisection CT, the coverage in the z-axis depends on the number of data channels, pitch, section thickness, scanning time, and gantry rotation time.

Although single-slice helical CT has improved over the past 8 years with faster gantry rotation, more powerful X-ray tubes, and improved interpolation algorithms, in practice the spiral data sets from single-slice systems suffered from a considerable mismatch between voxel dimensions; the transverse (in plane) and the longitudinal (axial) spatial resolution were unequal so an isotropic 3-D voxel could not be realized.

Most recent advances have increased multislice CT (MSCT) scanners from four channels of helical data simultaneously to 8 and then 16. For example a CT scanner with a 0.5 s rotation time and the simultaneous acquisition of four slices offers an 8-fold increase of performance compared to previous 1s, single-slice scanning, and more detectors further improve on the speed of volume acquisition. Fundamental advantages of MSCT include:

- Shorter acquisition times with improved temporal resolution (fewer motion artifacts)
- Retrospective creation of thinner or thicker sections from the same raw data
- Improved 3-D rendering with diminished helical artifacts

- Increased volume coverage per unit time
- High axial resolution; examination can be performed with thinner sections, leading to higher spatial resolution along the longitudinal axis
- Intravenously administered iodinated contrast material can be delivered at a faster rate, increasing contrast enhancement in the images

These factors combine to improve the spatial, temporal, and contrast resolution of the images, significantly increasing the diagnostic accuracy of the examination.

X-RAY TUBE AND GENERATOR

Shorter scan times lead to diminished X-ray tube heating, decreasing or eliminating delays for X-ray tube cooling between scans; reducing such delays is critical in multiphase examinations. More images are produced during the lifetime of a tube, decreasing operating costs.

14.4.1 Detector materials

The design of multislice CT scanners demands X-ray systems with extremely short response times to deliver sub-second spiral scanning. Extremely high mechanical stability and precise multisection geometry are required.

Gas detectors are not suitable, especially in terms of overall spatial resolution although these X-ray detectors have simple construction and provide uniform properties. Their major limitation is the low quantum detection efficiency of <50%, caused primarily by low X-ray absorption in the xenon gas and by the absorption of X-rays in the thick container housing the pressurized gas.

The new ceramic detector materials give high effective quantum efficiency and a potential reduction in patient dose. It is also possible to increase axial resolution and speed up spiral examinations without placing additional demands on the X-ray tube. This permits higher patient throughput, prolongs tube life, and thus increases cost effectiveness for the user.

MECHANICAL PROPERTIES

The mechanical property requirements are also important because scintillators must be precisely machined to dimensional tolerances of better than 5 μm and assembled into high-density scintillator/photodiode arrays.

X-RAY PHOTON ABSORPTION

A high X-ray absorption coefficient is essential for good signal-to-noise ratios and high luminescent output so that in 2 to 3 mm of stopping length the scintillator will absorb >95% of all X-rays, so scintillator materials should contain elements with high atomic numbers. Compounds containing yttrium, cesium, lanthanum, cadmium, tantalum, gadolinium, and tungsten are commonly used and have a high density (>5 g/cm^3). The **spectural linearity** must be good and requires scintillator response to be linearly proportional to the X-ray energy changes between 90 and 140 keV.

INTRINSIC QUANTUM EFFICIENCY

The absorption of an X-ray by the scintillator host lattice results in the generation of numerous free electrons and holes in the conduction and valence bands, respectively. Once the electron–hole pairs are captured and bound to a selected site, the recombination energy of these pairs is transferred to that site where radiative (**luminescence**) energy is emitted. Ideally there is a fast recombination of electron–hole pairs at the activator sites (**luminescent centers**). In this way a useful scintillator will produce several thousand visible photons from the absorption of one X-ray photon.

LUMINESCENT EFFICIENCY

This is the ratio of the total energy of visible emission to total X-ray energy. After X-irradiation the intensity of the visible emission quickly decreases with time. Once the luminescent intensity drops to a few percent of the luminescent light, further decay proceeds much slower; this is called **afterglow**. Luminescent afterglow is caused by the trapping of electrons and/or holes in crystal imperfections. The intrinsic luminescent efficiency should be >5% (signifying efficient recombination of electron–hole pairs at the activator sites) so producing a good signal. The strongest peak emission should be at wavelengths between 500 and 900 nm where silicon photodetectors have highest sensitivity. Optical transparency at the peak emitting wavelength should be high to permit good optical light collection efficiency at the photodetector.

AFTERGLOW

Temporal signal decay after a short radiation pulse is determined by (a) its decay and (b) its afterglow. The sintered ceramic composite phosphor, chosen for multislice detectors, has a rapid decay time of 10^{-6} s. A short primary decay time of <1 ms is essential because signal readout occurs within this time span during a typical CT scan of 1s duration. Luminescent afterglow should be <0.1% at 100 ms after X-ray cessation; if this value is too high then afterglow results in image blurring. The new ceramic detector materials do not need afterglow correction (unlike earlier scintillators) so high effective quantum efficiency is maintained without losses.

PRACTICAL DETECTOR MATERIALS

Early crystal scintillators used for CT detectors were thallium activated CsI and self-activated $CdWO_4$. They have a high relative light output (luminescent efficiency) giving high signal-to-noise ratios; however, they exhibit high values of afterglow (>0.3%). Yttrium gadolinium oxide ceramic scintillators doped with rare earth elements can be processed into a cubic, transparent form and exhibit luminescence in the 600 to 900 nm range. These phosphor materials can be manufactured with high purity >99.99% and have high stopping power for X-rays in the 90 to 140 keV range. For gadolinium approximately 99% of the X-ray photons are stopped in a 3 mm thick scintillator.

High luminescent efficiency of >10.3% and a major peak emission occur at a wavelength of about 610 nm and high light transmission in the 550 to 700 nm region. Various dopants have been used to reduce luminescent afterglow below 0.1% at 100 ms without adversely affecting the other key scintillator properties.

The ceramic scintillator $Y(x)$ $Gd(y)$ $Eu^{2+} O_3$ is a transparent, cubic rare-earth solid solution with a density of 5.92 g cm^{-3} and the main europium emission peak at 610 nm matched for higher spectral response by a Si photodiode. The X-ray absorption coefficient for the ceramic scintillator is identical to that of CsI(Tl). The light output of $Y(x)$ $Gd(y)$ $Eu^{2+} O_3$ is 2.5 times higher than that of $CdWO_4$ but about 30% lower than that of CsI:Tl. It is this moderately high light output combined with the lower values of luminescent afterglow that gives ceramic scintillators superior performance over other X-ray scintillators. The luminescent decay time of <1 ms also meets requirements.

The specifications for a detector suitable for a multislice CT machine are given in Table 14.6. The

Table 14.6 *Specifications for a multislice detector.*

Requirements of a computed tomography detector system	Acceptable values
Large dynamic range	10^3 to 10^6
High quantum absorption efficiency	>90% (ideally 100%)
High luminescence efficiency	>5% (ideally 100%)
Good geometric efficiency	80 to 90%
Small afterglow	<0.01% 100 ms after end of irradiation
Good homogeneity	purity >99.99%
Uniform response of all detector elements	<0.1% difference
High precision machineability	± 10 μm

mechanical tolerances are most important if the highest pixel resolution and uniformity are to be achieved.

14.4.2 Detector geometry (4, 8, 16, 64 slices)

The conventional single-section helical CT scanner has one X-ray tube and a single row of detectors. This detector row contains 500 to 900 detector elements, which describe an arc in the transverse (axial or x,y) plane, providing one channel of spatial data. Multislice CT scanners with more than one detector row have longer z-axis coverage and show problems due to the geometry of the greater cone angle employed (Fig. 14.26a).

MULTISLICE DETECTOR DESIGN

The multislice CT machine has its focal spot-to-isocenter and so focal spot-to-detector distances shortened in order to cover patient anatomy; the number of detector elements along the detector arc is increased. The multislice detector is divided into many elements along the z-axis. Figure 14.26b identifies the x-, y-, and z-axis orientation of a multislice machine. The number of slices currently on offer is 4, 8, 16 or 64 simultaneous axial slices. Table 14.7 shows the evolution of present day multislice options on offer.

Typical detector configuration choices for multislice spiral imaging have a z-axis length of 20, 32 and 48 mm with a total active detector length of 10, 15 or 20 mm, respectively (referenced to the isocenter).

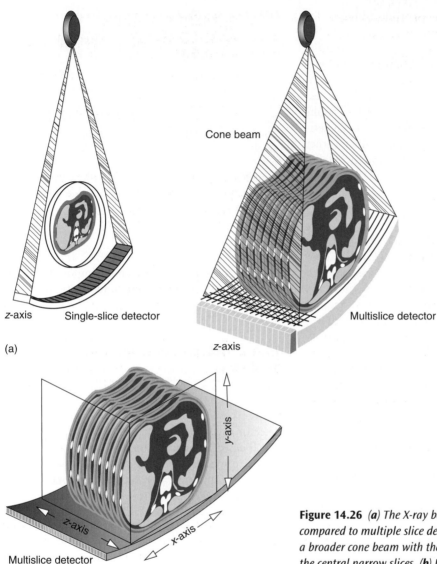

Figure 14.26 (**a**) The X-ray beam geometry of single-slice compared to multiple slice detector and X-ray beam, showing a broader cone beam with the central beam positioned over the central narrow slices. (**b**) Detector axis geometry of detector (x,y,z).

For spiral scanning, the multislice reconstruction algorithm uses data from all four interleaving spiral data sets. In contrast to single-slice spiral CT scanners, multislice models allow retrospective reconstruction of thinner or thicker scan widths in the axial acquisition mode.

The multislice CT scanner has its X-ray tube directed at multiple rows of detectors along the longitudinal (z) axis of the patient. Each row has many hundreds of separate elements and these combined rows create a two-dimensional curved array containing thousands of detector elements, sometimes exceeding 35 000 detector elements, each connected

to separate data acquisition channels that generate the multiple channels (4, 8, 16, 64) of spatial data.

FOUR SLICE MACHINES

The quad-section CT scanner has one X-ray tube covering multiple rows of detectors along the longitudinal (z) axis of the patient. The general arrangement is shown in Fig. 14.26a. Each detector together creates a two-dimensional curved detector containing thousands of detector elements, which are connected to four data acquisition systems that generate four channels of axial image data. In order to obtain

Table 14.7 *Fan beam development from single-slice to multislice arrays. Typical z-axis dimensions in brackets.*

Basic single detector
Sequential (2 mm)
↓
Single detector, helical (1 to 2 mm)
↓
Dual detector, helical (2 mm)
↓
Multidetector CT
↓
Adaptive array (4 slices) (20 mm)
Linear designs
↓
4 Slices linear array (32 mm)
8 Slices linear array (32 mm)
16 Slices linear array (32 mm)
64 Slices linear array (48 mm)

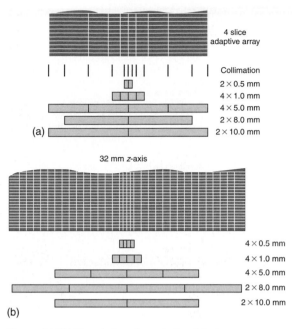

Figure 14.27 labels:

4 slice adaptive array

Collimation
2 × 0.5 mm
4 × 1.0 mm
4 × 5.0 mm
2 × 8.0 mm
2 × 10.0 mm
(a)

32 mm z-axis

4 × 0.5 mm
4 × 1.0 mm
4 × 5.0 mm
2 × 8.0 mm
2 × 10.0 mm
(b)

Figure 14.27 *Two designs for a 4-slice detector array. (a) An adaptive array detector with unequal size detector groups. (b) A linear array with 0.5 mm central detectors and 1.0 mm outer groups.*

several section thicknesses, separate detector elements along the z-axis are summed.

Commercial detector array designs may be divided into two groups: those with detector elements of unequal width (the **adaptive array detector**), which has now been superseded by detector banks having elements of equal width along the z-axis (the **linear or matrix detector**) (Fig. 14.27a and b).

Multislice CT does not necessarily mean that the same number of slices will be produced for every examination. This is true for most multislice configurations but is a major drawback with the **adaptive array** design. The evolutionary pathway for this detector design is shown in Table 14.7 and the detector configuration is shown in Fig. 14.27a. Narrow detector elements are close to the center; the width of the detector rows increases with distance from the center. Unnecessary dead spaces are avoided and with the corresponding pre-patient collimator and the proper readout schemes the following combinations of collimation can be achieved:

2 × 0.5 mm
4 × 1 mm

4 × 2.5 mm
4 × 5 mm
2 × 8 mm
2 × 10 mm

In contrast the **linear** multislice systems can produce four slices in each arrangement of detectors along the z-axis giving a selection of widths. Figure 14.27b shows how the various slice combinations are achieved by combining signals from the 0.5 and 1.0 mm separate detectors. The z-axial direction of the four-slice detector (32 mm wide) consists of four central 0.5 mm detectors with 15 detectors each side of 1 mm. The signals are from these outer rows are summed to give thick slices (four slices of 1, 5, 8 or 10 mm each). The mechanical cuts, collimation, and optical separations between the small elements reduce the geometrical efficiency and therefore the dose efficiency of the system.

MULTISLICE 8, 16, AND ABOVE

The linear array configuration is easily developed to provide more than four slices per rotation. The dimension of the z-axis is enlarged by increasing the

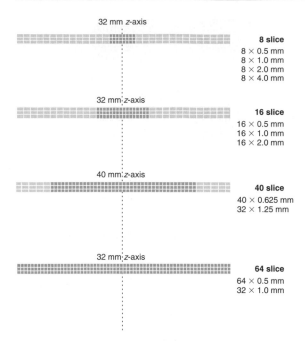

32 mm z-axis

8 slice
8 × 0.5 mm
8 × 1.0 mm
8 × 2.0 mm
8 × 4.0 mm

32 mm z-axis

16 slice
16 × 0.5 mm
16 × 1.0 mm
16 × 2.0 mm

40 mm z-axis

40 slice
40 × 0.625 mm
32 × 1.25 mm

32 mm z-axis

64 slice
64 × 0.5 mm
32 × 1.0 mm

Figure 14.28 *The detector arrangement for 8-, 16-, 40-, and 64-slice machines. Typical dimensions of available slice widths are given for each detector.*

width of the detector. Table 14.7 shows the increase in the z-dimension between 4, 16, and 64 slice machines, allowing a much wider coverage of the anatomy for each rotation. The number of centrally placed submillimeter detectors is increased significantly allowing faster coverage at finer resolutions. The cone beam geometry (Fig. 14.26a) is extended to cover the increased z-axis dimension. Some common multislice detector designs for 8, 16, 40, and 64 slice machines are shown in Fig. 14.28.

These machines can collect the full lung field in a single breath hold and display high definition 3-D images (HDCT). Submillimeter slices (0.625 or 0.5 mm) are commonly used for cardiac studies or examinations of the head. The thicker sections (1.25 or 2.0 mm) are used for the body. A more efficient isotropic data set can be collected.

Thicker slices (less noise and better contrast) can be obtained, post-acquisition, by combining thinner slices. Whenever slice thicknesses larger than the minimum thickness given by the array pitch are selected, the signal from several elements can be combined in the z-direction. Therefore the slice width can be defined by an electronic signal summation.

In conclusion, image quality in multislice spiral scanning must be optimized with respect to several factors:

- The narrowest collimation, consistent with the coverage of a certain volume and with a certain scan time, to minimize partial volume effects and to optimize image quality
- Fastest rotation time to maximize z-coverage and to minimize motion blurring
- Pitch values preserving temporal resolution and to minimize motion blurring (see Section 14.4.4)
- The exploitation of flying focal spot technology to avoid artifacts at high spatial resolution

GEOMETRIC EFFICIENCY

High geometric efficiency is a requirement for detectors which has particular importance for multislice detectors. This implies that dead spaces should be as small as possible. The antiscatter collimators between the individual detector elements which are oriented towards the focus have a width of typically 0.1 to 0.2 mm, while the separation of elements in the z-direction is approximately 0.1 mm. Values of geometric efficiency of 80 to 90% are typical. For arrays with a finer separation of detector elements in the z-direction a stronger reduction of geometric efficiency must be accepted.

ISOTROPIC SAMPLING COORDINATION SYSTEM (EQUAL X,Y,Z-AXIS)

This refers to the situation in which images can be created in any plane with the same spatial resolution as the original sections. The x,y-axis represents the normal transversal CT view of the body with the x-axis in a lateral direction and the y-axis in an anterior–posterior direction. The perpendicular to the x,y-axis oriented z-axis is parallel to the longitudinal axis of the body and the system axis (Fig. 14.26b). An isotropic data set is achieved by using the small focal spot with thin section collimation (0.5 mm); this gives a longitudinal resolution (z-axis) nearly identical to the in-plane (x-, y-axes) resolution. Figure 14.29 compares isotropic and non-isotropic data sets.

Coronal, sagittal, and axial images can be reconstructed from one multislice acquisition and will have the same spatial resolution as sections from the original acquisition. The examination can be done faster, with improved patient comfort. **Isotropic**

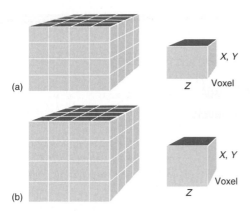

Figure 14.29 *(a) Non-isotropic and (b) isotropic dimensions.*

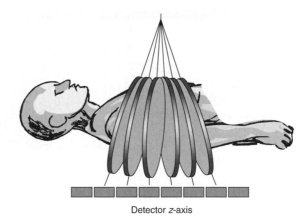

Detector *z*-axis

Figure 14.30 *The principal problem inherent in cone beam geometry. Details in the object are projected onto different detector rows for different projection angles, depending on their distance from the central plane. The data recorded in a 360° rotation by an off-center detector row (R1 and R2) no longer represent a planar slice, as expected for a single-row detector.*

viewing refers to image reconstruction created in any plane with the same spatial resolution as the original sections. The examination can be done faster, with improved patient comfort, and with less radiation.

14.4.3 Cone beam

The transition from scanning one or only a few slices to data acquisition for an entire field requires the transition from fan beam to cone beam geometry. With single-detector scanners, the beam is always central to the detector and encounters the same tissue section. Increasing the number of detectors in the *z*-axis increases the angular volume and the beam dimension resembles a cone rather than a flat plane. Cone beam CT is very different from sequential or single slice spiral CT, as the relation between the source and individual detectors is variable (Fig. 14.30). Detector elements in the periphery of the array are exposed more obliquely to those of the center. This and related geometric effects in spiral/helical multislice scanning have a major impact on noise, dose requirements, efficiency, image quality, and speed. The data sets recorded by any single row in cone beam geometry will become increasingly inconsistent with increasing distance from the central plane. If this is ignored, artifacts will result whenever the cone angle exceeds a few degrees. This leads to image distortion that is most pronounced for the outer regions of the cone and detectors. Beyond four detectors, image distortion becomes pronounced and reconstruction algorithms are needed to correct for the divergent beam angles. This solution works quite well for multislice scanners, with very little image distortion.

MULTISLICE COLLIMATION/SLICE WIDTH

Selection of a particular section thickness causes (1) movement of the pre- and post-patient (if available) collimators and (2) selection of detector rows. Activating or deactivating the detector elements can create all available section thicknesses for the linear detector design. For adaptive detector designs of unequal width, post-patient collimation is not needed to create the wider section thicknesses (5.0 mm and 2.5 mm). However, the narrower section thicknesses (1.0 mm and 0.5 mm) require precise post-patient collimation to cover portions of the detectors, which are exposed to radiation in the penumbra (Fig. 14.26a). The nominal slice thickness (width) is the full width at half maximum of the slice sensitivity profile. This is usually meant by the term **slice thickness**.

14.4.4 Pitch

For discussion of single detector spiral imaging the following definition of pitch is commonly used (see Section 14.3.4):

$$\text{single detector pitch} = \frac{\text{table travel per rotation}}{\text{slice width}}$$

$$(14.8)$$

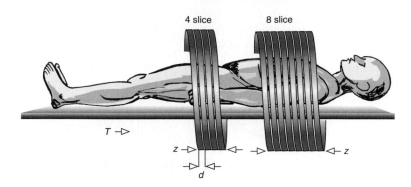

Figure 14.31 *Defining the pitch parameters used for Table 14.8.*

Pitch is of great importance for image quality and dose considerations. Some manufacturers use a variety of pitch definitions but the generally accepted definition of pitch should be in agreement with IEC 60601 regulations for computed tomography. Manufacturers of multislice CT systems use two different definitions of pitch. The terminology **pitch$_z$** (X-ray beam width or z-dimension) and **pitch$_d$** (detector width) differentiates between the two definitions used by commercial vendors of multislice CT scanners. Pitch$_z$ is determined by X-ray collimation determining the number of active detectors in a multislice machine, while pitch$_d$ will depend on the individual detector dimensions (d) as shown in Fig. 14.31.

$$\text{pitch}_z = \frac{\text{table travel per rotation}}{\text{X-ray beam collimation}} \quad (14.9)$$

$$\text{pitch}_d = \frac{\text{table travel per rotation}}{\text{single slice detector aperture}} \quad (14.10)$$

so

$$\text{pitch}_d = \text{pitch}_z \times \text{number of slices per rotation} \quad (14.11)$$

SINGLE VERSUS MULTISLICE PITCH

For any given exposure time, pitch, and collimation, multislice CT can cover a distance many times longer than single-slice helical CT. To enable the same coverage in a given interval with single-section helical CT, the pitch must be increased. Increasing the pitch creates a coarser spiral and image quality will deteriorate due to increasing effective section thickness. For single-section helical CT to cover the same distance as multi-slice CT in a given interval at the same pitch, an eightfold increase in section thickness would be necessary. To keep the section thickness and pitch constant,

the scanning time for single-section helical CT would need to be eight times longer, as indicated by eqn 14.11. For a single-slice CT scanner pitch$_d$ = pitch$_z$. The value of pitch$_z$ is determined solely by hardware parameters such as beam collimation and table speed, whereas pitch$_d$ will vary depending on the number of slices per rotation. These two pitch definitions are used differently by manufacturers. Confusion is caused because some manufacturers of multisection CT scanners use the original definition of pitch (see Section 14.3.4), and others use the value pitch$_d$. The use of pitch$_d$ is confusing because it alters the basic relationship between radiation dose, X-ray beam overlap, and pitch already established in single-section helical CT. The original definition of pitch is preferred because it can be unambiguously applied to both single-section and multisection scanning (two channels, four channels, eight channels, etc.).

For spiral scans one additional parameter has to be chosen: the table feed d in mm per 360° rotation. For single-slice scanners with a rotation time of 1 s, which represented the standard in single helical scanners, this corresponded exactly to the table speed in mm s^{-1}. For multislice CT scanners with variable rotation times between 0.5 s and 1.0 s this simple relation no longer applies. More importantly, the number of scanned slices has to be taken into account. The ratio of table feed to total slice width is generally termed the **pitch factor**:

$$\text{pitch factor} = \frac{\text{table feed}}{\text{number of slices} \times \text{slice width}} \quad (14.12)$$

A four- or eight-slice CT design with a nominal slice width of 1 mm and a table feed of 4 to 8 mm per rotation, respectively, gives a pitch factor of 1.0. The generally accepted definition of pitch according to

Table 14.8 *The different values obtained for pitch when changing between different multislice machines (4 and 8 slices in the example shown in Fig. 14.31). The calculation in eqn 14.12, however, gives them both a pitch of 1.0.*

Measure	4-slice	8-slice
Detector (d)	1 mm	1 mm
Collimation (z)	4 mm	8 mm
Table feed (T) per rotation	4 mm	8 mm
Pitch$_z$ (eqn 14.9)	4/4 = 1	8/8 = 1
Pitch$_d$ (eqn 14.10)	4/1 = 4	8/1 = 8
The pitch factor (eqn 14.12)	4/4 = 1	8/8 = 1

Box 14.3 Clinical examples

Thorax (30 cm in 10 s; low dose study)

Slices: 4×2.5 mm; feed/rotation: 17.5 mm

$$p = \frac{17.5}{4 \times 2.5} = 1.75$$

Thorax (30 cm in 39 s; high resolution study)

Slices: 4×1 mm; feed/rotation: 6 mm

$$p = \frac{6}{4 \times 1} = 1.5$$

Head ($\sim$25 cm in >100 s; inner ear study)

Slices: 2×0.5 mm; feed/rotation: 1 mm

$$p = 1.0$$

Pelvis (20 cm in 11 s; routine study)

Slices: 4×2.5 mm; feed/rotation: 10 mm

$$p = 1.25$$

Virtual colonoscopy (covering abdomen in 11 s)

Slices 16×0.75 mm; feed/rotation: 8 mm s^{-1}

$$p = \frac{8}{16 \times 0.75} = 0.6$$

---

eqn 14.12 is in agreement with the IEC 60601 regulations for computed tomography. Table 14.8 uses the dimensions in Fig. 14.31 to demonstrate the variation given by earlier pitch definitions and shows how eqn 14.12 provides the correct value for multislice scanners of any dimension. Examples are given in Box 14.3 for a variety of clinical studies; the virtual colonoscopy example shows oversampling with a pitch factor less than 1 in order to provide low noise, high quality, thin slices.

In practice pitch values between 1 and 2 are chosen to cover a given scan volume in the shortest time at optimum dose. To exclude gaps in sampling the object along the z-axis, pitch values should not exceed 2. The choice of the pitch factor is mostly determined by clinical requirements: the examination time t (in seconds) and a given scan range R (in millimeters). The desired table speed T_S (in mm s^{-1}) can be obtained if the selected slice width S, pitch factor p, and the number of slices per rotation M are known:

$$T_S = \frac{p \times M \times S}{\text{rotation time}} \quad (14.13)$$

The capability of the most modern scanners to acquire several slices simultaneously, where M is 4 or greater, gives the advantage of being able to achieve thin slice volume data sets at high scan speeds, allowing effective bolus chasing and breath hold.

GANTRY ROTATION TIME

This is the time for a full 360° rotation of the gantry around the patient table. Single-section helical CT scanners typically have a 360° gantry rotation speed of about 1 s. With multislice CT gantry rotation speeds of 0.4 or 0.5 s are possible; twice as fast as that of single-section helical CT. The product of the increased z-axis coverage and the faster rotation times lead to study times that are many times faster than for a single-slice scanner. Faster study times reduce motion artifacts due to voluntary and involuntary movement, i.e. intestinal peristalsis, cardiac movement, respiration etc. Breath-holding times are considerably reduced allowing high resolution pictures of lung parenchyma. So multislice machines achieve higher image quality by reducing movement unsharpness. Increased scanning speeds can be used to reduce scan time, or the increased scan speed advantage exchanged for thinner collimation and higher spatial resolution. Further speed increases will be limited physically by the high *g*-forces of the heavy gantries (see Section 14.3.2).

14.4.5 Efficiency

Particular attention is paid to ensuring that the most appropriate dose is used for infants and children. Dose reduction in pediatric patients is critical, due to the relatively high absorption in the small body volume, the greater sensitivity of rapidly growing tissue to radiobiological damage and, of course, the longer period of time over which damage can manifest itself.

The overall dose efficiency of a CT scanner can be simply described as the product of three factors:

- Geometric efficiency of the detector array
- Detector efficiency
- X-ray beam z-axis efficiency

GEOMETRIC EFFICIENCY

Geometric efficiency (G_{eff}) is a measure of the scanner's dose utilization in the z-axis. This is expressed as the ratio of the imaged slice section thickness relative to the z-axis dose profile. For optimum imaging, the geometric efficiency should be 100%, but it is often less, especially for narrow beam collimations where post-patient collimation may be necessary to bring the imaged slice thickness closer to the chosen value. The geometric efficiency (G_{eff}) of the detector array can be calculated by comparing the FWHM of the SDP with the SSP:

$$G_{eff} = \frac{\text{FWHM}(z - \text{sensitivity profile})}{\text{FWHM}(\text{dose profile})} \times 100\%$$

$$(14.14)$$

Where the SSP and SDP dimensions are identical, as in the case of sequential CT, the geometric efficiency is 100%. For single-slice and multislice spiral CT the geometric efficiency can fall as low as 60%. The geometric efficiency is influenced by the slice thickness so

$$G_{eff} = \frac{z - \text{sensitivity}}{\text{slice width}} \quad (14.15)$$

Multislice scanners will have a poorer geometric efficiency than single slice (Fig. 14.32). The geometric efficiency is an indication of the best utilization of patient radiation dose. As the number of slices increases the excess dose not contributing to the image ('wasted dose') becomes less. The value for a quad slice scanner having 1.25 mm slice thickness is

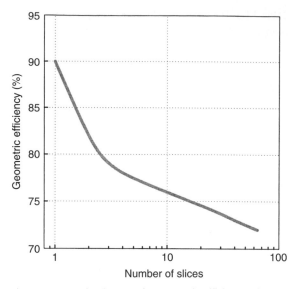

Figure 14.32 *The decrease in geometric efficiency with increasing slice number.*

about 78% (Table 14.9) whereas a 64-slice scanner with the same slice width gives a figure closer to 72%.

X-RAY BEAM Z-AXIS EFFICIENCY

The X-ray beam z-axis efficiency is the fraction of the dose profile seen by the detector element in the z-axis as

$$\frac{\text{FWHM}_{SSP}}{\text{FWHM}_{SDP}} \quad (14.16)$$

Typical z-axis dose efficiencies for three model scanners are shown in Table 14.9. The highest z-axis efficiency is given by 16-slice for thin slices of 1.5 mm and less.

DETECTOR EFFICIENCY

The detector efficiency is the product of the absorption efficiency for the photon energy used and conversion efficiency (X-ray photon to light photon conversion). This is approximately 98% for a 120 kV$_p$ X-ray spectrum.

DOSE EFFICIENCY

Since noise increases with smaller slice widths the dose must be increased (higher photon density) to maintain the same image quality. This dose increase reduces with the number of slices. Figure 14.33 compares a

Table 14.9 *Dose profile (full width at half maximum), total z-axis efficiency and geometric efficiency for three multislice machines.*

Scanner	Slice number (mm)	Geometric efficiency (%)	z-axis efficiency (%)	Overall dose efficiency (%)
Dual	2×1	80	63	50
Quad	4×1	78	72	54
Sixteen	16×1	75	93	65

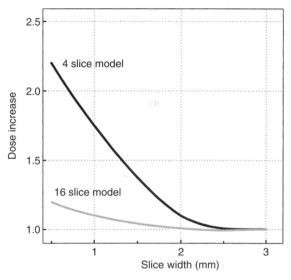

Figure 14.33 *The relative decrease in dose as slice width increases and noise drops. The dose variation is made to maintain the same image quality.*

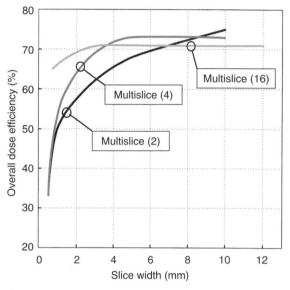

Figure 14.34 *The overall dose efficiency for dual, quad and 16-slice computed tomography models. The 16-slice machine makes better use of the beam and so reduces the full width at half maximum of the dose slice profile.*

4- and 16-slice model. The overall dose efficiency (see Table 14.9) is the product of all three efficiencies:

$$G_{eff} \times \text{detector detection efficiency} \\ \times \text{X-ray beam z-axis efficiency}$$

The results plotted in Fig. 14.34 expand the data given in Table 14.9 and show an improvement in the overall dose efficiency for thin slices when progressing from the 2-slice, 4-slice and 16-slice scanner. This improvement is mainly due to the wider beam width used to acquire the thin slices in the 4- and 16-slice scanners.

14.4.6 Image reconstruction

RECONSTRUCTED SLICE THICKNESS

Any nominal slice thickness can be reconstructed after acquisition providing that it is thicker than the original single detector configuration (scanned nominal slice thickness). The reconstruction of thicker slices than originally obtained is useful since it reduces the number of images to be viewed and decreases image noise.

HELICAL INTERPOLATION ALGORITHMS

To reconstruct an axial image from a helical data set, single-slice scanners have commonly used 180° linear interpolation algorithms. With this type of algorithm, the z-sensitivity profile (imaged slice width) for the helical scan, with a $\text{pitch}_x = 1$, is similar to that of an axial image. On multislice scanners, the use of a 180° linear interpolator, in conjunction with $\text{pitch}_x = 1$, results in wider z-sensitivity profiles, and increased artifacts, in comparison to single-slice systems.

Helical interpolation algorithms for multislice CT are different than those for single-section CT but in general do not cause any increase in image artifacts compared with the algorithms for single-section helical CT and are generally much less noticeable in multislice CT because most scanning is performed at lower pitch values than was practical with single-section systems.

The pitch can be optimized for multislice systems, in order to make best use of the data from the multiple detector banks. **Pitch optimization** improves distribution of projection data along the z-axis and a reduction in helical interpolation artifact. Generally a $pitch_x$ less than 1 gives an image quality similar to that of a single-slice scanner operating at $pitch_x = 1$.

DATA STORAGE

Multiple spiral acquisitions and the clinical requirement for reconstructing overlapping slices require very large memory storage (RAM) in the range of 512 MB to over 1 GB.

14.4.7 Image quality

In multislice systems, as in single-slice scanning, image quality decreases as pitch increases. The relationship is not straightforward in the case of multislice systems, however, and certain pitches will result in reduced helical artifacts. Whether slice width or noise increase with pitch depends on the interpolation method adopted by the CT machine but generally there will be some detriment in either noise or z-sensitivity with increased pitch, but with lower dose level.

Thinner sections improve resolution in the z-axis (along the table), reducing partial volume artifacts, and increase diagnostic accuracy.

In axial mode, multislice systems produce about the same image quality as equivalent single-slice scanners. The efficiency of individual detector arrays may vary, however, resulting in different noise levels between the slices. The cone beam geometry may lead to unequal z-axis sensitivities for different slices.

The increased examination speed of a multislice scanner should produce fewer patient movement artifacts, however.

COLLIMATION

The width of the X-ray beam is determined by collimators mounted in front of the X-ray tube. Geometric effects (distance between X-ray tube, center of rotation, and detector; height of the focus; position and setting of the collimator) lead to a more or less gradual increase and decrease of the quantity of radiation around the edges of the slice. In conventional scanning, the **slice sensitivity profile** and the **dose sensitivity profile** coincide precisely. The width of this profile, measured at full width; half maximum, FWHM is then the collimated slice thickness.

EFFECTIVE SLICE THICKNESS

The total effect of the collimation, pitch, and interpolation is described by SSP. The FWHM of this profile is commonly used as a measure for the effective slice thickness. With the 180° interpolation the FWHM of a pitch 1 acquisition is similar to that of a conventional scan with the same collimation. For larger pitches the FWHM increases linearly. While the SSP of the conventional scan has very steep edges, the SSP of the spiral multislice scan is more bell shaped as already seen in Section 14.3, so the area of anatomy that contributes to the image is wider.

NOISE

Data acquisition using multislice systems covers more patient length per rotation, so for extended-length studies X-ray tube current can be increased compared to single-slice machines. The higher current reduces image noise and improves image quality, which is critical for thin-section extended-length studies, but at the expense of increased patient dose.

In axial mode, multislice systems produce about the same image quality as equivalent single-slice scanners. The efficiency of individual detector arrays may vary, however, resulting in different noise levels between the slices. The cone beam geometry may lead to unequal z-axis sensitivities for different slices.

SPATIAL RESOLUTION

The spatial resolution in the scan plane is referred to as the **axial spatial resolution**. Resolution in the coordinate perpendicular to the scan plane (the z-direction) is referred to as the **longitudinal spatial resolution**. **Axial spatial resolution** is principally determined by the distances between the X-ray tube, the center of rotation, and the detector, as well as by the width of the focus and the detector elements, and the number of measurements made per rotation. These factors are determined by the construction of the scanner. **Longitudinal spatial resolution** is principally determined by the dimension of the cone beam angle and the selected protocol. In conventional CT, the longitudinal spatial resolution is entirely determined by the slice thickness.

CONTRAST

The choice of a thin slice is always associated with relatively low contrast resolution, long acquisition times, and relatively small section volumes; choices between slice dose and slice width must be made in order to optimize image quality.

SUMMARY

In conclusion, image quality in multislice spiral scanning must be optimized with respect to several factors:

- The narrowest collimation, consistent with the coverage of a certain volume and with a certain scan time, to minimize partial volume effects and to optimize image quality
- Fastest rotation time to maximize z-coverage and to minimize motion blurring
- Pitch greater than 4 to preserve temporal resolution and to minimize motion blurring
- The exploitation of flying focal spot technology to avoid artifacts at high spatial resolution

14.4.8 Multislice artifacts

Spiral interpolation artifacts, especially in structures that change rapidly in the z-axis, are an important issue for multislice scanners. Anatomical structures that generate spiral artifacts in multislice machines are mostly already seen in single-slice spirals. The most difficult situations arise from bony structures (high contrast) which are strongly inhomogeneous in axial direction. A typical example is the base of the skull with bony structures abruptly ending in an image plane. It is recommended that a larger pitch and narrower collimation is more successful for suppressing artifacts than a lower pitch and wider collimation for equal z-coverage; the main reason being the better elimination of partial volume artifacts.

Multislice machines are able to cover anatomical volumes with narrowest collimation and so minimize partial volume effects. This is only a matter of scanning technique (collimation) and is independent of the selected slice width. For optimization of image quality the narrowest collimation should be selected which is consistent with volume coverage and scan time.

In axial mode, multislice systems produce about the same image quality as equivalent single-slice scanners. The efficiency of individual detector arrays may vary, however, resulting in different noise levels between the slices. The cone beam geometry may lead to unequal z-axis sensitivities for different slices (see 'Cone-beam artifact' below).

In spiral mode on multislice systems, as in single-slice scanning, image quality decreases as pitch increases. The relationship is not straightforward in the case of multislice systems, however, and certain pitches will result in reduced spiral artifact. Whether slice width or noise increase with pitch depends on the interpolation method but there will be some detriment in either noise or z-sensitivity with increased pitch, but at a lower resultant dose. Spiral interpolation artifacts, especially in structures that change rapidly in the z-axis, are an important issue for multislice scanners. The increased examination speed of a multislice scanner produces fewer patient movement artifacts.

PARTIAL VOLUME EFFECT

In a CT scan, every part of the patient is represented by a pixel in a reconstructed image. If the slice is relatively thick, each pixel in the CT image will represent a larger quantity of tissue. If this quantity of tissue has different components, e.g. kidney parenchyma and fat, the pixel will be allocated a Hounsfield number somewhere between those of the two types of tissue. Consequently, the outlines of structures in the scan will appear to be vague, while this may not really be the case. The effect is most marked when structures vary in shape or position along the patient's longitudinal axis. Because spiral CT increases the width of the SSP, the partial volume effect will also increase.

SPIRAL ARTIFACTS

The interpolation algorithm is meant to overcome artifacts due to data inconsistency. This is only successful to some extent. The remaining effects can be divided in two groups.

CONE-BEAM ARTIFACTS

A spiral scan acquisition using a cone beam causes diameter decrease towards the top of the cone. These projections are treated the same in the interpolation process prior to reconstruction. The conic profiles, however, are not treated in the same way during interpolation and this generates an artifact similar to a partial-volume effect.

Instead of a perfect circle an ellipse-like reconstruction is displayed. This artifact is more apparent when the cone has a large top angle, or when large pitches are used; the top of the skull is a typical example. Because the X-ray beam diverges slightly along the z-axis of the patient in a four-section scanner, the data from the first section are acquired at a slightly different angle than the data from the fourth section. These cone beam artifacts in four-section systems are negligible compared with other causes of image degradation in CT and can safely be ignored.

The inclining surface of the skull acts like a cone and the cone-beam artifact can be seen as two crescent shaped bands of increased density along the skull–brain interface, mimicking a subdural hematoma. When three or more structures are present per rotation then these bands rotate around the brain in the same direction as the X-ray tube rotation.

ROD ARTIFACTS

This artifact is seen if a spiral scan of a cylinder or rod is made, angulated with respect to the scan plane, while the table holding the rod is moved during acquisition. Every subsequent projection locates the rod at a different position. Without table movement, i.e. in a conventional scan, the image would show an ellipse. With table movement, the variation in the registered position of the rod, together with the interpolation scheme, gives a distortion of the ellipse. These rod artifacts are especially seen in the liver in the area of the ribs.

14.4.9 Clinical advantages and application

The clinical advantages of multislice technology can be attributed to its increased speed and volume coverage. Multislice systems provide improved z-resolution and higher volume coverage speed, compared to single slice machines. The longer coverage is due to the simultaneous registration of 4, 8, 16 or more sections during each rotation and the increased gantry rotation speed. It is sometimes necessary to combine thin section multislice studies into broader slices and so reduce partial volume artifacts and noise content.

Since multislice systems acquire a very large number of thin slices quickly with improved z-axis resolution and isotropic voxels this allows accurate anatomical 3-D reconstruction for applications such as angiography and **virtual endoscopy**. Narrow collimation, low pitch, and a high mAs result in detailed multi-planar reconstruction (MPR) images. The amount of contrast material can be substantially reduced in all vascular studies.

CARDIAC

Fast rotation times allow ECG-gated cardiac studies. Measurement of coronary artery calcification in narrow slice acquisition provides a quantitative noninvasive means to evaluate the presence and extent of atherosclerotic change and give some method of **cardiac calcification scoring**. Cardiac imaging with fast multislice CT and retrospective ECG-gating provides 3-D image data sets displayed in a user-defined period of the heart cycle (systolic or diastolic phase). A spiral data set of the entire heart volume may be acquired within a single breath-hold.

LUNG

The fast acquisition significantly improves image quality and patient comfort for chest studies. A complete study of the lung fields takes only a few seconds so movement artifacts are no longer a problem and with narrow collimation fine lung detail can be resolved and the detection rate of small peripheral emboli increased.

14.5 COMPUTED TOMOGRAPHY: RADIATION DOSE

The number of CT examinations has increased as a consequence of the growing number of scanners installed. A typical annual number of CT examinations per machine varies between 3500 and 7000 in any one hospital. The total number of CT slices is the same order of magnitude as the sum of all the images produced using conventional projection radiography in the developed countries. This figure is still increasing significantly since multislice CT scanners have been introduced. An estimation of the contribution from CT to the radiation exposure of patients is shown in Fig. 14.35 based on data from various clinical surveys. The result is surprising in that such a relatively small fraction of only 4 to 5% of all CT examinations can give rise to a percentage contribution to the collective effective dose of over 40% (total dose delivered by the radiology department). CT therefore constitutes by far the largest proportion of radiation exposure to the population from diagnostic medical sources.

This is a serious development and the general trend is clear. Savings in collective dose over the past few years by introducing other radiation protection measures (most recent X-ray film-screen combinations of higher efficiency, use of radiation-free ultrasound or magnetic resonance imaging) will have been negated by the increasing contribution resulting from CT examinations, and CT examinations are still increasing because of their impressive image

quality and radiologists are complying since they earn most money by using this imaging technique. The expense of installing CT machines must also be justified by their increasing use.

Image quality is the major driving force behind machine development and consequently X-ray tube output has been necessary in order to deliver low noise thin sections (Fig. 14.36a). The slice dose to head and body has also shown inexorable rises (Fig. 14.36b)

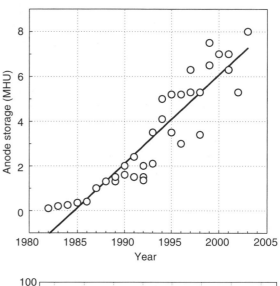

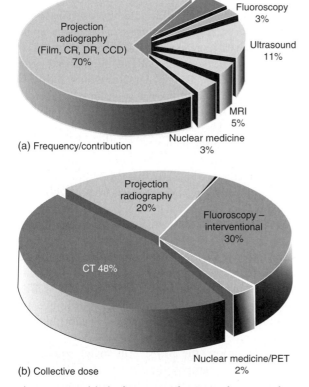

(a) Frequency/contribution

(b) Collective dose

Figure 14.35 (**a**) The frequency of computed tomography examinations (8%) is growing between 4 and 10% per year. (**b**) The patient collective dose (48%) reflects the high radiation dose per examination when compared to other radiographic techniques.

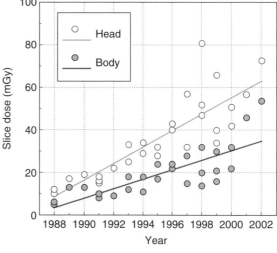

Figure 14.36 (**a**) The X-ray tube rating, and therefore output, measured in mega heat units (MHU). Data have been obtained from manufacturers' brochures from 1981 to 2003. (**b**) Head and body doses as reported over the period 1988 to 2002 showing consistently higher dose levels in head sections but with the introduction of new designs the body section doses have caught up.

particularly in latter years when spiral and multislice designs have been introduced. The referring physician and radiologist have responsibility for reducing this patient radiation burden; this can best be achieved by:

- Justifying each patient examination
- Automatic adjustment of scan parameters to patient size
- Choice of diagnostically adequate image quality
- Development of reference dose levels which should not be exceeded
- Particular attention to pediatric dose levels
- Improved radiology training for CT

Publication of reference dose values for a number of standard CT examinations should automatically lead to the optimization of scan protocols particularly for children. The education of CT users by the training staff of CT manufacturers and dedicated training courses will most probably result in a more significant reduction of doses in CT. Every machine must display the accurate radiation dose delivered to the patient for the total exam so that comparisons and improvements can be made.

14.5.1 Factors influencing dose

BEAM ENERGY

Energy of the X-ray beam in CT has a direct effect on dose. The higher the beam energy for an otherwise constant exposure, the higher the dose. Most CT scanners operate at 120 to $140\,\mathrm{kV_p}$. The most appropriate peak kilovoltage reduces patient dose.

FILTRATION

The type of filter placed in the X-ray beam also plays a major role in the resulting beam energy in CT. These filters may be shaped to present different thicknesses at different points across the X-ray beam. The filter used for a specific CT examination is usually determined by the manufacturer and can reduce the ratio of surface dose to midline dose.

COLLIMATION (SECTION THICKNESS)

Collimation of the X-ray beam plays a significant role in determining patient dose in CT. Effective methods of using pre-patient collimators are available to confine the beam to the section thickness intended at the area of interest. By restricting the beam in this manner,

the amount of radiation absorbed by tissue adjacent to that being imaged is kept to a minimum. Another set of collimators may be positioned post-patient or pre-detector to reduce the amount of scattered radiation that reaches the detectors. This technique produces images with better contrast resolution and may indirectly affect patient dose.

Multislice CT detector geometry alters radiation dose to patients for two reasons, as in section technology there are thin septa between detectors along the z-axis of the patient that absorb radiation and produce no data. These septa are about 0.06 mm thick. The umbra-to-penumbra ratio is also higher in multislice systems because the ratio of beam collimation to focal spot size is four times higher (for quad-section systems). This fact means that multislice systems produce less unusable radiation (in the penumbra). In summary, multislice CT has dose efficiency about equal to that of single-section CT.

SLICE NUMBER AND SPACING

Patient dose is affected by the number and spacing of adjacent slices. A greater number of slices in a single study irradiate a greater volume of tissue. The combined radiation dose expressed as the **multiple scan average dose** (**MSAD**) will increase because of widening penumbra resulting from scattered radiation and possible beam divergence. Figure 14.37a shows how the total dose, accumulated over a series of slices, increases due to the increased overlap between slices. As the ratio between section thickness and section interval increases (Fig. 14.37b), the MSAD increases because of increasing contributions from neighboring sections.

MSAD is the average dose across the central slice from a series of N slices of thickness T, with a constant increment I between successive slices. The MSAD represents the dose to a specific section location resulting from the scan at that location as well as contributions from adjacent scan locations since the penumbra from adjacent sections may contribute to the dose received by the section of interest.

By definition, the MSAD (in mGy) equals the computed tomography dose index (CTDI) for the seven contiguous sections above and below the section of interest (see CTDI below).

$$\mathrm{MSAD} = \frac{1}{I} \int\limits_{-\frac{1}{2}}^{+\frac{1}{2}} D_{N,I}(z)\,\mathrm{d}z \qquad (14.17)$$

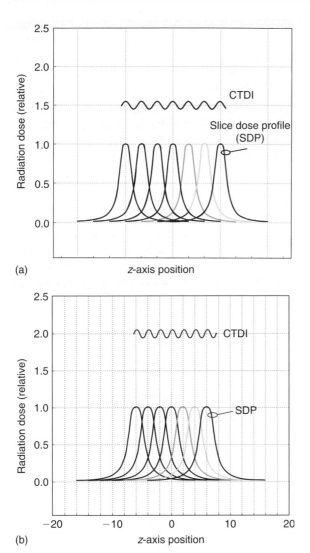

(a)

z-axis position

(b)

z-axis position

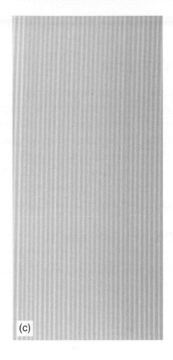

(c)

Figure 14.37 (*a*) *Slice overlap contributes to the final value of overall patient dose.* (*b*) *The overall computed tomography dose index (CTDI) increases as the pitch factor gets smaller and adjacent slices overlap resulting in a higher multiple scan average dose (MSAD) figure.* (*c*) *A film exposure of a multislice computed tomography machine showing uneven striped exposure due to the MSAD effect.*

where $D_{N,I}(z)$ is the multiple scan dose profile along the central 100 mm detector. If a sufficient number of slices are taken then:

$$MSAD = \frac{T}{I} CTDI \qquad (14.18)$$

MSAD is equal to CTDI when the distance between scans is equal to the slice thickness. In general MSAD ranges are 40 to 60 mGy for head scans and 10 to 40 mGy for body scans. If the CT scanner is used to acquire a scout or toposcan planar image similar to that obtained in radiography it gives a surface dose of approximately 1 mGy.

Figure 14.37c illustrates the uneven striped exposure given by a multislice CT machine; this was captured on a plain X-ray film. The radiation exposure is not uniform even at pitch 1 since the shape of the dose sensitivity profile (DSP) is not rectangular and so there is a peak value separated by lower interslice values.

IMAGE QUALITY AND NOISE

Two of the most significant factors affecting image quality are statistical noise and the loss of image contrast as a result of scattered radiation. If a decrease in noise is desired, the dose used to acquire the image will increase. Although detector collimators help increase image contrast, this improvement usually comes at the cost of increased patient dose. To maintain acceptable levels of noise, the peak kilovoltage and tube current used to acquire the image may need to be increased.

SCAN PITCH FACTOR

For a spiral CT examination performed with a pitch of one, the dose to the patient should be comparable with that delivered in a traditional CT study of the same volume of tissue. Patient dose is proportional to 1/pitch, so increasing the pitch decreases the dose at any point along the volume of tissue being imaged. Similarly, if the pitch is decreased, the dose will increase due to slice overlap, shown by the MSAD values given above.

14.5.2 Dose measurement

Dosimetry for a multislice scanner is similar to a single-slice scanner with some important differences. As mentioned above studies performed at a higher pitch value (greater than 1) give a lower patient dose but they also give more image noise. With a pitch less than 1, there will be some overlap between one rotation of the tube and another. This is not normally practiced on a single-slice spiral scanner because it increases patient dose with little increase in image quality. However, on multislice systems, all the information from the overlapping spirals is used to form an image, so improved image quality (with lower noise) can be obtained using lower mA per rotation, so keeping the dose to the patient constant.

When comparing dose values between multislice systems it is important to ensure that comparisons are made with equivalent definitions of pitch. Some studies quote pitch 1.4 as the optimum compromise between spatial resolution, contrast resolution and dose.

PATIENT SIZE

The dose that a patient receives is strongly dependent on the patient's size. If the same protocols are used for all patients, the center dose will be lower in obese patients due to the attenuation of the surrounding tissue. As an example taken from a typical spiral scanner, using a whole body phantom with a diameter of 30 cm, exposed to 120 kV at 100 mAs, with a slice thickness of 5 mm, this would give a central dose of 5 mGy and a peripheral dose of 10 mGy. Using the same exposure factors but this time on a 16 cm phantom the central dose would be 15 mGy and the peripheral dose very similar at 15.5 mGy. For this reason children's CT scan protocols, due to their smaller body and head size, should use a fraction of the adult exposure parameters. They are commonly ⅓ of the adult exposure settings.

DOSE, SCANNER GEOMETRY, AND KILOVOLTAGE

Due to differences in the geometry and construction between various scanners, and the use of different shapes and materials for filtering the X-ray beam, the dose to the patient at the same mA and kV values can vary by as much as a factor 2. In general CT machines with a short beam geometry have a reduced X-ray tube current (mA) value to give the same central dose to the patient. The skin dose in these machines is relatively high. Consequently, CT performance figures cannot easily be compared.

The voltage applied to the X-ray tube determines the energy of the X-ray spectrum. Radiation dose to the patient increases roughly as kV^2 but dose increases in a linear relationship to the tube current and the scan time. The total effect of voltage, current, geometry and filtration is expressed in the computed tomography dose index (CTDI).

DOSE AND SLICE THICKNESS

In the simple sequential CT machine, with a table index equal to the slice thickness, or a spiral machine with pitch = 1, the dose to the patient is, in principle, independent of the slice thickness. The amount of radiation emitted by the source is not affected by the subsequent collimation but the collimation prevents a certain proportion of the emitted photons from reaching the patient.

The number of photons reaching the patient for a 2 mm slice is one third of the number of photons for a 6 mm slice. Differences only occur due to the use of post-patient collimation, different focus sizes, and geometric effects.

The performance of a multislice CT machine, compared with a single-slice spiral machine, should consider:

- Radiation and slice sensitivity profiles
- Low-contrast and limiting spatial resolution
- Image uniformity and noise
- CT number
- Geometric efficiency
- Dose

In general for a typical abdomen and pelvis study, central and entrance doses for 5 mm helical scans would be higher on the multislice system by about 50%. The multislice system provides better image quality and a substantial reduction in study time and tube loading but at increased patient dose relative to the single-slice scanner.

14.5.3 Practical equipment for estimating patient dose

The majority of the dose from a single scan is delivered to the thin volume of tissue (usually 1 to 10 mm thick) exposed to the primary beam. Tissue outside the defined volume also receives dose from scattered radiation, as well as from any part of the primary beam that diverged from the intended thickness.

The two main variables used to describe doses received from CT are:

* Computed tomography dose index (CTDI)
* Dose–length product (DLP)

Both variables may be reported as a surface dose, at a depth no less than 1 cm, or at some point inside the patient, usually the midline.

The two doses most commonly reported for CT are those delivered during head scans and body scans. The US Food and Drug Administration (FDA) requires manufacturers to report CTDI derived from imaging 16 and 32 cm diameter phantoms for head and body scans, respectively. These standards are also used to report MSAD.

TLD MEASUREMENTS

The patient's surface dose can be measured using small thermoluminescent chips contained in sachets. This method has several drawbacks, perhaps the major one being the inability to separate slice exposure to a single chip. Measuring the dose for a single slice is therefore extremely uncertain in single-slice or multislice spiral machines.

PHANTOM MEASUREMENTS USING AN ION CHAMBER

The CT dose phantom was designed in accordance with the US Food and Drug Administration's performance standard for diagnostic X-ray systems, which includes regulations specifically applicable to CT systems (21 CFR 1020.33). A solid polymethylmethacrylate (PMMA) phantom design is described

for both 16 cm (head) and 32 cm (body) diameters, each 15 cm deep. Each body and head phantom has one central hole 1 cm in diameter. Four holes of the same dimension are placed 1 cm from the periphery to measure surface dose. The design in Fig. 14.38a and b

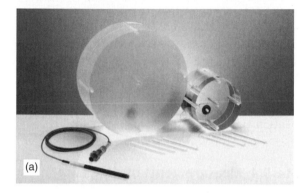

(a)

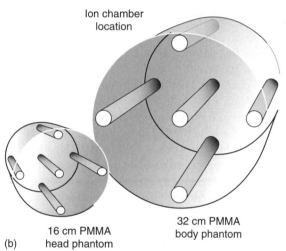

Ion chamber location

16 cm PMMA head phantom

32 cm PMMA body phantom

(b)

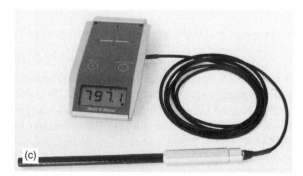

(c)

Figure 14.38 (*a*) *Typical PMMA CTDI phantom for head and body dose measurements. (Courtesy PTW Freiburg.)* (*b*) *Dimensions for body and head phantom.* (*c*) *A 100 mm pencil ion chamber used for making the measurements within the head/body phantom.*

shows that each phantom contains five probe holes: one in the center and four around the perimeter, 90° apart and 1 cm from the edge. Each hole can take a 100 mm long ion chamber (Fig. 14.38c). PMMA rods are used for filling unused holes in the phantom.

The integration of the radiation exposure profile in a head or body phantom produced by a CT scanner along a line normal to the slice, divided by the table increment, is equal to the exposure to a central slice at that point produced by a series of scans (CTDI). The line of integration must be of sufficient length to intercept not only the primary beam, but also the Compton scatter produced in the phantom. This integral is then expressed in mGy cm^{-1}.

14.5.4 Measurements of slice dose

COMPUTED TOMOGRAPHY DOSE INDEX

The basic CTDI measurement as defined by the US Federal Regulation 21CFR 1020.33(C) represents the dose at the center or peripheral point on a head or body phantom from a single scan and results from absorption of the X-ray beam over a distance of ±7 slices and the section thickness, centered on the location of interest. The dose is integrated over the 14 slices by a 100 mm ion chamber (Fig. 14.38c). The dose profile from a single CT scan spreads beyond the intended section thickness. The area beyond the section thickness is referred to as the penumbra. The CTDI attempts to represent the dose distribution outside the section thickness, taking a representative 14 slices in air or the phantom as:

$$CTDI = \frac{1}{nT} \int_{-7}^{+7} D_{(z)} \, dz \qquad (14.19)$$

This equation represents the dose $D_{(z)}$, for a single section at a given position z along the scan axis. This value is then divided by the intended section thickness per image (T) and the number of image slices per scan n to obtain the CTDI. This quantity is simple and can easily be determined free-in-air on the axis of rotation of the scanner for a single scan $CTDI_{(air)}$. By itself the $CTDI_{(air)}$ is only a coarse indicator of patient exposure for an examination, and is not well-suited for use as a reference dose quantity for all types of scanner. Table 14.10 gives typical values of CTDI for sequential, spiral, and multislice machines.

COMPUTED TOMOGRAPHY DOSE INDEX OVER A FIXED 100 MM LENGTH (CTDI$_{100}$)

A better, more representative dose measurement measures the CTDI over a fixed 100 mm length instead of the 14 arbitrary slices. The value of CTDI$_{100}$ is made over a fixed length of integration using a pencil ionization chamber with an active length of 100 mm. It provides a measurement of the basic CTDI, integrated over a standard 100 mm length expressed in terms of absorbed dose to air (mGy):

$$_{(mAs)}CTDI_{(100,\,a/p)} = \frac{1}{S} \int_{-50\,mm}^{+50\,mm} D_{(z)} \, dz \qquad (14.20)$$

where S is the slice width, the dose $D(z)$ being integrated over ±50 mm by the 100 mm pencil detector. The subscripts for the CTDI measurement include (mAs) to indicate the exposure value used to normalize the result (typically doses are stated for a 100 mAs value); the subscript 100 denotes a 100 mm scan length and a or p indicates that measurements were made in air or a PMMA phantom. In addition, the phantom size 16 or 32 cm should be stated depending on either head or body values. In some instances scattered radiation may fall outside the 100 mm detector length. In order to overcome this problem the FDA require acquisition of 14 nominal slice widths. In **multiple slice machines** it is necessary to modify the calculation of eqn 14.20 to take account of the number of simultaneously acquired slices (M) so

$$_{n}CTDI_{(100,\,a/p)} = \frac{1}{S \times M} \int_{-50\,mm}^{+50\,mm} D_{(z)} \, dz \qquad (14.21)$$

This formula allows comparison between machines acquiring simultaneous slices of 2, 4, 8 or more.

WEIGHTED VERSION OF THE COMPUTED TOMOGRAPHY DOSE INDEX (CTDI$_w$)

A weighted version of CTDI taking surface and center dose readings of the head or body phantom gives an adequate basis for specifying reference doses for CT. These measurements of a weighted CTDI$_w$ represent the average dose to a single slice:

$$CTDI_w = \frac{1}{3}CTDI_{100c} + \frac{2}{3}CTDI_{100p} \qquad (14.22)$$

Table 14.10 *Published values of computer tomography dose index for different detectors at various values of kV_p or kV.*

Position	CTDI at various values of kV_p or kV					
	125 kV_p	80 kV	110 kV	120 kV	130 kV	140 kV
Sequential single slice, xenon detectors						
16 cm, Center	8.0					
Periphery (1 cm)	11.0					
32 cm, Center	3.0					
Periphery (1 cm)	9.3					
Spiral single slice, ceramic detectors						
16 cm, Center		6.9	16.6		24.7	
Periphery (1 cm)		8.5	19.2		27.5	
32 cm, Center		1.9	5.4		8.3	
Periphery (1 cm)		4.9	11.8		17.4	
Multislice (4 images per slice)						
16 cm, Center		3.7		12.5		18.2
Periphery (1 cm)		4.3		13.8		19.6
32 cm, Center		1.1		4.3		6.4
Periphery (1 cm)		2.5		8.1		11.7
Multislice (16 images per slice)						
16 cm, Center		6.3		18.8		26.4
Periphery (1 cm)		8.0		21.9		30.6
32 cm, Center		1.2		4.6		7.0
Periphery (1 cm)		2.9		9.5		14.1

where subscripts c and p denote central or peripheral measurement from the phantom. The value is normally given as $_n$CTDI$_w$ where n denotes a normalized mAs value (typically 100 mAs). The true CTDI$_w$ figure per slice is given by $_n$CTDI$_w \times C$, where C is the mAs multiplier relative to 100 mAs. Manufacturers can choose either the normalized or full CTDI$_w$ value in their literature. An example of a CTDI$_w$ calculation is given in Box 14.4. The CTDI$_w$ will vary with slice width (Table 14.11).

THE FDA DEFINITION OF COMPUTED TOMOGRAPHY DOSE INDEX (CTDI $_{(FDA)}$)

This is the particular definition of CTDI given by the Food and Drug Administration (FDA), for the purposes of compliance testing of CT systems in the USA. It involves the integration of dose over a distance of 14 times the slice thickness. Manufacturers

of CT scanners are obliged to report values of CTDI$_{(FDA)}$ for all modes of operation. CTDI$_{(FDA)}$ is not ideal for practical dosimetry since a 14 slice dose integration depends on machine settings. CTDI$_{100}$ values are larger than corresponding values of CTDI$_{(FDA)}$ under similar conditions of exposure.

DOSE–LENGTH PRODUCT

The associated dose–length product (DLP) for a complete examination can be derived as

$$DLP = \sum CTDI_w \times T \times N \times C \qquad (14.23)$$

The summation $\sum$ denotes that all CT scan patient procedures should be included in the DLP value (i.e. before and after contrast studies etc.). N is the number of slices of thickness T, in cm, and C the exposure, in mAs (as fractions of 100 if the CTDI$_w$ was

Box 14.4 Calculation of CTDI$_w$

From measurements made using a PMMA head and body phantom the following readings are obtained:

	CTDI head (16 cm)		CTDI body (32 cm)	
	Center	Peripheral	Center	Peripheral
110	16.2	18.1	4.9	10.9
130	25.2	27.7	7.8	16.4

Using the formula

$$CTDI_w = \frac{1}{3} CTDI_{100c} + \frac{2}{3} CTDI_{100p}$$

the weighted dose figures are obtained:

	CTDI$_w$ head (16 cm)	CTDI$_w$ body (32 cm)
110	17.2	8.8
130	26.6	13.4

Table 14.11 *Dose variation (mGy) with slice width CTDIw/100 mAs for the head and body.*

Slice width (mm)	Dose		
	80 kV$_p$	120 kV$_p$	140 kV$_p$
Head			
1	3.8	13.2	17.5
2	3.2	11.1	14.8
3	3.3	11.3	15.1
5	3.3	11.9	15.3
8	3.3	11.9	15.3
10	3.5	12.0	16.3
Body			
1	2.1	7.5	9.9
3	1.8	6.5	8.6
10	2.0	6.9	9.3

standardized to 100 mAs). For spiral acquisition the formula changes to:

$$DLP = \sum CTDI_w \times T \times A \times t \quad (14.24)$$

For each study or scan sequence A is the tube current (mA) and t the study acquisition time. It is also convenient to modify this formula to accommodate

Table 14.12 *European dose guidelines per slice.*

Organ	CTDI$_w$ (mGy)	DLP (mGy cm^{-1})
Head	60	1050
Face & sinuses	35	360
Vertebral trauma	70	460
Chest	30	650
HRCT of lung	35	280
Liver	35	900
Abdomen	35	800
Pelvis	35	600

CTDI$_w$, weighted computed tomography dose index. DLP, dose–length product. HRCT, high resolution computed tomography.

Table 14.13 *Multiplying factors for obtaining the effective dose H$_e$ from the values for dose–length product (DLP).*

Body region	E$_{DLP}$ (mSv mGy^{-1} cm^{-1})
Head	2.3×10^{-3}
Neck	5.4×10^{-3}
Chest	1.7×10^{-2}
Abdomen	1.5×10^{-2}
Pelvis	1.9×10^{-2}

multislice scanners in the same way as CTDI$_{100}$ in eqn 14.21, where M is the number of simultaneously acquired slices, so

$$DLP = \sum CTDI_w \times T \times M \times N \times C \quad (14.25)$$

The scattered radiation component increases slightly with multislice machines increasing the overall dose. European guidelines for CTDI$_w$ and DLP values obtained as 75th percentile figures from a Europe-wide CT survey are given in Table 14.12.

EFFECTIVE DOSE (H_e) (WHOLE-BODY EQUIVALENT DOSE)

This is a useful indicator of patient radiation risk, although it is also not particularly suitable as a reference dose quantity since it can not be measured directly and its definition may be subject to further changes. Broad estimates of the effective dose may be derived from the DLP as

$$H_e = E_{DLP} \times DLP \quad (14.26)$$

where E_{DLP} is the region or tissue specific normalized effective dose, in mSv mGy^{-1} cm^{-1}. General values for E_{DLP} are given in Table 14.13 and a calculation of effective dose is given in Box 14.5.

Box 14.5 Calculation of effective dose H_e for European dose limits

From Table 14.13 the effective doses from the dose–length product (DLP) values can be calculated using the formula

$$H_e = E_{DLP} + DLP$$

The weighted dose figures are obtained as follows:

Organ	DLP	E_{DLP}	H_e (mSv)
Head	1050	2.3×10^{-3}	2.4
Chest	650	1.7×10^{-3}	1.1
Abdomen	800	1.5×10^{-3}	1.2
Pelvis	600	1.9×10^{-3}	1.1

14.5.5 Automatic dose control

During a scan sequence in single-spiral or multislice machines a considerable saving in patient dose can be achieved by varying or modulating the X-ray tube output according to the shape of the anatomy. At the shoulder region for instance more photons are needed to penetrate across the chest than perpendicular to it, owing to more attenuation in the broader dimension. A uniform photon fluence can then be presented to the detectors. Similarly, in other regions of the patient's body the tube output can be modulated so that a constant photon density, optimum for image quality, can be obtained. The two methods chosen by manufacturers for modulating the X-ray beam are essentially:

- A prior scoutview of the scanned area to alter a look-up table for modulating the X-ray beam during the intended scan
- A continuous slice by slice sampling and modulation of the X-ray beam

WHOLE-BODY DOSE MODULATION

This uses a scoutview to vary mA along the patient and during rotation. Prior to the axial scan a look at attenuation along one or two scoutviews is made and this prior mapping used to vary the mA in each acquired slice.

SLICE BY SLICE DOSE MODULATION

This uses feedback during the scan study to vary X-ray tube mA along the patient and during rotation, according to the attenuation seen in the previous rotation. The tube mA gradually changes in response to anatomy in real time.

14.5.6 Patient dose levels

With earlier spiral systems it was possible to claim a reduction in patient dose but this is no longer the case when pitch = 1 is employed with the same mA value as that for sequential slice acquisition; patient dose is reduced when table pitch is increased. The ability to reconstruct slices at any arbitrary table position within the scanned volume eliminates the need to produce additional scans with subsequent extra patient dose. Since X-ray output has been increased to accommodate larger scanned volumes and reduce image noise (Fig. 14.36a) the dose rate has increased particularly for studies using a table pitch of 1, where thin slices are required for multi-planar reconstruction (3-D). Figure 14.36b shows the increase in slice dose as CT models have changed from sequential, spiral, and multislice, over successive years; the data obtained from head and body phantoms using either TLD or ion chamber measurements. The slice dose for head scans shows the highest dose and the fastest increase due to the demands of image quality. Both head and body scans have shown a significant increase since the introduction of spiral and multislice acquisition.

Patient dose can be reduced when a higher pitch value is selected but this gives a reduced image quality. The geometric efficiency of the CT design can contribute to increased patient dose. Figure 14.34 showed that the 16-slice machine, being more dose efficient, can potentially give less dose than the 4-slice machine for narrow slice widths.

CHILDREN'S DOSE LEVELS

The head dose example shown in Fig. 14.36b shows the importance of careful reduction in exposure values when scanning the smaller body diameters of children.

DOSE AND TABLE INCREMENT/PITCH

The dose values indicated by CTDI always refer to 'contiguous' scanning. In spiral CT, contiguous scanning is equivalent to scanning with pitch 1. The greater the selected pitch at any given nominal slice thickness, the faster the patient will move through the X-ray beam. The dose along the longitudinal axis of the patient is thus in inverse proportion to the pitch. The situation with the skin is somewhat different. If the selected pitch is greater than 1, some square centimeters of the patient's skin will not receive the entrance dose, and will therefore be exposed to less radiation. Other areas will receive the same dose as with pitch 1. Some studies quote pitch 1.4 as the optimum compromise between spatial resolution, contrast resolution and dose.

14.5.7 Computed tomography environmental radiation

During a CT examination of a patient in a CT scanner, the X-ray tube rotates around the body. Beam energies of 120 to 140 kV$_p$ are commonly employed which give high levels of Compton scattered radiation from the detector assembly and particularly from the patient (hard and soft tissues). The exposure geometry of the fan-beam is fixed so the pattern of scattered radiation is consistent. The in-built gantry shielding provides protection against the primary beam so the scatter radiation pattern is decided by the volume of absorber irradiated, patient size, and intervening absorber in the form of the gantry.

The resulting pattern of scattered radiation has a 360° symmetry about the axis of rotation and has a conical shape in the front and rear of the gantry (Fig. 14.39a and b). The dose contour depends on study parameters, beam collimation, and filtration, and is characteristic for each type of scanner model.

Since the magnitude of the dose contours varies with CT gantry position within the room so the scanner orientation must be decided before room shielding requirements are finalized.

The calculation of scatter radiation levels is important for radiation protection purposes affecting both staff and other workers adjacent to the CT facility, including the control room.

Clinical personnel, who must be present in the examination room as part of an interventional procedure or patient care, must be aware of the radiation boundaries. A PMMA body or head phantom can be used when scatter radiation dose measurements are being taken and the relevant contour limits marked

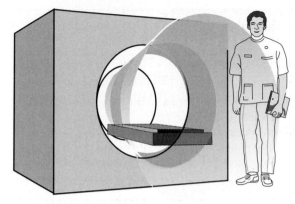

(a) 3D DOSE CONTOURS

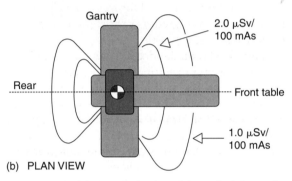

(b) PLAN VIEW

Figure 14.39 *(a) A representation of the conical shape of the scatter distribution from the gantry. (b) A plan view of the radiation dose contours.*

on the floor of the CT room. In particular, the dose rate values are quite low when the person remains in the shadow of the gantry.

An estimation of scatter dose can be gained from the total mAs product of the expected patient workload. For a position within the room at a contour point with a scatter radiation value of 1.0 μSv/100 mAs, for example, a patient study requiring 50 slices at 250 mAs would give a scatter radiation value of 125 μSv. As can be seen from the conical shape of the scatter distribution in Fig. 14.39a protection must be considered for rooms above and below the CT installation.

REFERENCES

US Federal Regulations 21CFR1020.33(C)
European Guidelines on QC for Computed Tomography. EUR 16262 (Available on www.drs.dk/guidelines/ct/quality)

Tsapaki *et al*. Reference dose levels in CT. *Br J Radiol* 2001; 836–840.

RECOMMENDED READING

Impact Technology Update (Available on www. impact.org.uk)

Kalender W. *Computed Tomography*. Publicis MCD-Verlag, 2000. (ISBN 3-89578-081-2)

KEYWORDS

back-projection: a method for reconstructing a sectional display from a series of radial projections

CT number: (see Hounsfield unit)

effective focal spot: this decides the size of a point at the iso-center as projected onto the detector

fan beam: the geometry of a third generation machine describing the fixed assembly between X-ray tube and detector array which rotates together.

helical scan: continuous rotation of a fan beam assembly while the scan bed moves incrementally

Hounsfield unit (H): the CT value or number relating $\mu_{unknown}$ to μ_{water}

iso-center: center of gantry

kernel: a discrete filter for image reconstruction

look-up table (LUT): controls displayed gray scale. Either linear or nonlinear

magnification: image enlargement re-displaying to full display dimensions. No improvement in resolution

pixel: picture element matrix holding a narrow range of CT numbers. Can be 4 to 8 bits deep

topogram/scoutview: longitudinal scan with the fan beam assembly fixed in AP, PA or lateral position

system magnification: focal spot to detector distance divided by focal spot to iso-center distance

voxel: volume element matrix holding the complete range of CT values from -1000 to $+3000$

windowing: displaying a selected range of CT numbers stored in a voxel array

zooming: image enlargement with reconstruction giving improved resolution

Nuclear medicine: basic principles

15.1 NUCLEAR PARAMETERS

15.1.1 Nuclear structure

The nucleus of any atom consists of a mixture of protons and neutrons (see Chapter 2); a simple nuclear model therefore consists of Z protons and N neutrons, making a total of A **nucleons**. Each element 'X' can therefore be defined uniquely in terms of these three components:

$$^A_Z X_N$$

where Z is the atomic number (proton number), N the neutron number and A the mass number ($Z + N$). Some common elements – iodine, potassium, and carbon – are described below using this coding:

$$^{131}_{53} I_{78} \quad ^{40}_{19} K_{21} \quad ^{14}_{6} C_8$$

In practice a nucleus can be identified by reducing these parameters to only Z and A. The atomic number Z is redundant, since the element name defines the value of Z; change the number of protons and the element changes. Therefore the mass number A is commonly used as a single identifier: ^{131}I, ^{40}K, ^{14}C. This is sufficient to identify a nuclear species or **nuclide** exactly. This model of the nucleus, using only neutrons and protons, fits all practical requirements in nuclear medicine. In the early days of chemistry most naturally occurring elements, e.g. iron, were found to have atomic mass values that were not whole numbers. This problem was solved when it was found that most chemical elements consist of a mixture of two or more species having different neutron numbers; iron has four stable species making up the common metal. These are shown in Fig. 15.1.

Since the Z value remains constant the chemical element itself does not change. The increasing number of neutrons, having no electrical charge, just adds mass without changing the element.

The percentages shown in this series are the relative abundance of each species in the natural element mixture but ^{59}Fe is unstable with a half-life ($T_{1/2}$) of 45 days. Figure 15.1 shows a section of the nuclide chart from the more familiar periodic table. This particular section identifies three stable isotopes of iron showing

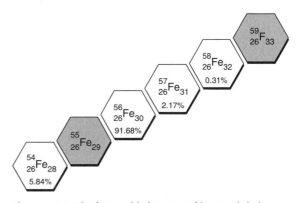

Figure 15.1 *The four stable isotopes of iron and their percentage abundance. The shaded hexagons indicate unstable (radioactive) members of the series.*

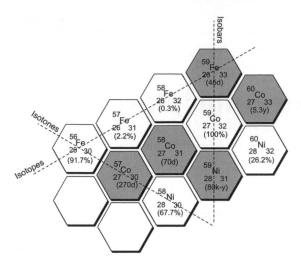

Figure 15.2 *Examples of isotope, isotone, and isobar series, identified for cobalt, iron and nickel.*

their percentage abundance and the unstable isotope ^{59}Fe. Stable and unstable isotopes of cobalt and nickel are also shown.

Nuclides with a constant Z (proton number) but varying N (neutron number) are called **isotopes**. The iron series shown above are isotopes. Nuclides with a constant N but varying Z are called **isotones**. The diagonal line in Fig. 15.1 indicates the series:

$$^{57}_{26}\text{Fe}_{31} \qquad ^{58}_{27}\text{Co}_{31} \qquad ^{59}_{28}\text{Ni}_{31}$$

Nuclides having a constant mass but varying Z and N values are called **isobars** or isobaric nuclides identified by the vertical line:

$$^{59}_{26}\text{Fe}_{33} \qquad ^{59}_{27}\text{Co}_{32} \qquad ^{59}_{28}\text{Ni}_{31}$$

Three of the stable iron isotopes are shown in Fig. 15.1 but the other iron isotope ^{59}Fe is unstable having a stated $T_{\frac{1}{2}}$ of only 45 days. Similarly, other unstable isotopes or **radionuclides**, indicated by their decay rate as half-lives ($T_{\frac{1}{2}}$), in brackets, are:

$$^{60}\text{Co} \quad ^{58}\text{Co} \quad ^{57}\text{Co} \quad ^{59}\text{Ni}$$

^{59}Ni has a very long $T_{\frac{1}{2}}$ of 80 000 years. Examples of isotope, isotone and isobar series for cobalt, iron, and nickel are shown in Fig. 15.2.

15.1.2 Nuclear decay rate

The decay, or transformation, of an unstable nuclide is a statistical process which is expressed in mathematical form as the rate of transformation of N nuclei changing per unit time (dN/dt) and is proportional to the number of nuclei N present at that moment: $dN/dt = \lambda N$ where λ is the decay constant. The rate or activity A at which the nucleus decays is measured in disintegrations per second (dps); this is the **becquerel** (Bq), which is a measure of activity: $A = dN/dt$. It is named after Henri Becquerel (1852–1908; French physicist) who, in 1895, discovered radioactivity. Prior to the adoption of the becquerel as the Systèm Internationale (S.I.) unit of activity, the common measurement was the **curie** (Ci); this is 3.7×10^{10} dps and was related to the activity of 1 mg of pure ^{226}Ra, named after Marie Curie (1867–1934; Polish-born French chemist), the discoverer of radium. Since the adoption of the SI Units this measure has been superseded by the becquerel. The becquerel, since it is a small unit, carries the common prefixes of: giga (G), mega (M) and kilo (k). The relationship between the curie and becquerel is:

1 curie	37×10^9 dps	37 GBq
1 millicurie (mCi)	37×10^6 dps	37 MBq
1 microcurie (μCi)	37×10^3 dps	37 kBq
1 nanocurie (nCi)	37 dps	37 Bq

THE HALF-LIFE

Since unstable nuclides decay exponentially their total life-span cannot be measured. The rate of decay is therefore measured as a half-life. Half-lives of radionuclides are determined by measuring the amount of activity in a sample over a period of time; since radionuclides emit ionizing radiation, the intensity of this can be measured by a radiation detector. The semi-log plot in Fig. 15.3a shows the decay with time for ^{131}I over a 30 day period. The slope shows that the intensity decreases as an exponential and since it is an asymptote the total life-span of a radionuclide cannot be given exactly (see Chapter 1). The stability is thus expressed as a **half-life**, 'the time taken for a given activity to reach half its initial value'. Examples of half-lives for various isotopes used in nuclear medicine are given in Table 15.1.

BIOLOGICAL AND EFFECTIVE HALF-LIFE

The time taken for a substance (chemical, drug, radiopharmaceutical, isotope, etc.) to undergo biological excretion often follows an exponential pattern, so the

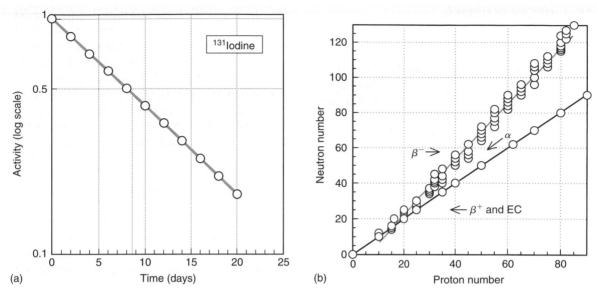

(a)

(b)

Figure 15.3 (**a**) Decay graph plotted on semi-log scale for ^{131}I. Half the initial activity remains at about 8 days. (**b**) Some of the nuclides plotted according to neutron and proton number. The stable nuclides have excess neutron numbers and breakaway from the 1:1 relationship. Beta negative decay gains proton number, beta plus loses protons. Alpha decay loses equal numbers of protons and neutrons.

Table 15.1 Physical half-lives of common clinical nuclides.

Isotope	Half-life	Clinical use
^{191m}Ir	5 s	Vascular imaging
^{81m}Kr	13 s	Lung ventilation
^{82}Rb	1.3 min	Cardiac imaging
^{99m}Tc	6 h	Universal imaging
^{111}In	2.8 d	Imaging sepsis
^{125}I	60 d	In vitro analysis
^{241}Am	500 y	Marker source

biological retention of an isotope or labeled compound is also expressed in terms of its half-life. The overall or **effective half-life** of a substance in a patient's body depends on both its **physical half-life** and its **biological half-life**. The effective rate constant is the sum of rate constants for physical and biological disappearance so that:

$$\text{effective half-life} = \text{physical half-life} + \text{biological half-life}$$

The biological half-life of a substance is difficult to measure; it is commonly derived from the measured effective half-life (excretion rate) and the known physical half-life of the nuclide.

15.1.3 Energy of emissions

There are three basic modes of decay associated with unstable nuclei, these decay processes are:

- Alpha (α)
- Beta (β^- and β^+)
- Gamma (γ)

Each decay process involves the expenditure of energy and in all three cases this is measured in **electron volts** (eV) (see Chapter 2). Since the energy emitted from radioactive materials usually involves energies of thousands or millions of eV the common prefixes are kilo-electron volts (keV) or mega-electron volts (MeV). Alpha emissions are always given in MeV. This is mostly true for β^- and β^+ radiation also, except for very low energies, e.g.

Tritium (^{3}H) 18.6 keV β^-
^{14}C 156.0 keV β^-

Gamma radiation, from radionuclides, used in nuclear medicine, mostly has energies measured in keV.

15.2 DECAY SCHEMES

Figure 15.3b plots a succession of nuclides according to their **neutron:proton ratio**. The straight line indicates equal numbers of neutrons and protons but since the stable nuclei have more neutrons than protons these form a distribution curve above this line. Alpha decay results in a loss of an equal number of neutrons and protons; the nuclear mass therefore decreases down the nuclide curve. Beta negative decay occurs only in 'neutron excess' isotopes so a neutron is lost and the decayed nucleus will take up a position to the right of the line. Beta positive decay and electron capture position the nucleus to the left of the line.

15.2.1 Alpha decay

This mode of decay involves an alpha particle or helium nucleus and causes the greatest loss of energy from an unstable nucleus since it loses four nucleons in the form of two neutrons and two protons. All naturally occurring helium is formed from alpha-particle decay; the alpha particle eventually captures an electron to form an atom of helium gas. The formula for alpha decay is

$$_Z^A X \rightarrow {}_{Z-2}^{A-4}Y + {}_2^4\alpha$$

where X and Y represent the parent and daughter elements respectively. Since the proton number changes so does the element. A particular alpha decay may involve the simultaneous emission of gamma radiation. Common examples of alpha decay are shown by sections of the natural ^{238}U decay series. This is a very complex decay chain involving many different elements. Radium decaying to radon gives a short half-life gas ($T_{1/2} = 3.8$ days) that is a natural radioactive contaminant of buildings:

$$_{88}^{226}\text{Ra} \rightarrow {}_{86}^{222}\text{Rn} + \alpha \ (4.78\,\text{MeV}) + \text{gammas}$$

In this equation the alpha particle energy is shown in brackets, 4.78 MeV. The ^{222}Rn decays further in the lung tissue to ^{218}Po and ^{214}Pb each giving an alpha emission:

$$_{86}^{222}\text{Rn} \rightarrow {}_{84}^{218}\text{Po} + \alpha \ (5.49\,\text{MeV})$$
$$\rightarrow {}_{82}^{214}\text{Pb} + \alpha \ (6.0\,\text{MeV})$$

This decay scheme is part of the ^{238}U decay series, a section of which is shown in Fig. 15.4 starting from ^{226}Ra. Following accepted convention α-particle emission is illustrated in decay schemes by showing arrows sloping to the left. Beta decay from ^{214}Pb is represented by right sloping arrows. Many alpha emitters decay in chains shown in Fig. 15.4: these are called **collateral series**. Table 15.2 shows some natural alpha emitters; their alpha energy decreases as $T_{1/2}$ increases.

CLINICAL VALUE OF ALPHA DECAY

Alpha emitters are rarely met in clinical work. They sometimes form useful therapy sources; e.g. ^{211}At with a half-life of 7 h and an alpha energy of 5.8 MeV has been used for labeling monoclonal antibodies for tumor therapy. The common anatomical marker source for gamma cameras is ^{241}Am, an alpha emitter that also has a useful 60 keV gamma ray emission.

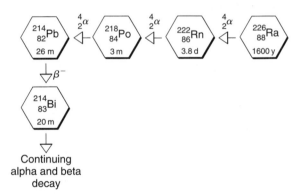

Figure 15.4 *Alpha and beta decay from radium which is part of the natural ^{238}U decay series.*

Table 15.2 *Alpha nuclides from the natural decay chain of uranium.*

Nuclide	Energy (MeV)	Half-life	Remarks
^{222}Rn	5.4	3.8 d	Radon gas from ^{232}Th
^{240}Pu	5.1	6537 y	Nuclear fall-out
^{239}Pu	4.9	2.4×10^4 y	Nuclear material
^{226}Ra	4.8	1600 y	Natural radium
^{235}U	4.6	7×10^6 y	1% Natural uranium
^{238}U	4.2	4.5×10^9 y	99% Natural uranium
^{232}Th	4.0	14×10^9 y	Natural thorium

15.2.2 Beta decay

The unstable nucleus can lose energy by neutron decay, proton decay or electron capture. A beta particle, or high-energy electron is ejected. The beta particle can carry either a negative or a positive charge.

$$n \rightarrow p + e^- \ (\beta^- \text{ decay})$$
$$p \rightarrow n + e^+ \ (\beta^+ \text{ positron decay})$$
$$p + e^- \rightarrow n \ (\text{electron capture, EC})$$

These nuclear transformations are accompanied by an electrically uncharged neutrino or anti-neutrino. This particle was initially postulated to explain the continuous beta spectrum; it plays no part in nuclear medicine imaging or dosimetry.

NEGATIVE BETA PARTICLE EMISSION

(β^-) For those unstable nuclei with excess neutrons a negative β^- particle is produced by neutron decay forming a proton; the nucleon number (atomic mass) does not change:

$$^1_0 n_1 \rightarrow ^1_1 p_0 + e^-$$

The equation for β^- decay is

$$^A_Z X \rightarrow ^A_{Z+1} Y + \beta^- + \bar{\nu} + \text{gammas}$$

An example is

$$^{99}_{42} Mo \rightarrow ^{99m}_{43} Tc + \beta^- + \bar{\nu} + \text{gammas}$$

Since the mass number A does not change the parent and daughter nuclei are **isobars**. The proton number Z increases so the element changes from X to Y. Gamma emission commonly accompanies β^- decay although pure β^- emitters do occur. The decay scheme of a negatron emitter is depicted by an arrow drawn sloping to the right. Figure 15.5a shows two important pure beta emitters commonly employed in nuclear medicine as therapy agents.

During beta decay a further small energy loss is observed in the form of an **anti-neutrino** ($\bar{\nu}$) (a neutral and mass-less emission similar to a photon). The random nature of neutrino ejection (angle of emission) gives a variable small energy loss for each beta decay so β^- particles from the same decay process have a range of energies and are therefore seen as a continuous spectrum. The curve plotted in Fig. 15.5b shows

the beta spectrum for ^{32}P which has a maximum β^- particle energy of 1.7 MeV. The continuous energy distribution of β^- emissions is of importance when calculating the radiation dose delivered to the patient from a β^- emitter.

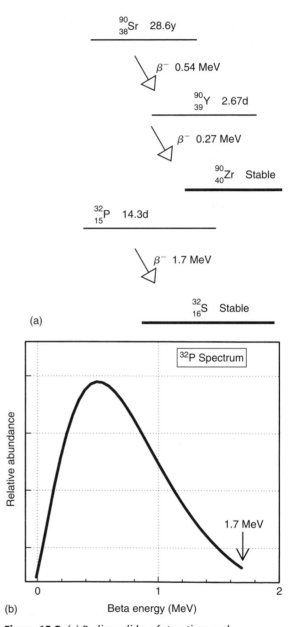

(a)

(b)

Figure 15.5 (**a**) Radionuclides of strontium and phosphorus showing pure β^- decay to a stable isotope. (**b**) Plot of the ^{32}P β^- spectrum showing a spread of energies rather like an X-ray spectrum with a peak or maximum energy point.

CLINICAL VALUE OF β^- DECAY

Very few β^- emitters are used for imaging since the β^- particle contributes a high patient radiation dose. The pure β^- emitters ^{90}Y and ^{32}P are commonly used for therapy. Thyroid investigations sometimes use ^{131}I for imaging as well as therapy since its β^- decay is accompanied by a gamma emission (364 keV); it has also been used for labeling antibodies since iodine chemistry is mild and does not disrupt complex molecules. Lung ventilation is commonly performed using ^{133}Xe, which is a gamma emitter, and the β^- decay similarly increases the patient radiation dose. In spite of their increased patient radiation burden these two isotopes continue to be used since they are cheap and readily available.

POSITIVE BETA PARTICLE (POSITRON, β^+)

A positive beta particle is produced by proton decay in the nucleus:

$$_1^1\mathrm{P}_0 \rightarrow \,_0^1\mathrm{n}_1 + \mathrm{e}^+$$

$$_Z^A\mathrm{X} \rightarrow \,_{Z-1}^A\mathrm{Y} + \beta^+ + \nu$$

$$_9^{18}\mathrm{F} \rightarrow \,_8^{18}\mathrm{O} + \beta^+ + \nu$$

As with negatron (β^-) decay the total number of nucleons remains constant; parent and daughter are **isobars** (Fig. 15.2). The proton Z has decreased by 1, so the element changes and again a continuous β^+ energy spectrum is seen since simultaneous neutrino (ν) emissions are also involved. The positron (a member of the antimatter world) can exist only as long as it has kinetic energy. At rest it undergoes mutual annihilation with any nearby electron. This electron reacts with the β^+ forming a positron/negatron pair; the two masses each having an equivalent rest mass of 0.511 MeV disappear, releasing two gamma photons of this energy. The two γ photons are ejected from the center of the reaction at 180°:

$$\beta^+ + \beta^- \rightarrow \gamma + \gamma \,(0.511\,\mathrm{MeV\ each})$$

This reaction has important applications in **positron emission tomography** (PET), described in Chapter 16. Positron decay for ^{13}N and ^{18}F, used in PET studies, is shown in Fig. 15.6a; β^+ decay adopts a left pointing arrow similar to alpha-decay schemes. Positron annihilation is a practical demonstration of Einstein's equation relating energy and mass: $E = mc^2$ (see Box 15.1).

CLINICAL VALUE OF β^+ DECAY

Positron emission tomographic imaging relies on β^+ decay which produces opposed 0.511 MeV gamma radiation. The physiologically important elements have isotopes that are pure β^+ emitters. The two isotopes ^{13}N and ^{18}F shown in Fig. 15.6a must be produced by an on-site cyclotron because of their short half-lives. The other two nuclides used in PET are:

^{11}C $T_{1/2}$ 20 min β^+ 1.97 MeV
^{15}O $T_{1/2}$ 2 min β^+ 1.74 MeV

15.2.3　Electron capture

In the neutron-poor region, below the line of stability seen in Fig. 15.3b nuclear instability can be satisfied by the capture of an orbital electron; this can be seen as the equivalent of positron emission since it achieves the same end result as a decaying proton:

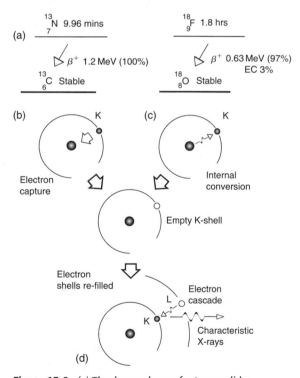

Figure 15.6 (**a**) The decay schemes for two nuclides produced by an on-site clinical cyclotron: ^{13}N and ^{18}F. (**b**) Orbital electron involvement with nuclear decay. The nucleus can either capture a K-shell electron or (**c**) K- and L-shell electrons absorb energy during internal conversion. Both interactions result in electron loss and subsequent filling of electron shells (**d**) producing characteristic X-radiation.

$$\,^{1}_{1}P_{0} + e^{-} \rightarrow \,^{1}_{0}n_{1} + \nu.$$

Figure 15.6b and c illustrates the two important interactions that involve the nucleus and closely bound electrons. Interactions with both K- and L-shell electrons are possible. Figure 15.6b shows the nucleus absorbing a K electron in **electron capture**. An alternative reaction is (c) where the K-shell electron absorbs all the energy during gamma emission resulting in photon loss due to **internal conversion**. Both electron capture and internal conversion result in electron loss from a K or L shell. The resulting vacancy in the K shell is quickly filled by an outer shell electron L; this vacancy in turn is filled by an electron from the M shell and

so on until all the electron vacancies are filled causing an **electron cascade** and the emission of characteristic X-radiation; they are characteristic of the daughter element (d).

Clinical nuclides that undergo electron capture are ^{201}Tl which produces X-rays characteristic of mercury and ^{125}I giving tellurium X-rays. The overall equation for electron capture is similar to β^{+} decay:

$$\,^{A}_{Z}X + e^{-} \rightarrow \,^{A}_{Z-1}Y + \text{characteristic X-rays}$$

For example,

$$\,^{123}_{53}I + e^{-} \rightarrow \,^{123}_{52}Te + \text{characteristic X-rays}$$

Electron capture by the nucleus produces a form of **Bremsstrahlung** radiation owing to the electron orbital disturbance. The resulting X-ray photons are termed **internal Bremsstrahlung** to distinguish them from similar X-ray tube radiation which is **external Bremsstrahlung**; these join the characteristic X-rays to produce a burst of X-ray photons.

CLINICAL IMPORTANCE OF ELECTRON CAPTURE

Common nuclear medicine isotopes that are not produced by a generator (see later) decay by EC. This mode of decay produces low patient radiation dose. Examples are ^{123}I, ^{201}Tl, ^{111}In, and ^{67}Ga. The decay schemes for the first three are shown in Fig. 15.7. Nuclides undergoing electron capture are represented by a left sloping arrow similar to alpha decay. ^{123}I and ^{111}In have useful gamma photons at energies suitable for imaging. The 520 keV of ^{123}I, however, only contributes to image noise. The nuclide ^{67}Ga has three useful gamma energies at 93, 185, and 300 keV. ^{201}Tl has poor gamma abundance but useful Hg X-rays for imaging.

Box 15.1 Positron annihilation

The creation of gamma radiation energy from matter (electron and positron) is given by the basic formula $E = mc^2$ where m is the sum of the rest mass of an electron and the rest mass of a positron, i.e.

$$9.1 \times 10^{-31} + 9.1 \times 10^{-31}\,\text{kg}$$
$$= 1.82 \times 10^{-30}\,\text{kg}$$

and c is the speed of light, i.e. $3 \times 10^{8}\,\text{m s}^{-1}$. Therefore, mc^2 is

$$(1.82 \times 10^{-30}) \times (9 \times 10^{16})\,\text{J}$$

Since $1\,\text{J} = 6.24 \times 10^{12}\,\text{MeV}$ then

$$E = 1.638 \times 10^{-13} \times 6.24 \times 10^{12}$$
$$= 1.022\,\text{MeV}$$

This energy appears as two opposed gamma rays each of **0.511 MeV**.

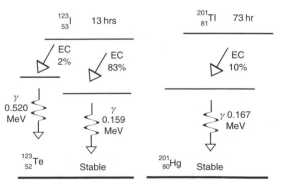

Te K X-rays 0.027–0.032 MeV Hg K X-rays 0.068–0.082 MeV

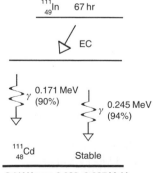

Cd K X-rays 0.023–0.027 MeV

Figure 15.7 *Electron capture in ^{123}I showing a useful gamma photon and ^{201}Tl which has a small (11%) abundance 167 keV gamma, not used for imaging; but the 93% abundant Hg K X-rays are useful. Electron capture in ^{111}In yields two useful gamma energies.*

Table 15.3 *Isomeric transitions giving metastable states.*

Parent	Mode of decay	Useful daughter	Gamma emission energy (keV)	Half-life of metastable nuclide	Decay product
^{99}Mo	β^-, 67 h	^{99m}Tc	140	6 h	^{99}Tc
^{81}Rb	Electron capture, 4.5 h	^{81m}Kr	190	13 s	^{81}Kr
^{195}Hg	Electron capture, 42 h	^{195m}Au	262	30 s	^{195}Au

15.2.4 Gamma radiation

Radionuclides emitting gamma radiation during their decay are potential imaging agents for nuclear medicine providing their gamma energies are between 80 and 200 keV. This is the ideal energy range for gamma cameras since lower energies undergo tissue absorption and higher energies are not absorbed by the thin NaI(Tl) detector used in gamma camera construction. Certain high energy gamma radionuclides (^{131}I; gamma energy 364 keV) are useful for non-imaging tracer studies where their activity levels are measured with thicker single crystal scintillation detectors (probes).

ISOMERIC TRANSITION

In the decay processes previously described for alpha- and beta-emitting nuclides, any gamma radiation that was emitted came from an excited nuclear state. These excited states usually last for extremely short times (pico-seconds) but others can last for relatively long periods (many seconds or even hours) and are called **metastable states**; these can be considered as transition processes. The transition from a metastable state involves the emission of a gamma photon and, since no other decay process (i.e. β^-) is involved, they impart a low radiation dose to the patient. Consequently, these nuclides have become most popular for imaging in nuclear medicine. Three examples of metastable states are listed in Table 15.3, the most widely used being ^{99}Mo/^{99m}Tc; its decay scheme is fully explored in Fig. 15.8 and discussed later.

Isometric transition can be represented by

$$^{A}_{Z}X^* \rightarrow {}^{A}_{Z}X + \gamma$$

where X* denotes an excited state. There is no change in proton or neutron number so X* and X are identical elements or **isomers**. An example is

$$^{99m}_{43}Tc \rightarrow {}^{99}_{43}Tc + \gamma \ (140 \ keV)$$

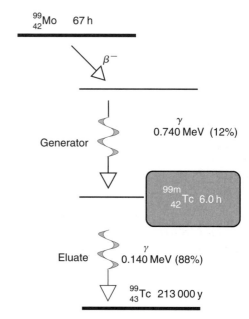

Figure 15.8 *Isomeric transition of molybdenum where ^{99}Mo decays to a metastable state. This then decays to give a pure gamma photon uncontaminated by beta decay.*

INTERNAL CONVERSION

A nucleus in an excited state may also interact with K- or L-shell electrons and transfer excess energy to these electrons. This is the process of internal conversion mentioned together with electron capture and illustrated in Fig. 15.6c where the converted electron is ejected from the atom with an energy minus its binding energy. This is a competing process with gamma ray emission and an **internal conversion coefficient** is used for describing the proportion of internal conversion events in a gamma decay process which blocks gamma emission and is measured as

$$\frac{\text{internal conversion process}}{\text{gamma emission}}$$

Table 15.4 *Summary of the radiation properties of alpha, beta, and gamma radiation.*

Property	Alpha	Beta	Gamma
Type	$[^4He^{2+}]$	High speed electrons	Electromagnetic
Specific ionization	4×10^7 for 5 MeV	6×10^4 for 1 MeV	
Range in air (cm)			
0.5 MeV	0.3	140	Infinite
2.0 MeV	1	840	Infinite
4.0 MeV	2.5	1600	Infinite
Range in tissue (cm)			
1.0 MeV	0.0006	0.42	Infinite
5.0 MeV	0.0037	2.2	Infinite
Range in Al (mg cm^{-2})			
0.5 MeV	0.5	111	Infinite
2.0 MeV	1.6	926	Infinite
Half-value in tissue (cm)			
1.0 MeV	–	0.04	10
5.0 MeV	–	0.4	24

This ratio can range from zero (all transitions result in gamma emission) to infinity (all transitions are internally converted: no gamma emission). The process of internal conversion makes the decay scheme for ^{99m}Tc more complex. It has been measured that 10.4% of all ^{99m}Tc nuclear transformations involve internal conversions by the K, L and, to a lesser extent, M shell electrons. Gamma emissions therefore occur in 89.6% of nuclear transformations and not 100%, which would seem likely from the ^{99m}Tc decay scheme. Similarly, 40% of transformations involve internal conversion in the decay of ^{81m}Kr.

CLINICAL VALUE OF GAMMA DECAY

Gamma radiation within the energies 90 to 200 keV is optimal for gamma camera imaging. Those isotopes that decay by isomeric transition provide a source of activity that is short lived yielding a pure gamma emitter; both points which lead to minimal patient radiation dose. A summary of alpha- and beta-radiation properties is given in Table 15.4, listing their range in various materials. In the case of β^- and gamma radiation a half-value layer is given for tissue; alpha radiation is stopped completely.

AUGER ELECTRONS

Since electron capture and internal conversion create electron vacancies in the inner orbits, an electron cascade starting from the outer electron orbits commences to fill the vacancies (Fig. 15.6d) causing characteristic radiation to be emitted. An alternative process is that instead of this energy being released as characteristic X-rays it can be transferred to another orbital electron ejecting it from the atom. These ejected electrons are Auger electrons and are important in patient dosimetry since they impart damage to surrounding tissue.

15.3 SPECIFIC ACTIVITY

Activity concentration can be used to describe several different terms in nuclear medicine but it commonly refers to the concentration of the nuclide, expressed as either activity by volume or activity by weight. This form of specific activity is measured in:

- becquerels per milliliter
- becquerels per mole
- becquerels per milligram

Since the becquerel is a small unit practical activities are expressed in mega- or giga-becquerels; the non-SI units are curies and millicuries as mCi mg^{-1}. In practice specific activity is commonly used for describing:

- Weight of a given activity
- Impurity concentration
- Residual activity

Descriptions of these and the formulas involved are given by the worked examples in Boxes 15.2 to 15.5.

Box 15.2 Weight of a given activity and toxicity

A patient professes to be iodine sensitive. What is the weight W of iodine in 550 MBq of ^{131}I used as a therapy dose?

Converting all parameters to seconds:

$$T_{\frac{1}{2}} = 8.04 \text{ days} = 6.94 \times 10^5 \text{ s}$$
$$\lambda = 9.985 \times 10^{-7}$$

The number of atoms in 550 MBq is

$$\frac{550 \times 10^6}{9.985 \times 10^{-7}} = 5.5 \times 10^{14}$$

Incorporating Avogadro's number k (see text)

$$W = \frac{131 \times (5.5 \times 10^{14})}{k}$$
$$= 1.2 \times 10^{-7} \text{ g}$$

Or approximately 120 ng, which is far below any toxicity level. Since the daily iodine intake is 150 µg, chemical toxicity and iodine sensitivity are not a problem. Similarly, 70 MBq of ^{201}Tl is equivalent to 9 ng, which is also way below the toxicity level.

15.3.1 Activity and concentration of a substance

It is sometimes necessary to calculate the activity of a known weight of radionuclide for contamination reasons. This is most often used for compounds containing long lived radionuclides (e.g. ^{238}U) but is sometimes required for clinical purposes. The weight of a known activity can also be calculated for toxicity reasons. If the weight W of a given activity A is required then the decay constant λ is $0.693/\lambda$, and if N is the number of radioactive atoms per gram of material then $A = \lambda N$ and A/λ. The **weight of a given activity** is then

$$W = \frac{M \times N}{k}$$

where M is the atomic mass and k is Avogadro's number: 6.0×10^{23}. Box 15.2 uses this formula in an example calculation.

Box 15.3 Activity per unit weight: contamination

Calculating the activity from certain naturally occurring nuclides, e.g. ^{40}K in sea water. The half-life of ^{40}K is 1.25×10^9 years or 3.942×10^{16} s, so $\lambda = 1.758 \times 10^{-17}$. Calculating the activity, A, of 1 g ^{40}K:

$$A = \frac{(6 \times 10^{23}) \times (1.758 \times 10^{-17})}{40}$$
$$= 2.34 \times 10^5 \text{ Bq}$$

The abundance of ^{40}K is 0.012% of the total natural potassium. Concentration of potassium in sea water is 380 mg L^{-1} of which 0.0456 mg is ^{40}K, which has an activity

$$(2.34 \times 10^5) \times (4.56 \times 10^{-5}) = 12 \text{ Bq}$$

The same calculation can be used to estimate the natural activity due to ^{40}K in the human body and the amount of activity introduced by spreading artificial potash fertilizer on agricultural land.

ACTIVITY PER UNIT WEIGHT

The above equation can be rearranged to give

$$A = \frac{k \times W \times \lambda}{M}$$

This formula is useful when considering contamination levels: an example is given in Box 15.3.

15.3.2 Residual activity after decay

SPECIFIC ACTIVITY PER UNIT VOLUME

This is given by the basic formula

$$A_t = A_0 \exp\left(\frac{-0.693T}{T_{\frac{1}{2}}}\right)$$

where A_t is the activity after time T and A_0 is the original activity. An example of its use is given in Box 15.4. Certain radiopharmaceuticals are sensitive to aluminum whose concentration reduces labeling effectiveness or when acidity (low pH) will be a biological hazard (i.e. white cell labeling). In both instances

Box 15.4 Specific activity per unit volume

Consider a solution of ^{131}I that on day 1 has an activity of 4.22 GBq (100 mCi) per 10 mL. On day 13 a 600 MBq (13.5 mCi) aliquot is required, so we need to calculate what volume will contain this activity. The half-life of ^{131}I is 8.05 days, and the amount remaining at day 13 can be calculated from the equation

$$\frac{A_t}{A_0} = e^{-\lambda t}$$
$$= 0.356$$

So 35.6% of the original activity remains in 10 mL (150 MBq mL^{-1}). Hence the required activity of 600 MBq is contained in 4 mL.

Concentration levels

There is 185 MBq mL^{-1} (5 mCi) of ^{111}In chloride on day 1. The half-life is 2.8 days, and 20 MBq is used for labeling in 0.1 mL (i.e. 0.9 mL remaining). What volume will 20 MBq occupy on day 4?

The quantity $\exp(-\lambda T)$ is 37% so on day 4 there is 61 MBq in 0.9 mL. The volume required for 20 MBq would be 0.3 mL.

Note that this larger volume may require extra buffering when labeling white cells, etc. This equation is useful for calculating decayed levels of activity prior to disposal as low-activity waste. An example is given in Box 15.5.

Box 15.5 Residual activity for waste disposal

The permitted activity of ^{125}I for waste discharge is 4.5×10^4 Bq (45 kBq). A sealed bag of contaminated waste measures 185×10^6 Bq (185 MBq). How long must it be stored before safe discharge? $T_{1/2} = 60$ days; $\lambda = 0.0115$. Rearranging the basic formula (see Box 15.4):

$$\ln\frac{A_t}{A_0} = -\lambda t$$

Inserting the above values:

$$\ln\frac{4.5 \times 10^4}{185 \times 10^6} = -0.0115t$$

So,

$$t = \frac{8.3214}{0.01155} \text{ days}$$

Where t is 720 days or approximately 2 years.

high specific activities are essential so that contaminants are present in small concentrations. An example is given in the second half of Box 15.4.

15.4 RADIONUCLIDE PRODUCTION

Three methods are available for producing nuclear medicine radionuclides:

- Bombardment of stable elements with charged beams
- Irradiation of stable elements with neutrons in a nuclear reactor
- Generator production

The first method uses a considerable amount of electrical power so these isotopes are costly. As a nuclear reactor works continuously it is the cheapest method for nuclide production. Both charged beams and nuclear reactors can provide parent isotopes that decay to give short half-life daughters which may be removed or **eluted** from time to time; this forms the basis of the isotope generator. These three methods produce quite different products.

15.4.1 Production rate

The first two procedures mentioned above obey the same basic equation for the rate of isotope production:

$$A = C(1 - e^{-\lambda t})$$

where A is the amount of activity and C is a **saturation constant**, since it is the maximum amount of activity that can be produced for the given conditions; t is the irradiation time and λ the decay coefficient for the nuclide. At a certain time during irradiation a production limit is reached: the number of atoms being produced is balanced by those decaying. This point is the **saturation limit**. For short half-life isotopes the saturation limit is reached quickly (ideal for expensive cyclotron operation), or can take minutes, hours or days for high activity nuclides with long half-lives so production is only practical by using high current cyclotron or reactor production methods.

15.4.2 Cyclotron production

Charged particles (i.e. protons or ions) can be accelerated to sufficiently high energies so that when they collide with target materials nuclear reactions are induced. This is an important method for the commercial production of radionuclides for nuclear medicine. Since charged particles are used in these reactions the nuclides tend to be relatively **neutron deficient** and in order to gain a stable neutron:proton ratio they decay by creating a neutron from a proton by one of two reactions:

- **Positron emission (β⁺)** by proton decay:
  $p \rightarrow n + e^+ + neutrino$
- **Orbital electron capture** by a nuclear proton:
  $p + e^- \rightarrow n + anti\text{-}neutrino$

An electron gun acts as an ion source, similar in design to an X-ray or cathode ray tube. The ions produced are accelerated towards the target by a high voltage. The acceleration of the charged particles takes place in an evacuated chamber by an applied electric field; the design of the field depends on the choice of accelerator. Particle beams are commonly derived from a light gas; hydrogen, deuterium or helium which produce respectively **protons**, **deuterons**, and **alpha particles**. The primary gases are ionized by either an electron beam or a radio-frequency field. Several forms of linear accelerator were developed for the early investigation of nuclear reactions but they required a great deal of space and still remain essentially research tools. Accelerators having circular orbits are more popular: these are called **cyclotrons**. A practical cyclotron was developed at the University of California at Berkeley by Ernest Lawrence and M. Stanley Livingston in 1931.

CYCLOTRON DESIGN

The cyclotron design restricts a beam of accelerated charged particles within a circular orbit contained in a strong magnetic field. Figure 15.9a shows the basic cyclotron design and a plan view of the spiral beam path. The charged particles are generated from an ion source located in the center of the machine. From

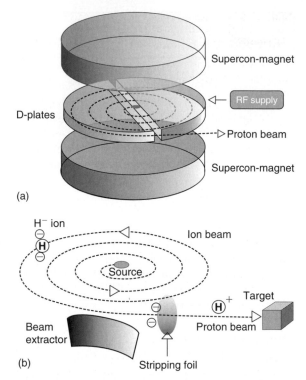

Figure 15.9 (**a**) Basic design of a clinical cyclotron showing superconducting magnets, D-plate electrodes in a vacuum housing and the alternating power supply for accelerating the charged particle beam. (**b**) The spiral path of the negative ions (H⁻) which are deflected then stripped of their electrons to give a proton beam which bombards the target.

here they are accelerated in a circular path by a high frequency field applied across two hollow metal D-plate electrodes placed in a strong perpendicular magnetic field. On each orbit the charged particles receive increments of energy which increase their orbit diameters until they reach the periphery of the D-plates. Here they are deflected from their spiral path by either a change in magnetic field or a momentary charge on a **beam deflector**. They are then steered through a thin, metal, **stripping foil** which removes electrons from the ions leaving a **proton beam** which bombards the target as shown in Fig. 15.9b.

Small cyclotrons are now available for a hospital environment and they can produce quantities of useful isotopes (positron emitters and electron capture isotopes, e.g. ¹⁸F and ¹²³I). They commonly use negative ion acceleration (H⁻) which is eventually stripped of electrons by a stripping foil to provide a proton (H⁺) beam. **Neutrons** can be generated by using a beryllium or lithium target.

Table 15.5 *Specifications of a small cyclotron.*

Parameter	Value
Proton energy	12 MeV
External beam current	100 μA
Ion source	H⁻
Magnet field strength	2.35 T
Beam radius	220 mm
Radio frequency	108 MHz
Concrete shielding	1 m thick

Table 15.6 *Cyclotron nuclide production for (a) small current (p,n) reactions and (b) large current reactions.*

Product	Target	Abundance (%)	Yield GBq (mCi)
^{15}O	^{15}N	0.36	90 (2500)
^{11}C	^{14}N	99	10 (270)
^{13}N	^{13}C	1.1	18 (500)
^{18}F	^{18}O	0.2	3 (66)

Product	Half-life	Target	Reaction
^{201}Tl	73 h	^{203}Tl	(p,3n)
^{67}Ga	78 h	^{68}Zn	(p,2n)
^{111}In	67 h	^{110}Cd	(p,γ)
^{123}I	13 h	^{127}I	*(p,5n)
^{81}Rb	4.5 h	^{82}Kr	(d,3n)

*See text.

CYCLOTRON PERFORMANCE

A compact hospital cyclotron can accelerate protons to 16 MeV and deuterons to 8 MeV energy. The extracted beam currents are between 50 and 100 μA. Typical specifications for a small superconducting cyclotron (Oxford Instruments) are shown in Table 15.5.

Clinical radionuclides that are manufactured by cyclotrons are listed in Table 15.6. Short-lived positron emitting isotopes can be produced using a small low current cyclotron on a hospital site.

The early production of ^{123}I relied on the reaction ^{122}Te(d,n)^{123}I but this was contaminated with long lived ^{124}I, giving radiation dosimetry problems. This reaction has now been superseded in the US by the reaction ^{124}Xe(p,pn)^{123}Xe → ^{123}I. (The ^{123}Xe has a half-life of 2 h and decays to ^{123}I.) In Europe the ^{123}Xe is obtained from the reaction ^{127}I(p,5n)^{123}Xe.

Both reactions yield uncontaminated ^{123}I. Typical production rates for radionuclides at 12 MeV using a low beam current of 50 μA are given in the table. The natural abundance of the stable target material and the half-life of the daughter nuclide are given. A dual particle feature (protons and deuterons) is advantageous since inexpensive target gases can be used. Radionuclides produced by large commercial cyclotrons with larger beam currents use more efficient higher energy reactions; a list is shown in the second part of Table 15.6. These are the commercially available nuclides with longer half-lives. Since parent (carrier element) and daughter are mostly different elements the daughter product can be separated chemically to give a **carrier-free state**.

RADIATION SHIELDING

If acceleration potentials are kept to within 10 to 12 MeV in a small hospital cyclotron then the cyclotron shielding can be easily manufactured to restrict surface dose rates to 25 μSv h⁻¹ (2.5 mR h⁻¹) which simplifies safety requirements.

15.4.3 Reactor production

Neutron bombardment of stable elements in a nuclear reactor produce radionuclides by two different reactions:

- **Neutron capture** where the nucleus accepts an additional neutron. The nucleus then has an excess of neutrons and decays as n → p + e⁻.
- **Fission** where a large nucleus accepts an additional neutron, becomes unstable and splits into two smaller nuclei.

REACTOR DESIGN

The basic design for a nuclear reactor is given in Fig. 15.10. This type of reactor is specifically designed for the production of medical radioisotopes and is smaller than the reactors used for power generation. The neutron field of a typical reactor would be 10^{14} neutrons s⁻¹. Nuclear reactions take place according to neutron energy. The energy bands are:

- Thermal neutrons with energies up to 0.025 eV
- Medium energy neutrons of up to 10 keV
- Fast neutrons up to 100 MeV

The moderator material is usually graphite, which slows the neutrons so that neutron capture reactions can take place.

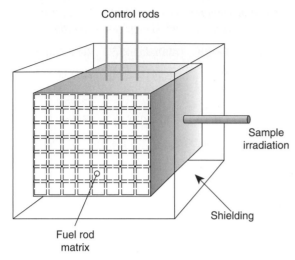

Figure 15.10 *Simplified reactor design for the production of radionuclides. In this design the enriched fuel $^{238/235}U$ is held in graphite blocks which act as the moderator. Cadmium control rods regulate the reaction (not shown) and the whole assembly is shielded with thick ferroconcrete. A sample tube holds the material for irradiation.*

NEUTRON CAPTURE REACTIONS

These involve a neutron/gamma (n,γ) reaction. The neutron is the bombarding particle and the gamma ray is emitted as a consequence. The gamma radiation from this event is called a **prompt gamma**.

Since the products of irradiation have excess neutrons these nuclides usually undergo β^- negative decay, converting a neutron into a proton: $n \rightarrow p + e^-$. Since parent and daughter elements are the same chemically, separation is not possible and reactor products contain small amounts of their stable parent (carrier) elements as impurities so they are not entirely carrier free. Nuclear medicine isotopes produced by neutron capture (n,γ) reaction are listed in Table 15.7.

FISSION REACTIONS

Fast neutron absorption can induce fission in such nuclides as ^{235}U which leads to a mixture of nuclides that can be chemically separated and then purified. Fission-produced radionuclides are carrier-free but small amounts of other radioactive contaminants are sometimes present. The fission reaction for ^{235}U is outlined in Fig. 15.11 and shows some of the products

Table 15.7 *Products from (n,γ) reactions.*

Target	Product	Comments
^{31}P	^{32}P	Therapy isotope
^{32}S	^{32}P	Therapy isotope
^{124}Xe	^{125}Xe	Decays to ^{125}I
^{74}Se	^{75}Se	Imaging
^{59}Co	^{60}Co	External therapy
^{112}Sn	^{113}Sn	Parent for ^{113m}In generator

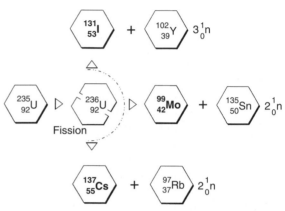

Figure 15.11 *The production of ^{131}I, ^{99}Mo and ^{137}Cs Mo from fission products. The individual elements are separated chemically.*

Table 15.8 *Nuclides from fission reactions.*

Isotope	γ (keV)	Half-life	Fission yield (%)
^{90}Sr	pure β^-	28.6 y	6.0
^{99}Mo	740	66 h	6.0
^{131}I	364	8.0 d	3.0
^{133}Xe	81	5.3 d	6.5
^{137}Cs	662	30 y	6.0

that are formed. Table 15.8 lists important medical nuclides manufactured by the fission process.

Originally, ^{131}I production was produced by a neutron capture reaction:

$$^{130}Te(n,\gamma)^{131}Te \rightarrow {}^{131}I$$

However, a fission process is now used:

$$^{235}U(n,F)^{131}Te \rightarrow {}^{131}I$$

where F indicates 'fission'. The ^{131}Te quickly decays to ^{131}I which now has a much higher purity and specific activity.

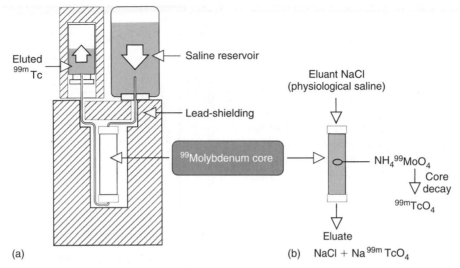

Figure 15.12 (*a*) *The basic components of a* ^{99m}Tc *generator showing the alumina core on which the [*^{99}Mo*]molybdate anion is absorbed. An evacuated vial sucks saline through the system so eluting the soluble [*^{99m}Tc*]pertechnetate. (*b*) Ammonium [*^{99}Mo*]molybdate adsorbed onto the alumina core decays to [*^{99m}Tc*]pertechnetate which undergoes ion exchange with* Cl^- *to form sodium [*^{99m}Tc*]pertechnetate.*

The early $^{98}Mo(n,\gamma)^{99}Mo$ reaction, which yielded ^{99m}Tc-generator grade molybdenum, has also been superseded by the fission reaction:

$$^{235}U(n,F)^{99}Mo$$

The fission sequence shown in Fig. 15.11 yields ^{99}Mo. The ^{99}Mo is 6% of the fission product and, after separation, is much cleaner than the (n,γ) reaction, which was used previously. It has a much higher specific activity; the (n,γ) production gives $400\,GBq\,g^{-1}$ ($10\,Ci\,g^{-1}$) whereas the fission product, after separation, gives $370\,TBq\,g^{-1}$ ($10^4\,Ci\,g^{-1}$). The radioactive gas ^{133}Xe is produced eventually from the second fission path in this reaction which is a clinical radionuclide used for lung ventilation studies.

15.4.4 Generator production

It has already been seen (Fig. 15.8) that radioactive decay can lead to the formation of intermediate or **metastable states**, which decay by **isomeric transition**. The metastable state can exist for periods of time covering seconds (^{81m}Kr and ^{185m}Au) to hours (^{99m}Tc and ^{113m}In). Metastable products form useful imaging nuclides if their gamma energies are in the range 100 to 200 keV and the parent isotope has a

sufficiently long half-life to allow for generator construction and shipment. The production of metastable isotopes by generator systems has been central to the growth of nuclear medicine. New generator systems are constantly under development and will form important future advances in nuclear medicine.

GENERATOR DESIGN

The basic design involves a long-lived parent which is adsorbed onto a column of alumina, silica or ion-exchange resin. As the parent decays the activity of the daughter rises. The carrier-free daughter is then eluted from the generator by passing a solvent over the column; the solvent is often saline (^{81m}Kr uses air). The basic construction of a typical generator system is shown in Fig. 15.12 which represents a $^{99}Mo/^{99m}Tc$ generator and is essentially a heavily shielded core holding the parent isotope ^{99}Mo with a system for eluting the daughter product ^{99m}Tc with saline.

BATEMAN EQUATION

The isomeric **parent:metastable daughter** transition is exploited to produce a radionuclide generator for clinical use. The parent has a longer half-life than the daughter in a clinically useful generator. The basic equation describing the ratio of parent:daughter activity in a generator is given by the Bateman equation, for which a simplified version is

$$A_d = \frac{\lambda_d}{\lambda_d - \lambda_p} \times A_p \times \left[\exp\left(-\lambda_p t\right) - \exp\left(-\lambda_d t\right)\right]$$

where A_d is the daughter activity at time t and λ_d is the decay constant for the daughter; A_p is the initial activity of the parent and λ_p is the decay constant of the parent. This equation can be applied to any parent:metatstable daughter system. Figure 15.13 gives two practical examples: ^{99m}Tc and ^{81m}Kr. The decay constants for these are given in Table 15.9.

TRANSIENT EQUILIBRIUM

When the parent has a longer half-life than the daughter and $\lambda_d > \lambda_p$ then the generator has a transient equilibrium. The example plotted in Fig. 15.13a: the ^{99m}Tc content grows to about half the ^{99}Mo content after 6 h (half-life of ^{99m}Tc). As time progresses the ^{99m}Tc activity is a function of the ^{99}Mo half-life only and at about 23 h in an uneluted generator there is actually more ^{99m}Tc activity than ^{99}Mo. This is shown as a crossover in Fig. 15.13a.

SECULAR EQUILIBRIUM

The second case demonstrates the condition where the half-life of the parent is much longer than that of the daughter: $\lambda_d \gg \lambda_p$. Ultimately, the activities of the parent and daughter are equal. This describes a generator having secular equilibrium. The example in Fig. 15.13b is a ^{91}Rb to ^{91m}Kr generator; the ^{91m}Kr, being a gas, is used for lung ventilation studies.

IMPURITY LEVELS

A certain concentration of chemical impurities is present in generator eluant; the list given in Table 15.10 is for the common ^{99m}Tc generator where a list of impurities and their acceptable levels is given. Significant quantities of aluminum can seriously influence the effectiveness of labeling chemistry so in order to reduce aluminum concentration fresh, high specific activity eluate should be used.

^{99}Mo 'breakthrough' from the core material into the elute also occurs and is calculated in Box 15.6. This should not be greater than 0.1% of the total

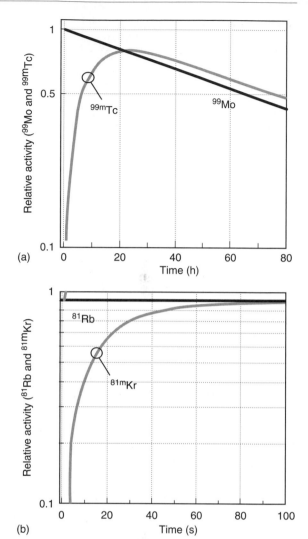

Figure 15.13 (a) Transient equilibrium shown by ^{99m}Tc where the daughter activity depends on the parent activity decay and (b) secular equilibrium demonstrated by the growth and decay of ^{81m}Kr and ^{81}Rb. The daughter activity reaches a maximum a very short time after elution and is virtually constant.

Table 15.9 Decay constants, λ, where λ=0.693/$T_{1/2}$.

Generator	Half-life ($T_{1/2}$)	λ
Technetium		
Parent, ^{99}Mo	67.2 h	0.0103
Daughter, ^{99m}Tc	6.0 h	0.1155
Krypton		
Parent, ^{81}Rb	16 488 s	0.000042
Daughter, ^{81m}Kr	13 s	0.0533

Table 15.10 *Impurity limits for* ^{99}*Mo/*^{99m}*Tc.*

Impurity	Typical level	Limit
pH	5.5	4 to 8
Aluminum	$<1\,\mu g\,mL^{-1}$	$10\,\mu g\,mL^{-1}$
^{131}I	0.0002 nCi	50 nCi
^{103}Ru	0.0001 nCi	50 nCi
^{99}Mo	3.0 nCi	*$1\,\mu Ci\,mCi^{-1}$ of ^{99m}Tc (see Box 15.6)
^{99}Tc	$0.3 \times 10^{-5}\,\mu Ci$	
H_2O_2	As a radiolysis product	

*< 900 Bq ^{99}Mo per 37 MBq ^{99m}Tc $\times$ 25 nCi per mCi.

Box 15.6 Molybdenum breakthrough

Two readings are taken with and without heavy lead shielding around the vial:

1. Shielded (S) 0.28 and background (B) 0.02 MBq
2. The unshielded (U) activity is 10 GBq

The ^{99}Mo activity is $k(S - B)$ where k is a constant specific to the generator (3.5 in this case). The percent ^{99}Mo breakthrough is

$$\frac{k(S - B)}{U} = \frac{0.91 \times 10^6}{10 \times 10^9} = 0.01\%$$

Recognized limits vary between 1 and 0.15 μCi ^{99}Mo per mCi ^{99m}Tc, equivalent to 0.1 and 0.015%.

---

eluate activity which is equivalent to $1\,\mu Ci/mCi$ or $1\,kBq/MBq$. Recent limits put this figure at 0.015%. Molybdenum breakthrough is measured by comparing eluate activity levels with and without 6 mm Pb shielding (shielded vial container).

Only about one millionth of the 140 keV gamma activity penetrates 6 mm of lead (HVL 140 keV is 0.25 mm Pb) so this can be ignored whereas 54% of the 740 keV gamma photon of ^{99}Mo can be counted (HVL 740 keV $\approx$ 8 mm). Box 15.6 gives an example.

NUCLEAR MEDICINE GENERATORS

Several potential generator combinations are listed in Table 15.11 where the half-life of the parent is long enough for shipment and the half-life of the daughter is short enough for low radiation dose imaging. Current commercially produced generators are marked. The gamma energies (except for ^{113m}In) are ideal for imaging. The beta generators would be useful for PET imaging.

15.4.5 Ideal clinical properties

These are listed in Table 15.12. The most common isotope used in nuclear medicine, ^{99m}Tc, satisfies most of the requirements but has a major drawback with its complex chemistry, which can damage sensitive substrates (hippuran, proteins etc.). The nuclide ^{123}I has a simpler labeling chemistry but has serious practical drawbacks of cost, transport, and shelf-life.

Some commonly used clinical radionuclides are listed in Table 15.13. Most of them have suitable gamma or X-photon energies for imaging various organs. The non-imaging nuclides are ^{51}Cr, which is

---

Table 15.11 *Clinically useful generators showing the properties of the parent and daughter nuclides.*

Parent $\rightarrow$ daughter	Production	Half-life of parent	Half-life of daughter	Gamma energy (keV)
^{81}Rb $\rightarrow$ ^{81m}Kr	Cyclotron	4.6 h	13 s	190
^{99}Mo $\rightarrow$ ^{99m}Tc	Reactor	66 h	6.0 h	140
^{113}Sn $\rightarrow$ ^{113m}In	Reactor	115 d	99 min	390
^{62}Zn $\rightarrow$ ^{62}Cu	Cyclotron	9.3 h	9.7 min	511 (β^+)
^{68}Ge $\rightarrow$ ^{68}Ga	Cyclotron	270 d	68 min	511 (β^+)
^{82}Sr $\rightarrow$ ^{82}Rb	Cyclotron	25 d	1.3 min	511 (β^+)
^{178}W $\rightarrow$ ^{178}Ta	Cyclotron	21 d	9.3 min	93
^{191}Os $\rightarrow$ ^{191m}Ir	Reactor	15 d	5 s	130
^{195m}Hg $\rightarrow$ ^{195m}Au	Cyclotron	41 h	30 s	190

Table 15.12 *The ideal medical nuclide.*

Requirement	Comment
Reasonable cost	Reactor made
Pure gamma	Generator or electron capture
Decays to stable state	Stable or long lived
Single gamma energy	Energy 120 to 200 keV
Good shelf life	Half-life of 2 days (or generator)
Short half-life	Generator produced
High specific activity	Generator produced
Easy chemistry	No damage to substrate
Robust labeling	Stable *in vivo*
Single target organ	Free isotope trapped
Rapid excretion	Low biological half-life

Table 15.13 *Clinical radionuclides.*

Nuclide	Half-life	Useful photons (gamma radiation) (keV)
^{18}F	1.83 h	511 (β^+)
^{51}Cr	27.7 d	320
^{67}Ga	78.2 h	93, 185, and 300
^{81m}Kr	13 s	159
^{99}Mo	66 h	740
^{99m}Tc	6.0 h	140
^{111}In	2.8 d	171 and 245
^{123}I	13.2 h	159
^{125}I	59.6 d	27 to 32 (X-rays)
^{131}I	8.0 d	364
^{133}Xe	5.2 d	81
^{201}Tl	73 h	68 to 82 (X-rays)

a red blood cell label for *in vitro* cell mass measurements, ^{125}I which is a radioimmunoassay label, and ^{131}I for therapy. ^{18}F produces 0.511 MeV gamma photons used for positron tomography.

SUMMARY

In isotope production techniques the choice of reaction depends on the nearest stable isotope, highest specific activity, contaminants, and cost.

15.5 LABORATORY INSTRUMENTATION

The emission of radiation from a radioactive source is **isotropic** so a planar (flat) detector surface can only capture a small proportion of the total activity

(see Chapter 2). The geometrical efficiency can be represented as:

$$\frac{\text{detector area}}{\text{area of a sphere}} = \frac{\pi r^2}{4\pi r^2}$$

where r is the detector radius and R the distance from the source. As the detector gets closer to the source the spherical area decreases, so more radiation is captured. Two types of counting geometry can be identified:

- 2π: a flat detector surface
- 4π: the detector surface surrounds the entire source

INVERSE SQUARE LAW

This describes the change in radiation intensity as a square of the distance D (see Chapter 2). As the detector moves away from the source the counts I decrease as

$$I = \frac{1}{D^2}$$

but this only applies to a point source of activity. If the distance is reduced to zero the count rate will not be infinite. A better law for flat detectors is the **cosine law** where the geometrical efficiency is represented as

$$\tfrac{1}{2}(1 - \cos\theta)$$

where θ is half the angle subtended by the detector surface. At zero distance θ becomes 90° and as cosine 90° is 0, the efficiency becomes 50%; a 2π detector will capture 50% of the activity placed on its surface.

15.5.1 Gas detectors

The ionization chamber is a gas filled detector and was described in Chapter 5. An important application is the isotope dose calibrator as used for measuring isotope activities.

DOSE CALIBRATOR

This is represented in Fig. 15.14a which shows the sealed plastic cylinder forming the first electrode and filled with an inert gas, either argon or xenon pressurized to about 10 atm. The high density gas improves radiation absorption efficiency. In the middle of the chamber there is a smaller cylindrical sample holder which forms the other electrode. The plastic material used in its construction is coated with a conductive surface.

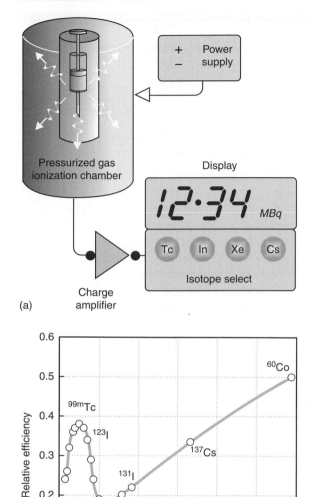

(a)

(b)

Figure 15.14 *(a) Dose calibrator. (b) Sensitivity curve.*

The radioactive sample is placed in this central hollow electrode and the emitted radiation (beta, gamma or X-ray) interacts with the gas atoms causing ionization. Both photoelectric and Compton interactions play a part, producing free ions and electrons. For beta radiation and low energy photons ($<200\,keV$) the photoelectric effect in the gas predominates. Above this energy the Compton process plays a more important role and the scattered electrons have sufficient energy for further secondary ionizations.

A voltage applied between the two electrodes (usually about 300 V) attracts the ions formed by the radiation event, the positive ions to the central negative electrode (cathode) and the free electrons to the positive outer electrode (anode). The current generated by the ionizing events within the chamber is proportional to the activity of the source. The current is very small: 40 MBq of ^{99m}Tc produces 1×10^{-10} A (0.1 nA) so is measured by a very high input impedance electrometer or charge amplifier. The time taken for the dose calibrator to reach 95% of its reading is typically 2 to 3 s and the detector achieves very nearly 4π counting geometry.

The dose calibrator, being an ionization chamber has a very slow response. It cannot separate individual events and distinguish different gamma energies so it can only be used for measuring single isotope activities.

The dose calibrator can measure activities from 4 kBq to 40 GBq (0.1 mCi to 10 Ci); the lower limit depends on the level of low-background activity, so the dose calibrator should be adequately shielded. The chamber sensitivity for different photon energies is plotted in Fig. 15.14b; low energies are efficiently absorbed by the photoelectric effect and the efficiency then decreases until the energies are sufficient to cause multiplication of electrons by the Compton process when the sensitivity is seen to increase. In order to adjust for this changing energy sensitivity the amplifier gain is varied in step with the photon energy; these settings are the calibration values for the detector; the values are pre-set for the most common isotopes. The dose calibrator is ideal for measuring ^{99}Mo breakthrough from the generator column.

15.5.2 Scintillation detectors

Unlike the dose calibrator, mixtures of nuclides can be separately analyzed since each nuclide energy in the mixture can be identified using the pulse height analyzer. There are count rate limitations since the NaI(Tl) detector **saturates** at high count rates owing to its finite decay time of 240 ns; pulses overlap from high activities causing pulse pile-up. The typical upper counting limit is 5000 cps; above this there is count loss and poor accuracy. The lower limit of this counter is decided by the interfering background activity.

Background activity can be reduced by ensuring the counter is placed away from other active sources (other samples and patients).

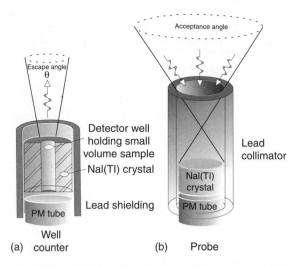

Figure 15.15 *(a) The well counter used for counting small samples. It is heavily shielded from background radiation with a lead castle. (b) A basic scintillation probe for organ uptake investigations. The crystal is typically 5 to 8 cm thick. The collimator is specifically designed to cover the appropriate organ area.*

WELL COUNTER

This is essentially a scintillation crystal with a hole or 'well' drilled to accept a sample tube. Figure 15.15a shows the basic design of a laboratory well counter commonly used for counting radioactive tracer samples having very low activity. Positioning the sample within the crystal achieves a high counting efficiency and 95% of photons emitted by a small (1 cm³) sample can be captured achieving nearly 4π geometry.

Good counting geometry and high sensitivity of NaI(Tl) allow activities of a few hundred becquerels (nano-curies) to be measured, depending on background activity, and surrounded by a lead-brick castle (5 cm thick) built up so the castle rim is about 1 to 2 cm above the well counter itself. The lead should be from an old stock since naturally occurring ^{210}Pb ($T_{\frac{1}{2}}$ 22 y) occurs in recently mined metal contributing to gamma background activity. For this reason lead-based paint should not be used in very low background environments.

EFFECT OF SAMPLE VOLUME

Counting geometry alters significantly with changing sample volumes for both dose calibrator and well counter. The escape angle becomes broader with larger volumes, and therefore the counter is less efficient.

Table 15.14 *Calibration isotopes for laboratory counters.*

Isotope	Half-life	Principal gamma energies (MeV)
^{129}I	1.57×10^7 y	0.03
^{241}Am	500 y	0.060
^{57}Co	271 d	0.122
^{133}Ba	11 y	0.356, 0.276, and 0.081
^{137}Cs	30 y	0.662
^{60}Co	5.3	1.173 and 1.332

Identical small volumes should consequently always be used.

Theoretically, any mixture of nuclides can be counted using a well counter but in practice this is restricted to four since good separation is required between gamma energies to minimize cross-talk between photopeaks and scatter.

Calibration of the well counter and other laboratory instruments is essential if accurate measurements are to be taken. A series of various gamma emitting calibrated sources are available for this purpose: a list is given in Table 15.14.

ORGAN UPTAKE PROBES

Single large scintillation detectors, from 5 to 8 cm diameter (3″ to 5″), are commonly used for measuring organ uptakes of various radionuclides. The most common detector probe is the thyroid uptake probe, used for measuring the concentration of radioiodine (either ^{131}I or ^{125}I) in the thyroid gland. The basic design is shown in Fig. 15.15b. It carries a specially shaped collimator which covers the area of the thyroid excluding other activities. It also serves as a sensitive personnel contamination monitor for measuring accidental iodine ingestion in laboratory workers. The overall efficiency for the NaI(Tl) detector depends on the crystal thickness; 5×5 and 8×8 cm NaI(Tl) crystal detectors are commonly available commercial sizes.

Several large probe assemblies can be used for low activity whole-body counting when placed in a specially shielded low background environment. Very small tracer activities of ^{40}K, ^{59}Fe, ^{57}Co etc. can be measured with this **whole-body counter**.

15.5.3 Dose rate constant (specific gamma ray constant)

The specific gamma ray constant, Γ, gives the dose rate in mSv h^{-1} from a gamma source at 1 m from a point

Table 15.15 *Specific gamma ray constants* *(mSv h^{-1} GBq^{-1} at m^{-1}).*

Nuclide	Gamma energy (keV)	Dose rate
^{241}Am	60	0.004
^{201}Tl	68 to 82 (X-ray)	0.012
^{57}Co	122	0.016
^{99m}Tc	140	0.017
^{99}Mo	740	0.041
^{131}I	364	0.057
^{111}In	171 and 245	0.084
^{137}Cs	662	0.087
^{60}Co	1.173 and 1.333	0.360

Box 15.7 Specific gamma ray constant

From Table 15.15 the constant for ^{99m}Tc is $17\,\mu\mathrm{Sv\,h^{-1}\,GBq^{-1}}$ at 1 m ($d = 100$ cm). What is the dose D for an activity A of 500 MBq at a new distance d_n of 30 cm?

$$D = \frac{G \times A \times d^2}{d_n^2}$$

or

$$94\,\mu\mathrm{Sv\,h^{-1}} \text{ at } 30\,\mathrm{cm}$$

emission. The **dose rate constant** replaces the specific gamma ray constant, Γ, according to ICRU33, although the two terms are not identical. For radiation therapy the dose rate constant G_d of a radionuclide emitting photons is the quotient $K_d \times r^2$ and the activity A. The symbol K_d is the air kerma rate which would be produced by all the photons of energy $E = d$ at a distance r from a spot radiation source of activity A, if the radiation were neither absorbed nor scattered at the source or in any other matter:

$$G_d = K_d \times \frac{r^2}{A}$$

The SI unit is $\mathrm{Gy\,m^2\,s^{-1}\,Bq^{-1}}$. The selection of the lower energy limit d, expressed in kV, depends on the application. The dose rate constant G_H is defined for radiation protection, where H_x is used in place of the air kerma rate K_d. The energy threshold is 20 keV for all nuclides: $G_H = H_x \times r^2/A$. The SI unit is Sv (or mSv) h^{-1} GBq^{-1} at 1 m. The dose rate constant for common nuclear medicine radionuclides is given in Table 15.15.

The calculation in Box 15.7 would be used for calibrating a gamma radiation monitor in terms of dose rate from a particular nuclide commonly used in the laboratory or clinic. The equation in Box 15.7 calculates the reading for different source distances.

CONTAMINATION MONITORING

Portable contamination monitors are an important accessory in the nuclear medicine department for detecting and localizing radioactive spills and contaminated areas.

The sensitivity of three typical contamination monitors is given in Table 15.16. It can be seen that

Table 15.16 *Specification and sensitivity of large area contamination monitors.*

Detector	^{125}I	^{57}Co/^{99m}Tc
100 cm^3 argon Al window (3 mg cm^{-2})	1.0	3.0
100 cm^3 xenon Ti window (5 mg cm^{-2})	3.5	5.4
100 cm^3 NaI(Tl) Al window (0.9 mg cm^{-2})	50	16

a large area scintillation detector has the greatest sensitivity.

In summary, monitoring equipment is used for measuring **absolute activities** of radioisotopes (in GBq, MBq, kBq or curies, millicuries, and microcuries) prior to radiopharmaceutical preparation or patient injection (a 4π **dose calibrator**). The slow response of the counter integrates the ionization events, giving an ion current measured by an electrometer. It cannot distinguish separate gamma energies so only single isotope activities can be measured.

Small activity samples use a well counter in the form of a small volume 4π scintillation detector. The fast response of the counter allows individual gamma events to be recorded; pulse height discrimination can be used to isolate multi-isotope samples.

Either a Geiger counter or scintillation detector or large field gas proportional counter can be used for identifying **contaminated areas** depending on isotope type and concentration. Alpha, beta, and gamma radiation can be monitored depending on design.

Organ uptake requires a suitably collimated scintillation detector. Examples are thyroid and kidney

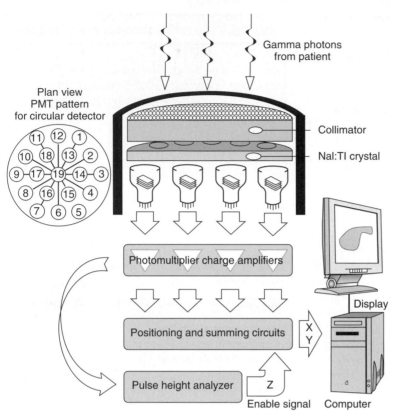

Plan view
PMT pattern
for circular detector

Collimator

NaI:Tl crystal

Photomultiplier charge amplifiers

Positioning and summing circuits

Pulse height analyzer

X
Y

Z

Enable signal   Computer

Display

Figure 15.16 *Basic gamma camera design. The collimator accepts orthogonal radiation from the patient which is detected by the positional sensitive detector. X and Y spatial information is computed by the positional and summing circuits. If the detected event is within the photopeak window a Z pulse enables the positional information which is then stored in an image matrix by the computer/array processor. The array pattern of the photomultiplier tubes on the surface of the crystal is shown top left.*

probes. Multiple large sized detectors, in a properly shielded environment, can measure whole-body uptakes of tracer isotopes.

For all these detectors shape, volume, and position of samples are critical parameters when comparing activities between different sources of radioactivity; this also applies to imaging systems as well as laboratory counting instrumentation.

15.6 THE GAMMA CAMERA

The basic design of a modern gamma camera shown in Fig. 15.16 identifies the major components and shows the detector crystal backed by an array of photomultiplier tubes which feed separate charge amplifiers. A collimator is fixed to the front of this assembly. The basic gamma camera was first constructed by H.O. Anger (US physicist/engineer) in 1956.

15.6.1 The scintillation crystal detector

A large NaI(Tl) scintillation crystal 300 to 500 mm (12 to 20 inches) in diameter and either 6 or 10 mm

Table 15.17 *Percent absorption for two gamma energies.*

Crystal thickness (inches)	Gamma energy	
	140 keV	500 keV
¼	75	8
⅜	84	12
½	90	18

(¼″ or ⅜″) thick forms the gamma camera detector. Radiation absorption for various energies (detector efficiency) versus crystal detector thickness is shown in Table 15.17. Thinner crystals give better spatial resolution at the cost of reduced absorption efficiency.

As the scintillator crystal is hygroscopic it is hermetically sealed using thin aluminum at the front and sides, and glass or transparent plastic at the rear; this transparent window acts as a light guide. Gamma radiation, absorbed by the sodium iodide scintillator, is converted to ultraviolet light events (see Chapter 5) the photons of which are then detected by a set of closely matched photomultiplier tubes (PM tubes) attached to the light guide.

15.6.2 Camera electronics

The PM tubes are arranged in 37, 61, 75 or 91 hexagonal arrays depending on the gamma camera model. A simple hexagonal PMT pattern is shown in Fig. 15.16 for a circular detector. Rectangular detectors typically have 55 or 59 detectors.

POSITIONAL OR SUMMATION CIRCUITRY

This receives the signals from all the PM tubes and is usually situated with the amplifiers in the camera head itself. Each photomultiplier signal contributes to the computation of the positional signal. The summation circuitry accepts signals from the PM amplifiers and computes the spatial coordinates (x and y) of the gamma event in the scintillator. The positional x,y signals can be further processed to correct for imperfections in both the crystal and photomultiplier interface and also the summing network itself.

SPATIAL INFORMATION

The light emitted by the gamma event in the detector crystal is dispersed throughout the large scintillator and is seen by all the photomultipliers. The diagram in Fig. 15.17a shows a simplified one-dimensional example where five PM tubes detect the light event with varying degrees of intensity. These signals undergo logarithmic amplification illustrated in Fig. 15.17b so that:

- Smaller photomultiplier signals, which carry very little positional information, are eliminated.
- Large signals are reduced so that the position of the light event on the photomultiplier face itself has only a small effect on PM signal amplitude.

The logarithmic response can be achieved using either analog or digital circuitry; the latter is now favored since digital processing can be specifically tailored to suit the camera.

PULSE HEIGHT ANALYSIS (ENERGY DISCRIMINATION)

This circuit accepts signals from all the PM tubes and measures the maximum signal height seen. If this is

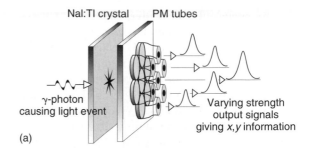

(a)

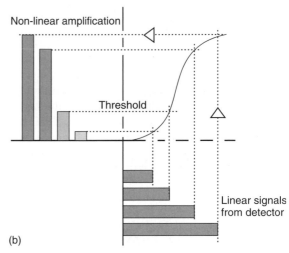

(b)

Figure 15.17 (*a*) A group of five photomultiplier tubes responding to a single light event. Their signal amplitudes and those of their surrounding neighbors determine the event position on the crystal surface. (*b*) Nonlinear amplification of these signals removes low amplitude signals that do not exceed a certain threshold. These do not carry important spatial information.

within the photopeak energy window, then a Z or energy signal is generated that enables (opens) the x,y signals and gates them to the image display computer shown in Fig. 15.16.

All the photomultipliers take part in the energy analysis. Efficient energy discrimination is essential for removing scatter events and maintaining optimum image quality.

DISPLAY

The final x and y signals, generated by the positional circuitry, are accepted by either an analog film formatter or digitized (analog-to-digital converter) to take part in a computer display system.

The analog film formatter, since it is a simple *x,y* recorder uses a cathode ray tube that has an extremely fine dot dimension. The light from this dot is recorded on the film directly to produce an image. On inspection the fine dots can be distinguished, each one represents a single gamma photon within the chosen energy window. A good quality image requires at least 1 million of these dots, equivalent to 1 million accepted gamma events.

SUMMARY

The gamma camera is an imaging device for nuclear medicine it consists of:

- A collimator accepting orthogonal gamma events from the patient. A large NaI(Tl) crystal is the scintillation detector and is usually ¼" or ⅜" thick.
- Photomultiplier tubes form a hexagonal (circular detector) or rectangular array on its surface.

- The signals from these go to charge amplifiers.
- The signals are logarithmically amplified and accepted by the positional circuitry which computes *x* and *y* axes of the gamma event.
- The pulse height analyzer enables this signal if the *x,y* signal is a photopeak event.
- The *x,y* signal forms the display.

15.7 CAMERA PERFORMANCE

The three graphs in Fig. 15.18a, b, and c compare camera spatial resolution and absorption efficiency for 6 and 10 mm (¼", ⅜") crystals with gamma photon energy. Combining (a) and (b) yields an overall performance curve (c) which peaks between 140 and 200 keV, confirming this as the optimum energy for gamma cameras.

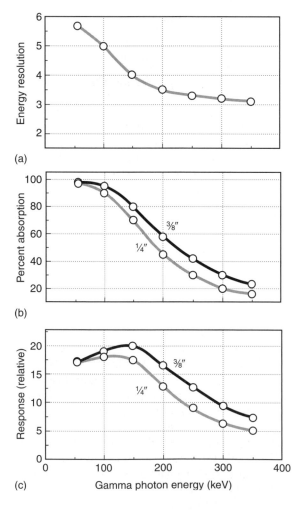

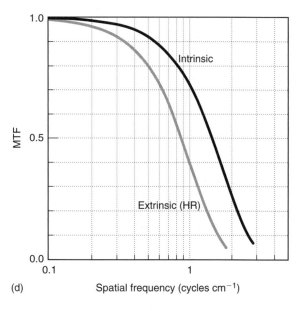

Figure 15.18 *Three graphs showing gamma camera performance versus photon energy for (**a**) camera resolution (FWHM), (**b**) photon absorption for two crystal thicknesses (1 cm or 0.6 cm; (⅜" or ¼", respectively)). (**c**) Graph combines the data revealing optimum efficiency for resolution and absorption in the energy range 100 to 200 keV. (**d**) The MTF for both intrinsic and extrinsic resolution taken with a high resolution collimator.*

15.7.1 Intrinsic resolution

The resolving power of the gamma camera system without any collimation is obtained by exposing the uncovered crystal to a point or line source of activity. In practice the crystal is covered by a lead sheet in which fine points or a thin single line have been cut.

A specially engineered source is then placed on these and a profile obtained. A modulation transfer function (MTF) is then obtained from the point spread or line spread function which gives the camera **intrinsic resolution**. An example is shown in Fig. 15.18d where the 10% MTF value is approximately 2.5 Lp cm^{-1} representing a FWHM value of 4 mm. The extrinsic MTF represents the system resolution which includes a high resolution collimator (HR).

The computer display also introduces distortions due to digitization errors placing random events into a fixed image matrix. Since nuclear medicine images are low resolution, when compared to other radiographic images, this is not a serious problem and fairly coarse matrices are acceptable, i.e. 64 × 64, 128 × 128 or 256 × 256, depending on detail required; larger matrices are not necessary except perhaps for large area whole-body imaging.

15.7.2 Energy resolution

This is measured as the full-width of the photopeak at half-maximum height (FWHM) and is about 10% for most current cameras (140 keV gamma). This setting directly affects spatial resolution of the camera since the accuracy of positional computation improves with decreasing photopeak width. In order to cover the majority area of the photopeak the energy window setting is typically 15%. Energy resolution is perhaps the most valuable fundamental measure of overall gamma camera performance.

Figure 15.19a represents a gamma camera photopeak displayed using the multichannel analyzer. From the channel measurements made from this spectrum the energy resolution can be calculated as:

$$\frac{\text{FWHM channel width}}{\text{keV per channel} \times 140}$$

The calculation requires a calibration 'keV per channel' which is derived from the number of analyzer channels representing 140 keV, which is 70 in this example giving 0.5 channel per keV. The photopeak

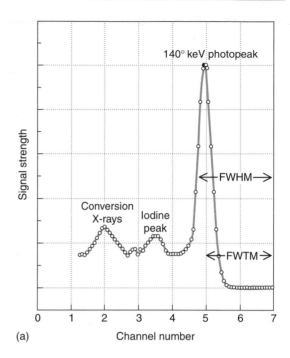

(a)

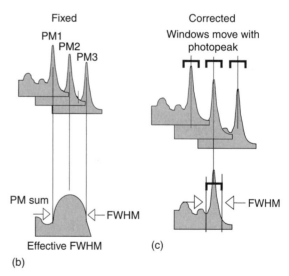

(b)　　(c)

Figure 15.19 (a) The spectrum for ^{99m}Tc collected over 100 channels. The 140 keV photopeak is centered over channel 70 and the FWHM is nine channels wide. The smaller peaks represent the conversion X-ray at 18 keV caused by the characteristic X-rays of Tc due to the internal conversion process. The iodine escape peak at 110 keV marks the escape of the K fluorescent X-ray of iodine (NaI detector). (b) Correction for energy window drift. A fixed window leads to loss of energy resolution. (c) A moving window follows the energy peak drift and overcomes this problem.

half-height width is 9 channels so the energy resolution (FWHM) is 12.8%. Since this percentage figure decreases as the photopeak energy increases both percentage and energy values should be stated when quoting FWHM. The full-width-at-tenth-maximum (FWTM) is also shown on the energy spectrum; this is a measure of scatter acceptance, commonly caused by collimator septa penetration and becomes very broad if higher gamma energies are experienced.

UNIFORMITY CORRECTION

Variations in sensitivity across the crystal face are mainly caused by the variation in the energy window placed over each PMT photopeak. This is due to small variations in photomultiplier gain together with drift. Variations in optical collection efficiency over the camera face can also contribute. If these variations are not corrected then:

- The energy resolution of the camera system will be the sum of the misaligned energy windows of all the PM tubes represented in Fig. 15.19b and will be subjected to continuous drift.
- Camera sensitivity will consequently vary over the camera face due to the energy window shifting from the photopeaks.
- Contrast and resolution performance will likewise vary.

Correction procedures have been introduced into recent camera designs (Siemens ZLC and GE Autotune); a simplified correction process is shown in Fig. 15.19c. Since the photopeak variations are quite slow the camera computer system can continuously alter individual PM performance during data collection. The varying position of the photopeak window is corrected by either moving the window or adjusting the PM supply voltage to shift the peak to the optimum position. This energy correction procedure can be used for a wide range of gamma energies. The correction process for detector/PM optical imperfections usually takes the form of a 64 × 64 matrix of correction values representing crystal areas seen by each PM tube.

15.7.3 Dead time

Owing to the detection dead time (see Chapter 5) the measured count rates from a gamma camera fall short of expected count rate. Gamma camera count rate is

therefore expressed as a figure representing a 10%, 20% or 30% count loss. The common value is taken at 20%. The count rate capability is limited by the decay time of the scintillator, about 240 ns for NaI(Tl), its charge amplifier and associated converter electronics. Figure 15.20 shows a typical gamma camera response to increasing count rate. The shape of the curve depends on the width of the energy spectrum and the scatter present; both of these factors should be minimized. If N_i is the incident number of gamma photons and N_a is the photon counts recorded then the dead time τ is given as

$$\tau = \frac{\ln \frac{N_i}{N_a}}{N_a}$$

The dead time calculated from this equation for a 20% loss at 200 000 cps in Fig. 15.20 gives a value of just over 1 μs. There are two types of detector dead time: **paralysable**, where further photon events serve to increase the total dead time and **non-paralysable** where further events are ignored, the detector operating again after a set time. Most gamma cameras behave as paralysable detectors over the clinical count range.

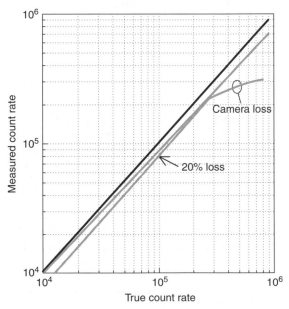

Figure 15.20 *System count losses plotting incident versus recorded count rate. The drop in recorded count rate is commonly measured at the 20% line. This camera has a maximum count rate of 200 000 for a 20% loss.*

FAST COUNT MODES

High activities of short lived isotopes and high bolus-activity heart studies require high count rate capabilities. Each gamma ray interaction with the scintillator requires about 1 ms for complete light collection. Since non-useful scattered radiation is similarly analyzed along with the photopeak events the total dead time for the camera is longer. Faster count rates can be handled if the positional computation uses only the first part of the light signal, but accepting only a fraction of the light output; the drawback is a small loss in resolution. So pulse shortening can increase count rate capability but with a corresponding reduction in intrinsic resolution.

15.7.4 Field of view

The **useful field of view** (UFOV) is defined as the practical or collimated area available for imaging. The uniformity and general response of a gamma camera deteriorates toward the edge of the crystal however and this can be seen as a bright periphery. The **central field of view** (CFOV) represents the central 75% of the camera field of view which commonly holds image clinical detail. Figures for resolution and uniformity are commonly quoted for both these areas; Table 15.18 lists typical values for two camera types along with spatial and energy resolution.

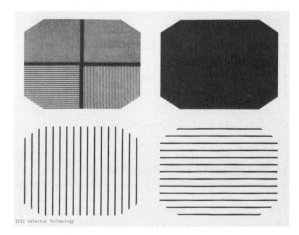

Figure 15.21 *A rectangular field of view camera showing a flood field uniformity picture and a multiple line source showing position linearity in both x and y directions.*

15.7.5 Field uniformity

The uniformity of camera sensitivity for both UFOV and CFOV is measured by placing a point source of activity at a distance at least ×5 the crystal diameter (2 m). This provides a photon flux with <1% variation. Any irregularities in the image obtained are caused mainly by variations in spatial linearity and energy response. The flood image should contain 10 million counts for planar work and 30 million for tomography; a uniformity image is shown in Fig. 15.21 together with a spatial linearity multiple line source. Camera non-uniformity of response for both UFOV and CFOV can be described as either **integral** or **differential**.

INTEGRAL NON-UNIFORMITY

This can be measured as the percentage difference between the maximum and minimum pixel counts in a sampling area (UFOV or CFOV). Table 15.19 gives

Table 15.18 *Intrinsic camera specifications.*

Parameter	CFOV (0.75 × UFOV)	UFOV
Spatial resolution		
FWHM	3.9 mm	4.1 mm
FWTM	7.6 mm	7.8 mm
Energy resolution		10.6%
Field uniformity		
Integral	±2.5%	±4.5%
Differential	±2.0%	±3.0%

CFOV, central field of view. UFOV, useful field of view.

Table 15.19 *Calculation of detector uniformity.*

Uniformity	Relevant equation
Integral non-uniformity	$U_i(+) = \dfrac{(C_{max} - C_x)}{C_x} \times 100\%$ $U_i(-) = \dfrac{(C_{min} - C_x)}{C_x} \times 100\%$
Integral non-uniformity (NEMA)	$\dfrac{C_{max} - C_{min}}{C_{max} + C_{min}}$
Differential non-uniformity	$\dfrac{\text{high pixel} - \text{low pixel}}{\text{high pixel} \div \text{low pixel}}$

NEMA, US National Electrical Manufacturers Association.

details of the formulas used in calculating integral and differential uniformities, where $U_i(+)$ and $U_i(-)$ are the measured extreme values for non-uniformity. C_{max} and C_{min} are the maximum and minimum pixel counts and C_x is the mean pixel count within the sampled area of an image matrix. The NEMA (1980) definition for integral non-uniformity (Table 15.19) gives the same result.

DIFFERENTIAL NON-UNIFORMITY

The percentage maximum difference between two adjacent pixels in an image matrix is the differential non-uniformity and is defined by NEMA as the high and low values obtained from image matrix pixel values measured over a range of five pixels in all rows and columns.

The uniformity quality control programs necessary for measuring integral and differential uniformities are commonly included in the gamma camera software along with error limits.

15.7.6 Spatial resolution

The intrinsic resolution described earlier is the best resolution that the camera is capable of giving without considering the degradation offered by collimation (extrinsic or system resolution). The total amount of light emitted by the crystal is proportional to the energy of the gamma ray and this influences the intrinsic resolution figure which increases with gamma energy, but since absorption decreases an optimum energy for gamma cameras is reached which is seen to be between 100 and 150 keV (Fig. 15.18). For high count rate acceptance **pulse shortening** or reduction in pulse density would reduce intrinsic resolution.

In summary, the two resolution measurements describing gamma camera performance: **energy resolution** and **spatial resolution** should not be confused. Energy resolution measures the ability of the detector system (crystal plus PM tube electronics) to resolve the small variation in photon signal events (pulse height discrimination) and is measured as the width of the photopeak spectrum at half its height (FWHM): this is a **percentage** figure. Spatial resolution describes the 2-D positional accuracy of the camera detector which is measured with a point of line source of activity placed directly on the crystal surface (intrinsic resolution) or collimator face (extrinsic resolution).

Table 15.20 *Typical performance specifications for current gamma cameras.*

Component or parameter	Specification
Detector size (rectangular)	60 × 45 cm
Useful field of view	53 × 38 cm
Photomultiplier tubes	59, each of 3″ diameter
Count rate	200 000 at 20% loss
Intrinsic resolution	
75 000 cps	5 mm
150 000 cps	5.7 mm

The point spread or line spread function also yields a FWHM measurement but this time it represents **distance** in millimeters.

SPATIAL DISTORTION

This is due to misregistration of an image event on the display so that its true position on the crystal is distorted. This is commonly due to unmatched PM tubes or variation over the face of the PM tube itself.

The overall effect produces positional deviations at regular positions on the crystal face. The visibility of the PM tube locations on a flood field picture is partly caused by this. A measure of spatial linearity as a deviation from a line source is typically 0.35 mm CFOV and 0.7 mm UFOV.

Typical performance specifications for current gamma cameras are shown in Table 15.20.

PERFORMANCE FACTORS

A number of factors have improved overall system performance:

- Increased number of photomultipliers (from 19, 37, 75, 91)
- Thinner crystals (1/4″ or 3/8″)
- Uniformity correction by continuous energy window adjustment
- Large field of view (from 10″ to 30″)

15.8 COLLIMATOR PROPERTIES

The collimator is a lead honeycomb plate containing a large number of holes (Fig. 15.22a). The plate can be constructed from either solid lead cast in a honeycomb pattern or made from lead sheet bent to form a honeycomb or cell-like system, illustrated in Fig. 15.22b.

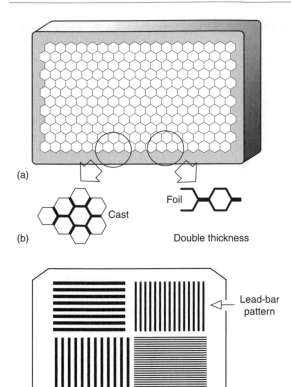

(a)

Foil

Cast

(b)

Double thickness

Lead-bar
pattern

(c)

Figure 15.22 *(a) A typical cast collimator design for a gamma camera showing honeycomb pattern for the holes. (b) A thumb-nail sketch shows the difference between cast and foil designs, the latter has non-uniform septa thicknesses (arrows). (c) Bar-phantom used for estimating the resolution of a camera/collimator system. Bar dimensions are typically 0.25, 0.19, 0.13 and 0.08 inches.*

The important directional properties of the collimator are responsible for rejecting oblique radiation and only accepting radiation orthogonal to the detector face. Without a collimator the camera would not be able to register spatial information since oblique radiation would saturate the detector. The collimator serves the same basic purpose as the antiscatter grid described in Chapter 8 although the radionuclide source is isotropic and not uni-directional like an X-ray source.

Common collimator designs use parallel hole patterns but degrees of image magnification or minification can be obtained from non-orthogonal collimators with angled holes. The hole dimensions and lead content decide the efficiency and resolving power of the collimator. With a collimator in place only a small photon fraction reaches the detector face (1 in 10 000 gamma events from the source). Collimator sensitivity

varies inversely with resolution so collimator design is always a compromise between these two factors.

15.8.1 Extrinsic resolution

This is a measure of the camera system resolution with the collimator in place, frequently referred to as the system resolution. Again a subjective measurement can be made with a bar phantom (an Anger or pie phantom used with the collimator would create Moiré or interference patterns with the collimator holes). Figure 15.22c shows a typical bar phantom with bar dimensions.

Resolution can be more precisely measured with a line source placed on the collimator face and a modulation transfer function derived (see Fig. 15.18d). The bar phantom or line source can be placed either on the collimator surface or at a distance with scattering medium (water or plastic) interposed to gain information about resolution with depth. From the original work by Anger an index of collimator resolution is given by

$$R = \frac{a + b + c}{a} \times d$$

where a is the collimator length or thickness, b is the distance from source to collimator, c is the distance from the collimator to the interaction within the crystal and d is the hole diameter. For the same camera and parallel LE collimator design both c and d can be ignored and the formula simplified to $R = (a + b)/a$. Some useful practical information can now be derived.

RESOLUTION CHANGE WITH COLLIMATOR LENGTH

If the distance from the collimator to the source (b) is constant then for collimator length $a = 2, 4,$ and 6 cm the resolution improves as 1.5, 1.25, and 1.16. Notice that the change from 2 to 4 cm improves the resolution by 16% but from 4 to 6 cm only a 7% improvement is obtained for the same hole density.

RESOLUTION CHANGE WITH DEPTH OF ORGAN

For a 2 cm collimator length (high sensitivity design) with the source 8 cm from the collimator face (b) then $R = 5$. If the source is now 12 cm from the face then $R = 7$; a 40% decrease in resolution. For a 6 cm

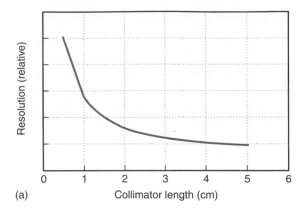

(a)

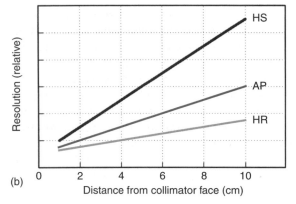

(b)

Figure 15.23 *The effect on system resolution by altering collimator depth **a** for the same value **b** (top graph) and using high sensitivity, an all purpose and a high resolution collimator to visualize an organ at various depths (varying **b**).*

collimator length (high resolution design) the resolution decrease is smaller, 28%. The camera should always be positioned as close as possible to the patient and a high resolution collimator used for imaging deep organs. Collimator properties are further demonstrated by the graphs in Fig. 15.23 showing that resolution is significantly affected by length of collimator or distance of source from the collimator face (value **b** in equations).

OVERALL RESOLUTION

An expression for system total resolution r_t combines intrinsic r_i and collimator r_c resolution so that

$$r_t = \sqrt{r_i^2 + r_c^2}$$

Crystal thickness alters r_i to some extent but these changes to intrinsic resolution have less effect than

changes in extrinsic resolution due to collimator design and position relative to the source. For instance an intrinsic resolution change from 4 to 5 mm will only have a small effect on the image resolution with a collimator resolution of 8 mm (r_t in the equation increases from 8.9 mm compared to 9.4 mm). If a scattering medium (the patient) is placed between the source and the collimator face the effect of small changes to intrinsic resolution would not be visible. When scatter is considered a third factor representing scatter resolution r_s should be added to the equation.

15.8.2 Collimator types

Collimator design optimizes sensitivity and resolution which are inversely related. **High sensitivity** collimators are used for high count rate studies when organ resolution is not important or unobtainable due to involuntary movement, for instance kidney or heart dynamic studies or lung ventilation perfusion. **High resolution** collimators are used when definition is important, e.g. for bone and brain studies, but patient movement must be controlled for best performance. Low energy all purpose or general purpose collimators (LEAP or LEGP collimators) try to combine the attributes of resolution and sensitivity for routine use.

Some common collimators are illustrated in Fig. 15.24a and b. A complete gamma camera installation should include high sensitivity and high resolution parallel hole collimators; and a low energy all purpose (LEAP) collimator for general static imaging (soft tissue pathology) and improved resolution dynamic studies.

PARALLEL

This is the most common design for collimators in nuclear medicine since it does not distort the source shape with depth having a 1:1 magnification. Designs for high sensitivity (Fig. 15.24a) and high resolution (Fig. 15.24b) cover all clinical applications.

CONVERGING

(Figure 15.24c) When a large field of view camera is the only one available in a nuclear medicine department a converging collimator is essential for providing

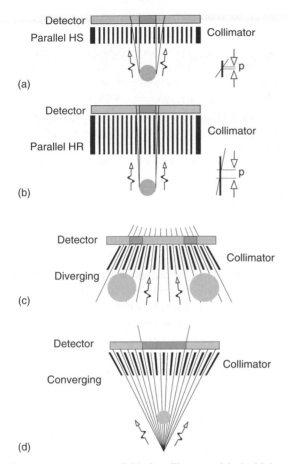

Figure 15.24 *Two parallel hole collimators. (**a**) The high sensitivity (HS) gives a large penumbra (unsharpness). (**b**) The high resolution collimator has a greater depth and smaller penumbra. (**c**) A converging collimator magnifies the image in the focal plane, since it is focused there is distortion with depth. (**d**) The diverging collimator minifies the image. Septa penetration by the gamma photon. The angular thickness* p *increases with hole length.*

practical-sized images of small organs including the brain, single kidney or thyroid, otherwise electronic zooming is the other option which will not improve image resolution which the converging collimator does. It will give magnification of about 3:1 but unfortunately since it has a focal point it will give distortion with depth. The extreme version of the converging collimator is the pin-hole collimator but this gives considerable distortion with depth and is difficult to align with the source and should be treated with the utmost caution.

DIVERGING

This collimator design is the converse of the previous collimator: it minifies the image, as shown in Fig. 15.24d. This is useful if a small field of view camera is required to image both lungs or kidneys. It also gives distortion with depth which causes problems with large areas of anatomy.

15.8.3 Collimator efficiency

SYSTEM SENSITIVITY

This is a measure of the ratio of count rate within the photopeak to the known activity of a source placed on the collimator and is commonly expressed as either counts per minute per μCi or counts per second per MBq. The conversion is cpm μCi^{-1} $\times$ 0.45 = cps MBq^{-1}. System sensitivity is influenced by collimator design and gamma spectrum. There is also a trade-off between collimator sensitivity and resolution; they are inversely proportional to each other. Table 15.21 lists the properties of some modern commercial collimators using a hexagonal design. In general LEAP collimators have sensitivity figures from 86 to 180 cps MBq^{-1}, LEHS from 180 to 290, LEHR from 51 to 145 and 'super' LEHR < 60.

COLLIMATOR SEPTA PENETRATION

Collimators for low energy radiation (^{201}Tl, ^{99m}Tc) are made of very thin lead. Septa penetration is not a problem and high resolutions can be obtained either by keeping the hole pattern the same and increasing the collimator depth (hole length) or maintaining a constant hole length but increasing the hole number (see Table 15.21). Increasing the collimator depth also increases the oblique angle p in Fig. 15.24a and b so high resolution collimators can have thinner septa with corresponding improvements in sensitivity for resolution.

Collimators for medium/high energy radiation (^{111}In, ^{131}I) suffer from septa penetration. The hole pattern is coarse and they give poor resolution. The thickness of lead separating the holes in a collimator depends on the energy of the gamma radiation being imaged. The septa thickness required to minimize penetration changes significantly over the energy ranges seen in nuclear medicine. Septa penetration makes the design of a high energy radiation collimators difficult since the hole pattern and septa thickness

Table 15.21 *Collimator specifications for ^{99m}Tc and performance: the source at three depths for low energy all purpose, high sensitivity, high resolution and HR (super).*

Type of collimator	Number of holes	Hole length (mm)	Septa thickness (mm)
LEHS	28	24	0.36
LEHR	148	24	0.16

Type of collimator	Full width at half maximum at			cps MBq^{-1}	Septa penetration (%)
	5 cm	10 cm	20 cm		
LEAP	6	9	15	148	0.8
LEHS	7	11	18	225	1.7
LEHR	5.5	8	13	103	0.4
LEHR(S)	5	6.6	10	63	0.2

could have a worse impact on image quality than the septa penetration that is being minimized. Septa penetration can be generally expressed as the penetration fraction f_p

$$f_p = \frac{\text{photons penetrating septa}}{\text{photons passing through holes}}$$

As the absorption of radiation is exponential a certain amount of radiation always penetrates the septa. Table 15.21 shows that high resolution collimators (LEHR and LEHR(S)) have much lower septa penetration figures since the oblique photon has a longer pathway p than the LEHS. However, because of their tighter scatter rejection the sensitivity (cps MBq^{-1}) decreases.

16

Nuclear medicine: radiopharmaceuticals and imaging equipment

16.1 CLINICAL NUCLIDES AND RADIOPHARMACEUTICALS

The parallel development of instrumentation and the chemistry of clinically useful isotopes has maintained nuclear medicine as a premier diagnostic imaging service. The distribution of labeled radiopharmaceuticals in the body allows imaging of organ function since these chemical substances are actively accumulated (e.g. MDP bone agents, liver colloid) or excreted (e.g. DTPA, EHIDA) by the target organ.

Although several radionuclides are available for nuclear medicine the predominant one is ^{99m}Tc; it complies with most of the requirements for an ideal clinical isotope. It is produced by a generator, which can be kept in the nuclear medicine radiopharmacy, and renewed at weekly intervals. It is immediately available, thereby allowing a nuclear medicine clinic to offer a continuous service.

16.1.1 ^{99m}Tc generator specifications

Basic information on generator construction was given earlier in Chapter 15, Section 15.4.4. The technetium generator used for routine nuclear medicine purposes is commonly eluted each morning; Fig. 16.1 shows the decreasing activity of available ^{99m}Tc A in equilibrium with ^{99}Mo and eluted ^{99m}Tc over a 3 day period (curves B and C).

Partial elution of the generator gives high activity in a small volume, which is useful for efficient labeling of small samples (white cells and complex molecules). Specific concentration for small volumes is plotted in Fig. 16.2.

Choice of the correct generator size is critical to the efficiency of a nuclear medicine department: if it is too small then not enough activity is available on a

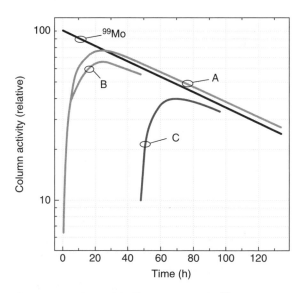

Figure 16.1 *The straight line represents the ^{99}Mo decay (T$_{1/2}$ = 67 h). Curve A is the ^{99m}Tc activity if the column is left undisturbed in equilibrium. ^{99m}Tc activity–time curves B and C reach a peak at about 23 h after each elution.*

day-to-day basis; too large and it is unnecessarily expensive. Box 16.1 calculates a specific generator size using the decay constants for ^{99}Mo and ^{99m}Tc in Table 16.1 which gives both ^{99}Mo and ^{99m}Tc decay

factors, ^{99}Mo decay factors (leftmost column) in days and ^{99m}Tc decay factors in hours with fractions of 15, 30, and 45 min. The calculation requires knowledge of:

- Patient numbers over the working week
- The type of investigations to be performed and their scheduling

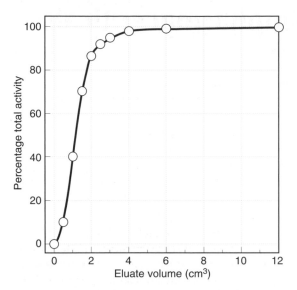

Figure 16.2 *Activity in a small volume elution (partial elution) gives a high specific activity: 5 cm³ contains approximately 90% of the available activity.*

Table 16.1 *Decay factors for ^{99}Mo and ^{99m}Tc.*

^{99}Mo (days)	Period	^{99m}Tc (h)	Time (min)		
			15	30	45
3.45	−5	1.78	1.83	1.89	1.94
2.70	−4	1.59	1.63	1.68	1.73
2.12	−3	1.41	1.46	1.50	1.54
1.66	−2	1.26	1.30	1.33	1.37
1.28	−1	1.12	1.16	1.19	1.22
1.00	0	1.00	1.03	1.06	1.09
1.00	0	1.00	0.97	0.94	0.92
0.78	1	0.89	0.87	0.84	0.82
0.61	2	0.79	0.77	0.75	0.73
0.47	3	0.71	0.69	0.67	0.65
0.37	4	0.63	0.61	0.59	0.58
0.29	5	0.56	0.54	0.53	0.51

Box 16.1 Calculating a suitable generator size

Choose the minimum size ^{99m}Tc generator that will fulfill the following requirements using ^{99}Mo and ^{99m}Tc decay factors in Table 16.1. The following points are noted:

1. The generator is for use on Monday morning
2. The generator referenced for 09:00 on the following Thursday
3. It is eluted once a day at 09:00
4. On the Wednesday before the reference day there should be activity for a clinic of eight patients. The following activities are required:
   - 2 × 550 MBq at 09:30 (total 1166 MBq eluted at 09:00)
   - 2 × 550 MBq at 10:30 (total 1309 MBq eluted at 09:00)
   - 2 × 75 MBq at 10:00 (total 168 MBq eluted at 09:00)
   - 2 × 500 MBq at 14:00 (total 1780 MBq eluted at 09:00)

The total activity required is then 1166 + 1309 + 168 + 1780 = 4423 MBq for 09:00 on Wednesday.

Size of generator: (see Table 16.1, ^{99}Mo decay)

Hence the **reference activity** for Thursday at 09:00 is

$$4423 \times 0.78 \text{ (24 h decay)} = 3449 \text{ MBq}$$

The minimum size of the generator that will supply the Wednesday activities can be calculated by using the ^{99m}Tc decay factors (Table 16.1). Available activities through the week are then:

Monday (RD − 3)	3449 × 2.12 =	7311 MBq
Tuesday	3449 × 1.66 =	5725 MBq
Wednesday	3449 × 1.28 =	4414 MBq
Thursday (RD)	=	3449 MBq
Friday (RD + 1)	3449 × 0.78 =	2690 MBq

(where RD means 'reference day').

The particular activities referred to in Box 16.1 require a standard generator of 3.7 GBq (100 mCi). Generators are sized according to their activity on a reference or calibration day; this is always quoted with their specification.

Typical commercially available generator sizes for most nuclear medicine department patient requirements are:

2	3.7	7.4	11	15	18	GBq
50	100	200	300	400	500	mCi

16.1.2 Oxidation states and labeling ^{99m}Tc

The chemistry of technetium involves seven oxidation or valency states. These are listed in Table 16.2 and play major roles in the labeling of radiopharmaceuticals.

Table 16.2 *Technetium oxidation states.*

Technetium(I)
Exists in certain organic complexes, e.g. ^{99m}Tc^{I}-(*t*-butyl-isonitrile), ^{99m}Tc^{I}-MIBI
Good *in-vivo* stability

Technetium(II)
Not important

Technetium(III)
Compounds labeled with Tc^{III} undergo *in-vivo* reduction: Tc$^{\text{III}} \rightarrow$ Tc^{II} giving liver activity
Tc^{III} may be the active form of ^{99m}Tc-HIDA

Technetium(IV)
This is the most stable state and is used for kit preparation
Tc^{VII} + 3E$^{2+} \rightarrow$ ^{99m}Tc^{IV}-'kit' + 3E^{3+}
E is commonly the stannous ion (Sn^{2+})
Oxidizes to Tc^{IV} + oxygen $\rightarrow$ Tc^{VII} (see Tc^{VII} below)

Technetium(V)
Modified reduction reaction: increasing the pH produces this oxidation state
Mostly seen as ^{99m}Tc^{V}-DMSA for tumor targeting

Technetium(VI)
Not important

Technetium(VII)
This is the most stable oxidation state represented by the eluted technetium
Labeled kits degrade to Tc^{VII} with atmospheric or blood-borne oxygen and disassociate producing free Tc^{VII} with the pharmaceutical

The eluted technetium has an oxidation state of (VII) and must interact with a reducing agent (Sn^{2+} stannous ion) in order to produce an oxidation state of (IV) which is necessary for radiopharmaceutical kit labeling. Other oxidation states are listed; some are important but others play a minor role in kit labeling. It is important to note that the reduced state of Tc(IV) is easily oxidized by atmospheric oxygen back to Tc(VII); the labeled compound (e.g. DTPA, MAA, MDP) becoming detached leaving free ^{99m}Tc which will concentrate in extraneous target organs (thyroid, stomach etc.).

16.1.3 Radiopharmaceuticals

The properties of an ideal isotope for nuclear medicine imaging have been described in Chapter 15. If ^{99m}Tc is accepted as a practical example of an ideal isotope (with some limitations) then the properties of an ideal radiopharmaceutical are listed in Table 16.3. Most of these points are satisfied by commercially available compounds and radiopharmaceuticals except the requirement for positive uptake in pathology (both liver colloid and lung MAA show pathology as a 'negative' uptake). Certain radiopharmaceuticals still need heating for optimum labeling (MAG3). All radiopharmaceuticals are nontoxic in the very low concentrations used although pediatric applications may need careful scrutiny. Some radiopharmaceuticals used in routine applications and their typical activities for each adult study are listed in Table 16.4.

16.1.4 Quality control

Tests for the *in-vitro* stability of labeled compounds should be carried out on a regular basis. Figure 16.3 shows a measuring cylinder fitted with a plastic

Table 16.3 *The ideal radiopharmaceutical.*

- Easy labeling: single procedure
- Short reaction time
- Single target organ
- Room temperature reconstitution: no boiling water bath
- Useful reconstituted life
- Multiple patients per vial
- No toxic or allergic response
- Good shelf-life (unreconstituted)
- Stable *in vivo* (minimum free isotope)
- Pathology seen as increased activity

Table 16.4 ^{99m}Tc radiopharmaceuticals in routine applications.

Organ	Agent	Application	Activity (MBq)
Bone	MDP	Metastases	500 to 700
	HMDP	Fractures	
Brain	DTPA	Tumor	500 to 700
	*HMPAO	Perfusion	400 to 600
Cardiac	**MIBI	Myocardium	400 to 600
	†Terfosmin	Infarct	400
	Pyrophosphate		
Kidney	DTPA	GFR	75 to 100
	††MAG3	Function	120
	DMSA	Function	80 to 200
Lung	MAA	Perfusion	80 to 100
	Aerosols	Ventilation	40 to 60
Liver/spleen	Colloid	Function	80 to 100
	EHIDA	Biliary	70 to 150
Bone marrow	¶Colloid	Metastases	200
Lymph	¶Colloid	Function	200 to 400
Whole body	*HMPAO	Infection	400 to 600
Whole body	White cells	Tumor sites	80 to 100
	Tc^v-DMSA		

*Commercially available as Ceretec®.
**Commercially available as Cardiolite®.
†Commercially available as Myoview®.
††Commercially available as MAG3®.
¶Commercially available as NanoColloid®.

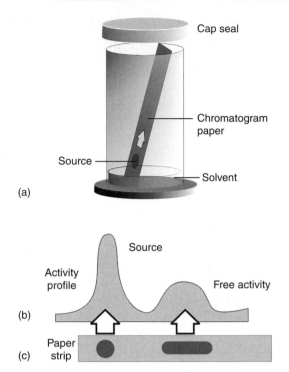

Figure 16.3 (*a*) Radiopharmaceutical quality control equipment consisting of a glass measuring cylinder holding a small volume of solvent. Detail of the activity profile (*b*) and the position of fractions on the thin-layer strip is shown (*c*).

sealing lid which is suitable for radiopharmaceutical quality control using chromatographic techniques.

A drop of the labeled radiopharmaceutical is placed onto a strip of absorbent gel (thin layer chromatography strips; Gelman Instrument Co.) approximately 0.5 cm from the bottom. The gel paper is carefully dried and placed upright in the solvent. For most ^{99m}Tc agents acetone is a suitable solvent. The cap is replaced to keep a saturated atmosphere in the container.

The solvent front advances up the paper quite slowly and when it reaches almost to the top it is removed, dried, and placed on a gamma camera with a high resolution collimator that is protected with a polythene sheet. A direct image is then obtained and activity profiles taken through the active areas on the strip. Alternatively, the paper can be divided and each half counted using a well-scintillation counter. The quality control result gives a measure of:

- Bound ^{99m}Tc
- Free ^{99m}Tc (i.e. TcO$_4$)
- Hydrolyzed ^{99m}Tc (i.e. TcO$_2$)

OTHER RADIONUCLIDES

Radionuclides other than ^{99m}Tc have less than ideal properties but they have either specific targeting (^{67}Ga, ^{201}Tl), easier chemistry (^{123}I) or longer half-lives for observing longer physiological phenomena (^{111}In). These are listed in Table 16.5.

16.2 DOSIMETRY

The exposure of nuclear medicine staff and patients to radiation is generally much lower than investigations using conventional X-rays. Staff experience most exposure to radiation either when in the radio-pharmacy or when in close contact with patients injected with high activities (e.g. as used for bone and cardiac investigations). In most nuclear medicine studies patient exposure is highest with isotopes

Table 16.5 *Other radionuclides and their applications.*

Nuclide	Half-life	Gamma energy (keV)	Compound	Target tissue or application
^{67}Ga	3.2 d	93, 185, 300	Citrate	Inflammatory lesions and tumor location
^{111}In	2.8 d	171, 245	Chloride	Biological labeling
			DTPA	Cisternography
^{75}Se	120 d	136, 265, 280	Norcholesterol	Adrenal cortex
			Methionine	Pancreas
^{201}Tl	3.0 d	*68 to 82	Chloride	Myocardium
^{133}Xe	5.3 d	81	Gas	Lung ventilation
^{127}Xe	36 d	172, 203, 375	Gas	Lung ventilation
^{81m}Kr	13 s	190	Gas	Lung ventilation
^{123}I	13 h	159	Hippurate	Kidney function
			MIBG	Adrenal medulla

*X-rays.

other than ^{99m}Tc so these activity levels are carefully controlled, as with ^{201}Tl and ^{131}I, for example.

16.2.1 External exposure

The limit for surface exposure levels in a controlled area from sealed sources is 7.5 μSv h^{-1}. Exposure levels, given as specific gamma ray constants, from gigabecquerel activities of common isotopes have already been introduced.

EXTERNAL DOSE LEVELS

Shielding and storage of radioactive substances must conform to international regulations (ICRP, NRPB) and feature in the hospital local rules for radiation safety. Some suggested limits for surface doses and dose rates 5 cm from the surface are:

- Surface activity, 7.5 μSv h^{-1}
- 5 cm distance (long-term storage), 0.2 mSv h^{-1}
- 5 cm distance (short-term storage), 2.0 mSv h^{-1}

These levels are constantly revised, the most recent limits should be observed. In the USA the areas containing radiation-producing sources must be labeled according to their exposure levels. A **radiation area** is defined as an area accessible to staff where radiation levels could approach 50 μSv h^{-1} at 30 cm, either from the source itself or any surface that the radiation penetrates. A **high radiation area** is an area where radiation levels to staff could approach 1 mSv h^{-1} at 30 cm.

GENERATOR SHIELDING

Radiation levels from a medium size technetium generator would be:

- Unshielded core of 18.5 GBq (500 mCi) generator 6 mSv h^{-1} at 0.5 m
- For 7.5 μSv h^{-1} this would require 6.8 cm Pb (HVL for ^{99}Mo 740 keV gamma, 7 mm Pb)
- A typical shielded core with 5.0 cm Pb plus additional shielding of 4.5 cm Pb, giving a total shielding of 9.5 cm Pb
- The total shielding supplied by the manufacturer typically exceeds the minimum levels.

SYRINGE SHIELDING

Lead or tungsten syringe shields of about 3 mm thickness reduce finger and body doses by about ×200 from syringe activities. The dose rate from an unshielded vial containing 4 GBq (100 mCi) ^{99m}Tc would be 800 μSv h^{-1} at 30 cm; the suggested shielding is based on an HVL of 0.25 mm Pb (140 keV). To maintain a surface dose level of 7.5 μSv h^{-1} it would require 1.67 mm Pb. A typical vial lead-pot supplies 3 mm to 10 mm.

RADIATION DOSE FROM PATIENTS

Close proximity to nuclear medicine patients contributes to staff radiation exposure and reasonable distances should be kept (Table 16.6). As a consequence waiting rooms for patients who have received a radionuclide injection should be separate areas in the department.

The reduction of staff exposure from nuclear medicine patients can be significantly reduced by taking sensible precautions. Table 16.7 lists the reduction possible if certain safety measures are maintained.

GUIDELINES OF ACTIVITY LIMITS FOR PATIENTS LEAVING HOSPITAL

Nuclear medicine offers a very useful outpatient service as the patient can normally be discharged. Certain precautions should be observed, however, depending on the isotope and activity used. Table 16.8 identifies **restricted** contact where the patient is likely to mix with children, so the activity levels are kept low. **No restriction** applies where children are unlikely to be involved so the patient activity levels can be higher.

Patients should be given an instruction leaflet detailing contact with other people and appropriate action if clothing becomes contaminated.

Table 16.6 *Staff exposure from patients.*

Nuclide	Half-life	Activity (MBq)	Exposure (μSv h⁻¹ at 1 m)
^{67}Ga	78 h	150	1.6
^{111}In	2.8 d	80	2.4
^{99m}Tc	6.0 h	800	6.0
^{131}I	8.0 d	40	0.9
^{201}Tl	73 h	80	0.3

Table 16.7 *Radiation reduction from a ^{99m}Tc study.*

Condition	Exposure
Patient activity (^{99m}Tc)	800 MBq (20 mCi)
Exposure to staff at 30 cm	160 μSv h⁻¹
Exposure to staff at 1 m	6 μSv h⁻¹
Complete 15 min study at 30 cm	20 μSv total
Complete 15 min study at 60 cm	5 μSv total
Wearing 0.25 mm Pb apron	10 μSv h at 30 cm
Natural radiation 2 to 5 mSv y⁻¹	8 to 20 μSv d⁻¹

Table 16.8 *Patient activity levels.*

Radionuclide	Restricted	No restriction
^{131}I	30 MBq	150 MBq
^{99m}Tc	80 MBq	400 MBq

16.2.2 Internal dosimetry

In order to maintain the patient radiation dose within acceptable limits various procedures have been developed for estimating dose to the patient from internally administered isotopes and radiopharmaceuticals.

MARINELLI FORMULA

This was an early attempt at calculating internal dosimetry estimating organ and whole-body radiation dose from beta, nonpenetrating radiation, D_β, and gamma, penetrating radiation, D_γ. It uses a rough geometric factor g allowing for simple variations in organ shape (liver, lungs, kidney etc.):

$$D_\beta = 21 \times C \times E_\beta \times T_e \qquad (16.1)$$

$$D_\beta = 0.3225 \times C \times \Gamma \times g \times T_e \qquad (16.2)$$

where T_e is the effective $T_{1/2}$ in days, Γ, in mSv GBq⁻¹ h⁻¹ at 1 m, is the gamma ray constant, and C is the percentage of activity retained by the target organ. E_β is the mean beta energy and the constants 21 and 0.3225 express D_β and D_γ in mSv. Box 16.2 calculates

---

Box 16.2 Use of the Marinelli formula to calculate radiation dose to an organ

A liver investigation uses 74 MBq (2 mCi) ^{99m}Tc-colloid. Eighty-five percent is trapped and the liver weight is 1.8 kg. The percentage retained, C, is given by

$$C = \frac{\text{total activity} \times \text{fraction absorbed}}{\text{weight of organ}}$$

The radiation dose to the liver from Auger electrons and gamma photons (eqns 16.1 and 16.2) where T_e is 6 h and Γ is 0.017:

$$D_\beta = 21 \times \frac{74 \times 0.85}{1.8} \times 0.016 \times 0.25$$
$$= 2.9 \text{ mSv}$$

$$D_\gamma = 0.3225 \times \frac{74 \times 0.85}{1.8} \times 0.017 \times 50 \times 0.25$$
$$= 2.39 \text{ mSv}$$

The total dose to the liver is therefore 5.29 mSv.

the radiation dose from a ^{99m}Tc liver colloid study using these equations. The limitations of the Marinelli method are:

- The geometry factor g only covers simple spheroids which do not relate to real organ shapes.
- No allowance is given for radiation exposure to adjacent organs from the target organ (liver or bladder to uterus, etc.).
- Unequal distribution of the tracer within the target organ cannot be included or distribution times within the organ.

THE MIRD FORMULA

A more accurate approach to internal dosimetry was proposed by the Medical Internal Radiation Dose (MIRD) Committee in the USA. The MIRD technique:

- Groups both penetrating and nonpenetrating radiations together
- Considers biological and physical data regarding distribution and residence time
- The irradiation of adjacent organs by the target organ

Dose calculations can be solved for:

- Radiotracers that accumulate mostly in one organ (liver colloid, lung perfusion)
- Tracers that are distributed in a number of organs (vascular, hepatobiliary system)
- Time varying distribution (bolus studies)
- Dose variations to selected organs (the bladder depending on voiding frequency)

The parameters used in the MIRD formula are listed in Table 16.9. Absorbed dose per unit of administered activity is therefore

$$\bar{D} = A_0 \times \tau \times S$$

where

$$\tau = \frac{\text{fraction retained by organ}}{\lambda}$$

and $\lambda = 0.693/6.02$.

A simple example is used in Box 16.3 to recalculate the liver investigation of Box 16.2. Contribution to other organs and irradiation of other organs would complete the dose calculation, i.e.

- Contribution from the spleen to the total liver dose: spleen $\rightarrow D_{\infty,\text{liver}}$
- Contribution from the skeleton to the total liver dose: bone $\rightarrow D_{\infty,\text{liver}}$
- Dose to specific organs from the liver: liver $\rightarrow D_{\infty,\text{uterus}}$

Since organ to organ radiation exposure values can be incorporated into the formula the MIRD dose rate

Table 16.9 *MIRD symbol definition.*

Parameter	Symbol	Non-SI	SI
Activity	A_0	1 mCi = 3.7 × 10^4 Bq	1 MBq = 27 μCi
Absorbed dose	D	1 rad = 10 mGy	1 Gy = 100 rad
Mean dose	$\bar{D}$	Same	Same
Mean dose per unit of cumulated activity	S	$\dfrac{\text{rad}}{\mu\text{Ci} \cdot \text{h}}$	$\dfrac{\text{Gy}}{\text{MBq} \cdot \text{s}}$
Residence time	τ	Hour	

Box 16.3 Use of the MIRD formula to calculate radiation dose to an organ

The details are the same as given in Box 16.2 but the MIRD equations are used to calculate the dose to the liver:

$$\bar{D}_{\text{liver}} = A_0 \tau S$$

where the activity A_0 is still 74 MBq and calculated residence time $\tau = 0.85/\lambda = 7.4$ h.

Using non-SI units, S is 4.6×10^{-5} rad mCi^{-1} h^{-1}, so

$$\bar{D}_{\text{liver}} = 2000 \times 7.4 \times 4.6 \times 10^{-5}$$
$$= 0.68 \text{ rad}$$

Using SI units, S is 1.2×10^{-5} Gy MBq^{-1} s^{-1}, so

$$\bar{D}_{\text{liver}} = 74 \times (1.2 \times 10^{-5}) \times 7.4$$
$$= 6.57 \text{ mGy}$$

Note that this is a higher value than the Marinelli result in Box 16.2.

is higher than the Marinelli formula. Other organs such as the spleen and bone marrow can also be included in the overall dose to the patient; a factor which is missing in other calculations.

LIMITATIONS

Although the MIRD calculations have solved a number of problems, there can be large uncertainty in some of the calculated parameters, e.g. absorbed fraction.

The coefficient of variation (a measure of uncertainty for the radiation dose) can be as much as 20 to 50% in some cases. Other weaknesses are:

- Models for certain organs, such as the kidney do not allow for cortex and medulla.
- Bone marrow is not well represented.
- The MIRD formula assumes a uniform distribution of activity within any organ, which is not always the case (e.g. transit of DTPA in the kidney, gas clearance in the lung).

PATIENT DOSE REDUCTION

When deciding radionuclide activities used for clinical studies the following points should be considered:

- Good counting statistics in laboratory tests (GFR etc.)
- A diagnostic image in a reasonable time
- Acceptable radiation dose to the patient from the target organ and excretion pathway
- Cost of expensive isotopes (^{123}I, ^{111}In)

The common activity levels used for various studies are listed at the end of this chapter. The activities listed in MBq give optimal results (best counting statistics or image quality); the ranges of whole-body dose (H_E) given by ^{99m}Tc-DTPA, MDP, EDTA etc. are due to variations in bladder retention/voiding times. World Health Organization (WHO) category groups approximate low, medium, and high radiation dose rates. As a comparison with conventional X-ray investigations a urogram using iodine contrast materials will give:

- Ovarian dose, 30 mSv
- Bladder wall dose, 43 mSv
- Whole-body dose (typical), 30 mSv

The patient radiation doses from nuclear medicine studies are therefore much lower than the equivalent functional radiology investigation and incidentally far less invasive.

16.2.3 Pediatric exposure

The injected activity level for determining adult radiation dose usually depends on the weight and age of the patient. Guidelines are given on the radiopharmaceutical package insert for a standard man. There are several different multiplication factors used for obtaining children's doses from the adult dose including:

1 Body surface area (BSA) ÷ 1.73
2 Child's age +1, divided by age +7 years
3 Child's weight divided by 70 kg
4 Child's height divided by 174 cm

For static studies multiplication factors based on 1, 2, and 3 are used. For dynamic studies where imaging time and image quality are of primary importance factor 4 is recommended. Box 16.4 gives an example of each for the same child size. Doses should be increased for 'large-for-age' children.

Most radionuclides used for nuclear medicine investigations are concentrated in breast milk (^{131}I and ^{99m}Tc particularly). A neonate thyroid gland can receive a high radiation dose from these nuclides in the mother's milk, therefore either nuclear medicine investigations should be voided or the mother instructed to bottle feed after the investigation for a suitable period. Over 90% of the ^{99m}Tc activity appears

> ## Box 16.4 The determination of the injected activity required for children
>
> The injected activity required for children is usually based upon the injected activity for an adult (see text). As an example, consider a 6-year-old child, weight 20 kg, and height 110 cm. An agent having an adult activity of 200 MBq is to be injected. Using the multiplication factors given in the text the injected activity for this child would be:
>
> Factor 1: BSA = 0.77/1.73 = 89 MBq
>
> Factor 2: 7/13 will give 107 MBq
>
> Factor 3: 20/70 will give 57 MBq
>
> Factor 4: 100/174 will give 126 MBq
>
> (Body surface area is given by the formula $W^{0.425} \times H^{0.725} \times 0.0072$ m^2 where W is the weight (kg) and H is the height (cm). For the child in this example the BSA is 0.77 m^2.)

in the breast milk over 24 h and breast feeding can continue after this term. The trauma imposed on the child and mother by restricting contact should be seriously weighed against the radiation risk.

16.2.4 Radiopharmacy

The management of radioactive materials is governed by local, national, and international regulations. The following recommendations are based on ICRP and IAEA reports detailed at the end of this chapter.

The classification of a laboratory space for a radiopharmacy depends on the expected workload and the isotopes used (group type). Table 16.10 lists the maximum activity levels that each radiopharmacy class should carry at any one time. Most radiopharmacies would be classified as medium, where the majority of work uses ^{99m}Tc for imaging (as the group 4 isotope), with small quantities of groups 2 and 3 isotopes.

In the USA areas containing radiation sources must be labeled according to possible radiation exposure levels. A **radiation area** is defined as an area where radiation levels could result in a dose equivalent in excess of 50 μSv h^1 at 30 cm from the source itself or from any surface that the source radiation penetrates. A **high radiation area** is one where the radiation levels could reach or exceed 1 mSv h^{-1} at 30 cm.

High levels of ^{99}Mo (group 2) contained in the ^{99m}Tc generator would require a separate location classified as a high radiation or controlled area. Suggested requirements would be:

- Isolated from radiopharmacy
- Dispensing bench shielded with 3 cm lead bricks
- Barrier essential (door)

Table 16.10 *Classification of nuclear medicine laboratories in terms of activity areas (ICRP 25).*

Classification	Low	Medium	High
Group 2 nuclides			
^{125}I, ^{131}I	<500 kBq	500 kBq to 500 MBq	500 MBq to 5 GBq
Group 3 nuclides			
^{51}Cr, ^{32}P, ^{99}Mo, ^{201}Tl	<5 MBq	5 MBq to 5 GBq	**5 GBq to 500 GBq
Group 4 nuclides			
^{99m}Tc, ^{133}Xe	<500 MBq	*500 MBq to 500 GBq	500 GBq to 50 TBq

*Supervised areas. **Generator room.

- 10 m^2 minimum area
- Hand monitoring (large area counter)
- Room monitoring (wall mounted TLDs)

A fume hood and extractor fan would not be essential since this radionuclide is not volatile. Disposable rubber gloves should always be used for preventing hand contamination. The radiopharmacy would also be treated as a **controlled area** and available access restricted to designated staff only.

DISPOSAL OF RADIOACTIVE WASTE

Radioactive waste may be identified as:

- Decayed sealed sources
- Spent radionuclide generators (^{99m}Tc, ^{81m}Kr, ^{185m}Au etc.)
- Laboratory solutions of low activity
- Low activity liquid washings from vials
- Liquid scintillants immiscible with water
- Biologically contaminated solid waste, e.g. syringes, vials
- Radioactive gases

Each of these requires special considcration since biological contamination (e.g. blood) may be a more serious hazard. Accepted levels for disposal of radioactive waste under controlled and noncontrolled conditions are given in Table 16.11; activities are given in becquerels (μCi in brackets).

Controlled disposal is defined as disposal with permission from the regulatory authority (government or state body). Records should be kept listing initial activities and recommended disposal dates for medium and long half-life nuclides. ^{99m}Tc waste

Table 16.11 *Discharged activity limits, in Bq (μCi).*

Classification	No control	Controlled
Group 1	Not used	Not used
Group 2		
^{125}I, ^{131}I	5×10^4 Bq (1.4 μCi) (USA, 1.0 μCi)	1×10^7 Bq (270 μCi) (USA, 10.0 μCi)
Group 3		
^{201}Tl, ^{32}P, ^{67}Ga, ^{51}Cr, ^{111}In, ^{57}Co, ^{58}Co, ^{99}Mo	5×10^5 Bq (14 μCi) (USA, 10.0 μCi)	5×10^6 Bq (140 μCi) (USA, 100 μCi)
Group 4		
^{99m}Tc, ^{133}Xe	5×10^6 Bq (140 μCi) (USA, 100 μCi)	5×10^7 Bq (1.4 mCi) (USA, 1 mCi)

should be kept for an appropriate decay period before disposal (24h); no records are normally required for decayed ^{99m}Tc contaminated items.

EXHAUSTED ^{99m}Tc GENERATORS

A 12.5 GBq (345 mCi) ^{99}Mo generator core decays to 5×10^6 Bq after 31 days so could undergo disposal under controlled conditions with proper authorization. Spent generators awaiting disposal should be removed to a separate store room or bunker for the requisite decay period. Shielding should be provided so that exposure does not exceed 7.5 μSv h^{-1}.

PATIENT WASTE

Special toilets should be available to nuclear medicine patients. The toilet should have direct access to the sewage system and should not run under the nuclear medicine department since high activities will affect the performance of counters and imaging devices by increasing background activity levels. Patient excreta are exempt from disposal restrictions. Urine and feces should be discharged using a toilet connected directly to a main sewer. Legislation exists which governs the handling, use, storage, administration, disposal, and transportation of isotopes and labeled radiopharmaceuticals. Local regulations and codes of practice should be consulted.

TRANSPORT OF RADIOACTIVE MATERIAL

Certain conditions have been defined by the IAEA for the packaging and transport of radioactive material. They include a transport index which is the maximum dose rate at a distance of 1 m from the package surface in μSv divided by 10. These transport indices are indicated on the three types of package label given in Table 16.12. The package category depends on both the transport index and the surface radiation level. An example label is shown in Fig. 16.4.

Table 16.12 *Package category.*

Category label	Surface dose (μSv h^{-1})	Transport index
I White		
Low level	5	0
II Yellow		
Moderate level	5 to 500	<1
III Yellow		
High level	500 to 2000	1 to 10

16.3 PLANAR IMAGING

Nuclear medicine planar images represent a volume activity so the activity from overlying tissue degrades image contrast from pathology within the organ volume. Circulating activity (blood) also adds background noise and also obscures pathology. Planar examples routinely collected in nuclear medicine are liver images (oncology), lung images (pulmonary embolism), DMSA (kidney function) and myocardial activity (^{201}Tl).

16.3.1 Static planar

This is the conventional procedure for following radiopharmaceutical distribution. Image acquisition normally provides anterior, posterior, and several lateral views with oblique views.

Table 16.13 lists common collimator types and their application for planar clinical studies. High sensitivity collimators are used where count rate is more important than resolution (moving organs, i.e. lungs, or dynamic studies). High resolution gives the best detail (bone). Converging gives magnified, detailed images but gives depth distortion.

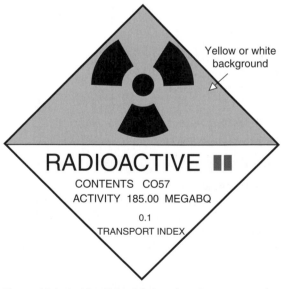

Figure 16.4 *An identifying label used on the transportation packaging of radioactive materials. The three types of labels are listed in Table 16.12.*

Table 16.13 *Collimator selection.*

Collimator	Application
Low energy (e.g. ^{99m}Tc ^{201}Tl ^{123}I)	
High sensitivity	Planar lungs, planar myocardium, dynamic renography, MIBG adrenals
All purpose (LEAP)	Planar liver, pediatric, ^{81m}Kr lungs
High resolution	SPECT brain, SPECT heart, planar DMSA kidney
Converging (magnification)	Planar brain, planar thyroid
Medium energy (e.g. ^{111}In, ^{67}Ga)	
All purpose	Labeled white cells, tumor marking
High energy (e.g. ^{131}I and positron emitters)	
All purpose	Thyroid metastases, PET (non-coincidence)

MATRIX SIZE

The gamma camera image is commonly represented as a matrix; common matrix sizes are 64×64, 128×128, and 256×256. It is recommended, for visual acuity, that the displayed pixel size should be smaller than the data pixel size and 256×256 would be used for displaying static images from present day gamma cameras; 64 gray levels seems optimum. Figure 16.5 illustrates three examples used in Box 16.5 where a circular field of view, holding a uniform 10^6 counts, is digitized to 64×64, 128×128, and 256×256 matrices; there is a drop in individual pixel counts for the same total count. Pixel depth would be 8 bits (256 decimal) although for clinical studies with high count rates 16 bits would prevent data overflow in a 64×64 matrix.

Noisy images will result if the pixel count density is not sufficient as Box 16.5 demonstrates, for 64×64, 128×128, and 256×256 matrices, assuming a required visible contrast difference 1.5 times the background activity. In order to maintain the noise equivalent of 6% seen in the 64×64 matrix (1), the total counts collected must increase for the three matrix sizes in (2) and (3); note the increased time necessary for a 256×256 matrix. **Time equivalent noise** is the increased time that must be spent to

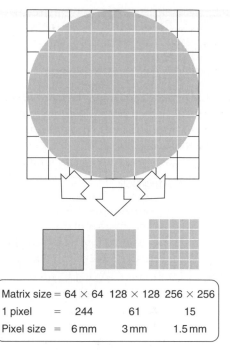

Figure 16.5 *Three sizes of matrix 64×64, 128×128, and 256×256, each holding a total of 1 million counts. The individual pixel count is given for the three matrix sizes along with the pixel size.*

achieve the same noise content of the reference matrix (64×64 pixels) for a fixed value of radioactivity given; for 256×256 this is $\times 16$.

The time taken to acquire a reasonably diagnostic image is a critical factor in a busy nuclear medicine department with a large patient load. A suggested maximum patient load for a single gamma camera facility, taking static images, would be about six to eight patients per day depending on study type. Beyond this a second camera should be considered or a multi-head camera installed. Speeding up image acquisition by increasing injected activity is usually not acceptable due to patient radiation dose restrictions.

CONTRAST AND RESOLUTION

Both contrast and resolution in a nuclear medicine image depends on whether the lesion shows as a negative or positive uptake, e.g. pulmonary emboli and liver metastases are identified as negative uptakes, a bony metastasis as a positive uptake. Figure 16.6 demonstrates that a 'cold' or negative lesion has a limited range whereas a positive uptake has no theoretical limit. As a consequence only large sized negative

Box 16.5 Relationship between matrix size and noise for three sizes of matrix

The matrix size M and count density N are taken from Fig. 16.5. The FOV is 38 cm, the pixel size is $380/M$, the pixel noise is $\sqrt{N}$, and the visible contrast difference is $1.5 \times \sqrt{N}$.

1. 64 × 64 matrix

This is the **equivalent noise** reference. The pixel size is 6 mm and the number of events per pixel is 244. The noise is therefore $\sqrt{244} = 6\%$, and Δcontrast limit is $1.5 \times \sqrt{244} = 10\%$. The **total counts = 1 million.**

Collimator used: high sensitivity
Suggested applications: renography, lung, cardiac (^{201}Tl), SPECT, MUGA, ^{111}In white cell scanning, ^{67}Ga tumor/infection studies

2. 128 × 128 matrix

The pixel size is 3 mm and the number of events per pixel is 61. The noise is therefore 12.5%, and the Δcontrast limit is 20% difference. The **total counts (equivalent noise) = 4 million.**

Collimator used: high sensitivity LEAP
Suggested applications: liver, cardiac (^{99m}Tc agent), MUGA, white cell scanning (^{99m}Tc label)

3. 256 × 256 matrix

The pixel size = 1.5 mm and the number of events per pixel is 15. The noise is therefore 25% and the Δcontrast limit is 40% difference. The **total counts (equivalent noise) = 16 million.**

Collimator used: high resolution LEHR
Suggested applications: bone detail, vascular blood pool, ^{99m}Tc-RBC intestinal blood loss, kidney DMSA

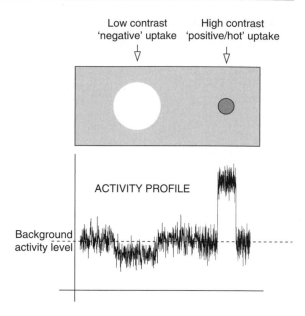

Figure 16.6 *The detectability of a negative uptake or 'hole' compared to a positive uptake or 'hot spot'. The contrast difference is limited for negative uptakes and sensitivity for hole detection is dependent on image background noise (high count density required) and size of lesion.*

sequence. A general equation describing the low count difference detectability ΔC for a known signal S and background activity B uses the signal-to-noise ratio S/B:

$$\Delta C = \gamma \log\left(1 + \frac{S}{B}\right) \qquad (16.3)$$

For the imaging chain in Fig. 16.7 the signal is high at the detector (a) but digitization (b) reduces $S{:}B$ which can be improved slightly by using emphasis in the display (c) such as a color scale.

The display contrast is demonstrated in Fig. 16.7d where increased display contrast shows that small count differences (y-axis) are more easily seen with a high signal to background ratio and high contrast (gamma values). A color display gives a higher contrast than a gray scale and film contrast will also play a significant role.

16.3.2 Dynamic planar

Dynamic studies almost always use high activities of ^{99m}Tc labeled agents. Rapidly changing distributions of this radionuclide (kidney studies) or moving

lesions are visible whereas very 'hot' lesions can be quite small.

Figure 16.7 shows a gradual degradation of contrast as the data passes through the imaging

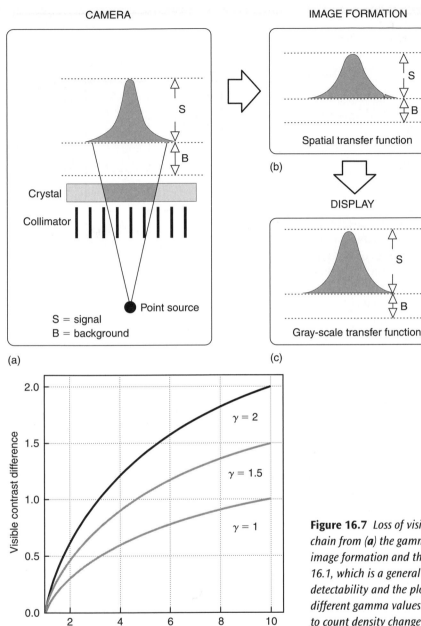

CAMERA

Crystal
Collimator

Point source

S = signal
B = background

(a)

IMAGE FORMATION

Spatial transfer function

(b)

DISPLAY

Gray-scale transfer function

(c)

Visible contrast difference

$\gamma = 2$

$\gamma = 1.5$

$\gamma = 1$

Signal to background ratio (S/B)

(d)

Figure 16.7 *Loss of visible contrast through the imaging chain from (a) the gamma camera detector through to (b) image formation and then (c) the display system. Equation 16.1, which is a general equation, describes low contrast detectability and the plot of contrast differences in (d) uses different gamma values. Gamma is a measure of response to count density change; a color display would have a high gamma value.*

organs (heart) can be captured as a sequence of image frames (frame mode).

The kidney renogram, as an example, is usually a series of at least 60 image frames (byte mode 64×64), each frame taking between 10 and 20 s. Multiphase studies are possible where the fast vascular phase of the bolus through the kidney is captured at 0.5 or 1.0 s intervals for say 30 frames then the clearance phase is captured at a slower 10 s frame rate,

ending with the excretion phase of 60 frames at 20 s per frame.

Very rapid sequences can be captured in list mode where the individual counts (coded for positional information) are stored directly in memory or disk and are reconstructed into matrices after the study. Matrix timing (0.5 s 5.0 s 30 s etc.) can be chosen after the study, unlike frame collection. Table 16.14 lists common protocols for frame mode dynamic studies.

Table 16.14 *Dynamic protocols.*

Study	Frame rate	Activity
Fast		
Lung transit (vascular)	100 at 0.5 s	800 MBq
Kidney transit (vascular)		
Medium		
Renography (vascular)	30 at 5 s	100 MBq
Renography (excretion)	60 at 20 s	
Slow		
Gastric emptying	60 at 60 s	40 MBq

REGIONS OF INTEREST

Regions of interest (ROIs) are used for identifying whole organs (kidneys) or specific regions (lung transit studies). Having selected a single or series of ROIs the computer program then sums all the counts over these regions for all the frames collected in the study (see Fig. 16.8a). The results are then presented as a time/activity curve which is the renogram shown in (b).

ROIs can cause major problems since the organ itself represents a 3-D volume source over which the 2-D ROI area is placed for quantification. This is not serious in the case of homogeneous organs (liver, lung) but can cause errors in non-uniform distributions (heart, brain).

16.3.3 First pass and gated acquisition cardiac studies

The problem of capturing the motion of the moving heart and measuring wall motion and ejection fraction can be solved by either:

* A first pass bolus study
* Gating the cardiac cycle

FIRST PASS BOLUS STUDY

This involves collecting fast dynamic frames while a bolus is in transit through the major heart chambers. Figure 16.9a represents a time–activity curve for a 'first-pass study', showing the swings between end diastole and end systole. The left ventricular mean point is used to calculate left ventricular ejection fraction (LVEF). A normal value would be 30 to 50%.

CARDIAC GATING

The data acquisition is gated with the ECG (EKG) giving a multiple gated acquisition (MUGA). Figure 16.9b shows how the image count data from the

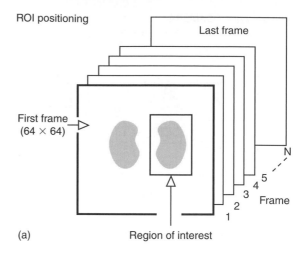
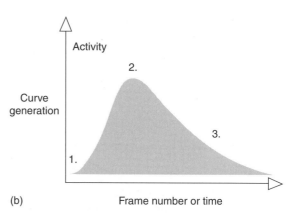

Figure 16.8 (**a**) A dynamic study showing several frames and a single region of interest (ROI) placed over the organ (kidney) which gives a time–activity curve in (**b**). Point 1 on the curve marks the injection time. Point 2 shows peak activity and point 3 indicates wash-out.

gamma camera is steered by the timing pulses (1 to 8 for simplicity) from the ECG, into the 8 image matrices (64 × 64) initiated by each QRS complex. About 500 to 600 QRS events are necessary to give a good series of diagnostic quality images.

In practice between 14 and 32 frames are collected. Irregular timing due to ectopic heart beats leads to data steering problems in MUGA programs but a certain amount of ectopic rejection tolerance is built into the program and gated list-mode acquisition can overcome errors associated with ectopic beats by rejecting these count data when reformatting.

The first-pass dynamic acquisition gives information on both left and right heart ejection fractions which is not usually available in gated studies.

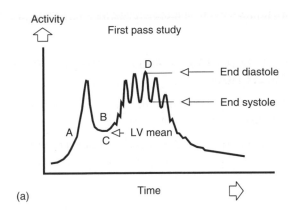

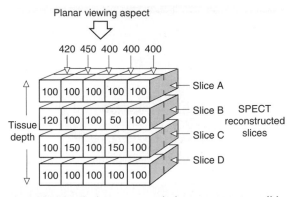

Figure 16.10 *The improvement in image contrast possible with tomographic sectioning. A planar view of this volume distribution of activity (420, 450, 400, 400, 400 in arrow direction), but separate slices will indicate the obscured contrast differences.*

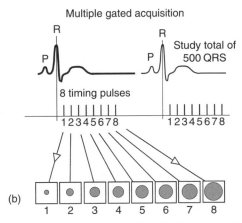

Figure 16.9 *(a) A representation of a first pass bolus study showing (A) bolus entry into the right ventricle (B) wash-out from right ventricle (C) pulmonary activity (D) left ventricular peak activity with end systole and end diastole. (b) The timing sequence for a multi-gated acquisition (MUGA) study. In this example eight cardiac images are stored in computer memory representing a phase of the cardiac cycle. About 500 QRS events are required for a complete study.*

16.4 SINGLE PHOTON EMISSION TOMOGRAPHY

The first single photon emission computed tomography (SPECT) images were obtained in the early 1960s using separate scanning detectors (David Kuhl, USA); this was before the development of X-ray computed tomography. In the 1980s improvements to gamma camera design (field uniformity) confirmed these as the tomographic machines of choice, since they gave multiple slices in multiple orientations (axial, sagittal, coronal, and oblique sectional views).

SPECT has many advantages; perhaps the main one is the separation of overlapping interference that is the problem on planar views. By removing overlying background activity image, contrast can be significantly improved. Figure 16.10 illustrates how contrast can be improved by viewing separate slices rather than a volume source given by the planar image.

In this example the differences between planar image counts of 420, 450, and 400 would only just be visible ($1.5 \times \sqrt{400} = 30$) but pixel differences in the separate slices would be easily visible ($1.5 \times \sqrt{100} = 15$).

16.4.1 Principles of operation

Single head rotating gamma camera tomographic systems are mounted on special gantries that allow the detector head to rotate 360° around the patient (Fig. 16.11a). The camera takes a series of images at equal angular spacing called projections during its rotational movement. The detector usually stops at each projection during data collection using a step-and-shoot mode. Either a complete 360° or partial 180° rotation can be chosen. Image quality is improved by reducing the camera/patient distance so elliptical or noncircular orbits which follow patient contours improve image quality. Improvement in sensitivity can be significantly increased by using a 2- or 3-head camera (Fig. 16.11b).

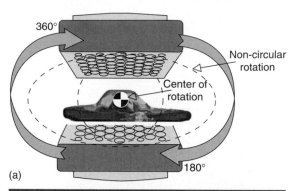

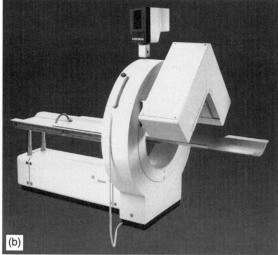

Figure 16.11 (*a*) *A single head rotating camera SPECT system using either a complete 360° or 180° collection. Circular and noncircular rotation is represented and the center of rotation.* (*b*) *Commercially available dual head SPECT system showing V opposed detectors for cardiac studies (courtesy GE Medical Inc.).*

DEDICATED SYSTEMS

These use multiple fixed detectors and have been exclusively developed for head scanning, giving single or multislice axial images. They have superior resolution to the rotating gamma camera but are restricted to axial tomographic planes. Some designs have four banks each of 16 NaI(Tl) detectors, the entire array rotates giving 40 projections in 180° rotation; this takes about 5 s and three slices are usually obtained simultaneously.

16.4.2 Machine requirements

Machine performance is critical for acceptable SPECT images. Careful choice of acquisition programs for

each organ study is necessary before embarking on a clinical study.

STEP-AND-SHOOT VERSUS CONTINUOUS DATA COLLECTION

There are two methods for collecting data from a rotating gamma camera:

- **Step and shoot** The camera indexes around the patient (stops to collect counts over a fixed time), then moves to the next projection and collects count data. It progresses around the patient until a full 360° (or 180°) data set has been collected. The data consists of 64 or 128 separate image matrices (size 64 × 64 or 128 × 128) which represent each projection.
- **Continuous rotation** The camera moves continuously collecting count data as it rotates for a complete 360°.

Step-and-shoot uses a considerable proportion of the scan time moving the camera between data acquisition points and waiting for the head to come to rest before collecting count data. Continuous rotation causes image blurring but as SPECT resolution is 10 to 15mm (at best), the blurring on a 64 projection 360° study is not significant. The speed of acquisition is much improved.

ANGULAR SAMPLING

This is determined by the resolution of the camera system. For gamma cameras with resolutions of 5 to 10 mm equivalent to a spatial frequency of $1\,cm^{-1}$ then the sampling frequency should be at least $2\,cm^{-1}$. An angular sampling interval of 3° should be maintained (120 projections). When a full 360° coverage has been made using an inadequate number of views the data distortion shows as image streaking due to aliasing problems. A sampling interval greater than 5° gives aliasing artifacts due to insufficient sampling points.

CENTER OF ROTATION

If a parallel hole collimator is positioned around an object first at 0° then at 90° and again at 180° then 270° the collimator at 0° should exactly align with the 180° position and again at 90° and 270°. The cells of the reconstructed matrix will then exactly coincide and a point source at the center of camera rotation will be situated exactly at the matrix center. In practice there

SPECT

FWHM

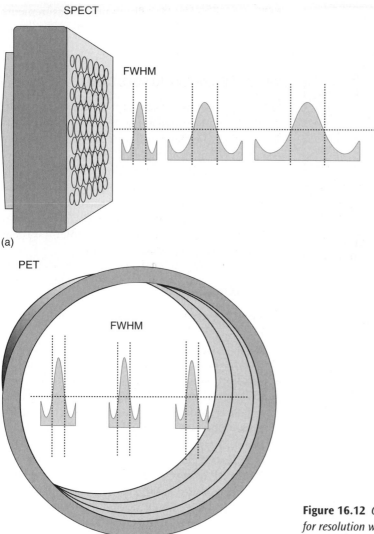

(a)

PET

FWHM

(b)

Figure 16.12 *Comparison between (a) SPECT and (b) PET for resolution with depth. A PET scanner maintains uniform resolution with depth.*

is always a slight misalignment due to mechanical errors and corrections must be made for this off-set error. Camera SPECT phantoms are available that allow the center of rotation to be identified before data collection.

NONCIRCULAR ORBITS

The patient in cross section is essentially ellipsoid so that the distance between the camera face and the patient will vary drastically with a circular camera orbit. Resolution deteriorates with distance, so the resulting tomographic image will show unsharpness. Noncircular orbits, illustrated in Fig. 16.11a, can be

achieved by either moving the detector in an elliptical path or by moving the table towards and away from the camera face while the camera itself traces a circular orbit. With the moving table technique image reconstruction is simpler than with elliptical orbiting of the camera head.

360° OR 180° ACQUISITION

Most SPECT imaging procedures collect data from a full 360° orbit. Cardiac studies, however, lend themselves to 180° data collection since the heart is partially shielded by the liver on the right side; this organ contributes a high activity particularly with ^{99m}Tc heart

Box 16.6 Quality control for SPECT field uniformity

SPECT field uniformity is related to matrix count density and noise. For a 64×64 matrix (4096 pixels):

    5 million total counts gives 1220 per pixel, and $\sqrt{\text{pixel}} = 35$; 3% variation
    10 million total counts gives 2441 per pixel, and $\sqrt{\text{pixel}} = 49$; 2% variation
    30 million total counts gives 7324 per pixel, and $\sqrt{\text{pixel}} = 85$; 1% variation

Note that a 30 million count density image matrix gives a noise figure suitable for SPECT calibration.

agents. Collecting data over 180° can save substantial time and improve image contrast; the camera can also be kept closer to the heart. Incomplete sampling can introduce artifacts and in the case of cardiac studies reduce information from the posterior wall of the ventricle.

UNIFORMITY

This is most important in SPECT imaging since a central non-uniformity of 3% can generate SPECT errors of 30%. Accurate non-uniformity correction must be applied before data collection, and measured for each collimator used. The reason for high count densities in the uniformity measurement is explained in Box 16.6 and in order to achieve the necessary accuracy when using a 64×64 matrix a total of 30 million counts must be collected.

16.4.3 Machine performance and image quality

The resolution given by SPECT images is worse than planar, due to count limitation. However, contrast levels are much improved.

RESOLUTION

This is simply measured by using a thin line source parallel to the image plane and measuring the full width at half maximum (FWHM) from this or the MTF (see Chapter 8). Resolution measurements should be taken at different distances from the detector face(s).

VARIABLE SPATIAL RESOLUTION

SPECT gives non-uniformity of resolution with depth; this is illustrated in Fig. 16.12a. Positron emission tomography has a uniform resolution across the detector field of view (Fig. 16.12b).

The loss of SPECT resolution with depth using two collimator types (general purpose and high resolution) is plotted in Fig. 16.13a and emphasizes the value of the high resolution collimator if resolution is to be maintained. A double headed SPECT system reduces this resolution loss still further.

SPECT CONTRAST

Using an asymmetric window over the photopeak set at 135 to 160 keV improves the image contrast by between 5 and 20% by decreasing scatter events. There are problems, however, with computing the attenuation correction for asymmetric windows which leads to additional image non-uniformity.

Different composite phantoms can be used for pictorial displays of both resolution and contrast performance. A typical QC phantom drawn in Fig. 16.13b has a series of hollow and solid rods of various diameters placed within a cylindrical plastic container filled with about 400 MBq ^{99m}Tc. The hollow rods can be filled with varying activities of ^{99m}Tc and give low contrast information.

SLICE THICKNESS

This can be measured by using a known dimension grid source. The minimum slice thickness will be determined by the camera resolution. Thin slices will have maximum noise so image quality can be improved by choosing an optimum slice thickness before reconstruction or summing slices together after reconstruction.

Choosing a large slice thickness will reduce image contrast and increase partial volume effects (see Chapter 14). Since the resolution of a parallel hole collimator decreases with distance the reconstructed slice thickness increases toward the center of rotation; multi-head camera SPECT designs reduce this effect.

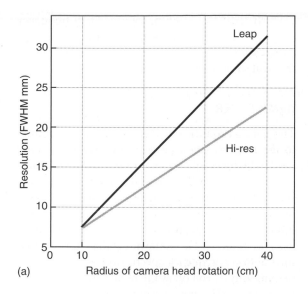

(a)

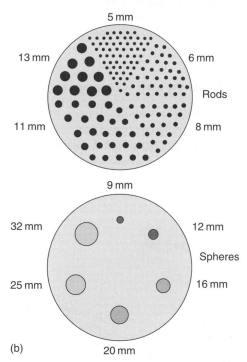

(b)

Figure 16.13 *(a) The loss of resolution from the face of the collimator in a SPECT study. A high resolution collimator maintains resolution but the study time is extended due to low sensitivity. (b) The test objects in a commercially available SPECT phantom. The rods are solid plastic which give negative 'holes' in an active background. The spheres are filled with different activities for high and low contrast levels.*

SPECT SENSITIVITY

This is defined as counts per second per MBq and is measured by imaging a 20 cm diameter cylindrical water phantom containing about 400 MBq ^{99m}Tc. It is important to quote the total number of axial slices being collected. Step-and-shoot systems show the poorest sensitivity, since they do not collect count data between projections. Long scan times using step and shoot improve sensitivity since more time is spent acquiring data than moving to the next projection.

16.4.4 Attenuation correction

Since the gamma camera collects data in a 2-D form calculation of a 3-D distribution from this data poses problems. A single slice through a volume source will present data as a single row of pixels across the camera face (ray-sum). Tissue activity near the surface contribute stronger signals than tissue of equal activity at the center of this row due to tissue attenuation. This leads to a cupping or depression of central values (similar to beam hardening in computed tomography).

If a uniform flood source is imaged without attenuation correction then this would show cupped images and profiles. In practice, attenuation leads to both spatial distortion in the final reconstruction and significant errors in quantitative accuracy. Correction is difficult and is commonly applied by assuming uniform distribution and knowing the dimensions of the object being imaged. Count data from opposing projections are averaged and to this modified projection a hyperbolic function is commonly added in order to boost the central regions of the projection. Attenuation distortion influences the image in the following ways:

- Surface detail emphasized while deeper detail in the center of the image is lost
- Pixel count density depends on position within the section preventing quantification of uptake
- Photon scattering from attenuation events destroys positional information
- Absolute uptake values cannot be obtained from a specific region of interest

Attenuation varies according to gamma energy; Fig. 16.14a compares 140 keV gamma photons (SPECT) with 511 keV (used in PET). Tissue attenuation is much less with the higher energy. **Transmission scans** (uniform activity on one side of the subject creating a shadow image on the camera) are useful for assessing true attenuation. Hardware and software are available for transmission correction and a commercial design is shown in Fig. 16.14b using a long lived nuclide (^{153}Gd; 97 and 103 keV; $T_{\frac{1}{2}}$ 242 d).

SPECT SCATTER PROBLEMS

Scattered photons can contribute to a significant number of events (up to 50%) and lesions which are seen as decreased areas of uptake (myocardial perfusion defects) suffer loss of contrast in the central regions of the image. Unless scattered correction is applied before attenuation correction an amplification of background noise will occur.

If scatter is assumed to be uniform then a background subtraction can be made before reconstruction. With a standard 20% photopeak window for ^{99m}Tc about 30% of the photons forming the image come from scattered events. Some compensation can be obtained by selecting an energy window that overshoots the photopeak by about 5% (asymmetric windowing).

16.4.5 Pre- and post-reconstruction filters

Pre-image filtration reduces noise content of the data set so preventing artifacts from appearing in the reconstructed tomographic images. High frequency noise in the projection image degrades the reconstructed image. Post-image filtration can be applied that will smooth or edge enhance images.

RAMP FILTER

This would produce a mathematically exact solution to the reconstruction problem but the data would need to be collected over an infinite number of angles with infinitely small pixels and maximum counts. It retains the highest spatial frequencies but, of course, would amplify any noise. Although this filter has very limited practical application it is basic to all filters used in SPECT. The following filters use a ramp for the lower frequency spectrum in the image and then modify or roll off at the higher frequency component by combining a second filter; this is called filter windowing. The window can be set to 'cut off' at a certain frequency so tailoring the filter to specific conditions.

BUTTERWORTH AND HAMMING FILTERS

These filters give varying degrees of smoothing with the Hamming filter giving the greater amount. Both the cut-off frequency and the slope of the roll off can be varied.

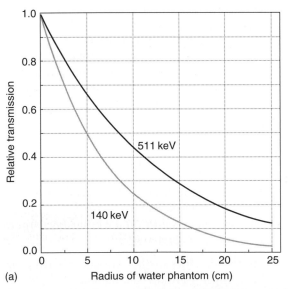

(a)

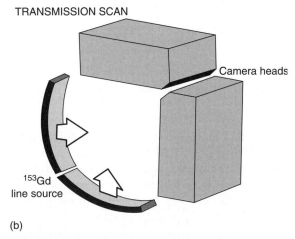

(b)

Figure 16.14 *(a) Photon transmission with depth in water for SPECT and PET imaging. Attenuation is less with 511 keV photons and correction is simpler since two photons are emitted. (b) Attenuation correction obtained by reference to a radionuclide source contained in the white rod which is scanned across the field of view.*

HANNING FILTER

This filter reduces higher spatial frequencies so fine detail is lost. The filter choice should reflect both the frequency content of the noise and the diagnostic frequency content of the organ. Figure 16.15 demonstrates how windowed filters differ from the basic ramp filter.

16.4.6 Practical aspects

Several important parameters must be considered before acquiring a SPECT study. A trial acquisition should be taken using a phantom holding about 200 MBq ^{99m}Tc. This can either be a commercially available phantom (seen in Fig. 16.13b) or a simple drum of uniform activity.

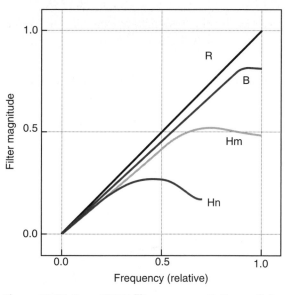

Figure 16.15 *Some SPECT filter responses: Butterworth B, Hamming Hm and Hanning Hn, compared to a simple ramp filter R.*

SUMMARY SPECT

The advantages and disadvantages of SPECT are summarized below.

Advantages

- Improved contrast
- Multi-planar reconstruction matching CT and MRI

Disadvantages

- Non-uniform sensitivity
- Slow so fast dynamic events cannot be followed
- Low photon density
- Poorer resolution
- Variable resolution with depth
- Accurate attenuation correction essential

RECOMMENDED PROTOCOLS

Common SPECT protocols are listed in Table 16.15. Before setting up a SPECT protocol the following choices should be made:

- Quality control
- Uniformity reference
- Center of rotation reference
- Size of image matrix
- Collimator choice
- Number of projections or angular increments
- 360° or 180° orbit
- Time per projection
- Total counts collected

During reconstruction the filter type should be selected and attenuation correction applied. Commercially available camera designs for SPECT are shown in Fig. 16.16.

Table 16.15 *SPECT protocols.*

Study	^{99m}Tc agent	Collimator	Projections	Counts per projection	Time projection (s)
Cerebral	HMPAO (700 MBq)	High resolution	64 to 128 over 360°	50k	20 to 10
Cardiac	MIBI (500 MBq)	High resolution	64 to 128 over 180°	30k	40 to 20
Lumbar spine	MDP	High resolution	64 to 128 over 360°	50k	40 to 20
Liver	Colloid	LEAP	64 to 128 over 180°	50k	40 to 20
Lungs	MAA aerosol	High sensitivity	64 over 360°	20k	20

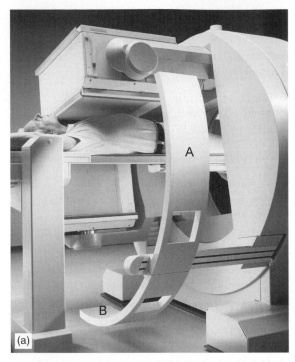

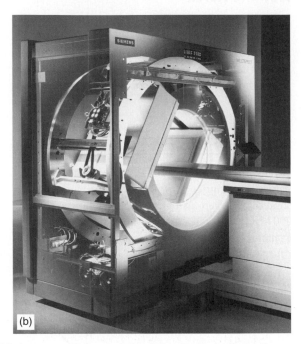

Figure 16.16 *Two rectangular field of view gamma cameras (**a**) ring gantry with a single head showing transmission line sources A and B and (**b**) double head SPECT design (courtesy Siemens Medical Inc.).*

16.5 POSITRON EMISSION TOMOGRAPHY

POSITRON FORMATION AND DECAY

Positron emission tomography (PET) uses cyclotron produced β^+ isotopes to provide an imaging procedure that takes advantage of the unique coincident gamma radiation. Positrons are emitted in the beta decay of nuclei which contain a proton excess for their mass (see Chapter 15):

$$_1^1\mathrm{P}_0 \rightarrow {}_0^1\mathrm{n}_1 + \left(\beta^+ + \nu\right)$$

$$\beta^+ \rightarrow \gamma + \gamma$$

where the gammas are 511 keV each, and opposed by 180°. The proton is converted into a neutron, and a positron and a neutrino are emitted. Because of the nature of the decay, sharing energy between the positron and the neutrino, the emitted positrons have a range of kinetic energies. After a period in thermal equilibrium the positron will annihilate with an electron (β^-) into two 511 keV photons emitted back-to-back (180° apart).

In an absorbing medium (e.g. soft tissue or bone), the emitted positron slows down to thermal energies in a few picoseconds (10^{-12} s) having traveled up to 1 mm (less in a denser medium).

POSITRON NUCLIDE PRODUCTION

Cyclotron production of positron emitting isotopes has been described in Chapter 15. Recent cyclotron models using super-conducting magnets have dramatically reduced cyclotron size so that small, department based positron imaging systems are now commercially available with their own integral shielding.

POSITRON IMAGING

Positron emission tomography (PET) is based on the existence of positron emitting isotopes of low atomic number elements such as carbon, nitrogen, oxygen, and fluorine. These elements can be used to make tracers with the same or similar chemical forms to naturally occurring biological substrates. PET offers the greatest sensitivity of all diagnostic imaging techniques. Table 16.16 indicates the tissue concentration of labeled compounds necessary for imaging;

Table 16.16 *Applications and concentrations.*

Target	Specific activity (MBq/mole)	Tissue concentration (g/g tissue)
Metabolites (e.g. glucose)	2.5×10^{-3} to 2.5×10^{-2}	0.2 to 1.0×10^{-3}
Neurotransmitters (e.g. adrenaline)	2.5 to 25	0.2 to 2.0×10^{-6}
Receptor sites (e.g. morphine, DOPA)	2.5×10^3 to 2.5×10^5	0.04 to 4.0×10^{-9}

they range through milli-, micro-, and nanogram amounts. The unique coincident gamma events, 180° opposed, provides 'self-collimation' which significantly improves detection sensitivity. Attenuation correction is also simplified, due to the paired gammas, and resolution loss with depth is much reduced. Resolution and contrast are superior to SPECT images and recent software developments have enabled both coronal and sagittal sections to accompany the familiar high quality axial images. More precise localization of positron events gives superior resolution (theoretically 3 mm); far superior to SPECT images. Accurate attenuation correction allows quantification of activity.

SENSITIVITY

PET has established an increasingly proven clinical role, primarily using 2-[^{18}F]fluoro-2-deoxy-D-glucose (^{18}F-FDG) in oncology, but also in cardiology and neurology. Extreme sensitivity (approximately $\times 1000$ that of SPECT) means that dangerous, addictive or toxic materials can be labeled and target organs and receptor sites identified with picogram quantities of agent. Figure 16.17 shows examples. Positron radionuclides can be incorporated into complex biological molecules without distorting them: glucose, DOPA, alkaloids etc. Short half-lives give very small patient doses but a cyclotron must be on-site for continuous delivery.

16.5.1 Clinical cyclotron specifications

Most hospital cyclotrons accelerate negative hydrogen ions (H^-) which are stripped to protons by a carbon stripper foil prior to bombarding the target.

$$H^- \rightarrow p + e^-$$

The general design was shown earlier (Chapter 15). Very heavy shielding is not required in small cyclotron installations and beam currents are intentionally restricted to 100 μA. Beam currents are commonly 50 μA which limits surface dose on the cyclotron surface to 25 μSv h^{-1}; this simplifies protective shielding requirements. The target area at the exit port of the cyclotron is surrounded by up to 90 cm of boronated polyethylene which is a very effective barrier to neutrons formed during the various reactions.

Table 16.17 gives typical specifications for a small cyclotron design, illustrated in Fig. 16.18. This has a 12 MeV proton beam designed to produce ^{11}C, ^{13}N, ^{15}O, and ^{18}F. Higher beam energies require larger shielding thicknesses. Most small cyclotrons use super-conducting magnets which give high intensity magnetic fields. This further reduces the size and weight of the installation and consumes less power. The whole cyclotron sits inside its own integral shielding forming a complete room sized unit.

CYCLOTRON DERIVED PET RADIONUCLIDES

Table 16.18 lists useful cyclotron derived positron emitters. Each one has a good yield but their half-lives differ considerably. Different positron isotopes can be chosen by selecting a particular target on a remote changer. In some instances less abundant (and so more expensive) stable isotopes are used as target material for (p,n) reactions.

16.5.2 Automated chemistry modules

These are provided by most small cyclotron manufacturers in order to simplify production of labeled compounds. Some common compounds that can be rapidly manufactured 'on-line' are listed in Table 16.19. Some of them are precursors for other more complex compounds while compounds such as carbon monoxide, carbon dioxide, and water are used directly for regional blood flow measurement.

Figure 16.18 gives a simplified design for a positron imaging facility complete with small cyclotron, radiopharmacy unit for preparing the labeled compounds and the dedicated PET scanner. The whole imaging suite can occupy the basement or ground floor of a diagnostic imaging department. The weight of the cyclotron and its shielding precludes low-weight-bearing floors.

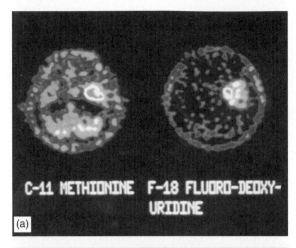

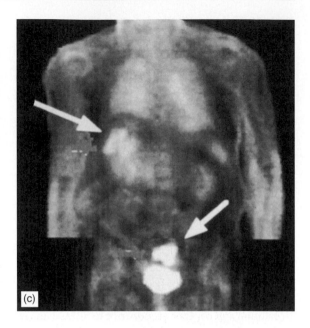

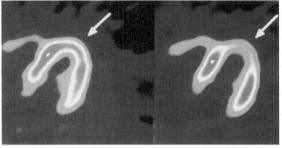

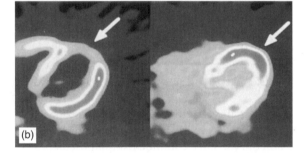

Figure 16.17 *Examples of PET scans. (a) Axial scan of brain using ^{11}C and ^{18}F compounds for the same high grade glioma (courtesy Tohoku University, Japan). (b) Heart sections demonstrating the value of ^{18}F-FDG for metabolism and $^{13}NH_3$ for perfusion studies. (c) Coronal section of the body showing ^{18}F-FDG used for oncology (courtesy Guy's & St. Thomas's Hospital, London, UK).*

Table 16.17 *Specifications for a small cyclotron.*

Energy (protons)	12 MeV
Beam current	100 μA
Ion source	H$^-$
Mean field strength	2.35 T
Orbit frequency	36 MHz
Radio frequency	108 MHz
Weight	3000 kg
Power consumption	25 kW

[^{18}F]FLUORODEOXYGLUCOSE

A significant development in the clinical value of positron imaging was the synthesis of 2-[^{18}F]fluoro-2-deoxy-D-glucose (^{18}F-FDG) at Brookhaven National Laboratory in 1976.

^{18}F-FDG is a glucose analog and gives an accurate picture of regional metabolism in brain, heart, body organs, and tumors (Fig. 16.17). ^{18}F has a half-life of 110 min which allows transport away from the cyclotron unit to local hospitals who have PET imaging facilities. The relatively long half-life also gives

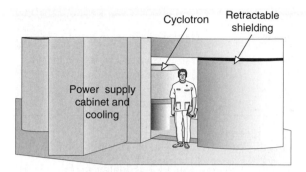

Figure 16.18 *Basic design for small clinical cyclotron that can be built into a room complete with concrete shielding.*

Table 16.18 *Positron radionuclides available from an on-site cyclotron.*

Nuclide	Half-life (min)	β^+ yield (%)	β^+ energy (MeV)
^{15}O	2.0	99.9	0.735
^{13}N	9.9	99.8	0.491
^{11}C	20.4	99.8	0.385
^{18}F	109.8	96.9	0.242

time for identifying tumors and metastases with whole-body scans. The imaging and quantification of ^{18}F-FDG in malignant or suspect space occupying lesions helps clinical management by indicating:

- Tumor site
- Whether the tumor is malignant, benign or scar tissue
- Effectiveness of any therapy
- Subsequent spread of the initial cancer site

BIOCHEMISTRY OF FDG

The mechanism of ^{18}F-FDG localization in cells metabolizing glucose is illustrated in Fig. 16.19.

Table 16.19 *Positron compounds.*

Positron emitter	Labeled compounds	Dose (H_E) (mSv per 40 MBq)	Clinical use
^{11}C	^{11}CO, $^{11}CO_2$, $^{11}CN-$, $^{11}CH_3I$, $H^{11}CHO$	0.05 to 0.2	Dopamine uptake sites, brain Opiate receptor sites, brain Amino acid metabolism Cellular proliferation
^{13}N	$^{13}N_2$, $^{13}NH_3$	0.002 to 0.05	Blood flow Myocardial perfusion
^{15}O	$^{15}O_2$, $H_2^{15}O$, $C^{15}O$, $C^{15}O_2$	0.02 to 0.2	Metabolism activity Cerebral blood flow
^{18}F	$^{18}F_2$, $H^{18}F$, $^{18}F-$, ^{18}F-FDG	0.5	Glucose metabolism Dopamine storage Cellular proliferation

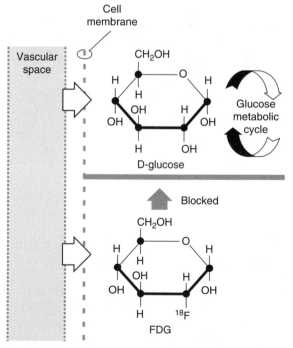

Figure 16.19 *Chemical formula for ^{18}F-FDG showing replacement of an OH^- group in glucose with a ^{18}F atom.*

Table 16.20 *Positron radionuclides available from generator sources.*

Generator	Half-life (min)	β^+ yield (%)	β^+ energy (MeV)	Clinical application
^{68}Ga	68.1	89	0.740	Transmission source, tumor imaging
^{82}Rb	76.4	95	1.409	Myocardial perfusion
^{62}Cu	9.7	97	1.280	Myocardial perfusion
^{122}I	3.6	77	1.087	Thyroid metastases

Following the intracellular transport, ^{18}F-FDG is phosphorylated to give ^{18}F-FDG-6-phosphate. This is a foreign analog of glucose-6-phosphate and since it is not recognized by the cell enzyme glucose-6-phosphatase it takes no further part in the glucose phosphorylation cycle and remains immobile, trapped within the cell.

Experimental and clinical studies have demonstrated that ^{18}F-FDG uptake in cancer cells correlates with growth rate and so is a good indicator for malignancy. The high uptake in these regions enables tumor sites to be easily localized. Evaluating the exact localization of the tumor for staging, treatment planning or follow-up requires an anatomic framework for the PET image.

GENERATOR DERIVED PET RADIONUCLIDES

A cyclotron is not an essential item for some studies since useful positron nuclides can be obtained from good shelf life generators. Table 16.20 lists some commercially available or prototype generators useful for clinical application.

16.5.3 Clinical applications

ONCOLOGY

To date the greatest developments in PET imaging have been in oncology. A number of PET radiopharmaceuticals have been utilized for oncological investigations. The majority of PET imaging centers on FDG labeled with ^{18}F. The 110 min half-life not only makes whole-body imaging practical but allows for multicenter distribution of the tracer.

The high aerobic glycolytic rate of most tumors means that there is a much higher uptake of FDG in malignant tissues than in normal tissue. Quantitative analysis techniques include dynamic studies which generate absolute glucose metabolic rates and simple relative quantitative ratios, known as standardized

uptake values (SUVs). The main applications are:

- **Tumor evaluation** PET is highly useful in non-invasively evaluating the size and grade of various types of tumors.
- **Determination of necrotic tissue** PET can differentiate recurrent tumor growth from necrotic tissue following radiation therapy.

CARDIOLOGY

Advantages of cardiac PET over SPECT imaging include higher spatial resolution, accurate attenuation correction, and the capability to perform quantitative measurements. In the detection of coronary artery disease, PET imaging has a sensitivity of 92%, a specificity of 89% (higher than SPECT, which is about 75%). The higher specificity is related to the capability of PET imaging in providing reliable attenuation correction that decreases the false positive rate. The main applications are:

- **Regional myocardial blood flow** PET, through the use of cyclotron produced [^{13}N]ammonia or generator produced ^{82}Rb, provides high sensitivity and specificity in the detection of coronary artery disease (CAD).
- **Myocardial tissue viability** PET, using metabolic agents, is unique in its ability to determine if myocardial tissue is metabolically alive or dead.

NEUROLOGY CNS IMAGING

PET is very sensitive in the early detection of epilepic foci. It is also valuable for imaging the regional distribution of cerebral blood volume (CBV). Cerebral blood flow (CBF) can be measured by using either [^{15}O]water, carbon [^{15}O]dioxide, or ^{11}C-butanol and either [^{18}F]fluorodeoxyglucose or ^{11}C-deoxyglucose can be used to determine cerebral metabolic rate for glucose.

In a normal resting brain, cerebral blood flow, glucose metabolism, and cerebral metabolic rate are linked by a constant relationship which is a useful indicator for localizing cerebral infarction. Major applications are:

- **Dementia** PET has been widely investigated in the diagnosis and differentiation of dementia types. Alzheimer's disease and multi-infarct dementia are readily diagnosed and differentiated.
- **Psychiatric disorders** PET has the capability to reveal functional changes in cerebral biochemistry associated with behavioral disorders.
- **Epilepsy** PET provides the ability to identify focal lesions, aiding in the diagnosis and treatment of epilepsy.
- **Cerebrovascular disease** PET has provided an understanding of the pathophysiology of transient ischemic attack (TIA) and acute infarction. It has proven to be a valuable approach for in-vivo studies of the localization, progression, and resolution of the associate cerebral injury in these disorders.

ADVANTAGES OF PET

PET provides quantitative in-vivo measurement of many functional processes: perfusion, metabolism, and receptors. PET can localize and measure the distribution of neuroreceptors by detecting sub-nanomolar concentrations of labeled drugs (see Table 16.16). The spatial resolution of the PET scanner is superior to SPECT. The high temporal resolution of PET (high count rate) also permits dynamic imaging. Figure 16.17 gives examples of PET images in cardiology, neurology, and oncology. The axial images acquired by the PET system can be reformatted in sagittal and coronal sections as well as any chosen oblique view.

16.5.4 Imaging principles/event location

The two major types of current clinical PET instrumentation are the dual-head gamma camera with coincidence detection and the dedicated PET with a full-ring of detectors. Brownell and Sweet at Massachusetts General Hospital made the first positron medical image in 1951. The first cyclotron dedicated to medical use was installed at Hammersmith Hospital, London, in 1955.

There are three major requirements for positron imaging:

- Distinguishing the opposed 180° gamma photons from background nonpositron derived gamma

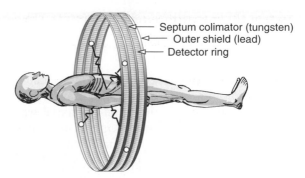

Figure 16.20 *Basic design of a PET scanner showing detector ring, collimators, and end shielding.*

photons, using geometry or time of flight information
- Identifying the angle of travel
- Reconstruction of the activity distribution

A basic dedicated PET machine for axial images is shown in Fig. 16.20. It contains opposed detectors in a ring formation for collecting 180° opposed gamma events in coincidence. Spatial resolution is independent of depth within the section provided the coincidence detectors are sufficiently far apart and occupy about 60% of the detector diameter. The probability of two noncoincident events occurring in opposing detectors is reduced by shortening the coincidence resolving time (usually 12 ns).

When an event is detected in coincidence the line passing through the site of annihilation can be identified as a **line of response** (LOR). A large number of events must be collected from which the spatial distribution of the tracer can be determined. True coincidence events can only be recorded from a positron annihilation that occurs within a boundary defined by the two opposing detectors. If the positron annihilation occurs outside this boundary, then only one detector can pick up a 511 keV photon in the annihilation pair.

16.5.5 Coincidence detection

Registering a coincident event depends on the two 180° opposed photons being detected by the system within a specified time interval known as the 'coincidence window' (typically 10 to 20 ns). All events (E) that are found in coincidence can be true (T), random (R) or scatter (S) coincident events. These events are related by the formula

$$E = T + R + S$$

The true events represent the good data. The random events can be estimated and corrected, and the scatter can be rejected. Depending on the crystal type and thickness a fraction of true events will be lost due to the lack of sensitivity and dead time of the detector material. The location of the coincident event (hence the location of the positron emitter) is assumed to be along the path between the two detectors, but this is complicated in practice since not all events found in coincidence are true coincidence events (Fig. 16.21a, b, and c).

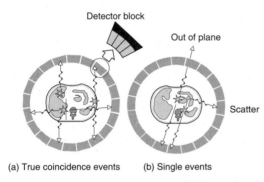

(a) True coincidence events   (b) Single events

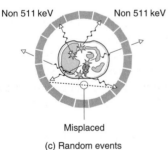

(c) Random events

Figure 16.21 *Event detection by a PET scanner. **(a)** True coincidence events where the 180° opposed photons are detected. A magnified detector block is shown comprising four separate PMT units shown in more detail in Fig. 16.22a and b. **(b)** Single events. Either an out-of-plane coincidence or one photon of a true coincidence is scattered. A scattered annihilation photon (with reduced energy) can be detected in coincidence with a true 511 keV photon within the 511 keV window and in the same coincidence time. **(c)** Two photons that are not 511 keV are detected separately or the detection of two 511 keV photons generated from annihilations of two separate positrons giving a misplaced line of response (see text).*

TRUE COINCIDENT EVENTS

A true coincidence is the simultaneous interaction of emissions resulting from a single nuclear transformation. Figure 16.21a shows two such events.

A typical complication occurs when two photons from separate annihilation events are found in coincidence due to close timing of the coincidence window. PET relies on the coincident detection of photons in two detectors. Pulses are considered to be coincident if they occur in two detectors within a specified resolving time τ of each other. Because of this finite resolving time there is the possibility of two independent pulses occurring by chance so as to produce a random coincidence. The resolving time τ for the coincidence window in the most recent PET scanners is typically 6 ns with a coincidence time resolution of $\approx$3 ns within the window.

RANDOM EVENTS

Simple probability provides that given singles rates S_1 and S_2 for a pair of detectors and a coincidence window of width 2τ then events will be found in coincidence due to random occurrence with a rate:

$$R = 2\tau \times S_1 \times S_2$$

These coincidences occur at random within the coincidence window (Fig. 16.21b). Since the detector's 'singles' rate is proportional to the imaged activity, then the 'random' rate is proportional to the square of the activity. This contrasts with the 'true' coincident events, which are only proportional to the activity. Random coincident events become a limiting factor at higher activities and may limit the activity which may usefully be imaged. Thus as the real coincidence count rate increases, the proportion of randoms also increases, eventually becoming unacceptable; this is particularly serious when the **efficiency** of the detectors is low.

It is possible to detect just the random coincidences by introducing a delay into one arm of the coincidence circuit, and these can then be subtracted from the full data. Usually 'randoms' measurement is done in parallel with the normal data collection. Theoretically, this enables an exact correction to be made for the presence of randoms but in practice because of limited statistics the quality of the data deteriorates dramatically once the number of randoms exceeds the number of real coincidences.

Minimizing the coincidence window is important as well as any optimization that increases the trues to singles ratio. If the singles rates for each detector pair are measured, randoms can be estimated either directly by the formula or by a second delayed coincidence window. A narrow event window is essential if false coincident randoms are to be rejected.

Random coincidences can be reduced by using a shorter coincidence timing and increasing the ring radius of the detectors. Random coincidences can occur when there are two simultaneous positron–electron annihilations. The opposing detectors simultaneously detect uncorrelated 511 keV photons. Acceptance of the random coincidence falsely records the event as arising from a line drawn between the two detectors.

SCATTER EVENTS

A scatter coincidence occurs when one or both gamma photons from an annihilation are scattered but both are detected within a single detector ring. Scatter coincidences are seen as true coincidences, so the correction for accidental coincidences does not compensate for them.

One or both of the photons from a single positron annihilation event may scatter in the object of interest (Fig. 16.21c). Annihilation radiations may undergo scattering while passing through the body tissue, and because of the high energy (511 keV), most of these scattered radiations move in the forward direction without much loss of energy (see Chapter 3 on X-ray scatter) so these will be accepted within the energy window of 511 keV and therefore be counted as true coincidences. The position information of the event is lost. In practice scattered events constitute a significant fraction of the events detected by the system (10 to 20% of total counts in a 2-D system and 40 to 60% of total counts in a 3-D system).

PET machines using **septal collimator rings** (Fig. 16.20) markedly reduce scatter events from being collected, due to improved geometric efficiency. If an annihilation occurs within a particular detector ring then if either of the photons scatters, it is most likely that the new trajectory of the photon will cause it to miss the detector ring, thereby preventing a scatter coincidence. Since loss of photon energy during scatter places the event below the energy window, most of these scatter events are eliminated. However, a scatter event having a 10° change in direction results

in an energy change of only 7.6 keV in 503.3 keV so places it within the coincident window and this could account for a radius error in the line of response (LOR) of over 85 mm (see misplaced event in Fig. 16.21c).

16.5.6 PET detector materials

The detection of 511 keV photons for PET scanners requires:

- High coincidence photopeak efficiency (41%)
- Good timing resolution (approximately 3 ns)
- Good energy resolution (approximately 13% FWHM)
- Fast scintillation decay constant (better than 300 ns)

The commonly used scintillation materials are bismuth germinate ($BiGeO_4$ or BGO), cerium activated lutetium oxyorthosilicate (Lu_2OSiO_4:Ce or LSO), cerium activated gadolinium oxyorthosilicate (Gd_2OSiO_4:Ce or GSO) and thallium activated sodium iodide (NaI:Tl). Table 16.21 lists the major properties of these scintillator materials.

BISMUTH GERMINATE

BGO crystals have a high stopping power (high efficiency), high spatial resolution, and are 50% more efficient than NaI(Tl) crystals. Most crystals are 3 to 6 mm thick and are not hydrophilic. The spatial resolution approaches 5 mm which nears the theoretical limit of resolution. The disadvantages of BGO crystals are that they have a much lower light output (15% of NaI(Tl) crystals), long photofluorescent decay times (decay constant of 300 ns which limits count rates/coincidence timing resolution), and poorer energy resolution than sodium iodide crystals. Energy resolution of BGO is normally worse than 20% in FWHM at 511 keV. This poor energy resolution makes it difficult to remove scattered events by energy discrimination. The coincidence time window is normally set for 10 to 20 ns. The inferior time resolution causes larger accidental detections and greater dead times. BGO detectors are best suited for imaging isotopes with long half-lives such as ^{18}F and [11]C. Detector material should have a high absorption coefficient for 511 keV gammas and BGO has over ×2 greater attenuation than NaI(Tl).

Table 16.21 *Properties of detector materials used in positron emission tomography.*

Property	Characteristic	Desired value	LSO	BGO	GSO	NaI
Density (g cm^{-3})	Define detection efficiency of detector and scanner sensitivity	High	7.4	7.1	6.7	3.7
Effective atomic number		High	79	75	59	51
Decay time (ns)	Defines detector dead time and randoms rejection	Low	40	300	60	230
Relative light output (%)	Impacts spatial and energy resolution	High	35	15	75	100
Energy resolution (%)	Influences scatter rejection	Low	15	20	10	7.8
Attenuation for 511 keV	Sensitivity	High	12	11	14	29
Nonhygroscopic	Simplifies manufacturing, improves reliability	Yes	Yes	Yes	Yes	No

LUTETIUM OXYORTHOSILICATE

LSO offers the best combination of properties for PET imaging. LSO has a higher effective Z (number of protons per atom) and density compared to BGO which results in a higher detection efficiency. It has a short decay constant for improved coincidence timing (decay constant 40 ns), and higher light output (compared to BGO). The crystal is rugged and non-hygroscopic and lends itself to precise machining.

GADOLINIUM OXYORTHOSILICATE

GSO gives a better energy resolution and higher light output than LSO. It also has better attenuation for 511 keV photons; its light decay time is slightly higher.

SODIUM IODIDE DOPED WITH THALLIUM

Although NaI detectors have a relatively low stopping power compared to other PET detectors, they demonstrate very good energy resolution (11%) and have excellent light yield. The better energy resolution permits lower energy thresholds approaching 435 keV (rather than 350 keV) to limit scattered events without reducing true events (the window has an upper threshold of 665 keV). The coincidence time window is typically 8 ns which is an improvement on BGO systems. A shorter coincidence time window should improve counting characteristics. The system has a long crystal decay time (230 ns) compared to LSO systems (40 ns), but this is shorter than the decay time for BGO (300 ns).

SUMMARY

Bismuth germanate (BGO) and lutetium orthosilicate (LSO) are currently the preferred materials for scintillation detectors in PET scanners because their higher densities and atomic numbers make them more sensitive than NaI(Tl) to higher energy 511 keV gamma photons.

The attenuation length for 511 keV photons in both BGO and LSO crystals is approximately 10 mm. The scintillation light yield of BGO (15%) is significantly less than that of NaI(Tl), but is sufficient for high-energy photon detection; LSO has an improved light yield (75%); both are nonhygroscopic, permitting the material to be cut into small sections and packed tightly into element arrays without a metal hermetic seal. Figure 16.22 shows a block of scintillator material (either BGO, LSO or GSO) backed by four matching photomultipliers. The scintillator block is cut to form an 8 × 8 matrix.

16.5.7 The gamma camera PET system

Dual-head gamma camera SPECT systems can be upgraded for coincidence imaging using thicker crystals of 5/8 or 3/8 inch (16 mm or 19 mm) than are used for ^{99m}Tc imaging; this increases the camera sensitivity to 511 keV photons. Even then the absorption fraction of 511 keV photons is 0.10, leading to an efficiency of only 0.01 for coincidence detection.

Since coincidence imaging is done with collimators removed, the gamma camera detectors must be able to operate at more than 1 million cps. Since conventional collimators are not present, the reconstructed resolution is solely determined by the intrinsic resolution of the gamma camera detector in coincidence mode, which is approximately 6 mm FWHM although in clinical practice this is usually nearer 10 mm.

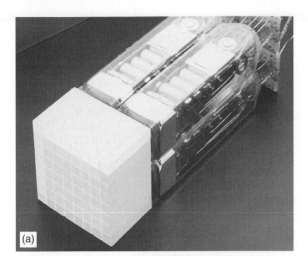

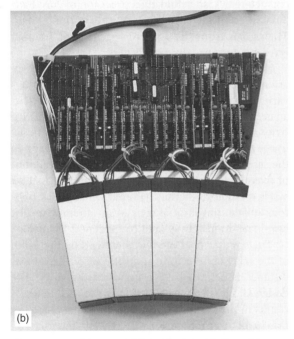

Figure 16.22 *(a) Group of four photomultipliers with a scintillator block. This can be the nonhydroscopic bismuth germanate (BGO), lutetium oxyorthosilicate (LSO) or gadolinium oxyorthosilicate (GSO). (**b**) A detector unit comprising four of the groups shown in (a).*

Table 16.22 *Comparison of gamma camera and dedicated PET scanner.*

Specification	Dual head 5/8″ camera PET	PET ring scanner BGO
Imaging times for whole body (min)	60	30
2-D mode sensitivity (kcps pCi^{-1} mL^{-1})	25	200 to 220
3-D mode sensitivity (kcps pCi^{-1} mL^{-1})	275	900 to 1225
2-D mode noise equivalent count rate (peak) (kcps)	2	97 to 159
3-D mode noise equivalent count rate (peak) (kcps)	4	88 to 261
2-D mode scatter fraction	24%	10% to 16%
3-D mode scatter fraction	37%	35%
Detection efficiency		
140 keV (^{99m}Tc)	94%	
511 keV	17%	92%
511 keV (in coincidence)	3%	85%
Intrinsic resolution (mm)	4 to 6	3.5 to 4
Clinical resolution (mm)	7 to 10	5 to 6

imaging and thus hold the prospect of cheaper PET imaging in a routine clinical department. In principle, all that is needed to allow a dual headed gamma camera to perform PET imaging is the addition of coincidence circuitry. Dual-head gamma cameras with coincidence detection have the advantage of their lower cost and their ability to perform SPECT and routine nuclear medicine studies using ^{99m}Tc. Their application to PET imaging however reveals serious limitations. The performance specifications for the two systems: gamma camera and dedicated scanner are compared in Table 16.22. They have much lower sensitivities resulting in noisy images; they also have high scatter and inaccurate photon attenuation correction. These disadvantages significantly reduce resolution and smaller lesions cannot be detected. So for this reason, PET imaging has switched almost entirely to the dedicated PET with a full ring of detectors, where sensitivity and count rate performance are much higher than those of dual-head gamma cameras and corrections for scattering and attenuation allow quantitative studies. Dedicated PET systems can perform whole-body imaging with ^{18}F-FDG where lesion size limitation is between 5 mm and 7 mm as against 10 mm for the best gamma camera system.

In noncoincident SPECT mode, using 511 keV collimators, only 20 mm resolution can be achieved. This is not satisfactory for capturing diagnostic information.

Although gamma camera PET systems, even in coincident mode, offer only poor quality images compared to dedicated PET systems, they retain the ability to perform conventional nuclear medicine

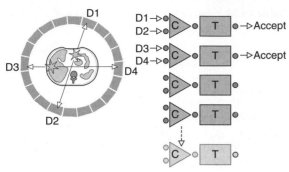

Figure 16.23 *The schematic of a basic positron section scanner with circular detector arrays showing coincidence comparators (C) and time windows (T). Two pairs of detectors are active (D1/D2 and D3/D4).*

16.5.8 The PET scanner

Current PET scanners have large fields of view, built-in attenuation correction and computerized whole-body techniques that allow images of the entire body to be acquired in approximately 30 min compared to 1 h for gamma camera PET systems. Resolutions are in the 5 to 6 mm range in all three planes, although smaller lesions with highly increased uptake can be easily identified. The best gamma camera systems give 7 to 10 mm resolution. A block diagram of a PET scanner with its associated coincidence detection circuitry is shown in Fig. 16.23. The performance specifications for a typical PET Scanner are listed in Table 16.23.

THE BLOCK DETECTOR

Current PET systems use large segmented block scintillators, each of which is coupled to four square photomultipliers. Each machined detector block is about 3 cm deep and grooved into 6 × 8, 7 × 8, or 8 × 8 elements (see Fig. 16.23); (a comparable LSO block is thinner). The nonhygroscopic detectors (BGO, LSO, and GSO) permit the material to be cut into small sections and packed into element arrays without the problem of supplying a hermetic seal (NaI).

The block detector design shown in Fig. 16.22 uses an encoding system with four photomultipliers viewing 64 scintillation detectors arranged in an 8 × 8 matrix. The position of the gamma ray interaction in a given element is determined by the combined light output from the four PM tubes in the same way as positional information is obtained in a gamma camera.

Table 16.23 *Specification for a typical PET scanner.*

Item	PET scanner
Block detectors	288
PMT per block	4
PMT total	1152
Segments	8 × 8
Size (mm)	4.05 × 4.39 × 30
Total detectors	18 432
Number of rings	32
Coincidence time resolution	6 ns
Ring diameter	82.7 cm
Field of view	15.5 cm

Each PMT is corrected for its own response time characteristics, so achieving a precision of 2 ns. Each block uses a time encoder with a resolution of 4 ns. The signals from the PMTs in each block are analyzed for position, time, and energy.

Many thousands of individual detectors are arranged as a circular array. The number of rings varies from 18 to 32. Coincidence detection between adjacent rings also is used, further increasing sensitivity and giving rise to an additional cross-sectional image situated halfway between the detector rings. In the case of a three-ring detector, the reconstructions of five cross-sectional slices are possible. Most PET systems employ collimating septa which block photons incident at large angles in an attempt to discriminate against unwanted coincidences (scatter).

The scanner field of view is defined by the width of the array of detectors, and the source-to-detector distance is defined by the radius of the array. The design of equally spaced crystal rows and columns results in the scanner's homogeneous spatial resolution in all three dimensions.

THE GANTRY

The gantry (see Fig. 16.20) houses the crystal scintillation units and electronics, septal ring assemblies, patient alignment lasers and rotating source mounts, which provide for mounting phantoms and ring sources for use in testing, calibrating, and imaging procedures.

SEPTAL RINGS

The septal collimator ring assembly consists of a series of 1 mm thick tungsten disks, spaced and positioned to align with the tiny gaps between the rings of detectors. The outside diameter fits close to the inside of the detector rings (see Fig. 16.20). The outside edges of the active region of the scanners are shielded with thicker disks of lead. The septal rings and edge shields are stationary. Septal assemblies reduce scatter from out-of-plane activity and in-plane scatter to the detector rings. This reduces single count rates and improves the ratio of coincident events to noncoincident events.

EXTERNAL SOURCE MOTION

A computer controlled gantry movement is 'detector wobble'. This is a two-detector wide orbit motion which more finely samples the spatial data acquired for image reconstruction (similar to focal spot movement in CT). The PET scanner commonly uses three eccentric cams driven by a variable speed motor to swing the physical center of the detector ring assembly in a circle. The ring assembly does not rotate nor move axially. Wobble is used to double the spatial sampling frequency and to decompress the angular sampling raster in sinograms. Wobbling during acquisition provides the finest resolution possible for delineation of small structures at the expense of increased memory utilization and reconstruction time. For high patient throughput the wobble is disabled and imaging performed in a stationary mode.

16.5.9 Data acquisition

Maximum data acquisition is typically 1 million events per second. Image processing typically takes less than 10 s. The signals are decoded for position, time, and energy of the detected event. The time encoder defines the time of the 511 keV event to within 2 ns of its appearance. The events recorded by the coincident detectors are used in a similar manner to computer tomography for reconstructing an axial slice of activity. The accuracy of reconstruction depends on the number of detectors in the detector ring; a typical PET system can contain 300 detectors.

The real-time sorter (RTS) receives 32 bit line-of-response (LOR) data produced by the image plane coincidence processor through a standard, double-buffered memory. These data, together with current wobble position, geometrically specify the line along which the annihilation event apparently occurred.

Each module is polled for output every 256 ns by the ring receiver. All combinations of module pairs

are checked by the image plane coincidence processor for events typically within 12 ns wide coincidence windows. These windows accept over 95% of all true coincidence events detected from annihilations within the entire patient port volume.

EVENT LOCATION

The distance traveled by the positrons before annihilation also adversely affects resolution. This distance is limited by the maximal positron energy of the radionuclide and the density of the tissue. A radionuclide that emits lower energy positrons yields superior resolution. Table 16.18 lists the maximal energies of positrons emitted by radionuclides commonly used in PET and the graph of β^+ energy versus mean distance traveled before annihilation is plotted in Fig. 16.24. Activity in bone yields higher resolution than activity in soft tissue, which in turn yields higher resolution than activity in lung tissue. Thus, the site of photon emission differs from the site of annihilation photons. The distance of the positron path increases with the positron energy, and this phenomenon degrades the spatial resolution. Therefore, high-energy β^+ emitters give poorer spatial resolution than low-energy β^+ emitters, myocardial perfusion imaging with

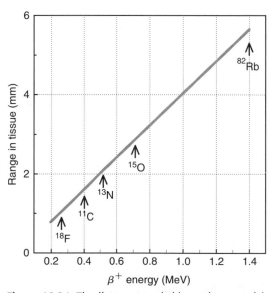

Figure 16.24 *The distance traveled by positron particles in tissue (in millimeters) produced from five clinically used radionuclides. This distance, before anhilation, will degrade image resolution since positron origin and eventual annihilation radiation will not coincide.*

[^{13}N]ammonia ($\beta^+ = 0.491$ MeV) will give better spatial resolution than that with ^{82}Rb ($\beta^+ = 1.409$ MeV). Furthermore, two annihilation photons are not always emitted at 180°, because the positron–electron pair is not completely at rest during annihilation. Such angular deviations may be of the order of 0.25° and can also degrade the spatial resolution of the image.

IMAGE ACQUISITION: 2-D VERSUS 3-D

Lead or tungsten septa are placed between the detectors for 2-D acquisitions to absorbed scattered radiation. The septa reduce the amount of scatter to 10 to 15% of the total counts acquired.

When the septa are removed (3-D acquisition), each individual detector is sensitive to radiations from a much larger area and the count rate increases 5- to 6-fold. Three-dimensional imaging can significantly reduce the tracer activity needed or shorten the acquisition time. Disadvantages of 3-D scanning are the counting rate limit of the scanner, increased random events, and increased scatter. Also 3-D scanning requires more computer memory and more time for image reconstruction.

For a given total counting rate, the fraction of random events recorded will be greater when scanning in 3-D mode. When scanning in a high counting rate environment, the random counting rate increases much more rapidly than does the true counting rate as a function of radioactivity in and near the field of view. The true counting rate scales linearly with radioactivity in the field of view, while the random rate scales as the square of the radioactivity in and near the field of view.

In the 3-D mode, the number of scattered events approaches half of all recorded events. Because of this, for proper quantification, a scatter correction must be applied to 3-D data. Three-dimensional scanning is advantageous when the count rate is much lower and the benefit from additional events far outweighs any loss attributed to increasing the fraction of random and scatter events.

TIME OF FLIGHT MEASUREMENT

Incorporating the time of flight into image reconstruction can significantly improve resolution. If the coincident radiation originates from the center of the source (patient's head) then the two gamma photons will reach the opposing detectors at the same time; however, if the positron annihilation is at the surface of the source then the coincident gammas will arrive at different times. Since they are traveling at the speed of light very fast timing circuits are needed. Commercial systems are capable of resolving events less than 200 ps apart (0.2 ns). Several detector materials are used for PET scanners.

Coincidence circuits check the simultaneity of the PMT pulses to within 7.5 ns. When coincident, a single coincident event is recorded; otherwise, the PMT pulses are rejected. The detector closest to the positron–electron annihilation event picks up the 511 keV photon first. Photons travel at approximately 30 cm ns^{-1} (speed of light) so for a 15 ns coincidence timing window, the detectors must be separated by more than 4.5 m before time-of-flight differences are a factor. Prototype PET scanners are available that use a 0.3 ns coincidence timing window, which allows the system to localize the annihilation event to within 10 cm. Instability of the timing circuits at such short time intervals can be a major problem.

'Time of flight' PET (TOF PET) imaging systems have very short resolving times and coincidence localization can be obtained to within a fraction of a nanosecond, permitting improved sensitivity and signal-to-noise ratio. The coincidence time window is normally set for 2 ns or less. The time difference between the arrival of the two events at the detectors is used to approximate the origin of the pair (see Fig. 16.25). The use of deeper detectors also degrades image resolution so LSO and GSO detectors have the advantage. The major function of TOF PET is to improve statistical data, not spatial resolution. TOF PET is best for imaging large objects with low contrast (due to the presence of less background noise) and for studying dynamic processes.

SINOGRAMS

These organize the data so that it can be examined more readily. Coincident events (line-of-response or LOR) for all projection rays are sorted and stored into sinograms. The LOR has a certain angular inclination and a radial distance from the central axis so it is convenient to adopt a cylindrical coordinate system for storing tomographic image data into these sinograms (Fig. 16.26). The illustration shows how sinograms are constructed by combining information from several LORs (Fig. 16.26a) and representing these as projected points on a sine wave (Fig. 16.26b). The collection of many such views can be presented as a 2-D plot or image; each is a 1-D profile of measured attenuation as a function of position, corresponding to a particular angle. This is the sinogram of the 2-D slice; a collection represents the entire image (Fig. 16.26c).

The phase and amplitude of the sine wave is unique to the **source location** in the tomographic plane. The intensity of the sine wave indicates **source**

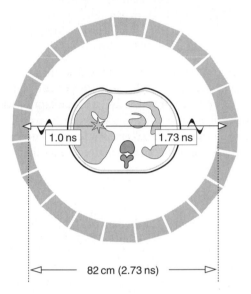

Figure 16.25 *Time of flight calculation for a gantry diameter of 82 cm. A very fast clock is required in the electronic timing if this information is to augment coincidence geometry in localizing the positron event.*

strength. The sinograms are transferred to the array processor and used for transaxial image reconstruction using a standard spatial filter (Shepp–Logan, Butterworth, Hann, Hamming, a simple ramp filter, or a specific user defined filter). Image construction from these sinograms then relies on filtered back-projection or iterative reconstruction.

16.5.10 Attenuation correction

The linear attenuation coefficient for 511 keV photons in soft tissue is $0.09\,cm^{-1}$, compared to $0.15\,cm^{-1}$ for 140 keV photons of ^{99m}Tc, but because coincidence detection requires two 511 keV photons to be detected, both photons must exit the patient. Therefore the total thickness of the patient cross section along each projection ray always enters into the photon attenuation problem. Fig. 16.14 compares photon transmission through a 25 cm water phantom for 140 keV (^{99m}Tc) amd 511 keV photons.

TRANSMISSION SCAN

The attenuation of the patient is determined by using a transmission acquisition, which is then used to generate transaxial maps which resemble CT images and provide sufficient information to define the various densities inside the thorax (lungs and heart). These maps, along with the emission data, are used to correct for attenuation using an iterative reconstruction method. It is usual to perform a coincidence–transmission study on the PET scanner by rotating a rod or pin source of

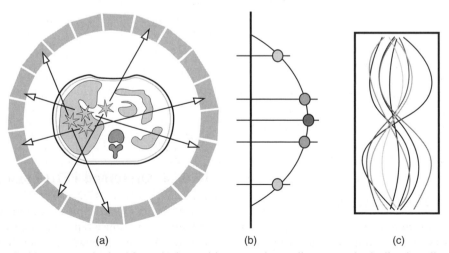

(a) (b) (c)

Figure 16.26 *Coincident events obtained from the image (**a**) are sorted according to angular inclination, distance and activity. (**b**) This information represented as a series of sinograms (**c**).*

^{68}Ge/^{68}Ga about the patient, and computing the linear attenuation coefficient map.

^{68}Ge (electron capture, $T_{1/2}$ 288 d) → ^{68}Ga (β^+ emission, $T_{1/2}$ 68 min)

The PET scanner is commonly equipped with ring source holders which are filled with ^{68}Ge. During a transmission scan, the patient is positioned as for an emission scan, usually with no internal positron activity present. The transmission source is placed just inside the septal ring and then data are acquired for several minutes; the time depends on the strength of the source. After removing the ring, internal activity can be administered to the patient and imaged as emission data.

16.5.11 Image reconstruction and image quality

RECONSTRUCTION METHODS

These can be grouped into two general classes: direct and iterative. Direct methods, such as filtered back-projection, have been used in most PET reconstructions. Iterative reconstruction algorithms offer much more flexibility and can correct for non-uniform attenuation. Attenuation, scatter, and the detector response function can be modeled in iterative reconstruction algorithms, so they are clearly the choice for attenuation correction.

SENSITIVITY

The sensitivity of PET systems depends on the detector material, slice thickness, and the diameter of the ring. Sensitivity is ultimately determined by many factors like the detection efficiency of the crystal, system geometry and acquisition mode (2-D or 3-D). Since two photons must be detected to record one coincidence event, coincidence sensitivity is proportional to the square of the detector efficiency.

Sensitivity increases with slice thickness at the loss of resolution along the depth. It also increases with decreasing ring diameter as an increasing number of coincidence events are detected. To increase the sensitivity of coincidence detection large energy windows are used, typically 50% wide. A significant portion of the interactions in the scintillator crystal are Compton interactions of unscattered 511 keV photons. Widening the energy window to include these interactions increases the probability of coincidence

detection. To minimize the detection of scattered photons at least one of the photons must be within the 511 keV photopeak.

High performance dedicated PET systems have evolved to provide a photopeak coincidence interaction probability of 85% at 511 keV.

SPATIAL RESOLUTION

Modern PET systems achieve a spatial resolution of about 5 mm FWHM of the line spread function. There are four factors that primarily determine the spatial resolution of PET scanners:

- The intrinsic resolution of the detectors
- The scattering of photons in the patient
- The distance traveled by the positrons before annihilation
- The annihilation photons are not emitted in exactly opposite directions from each other

The resolution limit in positron imaging is largely determined by the intrinsic detector resolution.

The resolution achievable by any PET imaging system is ultimately limited by the finite range of the positron prior to annihilation and the effect of the slight nonlinearity of the two photons (the paired photons not exactly at 180°). If a pair of detectors separated by 50 cm is used to detect the photons then the uncertainty in location arising from this nonlinearity is around 1 mm. However, in practice, detector systems never achieve this level of precision. For PET, the best resolution achievable is around 5 mm. This depends mostly on the imaged radionuclide and, to some extent, on the detector radius. For example, ^{18}F ($\beta^+_{max} = 0.6$ MeV) has better resolution (i.e. shorter distance before the positron annihilates into two photons) than ^{15}O ($\beta^+_{max} = 2.1$ MeV).

Several other factors will contribute to the final reconstructed image resolution. For PET on gamma cameras, the reconstructed resolution is about 10 mm. For premium dedicated PET scanners, this resolution can reach 5 mm.

16.5.12 Combined PET/CT systems

Combined positron emission tomography (PET) and computed tomography (CT) imaging was first used on patients in 1998. CT and PET images are acquired in sequence, one directly following the other and without the patient leaving the imaging table. This permits exact correspondence between the CT and PET axial image.

In some newer systems, a CT X-ray tube and a PET camera are mounted on a single gantry that rotates at a constant speed. They are mounted such that the centers of the PET and CT imaging fields are separated by a fixed distance. In a single imaging session, CT images are first taken with the region of interest at the center of the CT field of view. Then the imaging table with the patient lying in the same position is moved to the center of the PET field of view, and PET images are taken. Because the patient does not move, both CT anatomical images and PET functional images can be superimposed with accurate alignment. Furthermore, CT transmission data can be used to make attenuation corrections for PET images.

The idea of a hybrid imaging system is relatively simple: to incorporate two different but complementary modalities into a system that, in a single study, can produce images showing functional data mapped precisely on to the corresponding anatomy.

Diagnostic imaging can be divided into two broad categories: anatomical imaging and functional imaging, the former such as CT and MRI, which shows anatomical structure, and the latter functional imaging largely the domain of nuclear medicine (particularly PET) which shows physiological processes. MRI has entered the world of functional imaging but this is still in its infancy.

The ability of CT to produce high resolution, 3-D anatomical images is well established, but so are its functional limitations on the basis of anatomical changes: a dead person will give the same CT image as a healthy person! Early-stage disease can be difficult to differentiate from normal appearances. Radionuclide techniques identify disturbances in the body's biochemical processes that are often the first signs of pathology. Radionuclide images generally lack the anatomical detail needed to pinpoint the lesion. Although the PET image has improved resolution over SPECT images they still lack precision. Although CT and PET images can be reported separately interpretation is improved when they are overlaid.

16.6 COMPARISON OF OTHER TOMOGRAPHIC TECHNIQUES

Positron emission tomography, single photon emission computed tomography, and nuclear magnetic

Table 16.24 *Comparison of CT, MRI, SPECT, and PET.*

System	Specific details
CT	
Collimated source and detector	Multiple axes
	Fixed source to detector position
	No attenuation problems
	Good signal strength
SPECT	
Collimated detector	Multiple axes
Photopeak windowed	Attenuation corrected
	Good signal strength
	Poor resolution (10 mm)
PET	
Coincident detectors	Multiple axes
Internal source (β^+ nuclides)	No attenuation problems
	Good signal strength
Fixed energy (511 keV)	At least $\times 2$ sensitivity of SPECT
	Good resolution (5 to 7 mm)
	Radionuclides physiologically based (carbon, nitrogen, oxygen)
MRI	
General/local coils	Radio signals
Magnetic field	Multiple axes
^{1}H, ^{31}P, ^{23}Na images	RF signal attenuation
	Poor signal strength
	Functional information

resonance imaging have now reached a degree of maturity where it is possible to assess where, if at all, any overlap occurs in their clinical usefulness. The early expectations that MRI would provide similar information as SPECT or PET in measuring regional metabolic processes has not been realized. The sensitivity of these three imaging processes is given in Table 16.24. The normal composition of living tissues includes, in addition to hydrogen, other elements that can generate nuclear magnetic resonance (NMR) signals (see Chapters 19 and 20). Unfortunately, because of their low concentration in soft tissues and their lower NMR sensitivity (compared to hydrogen) their image gives a very high signal-to-noise ratio. At the present time the MRI image of ^{31}P is poorer than conventional nuclear medicine imaging.

The application of tracer techniques in MRI is severely limited by the low signal-to-noise ratio which requires high concentrations of a stable NMR isotope to give a good image. This invalidates tracer techniques in MRI for studying metabolic processes: compare the concentrations required for imaging drug receptor sites in PET and the use of sub-toxic levels of ^{201}Tl for cardiac imaging in nuclear medicine. The present MRI resolution for protons is about 1 mm. The best achievable PET resolution is 3 mm but with a sensitivity about 10^{12} times greater than MRI. SPECT has a best resolution figure of about 5 mm with a similar sensitivity as PET but over a much limited range of useful metabolic tracers. The usefulness of MRI has been recognized as a non-ionizing investigation and its ability to deliver multiple section planes (axial, sagittal, coronal, and oblique). Disadvantages are length of study time limiting good quality studies to the head and extremities at a distance from respiratory movement, cost, and lack of sensitivity. The usefulness of PET has become established mostly for investigating physiological processes.

A certain number of clinical investigations have been identified, particularly brain receptor sites of psychotropic drugs (morphine, LDOPA) and metabolic agents (glucose) for cardiac function (perfusion, metabolism, and blood pool). With a sufficiently large population of patient material the cost per examination decreases to the level of MRI and complex nuclear medicine studies (cardiac and labeled white cell imaging). The usefulness of SPECT is more varied. Its resolution and contrast is lower than PET.

Multiple section acquisition leads to section overlap and interference. The isotopes available are more limited but have become wider since the introduction of ^{99m}Tc labeled brain perfusion (HMPAO) and cardiac (MIBI) agents.

Other radiopharmaceuticals specifically developed for SPECT imaging would increase the usefulness and more routine application of SPECT. The complementary nature of MRI, PET, and SPECT seems to reduce competition among the three imaging methods. MRI gives superb morphological information which allows integration with the functional images of PET and SPECT.

CT images are purely anatomical in character with no physiological information but, because they provide valuable anatomical information, the combination of CT and PET or SPECT becomes a potentially powerful imaging set.

FURTHER READING

Institute of Physical Sciences in Medicine (1991) *Radiation Protection in Nuclear Medicine and Pathology*. Report No. 63. ISPM, York, UK.

International Commission on Radiological Protection (1977) *The Handling, Storage, Use and Disposal of Unsealed Radionuclides in Hospitals and Medical Research Establishments*. ICRP Publication 25. Pergamon Press, Oxford, UK.

Loevinger R, Budinger TF, Watson EE (1988) *The MIRD Primer for Absorbed Dose Calculations*. Society of Nuclear Medicine, New York.

Maisey MN, Britton KE, Gilday DL (1991) *Clinical Nuclear Medicine*. Chapman and Hall, London.

National Council on Radiation Protection and Measurements (1996) *Sources and Magnitude of Occupational and Public Exposures from Nuclear Medicine*. NCRP Report 124. NCRP, Bethesda MD.

National Electrical Manufacturers' Association (1986) *Performance Measurements of Scintillation Cameras*. NEMA report NUI-1986. NEMA, Washington.

KEYWORDS

alpha decay: nucleus loses two neutrons and two protons in the form of a helium nucleus

angular sampling: the sampling interval for SPECT imaging

Bateman equation: describes parent:daughter decay in a radionuclide generator

beta decay: the unstable nucleus loses a positive or negative beta particle

body surface area: this is computed for dose or GFR calculations. Combines an individual's weight and height as $W^{0.425} \times H^{0.725} \times 0.0072 \, m^2$

center of rotation: adjusted so that 0° and 90° and 180° and 360° positions align before the acquisition of SPECT data

collimator: the device in front of the camera crystal that accepts gamma photons only from a particular angle. Common collimators have a parallel hole design that only accepts, gamma photons perpendicular to the crystal face

collimator: a device which fits onto a probe or gamma camera accepting only gamma photons from a particular direction. Parallel hole gamma camera collimators only accept radiation perpendicular to the detector surface

controlled area: a room or location where the maximum exposure level is $7.5\ \mu Sv\ h^{-1}$

cyclotron: a charged particle accelerator where the beam travels in a circular path. Used for manufacturing short-lived positron emitters

dead time: the point at which measured count rates fall short of incident count rates for a detector

dynamic study: a study where a certain number of timed frames are collected (see renogram)

electron cascade: the successive filling of empty orbit locations after electron loss leading to characteristic X-ray photons

field uniformity: acceptable planar imaging non-uniformity in the central field of view is about 3% but SPECT requires a uniformity of <1%

filters: image data is filtered pre- and post-reconstruction to reduce noise. There are also smoothing and edge enhancement filters

first pass: a fast dynamic study which follows transit of a bolus of activity (e.g. heart/lungs)

gated acquisition: image data acquisition under the control of a gating signal either ECG or respiration

generator: a device for generating clinically useful daughter products from a long lived parent, e.g. $^{99}Mo/^{99m}Tc$ and $^{81}Rb/^{81m}Kr$

group classification: a radionuclide toxicity classification ranging from group 1 (most toxic) to group 4 (least toxic). Group classification determines the limits for safe disposal

half-life (biological): the time taken for half the activity of a substance to be excreted. A recommended symbol is $t_{1/2}$

half-life (effective): the sum of the biological and physical half-lives

half-life (physical): the time taken for a given activity of a radionuclide to reach half its initial value. A recommended symbol is $T_{1/2}$

internal conversion: excess nuclear energy is transferred to a K- or L-shell electron. This is a competing process with gamma emission and reduces the incidence of gamma photon emission

isobar: nuclides having a constant mass A (a constant) but varying proton Z and neutron N values, e.g. ^{201}Hg, ^{201}Tl, ^{201}Pb

isomeric transition: the decay of a metastable state yielding a single gamma photon only (pure gamma emitter), e.g. ^{99m}Tc and ^{99}Tc are isomers

isotone: nuclides with a constant neutron number N (a constant) but varying proton number. The stable isotones with $N = 1$ are ^{1}H and ^{2}H

isotope: nuclides with the same proton number (Z constant) but different neutron numbers. The three stable isotopes of oxygen are ^{16}O, ^{17}O, and ^{18}O. Radioactive isotopes of oxygen are ^{14}O ($T_{1/2} = 1.2\ min$) and ^{15}O ($T_{1/2} = 2\ min$)

Marinelli formula: an early method for calculating internal dose rates using a simple organ geometry estimation but with no organ to organ contribution

metastable state: a excited nuclear state existing after alpha or beta decay lasting for seconds, minutes, hours or days. Sometimes called isomeric state. Indicated as, e.g. ^{99m}Tc. (Some publications might use the previous notation of $^{99}Tc^m$)

MIRD formula: an improved internal dose estimation with better organ geometry factor and the addition of contributing organ activity

moderator: a material used in nuclear reactors to slow down neutron velocities. Typical moderators are graphite or heavy water (D_2O)

MUGA: multi-gated acquisition using the ECG for gating heart images according to their position in the cardiac cycle

multiphase study: a dynamic study using a mixture of frame timings

neutron capture: slow and thermal neutron reaction of the form (n,γ) indicating gamma photon emission. A common method for preparing clinical nuclides, e.g. ^{60}Co, ^{125}I

non-uniformity (differential): percentage maximum difference between two adjacent pixels. Typical value $\leq \pm 1.5\%$

non-uniformity (integral): the percentage difference between maximum and minimum pixel counts in a sampling area. Typical value $\leq \pm 2.0\%$

nuclide: a specific nuclear species identified by the form EQ where A is the atomic mass, Z the proton number and N the neutron number. Consists of stable and unstable nuclides

oxidation state: this is related to the valency state of an ion which influences chemical combination. Iron has two oxidation states, ferrous, Fe^{II}, and ferric, Fe^{III}, whereas technetium has seven

PET: positron emission tomography using the 180° opposed 511 keV gamma photons from positron annihilation

photopeak: the peak in an energy spectrum (e.g. scintillation detector) corresponding to complete photoelectric absorption

planar imaging: acquiring the volume activity image of an organ either as a static or dynamic sequence

Table 16.25 *Common investigations, the administered activity, and whole-body dose.*

Investigation	Radiopharmaceutical	Activity (MBq)	Whole-body dose, H_E (mSv)
WHO category I	(<0.5 mSv)		
Glomerular filtration rate	^{51}Cr-EDTA	3	0.01 to 0.03
Lung ventilation	^{81m}Kr gas	37	0.06
Effective renal plasma flow	^{125}I-hippuran	2	0.1 to 0.4
Thyroid uptake	^{123}I, oral	1	0.17
Renography	^{123}I-hippuran	12	0.2 to 0.4
Gastric emptying	^{99m}Tc-colloid, oral	12	0.3
Renography	^{99m}Tc-MAG3	75	0.2 to 0.3
	^{99m}Tc-DTPA	75	0.4 to 0.7
WHO category II	(0.5 to 5.0 mSv)		
Renography	^{131}I-hippuran	3	0.5
Thyroid imaging	[^{99m}Tc]pertechnetate	75	0.8
Lung perfusion	^{99m}Tc-MAA	75	0.9
Liver imaging	^{99m}Tc-colloid	75	1.0
Renal function	^{99m}Tc-DMSA	70	1.0
Thyroid imaging	[^{123}I]iodide	8	1.4
Plasma volume	^{125}I-albumin	0.2	1.5
Hepatobiliary	^{99m}Tc-EHIDA	100	2
Renal blood flow	^{99m}Tc-DTPA	400	2.0 to 4.0
Meckel's diverticulum	[^{99m}Tc]pertechnetate	200	2.2
Brain perfusion	^{99m}Tc-HMPAO	500	2.5
Myocardial perfusion	^{99m}Tc-MIBI	400	2.7
Thyroid uptake	^{131}I oral	0.2	3.2
Cisternography	^{111}In-DTPA	30	3.6
Bone imaging	^{99m}Tc-MDP	550	3.7 to 6.0
Bone marrow	^{99m}Tc-nanocolloid	300	3.9
WHO category III	(5 to 50 mSv)		
Abscess	^{111}In	30	5.0
Brain	[^{99m}Tc]pertechnetate	500	5.5
Gated MUGA	^{99m}Tc-labeled red blood cells	800	5.6
Haemodynamics	[^{99m}Tc]pertechnetate	600	7.0
Myocardial	^{201}Tl chloride	75	7.0
Abscess imaging	^{67}Ga citrate	80	9.0

positron: β^+, the antiparticle to β^- or negatron (electron). The two mutually annihilate producing 180° opposed 0.511 MeV gamma photons

pulse height analyzer: an electronic circuit that can threshold the lower and upper limits of the photopeak energy and accept signals just within these limits

radiation area (high): (USA) an area where levels approach 1 mSv h^{-1} at 30 cm from the source

radiation area: (USA) a staff area where radiation levels approach 50 μSv h^{-1} at 30 cm from the source

radionuclide: an unstable nuclide

reactor: a critical assembly of fissile material, e.g. ^{235}U, ^{239}Pu, capable of a sustained chain reaction

renogram: an example of a dynamic study using multi-phase acquisition where, for instance, the vascular phase is collected as 30 frames at 0.5 s, GFR phase as 30 at 1 s and excretion phase as 30 at 20 s

resolution (energy): the FWHM dimension of a photopeak, the energy spread at this level expressed as a percentage of the peak energy. A typical value for a single NaI(Tl) detector would be 8%. A gamma camera value would be 11%

resolution (extrinsic): the spatial resolution of a gamma camera with the collimator in place. Measured in millimeters. A typical high resolution collimator gives 5 mm FWHM

resolution (intrinsic): the spatial resolution of a gamma camera with the collimator removed and using a line source. A typical value would be 3 mm FWHM

resolution (spatial): see extrinsic and intrinsic resolution

secular equilibrium: a parent:daughter decay series where $\lambda_d > \lambda_p$

shelf life: a measure of radionuclide storage, related to half-life. ^{123}I has a poor shelf life ($T_{\frac{1}{2}} = 13\,\text{h}$) whereas ^{201}Tl has a good shelf life ($T_{\frac{1}{2}} = 3.0\,\text{d}$)

SPECT: Single photon emission computed tomography. Axial tomographic images acquired by rotating a gamma camera 180° or 360° around the patient and reconstructing multiple slices according to the camera field of view. Coronal and sagittal slices can be obtained from the axial information

step and shoot: as opposed to continuous rotation where the camera stops at each angular projection and acquires data

target organ: the organ receiving most activity. The thyroid is the target organ for iodine radionuclides and ^{99m}Tc

time of flight: improving PET resolution by including time of detection for the coincidence gammas

transient equilibrium: a parent:daughter decay series where $\lambda_d > \lambda_p$

WHO category: a segregation of labeled radiopharmaceuticals according to patient dose. There are three groups denoting high, medium, and low radiation dose (see Table 16.25)

Principles of ultrasound

17.1 PROPERTIES OF ULTRASOUND

Ultrasound waves have frequencies many times higher than the upper limit for human hearing. A comparative range of common sound frequencies is given in Table 17.1 along with the clinical ultrasound range for comparison.

High frequency ultrasound can provide information about tissues *in vivo* by producing a sound image. Rapid image formation can reveal organ movement in real time. Ultrasound differs from most conventional imaging methods in two important ways:

- The ultrasound beam is a non-ionizing longitudinal wave (unlike electromagnetic radiation).
- The signal is recorded in reflection rather than transmission mode (unlike X-ray imaging).

Table 17.1 *Frequencies and hearing range of common sounds.*

Hearing range, or sound	Frequency
Audible range	15 to 20000 Hz
Range for children's hearing	Up to 40000 Hz
Male speaking voice	100 to 1500 Hz
Female speaking voice	150 to 2500 Hz
Middle C	262 Hz
Concert A	440 Hz
Top C	2093 Hz
Bat sounds	50 000 to 200 000 Hz
Maximum sound frequency	6×10^8 (600 MHz)
Medical ultrasound	2.5 to 40 MHz

Ultrasound images are constructed by computing the time taken for an ultrasound beam to travel from a transducer, and return from a reflecting surface. Figure 17.1 shows an ultrasound pulse reflected from two surfaces at different depths. If the sound velocity in soft tissue is $6.7\,\mu s\,mm^{-1}$ ($1500\,m\,s^{-1}$) then from the time of arrival (round trip) the depth of the reflecting surface can be calculated.

The magnitude of the echo influences (modulates) the brightness of a display and is coded as a gray scale. An echo image is then built up to give an image of a body slice. Clinical ultrasound systems use computer methods for producing images continuously in 'real time' which has valuable clinical applications.

The ultrasound signal is produced by electrically stimulating a crystalline material to oscillate. Ultrasound waves obey all the conventional laws associated with light waves except they require a medium (gas, solid or liquid) for their transmission, which takes place by a sequence of compressions and rarefactions within the conducting medium (see Chapter 2).

17.1.1 Propagation

Sound waves are **longitudinal waves** and require a medium (gas, liquid, solid) for their transmission. The passage of ultrasound energy through a medium is illustrated in Fig. 17.2a; the material boundaries or molecules are represented as flat plates connected by massless bonds shown as springs. A longitudinal wave transmits its energy through material by causing the

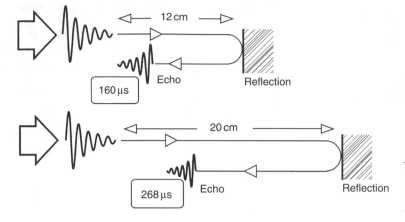

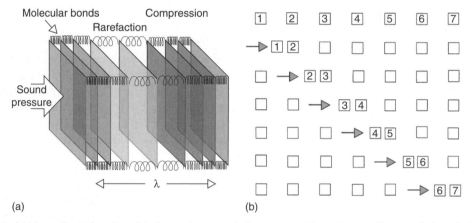

Figure 17.1 *Sound waves reflecting from two surfaces. Echo arrival is 160 μs and 280 μs for 12 and 20 cm depths, respectively. Speed of sound is 1.5 mm μs⁻¹ for soft tissue.*

Figure 17.2 *(a) Three-dimensional model of sound pressure being conveyed through a medium consisting of plates (molecules or particles) loosely connected by spring-like bonds. (b) Propagation of sound energy as elongation about a center of equilibrium (particle velocity about its center is v).*

molecules in its path to oscillate back and forth parallel to the direction of travel of the wave front; oscillations are shown as compressions traveling along the plates. Sound travel first involves molecular or particle vibration (elongation) at the excitation frequency. Sound particle velocity (elongation velocity v, in cm s⁻¹) is the velocity of a particle about its equilibrium position (v in Fig. 17.2b). The elongation disturbance **propagates** through the medium (tissue) at a specific propagation velocity c in m s⁻¹, the absolute speed depending on the medium.

A picture of ultrasound transmission is represented in Fig. 17.2(b) as a row of connected particles. The sound pressure applies a force from the left hand side to particle '1'. The force exerted on '1' causes it to acquire a velocity and be displaced to the right

both stretching and compressing the connecting bonds. Particle '2' now receives the force from '1' and '2' is now displaced.

The force having now been transferred, '1' now returns to its original position. The energy of the sound wave is contained in the compressed bonds or springs.

Ultrasound causes the particles in its path to oscillate back and forth at the particular frequency so mechanical energy is transported across the material. Particle '2' displacement is slightly smaller than '1' due to loss of heat energy within the bond, so the signal energy gradually decays.

This vibration phenomenon is repeated for the remaining particles, causing the original sound wave to be transported across the particles by compression and rarefaction events, as the particles move to and

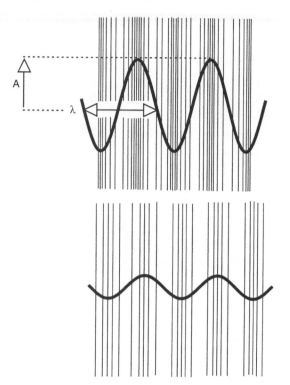

Figure 17.3 *Compression and rarefaction in a medium producing a sound wave with wavelength λ and amplitude* A *emulating a sine wave. A reduced power level is shown in the lower waveform.*

fro. This can be treated as a sine wave as shown in Fig. 17.3 which has wavelength λ, frequency f (cycles per second: Hz) and amplitude A depending on the sound pressure characteristics and transmitting medium.

17.1.2 Sound characteristics

SOUND PARTICLE VELOCITY, V

Sound particle velocity, v is the velocity of the material particles as they oscillate to and fro with the sound pressure. A typical value would be 35 mm s^{-1}.

ACOUSTIC PRESSURE, P

Acoustic pressure, p is caused by the pressure changes induced in the material by the sound energy measured in pascals (Pa). A typical value would be 0.06 MPa. Imaging pressures can be ×10 this value and Doppler pressures ×25, which has important safety associations.

FREQUENCY F AND WAVELENGTH Λ

These are identified in Fig. 17.3 where compression and rarefaction events in the medium are described as a sine wave having a frequency measured in cycles s^{-1} or hertz and a wavelength measured in millimeters (mm). Frequency and wavelength are related as λ = c/f where c is the speed of sound in the medium (tissue, bone, air etc.).

PROPAGATION VELOCITY

This is the speed with which the elongation displacement is transferred across the material and is measured in meters per second (m s^{-1}). The excitation in the medium propagates with a velocity specific to the material. The stiffer the springs in Fig. 17.2a and the smaller the molecular masses the greater the propagation velocity. The distance between repeated compression states is the wavelength of the propagation event. Propagation velocity, wavelength and frequency (Hz) are related as:

$$\lambda = \frac{v}{f} \qquad (17.1)$$

where λ is the wavelength, v is the propagation velocity, and f is the frequency. Propagation speeds increase from gases to liquids and are highest in solids. This is not directly related to material density but depends on increasing molecular bond stiffness or 'springiness'. A typical velocity for soft tissue (a mixture of connective tissue and fat) is between 1480 and 1568 m s^{-1}; a rounded value of 1500 m s^{-1} is used in order to simplify calculations. The magnitude of the force produced by each particle shown in Fig. 17.2b gradually decreases or **decays** as the wave travels across the medium.

From eqn 17.1 the propagation velocity is related to frequency of oscillation f in cycles s^{-1} (Hz) and its wavelength (λ, in meters) as:

$$c = \lambda f \text{ and } \lambda = \frac{c}{f} \qquad (17.2)$$

If the velocity of the ultrasound wave changes (traveling from one medium to another) then the wavelength and not the frequency changes (see Box 17.1). This is demonstrated in Fig. 17.4 for two different materials: soft tissue and bone for a frequency of

Box 17.1 Ultrasound wavelength change

Use eqn 17.2 to calculate the wavelength λ of a 2.0 MHz sound wave in

- soft tissue ($c = 1500\,\text{m s}^{-1}$)
- bone ($c = 4080\,\text{m s}^{-1}$)

For soft tissue:

$$\lambda = \frac{1500}{2 \times 10^6} = 7.5 \times 10^{-4}\,\text{m or } 0.75\,\text{mm}$$

For bone:

$$\lambda = \frac{4080}{2 \times 10^6} = 2.04 \times 10^{-3}\,\text{m or } 2.04\,\text{mm}$$

These values are represented by the waveforms in Fig. 17.4.

Table 17.2 *Frequency and wavelength for ultrasound in soft tissue.*

Frequency (MHz)	Wavelength (mm)
2.0	0.74
3.5	0.42
5.0	0.30
7.5	0.20
10.0	0.15

AMPLITUDE

The maximum amplitude coincides with the compression peak (*A* in Fig. 17.3). Reduced power levels give a reduced amplitude.

POWER

This is the rate at which work is done or the rate of sound energy transfer. It always contains a time period. Power is measured in watts (W = J s^{-1}).

INTENSITY

This is a measure of power per unit area and is commonly measured as W cm^{-2}. Comparative power and intensity are measured in decibels.

MODULUS OF ELASTICITY, *E*

The rate of transfer of the molecular displacement (the wave velocity) depends on the molecule's reluctance to motion and the density of the material. The material elasticity is measured as Young's modulus (Thomas Young, 1773–1829; British physicist/physician), measured as material stress under a given strain: E = stress/strain. Stiffer springs (higher modulus) and smaller molecular masses increase the propagation velocity *c* so that

$$c = \sqrt{\frac{E}{\rho}} \qquad (17.3)$$

where E is Young's modulus and ρ is the material density. As E increases, signifying stiffer springs, sound propagation velocity also increases.

The modulus of elasticity is inversely proportional to the **deformation** or compressibility $1/E$. The modulus of elasticity is measured in pressure units, gigapascals (GPa). Typical values of E are: fat 2.0 GPa, soft tissue 2.2 GPa, and bone 25 GPa. Bone has a larger

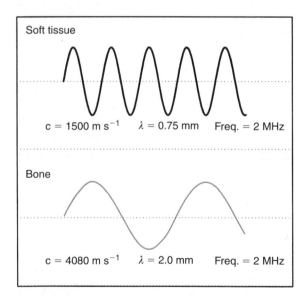

Figure 17.4 *Sound waves having the same frequency but different wavelengths when traveling in soft tissue and bone.*

2 MHz. Change of wavelength is an important consideration for imaging resolution. Examples of frequency and wavelength for ultrasound in soft tissue are given in Table 17.2.

Table 17.3 *Velocity, density, and acoustic impedance for clinical materials.*

Material	Speed of sound, c (m s^{-1})	Density, ρ (kg m^{-3})	Acoustic impedance, Z (kg m^{-2} s^{-1}, $\times 10^{-6}$)
Air	330	1.3	0.00043
Fat	1470	970	1.42
Castor oil	1500	933	1.40
Water	1492	1000	1.48
Soft tissue	1500	<1000	~1.45
Brain	1530	1020	1.56
Blood	1570	1020	1.60
Kidney	1561	1030	1.61
Liver	1549	1060	1.64
Muscle	1568	1040	1.63
Eye lens	1620	1130	1.83
Bone	4080	1700	6.12

value of E (less compressibility or deformation) so sound travels faster in bone than in soft tissue.

17.1.3 Acoustic impedance

When pressure p is applied to a molecule it will move exerting a pressure on an adjacent molecule and so setting up the sequence seen in Fig. 17.2b. Acoustic pressure increases with particle velocity v but it also depends on properties of the medium. The relationship between these parameters is characterized by the **acoustic impedance** Z so that

$$Z = \frac{p}{v} \qquad (17.4)$$

Acoustic impedance Z, sound pressure p and particle velocity v have certain similarities to electrical units of resistance R, voltage V and current I (see Chapter 2) so the following relationships exist:

$$v = \frac{p}{Z} \text{(analogous to } I = \frac{V}{R})$$
$$p = v \times Z \text{ (analogous to } V = I \times R)$$
$$Z = \frac{p}{v} \text{(analogous to } R = \frac{V}{I})$$

The acoustic impedance Z, which is measured in kg m^{-2} s^{-1} shortened to **rayl**, is also related to the **modulus of elasticity** E. The stiffer the bonding between molecules (springs) the greater the pressure exerted by a molecule moving at a particular velocity so sound pressure is related as $p = Zv$, thus acoustic impedance is directly related to sound pressure. A material having a great deal of springiness (low E value), and consequently high molecular motion, will absorb sound energy in the bonds and less will be

transferred to the next molecule so impedance Z and modulus of elasticity E are related as

$$Z = \frac{E}{c} \qquad (17.5)$$

Velocity of sound transfer depends on material elasticity E (modulus of elasticity) and density of the medium ρ, shown by eqn 17.3, and combining eqn 17.3 and eqn 17.5 gives

$$Z = \rho c = \sqrt{E\rho} \qquad (17.6)$$

Z is a material specific constant and is analogous to electrical resistance: as resistance increases it inhibits velocity (current) for a given pressure (voltage). Acoustic impedance is the product of density and propagation velocity: ρc. Acoustic impedances for various materials are given in Table 17.3.

17.1.4 Power and intensity

Sound energy is measured in joules. Sound power is measured as J s^{-1} or watts and since it is analogous to the respective electrical unit power can be derived from pressure and particle velocity and is transferred as kinetic energy from one molecule to the next since $P = pv$.

Increased energy drives the compression bands closer together, depositing more energy in the tissue and increasing the amplitude of the ultrasound oscillation. During travel through the tissue the oscillations lose energy as heat and the wave amplitude decrease, while frequency and wavelength are unaltered in the same tissue.

Sound or acoustic intensity is measured as W cm^{-2}; this is the instantaneous power passing through a unit area of material (tissue). A practical measure is mW mm^{-1} and the energy of medical ultrasound is typically between 0.01 and 1 mW mm^{-2} for imaging and 0.01 and 0.3 mW mm^{-2} for Doppler flow. Acoustic intensity across the ultrasound beam is not uniform but has a **spatial peak intensity** (SP) and **spatial average intensity** (SA) identified in Fig. 17.5. Common parameters used when describing ultrasound properties or specifying transducers are given in Table 17.4.

DECIBEL SCALE

Comparative sound intensity is measured using the decibel scale (described Chapter 1). The range of intensity values in clinical ultrasound extends over 100 dB. Power or intensity variations (I_1 and I_2) are compared as:

$$dB = 10 \log_{10} \frac{I_2}{I_1} \qquad (17.7)$$

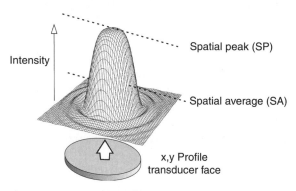

Spatial peak (SP)

Intensity

Spatial average (SA)

x,y Profile
transducer face

Figure 17.5 *Intensity profile across an ultrasound beam.*

So for an incident power of 1.0 W cm^{-2} and an echo power of 0.1 mW cm^{-2} the power loss would be

$$dB = 10 \log_{10} \frac{0.0001}{1}$$
$$= 10 \times -4.0$$
$$= -40 \, dB$$

The value -40 dB is termed '40 dB below'. The **half power distance** (a reduction of 50%) is the distance over which the power is reduced by 3 dB, derived from $10 \log_{10} 0.5 = 3.010$. From the diagram in Fig. 17.3 the maximum intensity coincides with maximum pressure in the medium (air). Pressure p and intensity I are related as

$$I = \frac{p^2}{2\rho c} \qquad (17.8)$$

where ρ is the density of the medium and c the speed of sound in that medium. Substituting eqn 17.8 in eqn 17.7 and canceling the common factor $2\rho c$ gives:

$$10 \log \left(\frac{p_2}{p_1} \right)^2 \text{ or } 20 \log \frac{p_1}{p_2} \qquad (17.9)$$

so pressure or amplitude (measured in volts) is described by eqn 17.9 and commonly describes amplification or **amplifier gain**.

The **half amplitude** value (a 50% loss of gain) would be -6 dB. Ultrasound **attenuation** is measured per unit length and frequency as dB cm^{-1} MHz^{-1} and will be used later to describe ultrasound absorption. For soft tissue it is approximately 1 dB cm^{-1} MHz^{-1}.

Table 17.4 *Common parameters used to describe ultrasound.*

Measurement	Symbol	Unit	Clinical range
Velocity	c	m s^{-1}	1500 m s^{-1} (soft tissue)
Wavelength	λ	mm	0.6 to 0.15 mm (soft tissue)
Frequency	f	hertz	2.5 to 10 MHz
Elastic modulus	E	pascal	25 GPa (bone)
Acoustic impedance	Z	kg m^{-2} s^{-1}	1.63×10^6 kg m^{-2} s^{-1}
Density	ρ	kg m^{-2}	water = 1000 kg m^{-2}
Power	W	watts cm^{-2}	typically 1 to 10 mW cm^{-2}
Elongation	ζ	mm	$\approx 2 \times 10^{-6}$ mm at 3 MHz
Pressure	p	pascal or bar	0.6 bar or 0.06 MPa
Elongation velocity	v	cm s^{-1}	<3.5 cm s^{-1}

7.2 INTERACTION OF ULTRASOUND WITH MATTER

When ultrasound waves interact with matter they exhibit the same phenomena as visible light. They can undergo:

- Reflection (specular and nonspecular)
- Refraction
- Diffraction
- Attenuation or absorption

17.2.1 Reflection

SPECULAR OR MIRROR REFLECTION

Specular or mirror reflection occurs when the ultrasound beam strikes a smooth boundary between two media having different impedance. The reflection of sound is the basis of ultrasound image formation. From Fig. 17.6a an ultrasound beam incident (I_i) on a smooth surface (that is, one where the irregularities are much smaller than the wavelength of the sound impinging upon it) has a proportion of the beam reflected (I_r) and the remainder is transmitted (I_t) through the surface or interface. The fraction that is transmitted (T) and reflected (R) depends on the acoustic impedances of the two media (Z_1 is acoustic impedance of the first tissue and Z_2 the acoustic impedance of the second).

When an ultrasound wave perpendicular to the surface crosses from one medium Z_1 to another Z_2 a change in **velocity** occurs. There is partial reflection of the **incident wave** at the interface between the two materials as shown in Fig. 17.6a. The wavelength of the reflected wave has not changed and remains in phase with the incident wave. The amount of reflection depends on impedance differences Z_1 and Z_2.

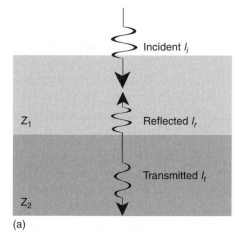

(a)

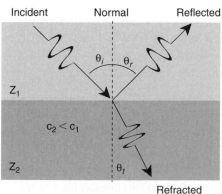

(b)

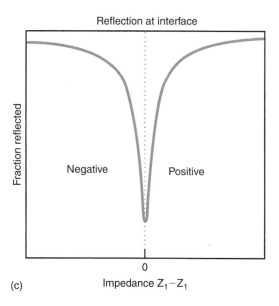

(c)

Figure 17.6 *(a) A sound wave perpendicular to a reflecting surface showing incident, reflected and transmitted rays and (b) at an angle to a smooth surface θ_i showing angles of reflection θ_r and refraction θ_r (c) Reflection from interfaces due to mismatch between Z_1 and Z_2 values. The null point (zero reflection) is where $Z_1 = Z_2$; to the left and right of the null point $Z_1 > Z_2$ and $Z_1 < Z_2$, respectively.*

For a sound wave perpendicular to a smooth surface, the amount of reflection is given by:

$$R = \frac{I_r}{I_i} = \left(\frac{Z_1 - Z_2}{Z_1 + Z_2}\right)^2 \times 100 \qquad (17.10)$$

where R is the percentage of the beam reflected. This relationship is only valid for incident radiation perpendicular to the surface of the medium. **Reflection** is greatest when the difference in acoustic impedance between materials, Z_1 and Z_2, is large, for example between soft tissue and air, or between bone and soft tissue. Only small reflections occur between different soft tissues, the echoes from these interfaces have a weak intensity. Box 17.2 gives some worked examples.

NONSPECULAR REFLECTION

If the beam strikes a boundary having irregularities or fine structures similar in size to the ultrasound wavelength then nonspecular reflection or **scatter** is produced. The same effect occurs when an ultrasound beam passes through a particulate medium, e.g. blood corpuscles, which are small compared with the wavelength and have a different impedance from the surroundings. This again gives scatter.

The scattered echoes from the incident beam form a cone about the reflection axis. The spread or the scatter (cone angle) depends on the wavelength of the ultrasound and the magnitude of the roughness. For rough surfaces and small wavelengths (higher frequency) then the scatter angle is wider. Ultrasound scatter assists in the imaging of curved surfaces and of boundaries which are not 90° to the direction of the ultrasound beam. Intensity of scattered ultrasound is related to frequency f decreasing as f^4. The echoes produced by scatter are much smaller than those produced by specular reflection but they can contribute useful information on tissue characteristics inside an organ. Scattering is responsible for a characteristic of diagnostic ultrasound imaging called **speckle** (not to be confused with speculation mirror reflection). Speckle is produced when scattered ultrasound waves from different sites interfere or add together constructively. The pattern produced does not correspond to anatomical detail but disruptions in the pattern may indicate pathology; liver pathology is an example that may be distinguished.

Box 17.2 Reflection and transmission of ultrasound

Use the acoustic impedance values Z given in Table 17.3 to calculate reflection and/or transmission at two different interfaces.

Interface A: air:fat

From Table 17.3, air $Z_1 = 0.0004 \times 10^6$ and fat $Z_2 = 1.42 \times 10^6$. The amount of sound reflected, R, is given by eqn 17.10, i.e.

$$R = \left(\frac{Z_1 - Z_2}{Z_1 + Z_2}\right)^2$$

Hence, $R = 99.9\%$, i.e. 99.9% of the incident radiation can be reflected from an air/tissue interface.

Interface B: liver:kidney

From Table 17.3, liver $Z_1 = 1.64 \times 10^6$ and kidney $Z_2 = 1.61 \times 10^6$. Using eqn 17.10 the reflection can be calculated as 8.5×10^{-5}, or 0.0085%. The amount transmitted, T, can be calculated by using eqn 17.11:

$$T = \frac{4 Z_1 Z_2}{\left(Z_1 + Z_2\right)^2}$$

Hence, $T = 99.9915\%$. Also, $T = 1 - R$, i.e. $1 - 0.0085$, or 99.9915%.

Conclusion: Over 99.9% of the incident radiation is transmitted through tissues having similar Z values.

Both specular and nonspecular reflection reduce the intensity of ultrasound traveling through different tissue types.

17.2.2 Transmission and refraction

TRANSMISSION

The unreflected ultrasound passes on as a transmitted beam, and the efficiency of transmission (T) of an incident sound beam at right angles to a smooth interface (Fig. 17.6a) is described by the equation:

$$T = \frac{I_t}{I_i} = \frac{4Z_1Z_2}{\left(Z_1 + Z_2\right)^2} \times 100 \quad (17.11)$$

and also $T = 1 - R$.

The response in Fig. 17.6c between Z_1 and Z_2 values graphically illustrates the rapid increase in reflection even with small mismatches between Z_1 and Z_2 reaching a null point when $Z_1 = Z_2$.

REFRACTION

When the incident wave strikes a surface at 90° (Fig. 17.6a) a reflected wave travels back along the incident path. The incident and reflected wave are superimposed additively since they have the same wavelength and phase. An ultrasound wave passing from one medium to another (Z_1 to Z_2) changes its velocity. As the frequency of the beam is not altered the wavelength must change to accommodate the new velocity in the second medium. The transmitted wave therefore has a longer wavelength in the denser medium Z_2.

If the incident beam strikes a smooth boundary at some oblique angle θ, then the reflected beam is projected at the same angle from the surface (Fig. 17.6b). A boundary is described as smooth if its surface roughness is small compared with the ultrasound wavelength. The nonreflected transmitted wave is now traveling at a new (faster) velocity and so the wavelength increases which changes the direction of the wave front in the second medium causing it to undergo refraction; the main beam deviates from its original pathway. Since the speeds in various soft tissues are very similar refraction only plays a minor role in diagnostic ultrasound imaging but refraction can be used deliberately in a transducer design to construct acoustic lenses which will focus the ultrasound beam.

SNELL'S LAW

Snell's law (W. Snell, 1591–1626; Dutch physicist) governs angles of reflection and refraction for ultrasound; if $\sin \theta$ is the angle the beam makes with the surface and v is the sound velocity then:

$$\frac{\sin \theta}{v} = \text{constant} \quad (17.12)$$

The **angle of refraction** θ_t in Fig. 17.6b is described by modifying eqn 17.12, so

$$\frac{\sin \theta_i}{\sin \theta_t} = \frac{V_i}{V_t} \quad (17.13)$$

where θ_1 is the angle of incidence, θ_2 is the angle of refraction, V_i is the wave velocity in the first medium and V_t is the wave velocity in the second medium. The change in direction depends on the change in velocity between the two tissues. When the wave moves from a material in which its velocity is higher to another in which its velocity is lower the angle of refraction is less than the angle of incidence and vice versa. Examples are given in Box 17.3.

DIFFRACTION

This is the bending of the ultrasound beam into the shadow of a strong absorber. It takes place at the

---

Box 17.3 Examples of Snell's law

Refer to the parameters in Fig. 17.6b and use the sound velocities listed in Table 17.3. From eqn 17.13 the refracted beam angle θ_t is related as

$$\sin \theta_t = \frac{\sin \theta_i \times V_t}{V_i}$$

A common incident angle of 20° where $\sin \theta_i = 0.3420$ is used.

Interface 1: water:saline

Where the velocity in water is 1492 and in saline is 1540, then $\theta_i = 20°$ and $\theta_t = 20.6°$.

Conclusion: For similar tissues there are only small differences between incident and refracted angles.

Interface 2: liver:fat

Where the velocity in liver is 1549 and in fat is 1470, then $\theta_i = 20°$ and $\theta_t = 18°$.

Conclusion: The refracted angle is smaller than the incident angle; conversely, if the velocity in the second medium is greater then the refraction angle is greater.

absorber edge and can be seen when a denser material (gall stones, bone, etc.) interrupts the sound beam and a shadow is cast behind the object. Although the ultrasonic intensity in this shadow is less than in the incident field it is not reduced to zero, due to diffraction around the edges of the dense material. This leads to image artifacts.

17.2.3 Absorption and attenuation

The decrease in the intensity of the ultrasound beam in the direction of propagation is called attenuation. There are two processes which produce attenuation:

- **Absorption** by the tissue. This is the main mechanism for the reduction of beam intensity (accounting for up to 80% of the power loss).
- **Beam divergence** by reflection or scattering.

ABSORPTION

Ultrasound absorption is the conversion of ultrasound energy to heat and is produced by the frictional forces which oppose the motion of the particles in the medium. The amount of absorption is determined by the viscosity of the medium, its relaxation time, and the frequency of the ultrasound. Increasing the viscosity of a medium decreases the molecular motion and increases the internal friction.

RELAXATION FREQUENCY

The rate of energy loss in a medium depends on the frequency of ultrasound. Ultrasound may be attenuated more strongly in one type of tissue than another if the relaxation frequency of that medium is near the ultrasound frequency. This is illustrated in Fig. 17.7a where, for a given tissue, maximum absorption occurs at the relaxation frequency ω.

The decrease of the ultrasonic intensity with increasing tissue thickness or path length x can be characterized by an exponential law which has already been used for gamma and X-radiation:

$$\frac{I_x}{I_0} = e^{-\beta x} \tag{17.14}$$

where I_0 is the initial value of ultrasound intensity (at $x = 0$) and I_x is the reduced intensity at depth x, and β is an **absorption coefficient** which is not unlike the linear attenuation coefficient in diagnostic radiology.

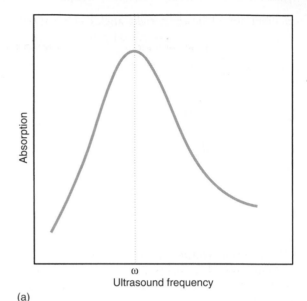

(a)

(b)

Figure 17.7 (**a**) Absorption of ultrasound with frequency for a particular tissue showing its relaxation frequency (ω). (**b**) Tissue depth for 50% loss of intensity for a typical frequency range assuming $1\,dB\,cm^{-1}\,MHz^{-1}$.

For water the value of β is proportional to frequency as f^2. Instead of the absorption coefficient β a measure of power loss α is often given:

$$\alpha = 10\log_{10}\frac{I_0}{I_x} \tag{17.15}$$

Table 17.5 *Sound absorption and acoustic impedance in various tissues and materials.*

Tissue or material	Absorption, α (dB cm^{-1} at 1 MHz)	Impedance, Z (kg m^{-2} s^{-1}, $\times$ 10^{-6})
Fat	0.6	1.38
Blood	0.18	1.61
Brain	0.85	1.55
Soft tissue	1.0	1.63
Liver	0.9	1.65
Muscle (along fibers)	1.2	1.65
Muscle (across fibers)	3.3	1.65
Eye lens	2.0	1.85
Bone	20.0	6.1
Plastic	2.0	3.2

where α is the attenuation in dB per unit length. Table 17.5 lists the reference absorption values (α dB cm^{-1} for 1 MHz) for some common tissues. There is an approximate linear relationship between attenuation α and frequency f as the ratio of α/f which is roughly constant for the diagnostic frequency range. In tissue the absorption of ultrasound increases almost linearly with frequency over the range 0.2 to 100 MHz. Doubling the frequency halves the beam intensity.

Higher frequency ultrasound is attenuated more strongly than lower frequencies; the sharp decline in tissue penetration at frequencies greater than 7.5 MHz is shown by the graph in Fig. 17.7b which shows image depth in millimeters for a 50% attenuation of the signal.

17.3 THE ULTRASOUND TRANSDUCER

Audible sound waves can be produced by hitting a piece of metal and making it ring. The same basic principle is used to produce ultrasound waves but in this case an electric pulse is used as the 'hammer' which causes deformation and vibration of special crystalline material.

A device which converts one form of energy to another is called a **transducer**. Transducers are used in the production and detection of diagnostic ultrasound and convert electrical energy into mechanical energy (producing sound); the returning sound echoes convert their mechanical energy to electrical energy (the signal). This is the **piezoelectric effect** and the materials are piezoelectric crystals. Ultrasound transducers are used in a variety of clinical applications:

- **A-scan**. This displays reflection patterns only as time/depth displays.

- **B-scan**. The transducer is scanned mechanically or electronically. Positional signals give x and y axes for the single slice display.
- **Real time scan**. The beam is swept electronically at fast frame rates. This is the most common form of transducer now available.
- **M-mode**. This transducer records the movement of organ walls, particularly cardiac chambers.

17.3.1 Piezoelectricity

Piezoelectric materials experience a change in shape upon the application of an electric field. They have **molecular dipoles** where positive and negative charges are separated. This is represented in the diagram Fig. 17.8. When an electrical pulse is applied across the crystal the orientation of these dipoles changes, causing a variation in the thickness of the crystal, **compression** or **expansion**. Conversely, if mechanical force is applied to the crystal the molecular dipoles change their orientation, altering the electric field and producing a small voltage signal. Due to the reciprocal property the same transducer can be used for producing ultrasound pulses (mechanical signal) and detecting the returning sound echoes (electrical signal). Quartz was the first material seen to have piezoelectric properties, but the most commonly used transducer materials in diagnostic ultrasound are synthetic materials e.g. ceramic lead zirconate titanate (PbZrTiO$_4$). These have replaced quartz in transducer manufacture.

17.3.2 Basic transducer design

Simple, individual transducers are now rarely used in medical ultrasound imaging, but the basic design of a

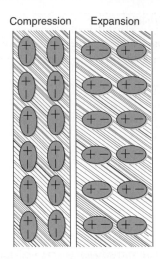

Figure 17.8 *Piezoelectric effect showing the electrically charged dipoles positioned during compression and expansion due to either electrical or mechanical effects.*

single transducer serves to illustrate the important parts that are common to multiple crystal (multi-element) transducers. The basic design illustrated in Fig. 17.9a shows a **transducer crystal** with electrical connections to front and back.

Damping material as a **backing block** behind the crystal is composed of a resin/metal powder composite (Z is 3×10^7 kg m^{-2} s^{-1}), damping reverberations in the crystal, absorbing backward radiation and maintaining a forward pulse direction through the tissue (a lower impedance path).

In **transmitting mode** a high voltage is applied to the transducer. The applied voltage V is related to intensity as:

$$V = \sqrt{\text{intensity}} \qquad (17.16)$$

Similarly, in **receiving mode** the crystal experiences changes in pressure from the returning echo signals producing the very small signal voltages.

17.3.3 Wavelength matching

When an ultrasound probe is applied to a patient it is desirable that the majority of sound energy produced in the crystal should penetrate the patient's skin, but there is a very large difference between the acoustic impedance of the transducer crystal and soft tissue. Major mismatch problems are solved by fixing a matching or **transmission layer** on the transducer crystal face. This is a plastic polymer layer which, for

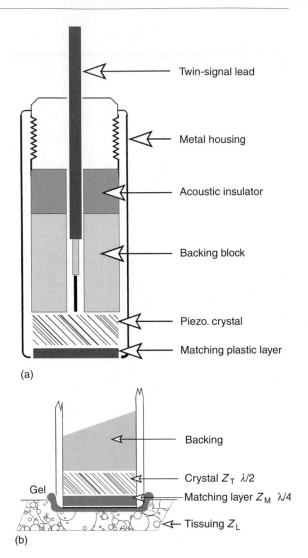

(a)

(b)

Figure 17.9 *(a) Basic single transducer design showing the component parts that are also common to transducers having multiple elements (crystals). (b) Half- and quarter-wave matching for the transducer crystal and matching layer.*

optimum transmission, has a thickness equal to a **quarter wavelength** of the sound ($\frac{1}{4}\lambda$ or odd multiples of this value). Its impedance is given by:

$$Z_M = \sqrt{Z_T \times Z_L} \qquad (17.17)$$

where the acoustic impedance is Z_M for the plastic matching layer, Z_T for the crystal and Z_L for the tissue. Figure 17.9b identifies the crystal and matching layer thicknesses used for optimum performance examples and examples are calculated in Box 17.4.

Box 17.4 Matching layer impedance

The basic formula is

$$Z_M = \sqrt{Z_T \times Z_L}$$

where Z_M is the required acoustic impedance for the matching layer, Z_T the transducer acoustic impedance ($30 \times 10^6 \, kg \, m^{-2} s^{-1}$), and Z_L the tissue acoustic impedance ($1.5 \times 10^6 \, kg \, m^{-2} s^{-1}$). Hence,

$$Z_M = \sqrt{30 \times 1.5} = 6.7 \times 10^6 \, kg \, m^{-2} s^{-1}$$

The matching layer is usually made from plastic material: for Perspex/Plexiglas $Z_M = 3.2 \times 10^6 \, kg \, m^{-2} \, s^{-1}$. This is commonly loaded with aluminum powder to exactly match the calculated Z value.

Box 17.5 Transducer crystal thickness

The basic formula is

$$\lambda = \frac{c}{f}$$

For PbZrTiO$_4$ material $c = 4000 \, m \, s^{-1}$, so in order to construct a 1 MHz transducer

$$\lambda = \frac{4000}{1 \times 10^6} = 4 \times 10^{-3} \, m \text{ (i.e. 4 mm)}$$

Therefore $\frac{1}{2}\lambda = 2$ mm for a 1 MHz transducer. For a 5 MHz transducer this would be: $\lambda = 8 \times 10^{-4}$ m (0.8 mm) $\frac{1}{2}\lambda = 0.4$ mm.

Matching layer thickness

The speed of sound in the plastic used for transducer lenses is typically $2680 \, m \, s^{-1}$. The wavelength for a 5 MHz transducer would be 0.536 mm. A $\frac{1}{4}\lambda$ matching layer would be 0.134 mm or odd multiples of this (i.e. $\times 3 = 0.402$ mm).

The primary function of the matching layer is to increase sound transmission into the soft tissues. Applying a layer which has a quarter wavelength thickness or an odd multiple known as 'quarter-wave matching' provides good transmission through the skin layer. A gel coupling medium, between the skin surface and transducer matching layer is used which removes air bubbles which would cause significant signal loss.

Due to a range of frequencies in the ultrasound pulse the matching layer cannot be exactly $\lambda/4$ for all wavelengths so matching is less than 100% efficient. Multiple matching layers are sometimes employed to improve efficiency. The frequency of the transmitted ultrasound pulse is determined by the crystal thickness d; the wavelength λ of the ultrasound is equal to twice the thickness of the crystal and from eqn 17.2 as $\lambda = 2d$ then

$$f = \frac{c}{2d} \tag{17.18}$$

where c the velocity of sound in the piezoelectric crystal. If crystal thickness is $\lambda/2$ then excitation stresses are reinforced and the crystal resonates at that frequency. These formulas are used in the design of ultrasound transducers and worked examples are shown in Box 17.5.

The output from the crystal should fall off quickly once the electrical stimulus is removed. The damping material provides this since the backing block behind the piezoelectric crystal is highly absorbent as it is made of fine tungsten particles suspended in epoxy resin. The tungsten particles act as scattering centers, while the resin absorbs the scattered ultrasound. The backing block should ideally have an acoustic impedance which equals that of the crystal so that no reflection occurs at the crystal/backing block interface.

The transducer and backing block are separated from the casing of the probe by an ultrasonic insulator, e.g. rubberized cork. This minimizes the transmission of the ultrasound energy to the casing vibrations that would be picked up by the transducer in receive mode and registering as image artifacts.

17.3.4 Pulse geometry

Once the crystal is pulsed the duration of its output is very short. Ideally, the pulse would rise and fall very rapidly and contain only one wavelength, but a pulse usually contains two to three wavelengths. A typical pulse shape is shown in Fig. 17.10a identifying wavelength λ, amplitude A and the pulse length.

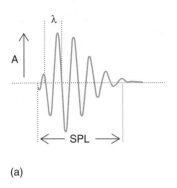

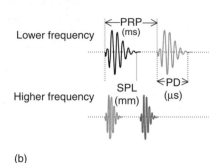

Figure 17.10 (*a*) *Ultrasound pulse shape showing 3 cycles having wavelength* λ *and amplitude* A *and spatial pulse length SPL.* (*b*) *Increasing the frequency shortens the SPL.*

Table 17.6 *Frequency, spatial pulse length, and pulse duration for 3*λ.

Frequency (MHz)	Spatial pulse length (mm)	Pulse duration (µs)
2.5	1.8	1.2
5.0	0.9	0.6
7.5	0.6	0.4
10.0	0.45	0.3

SPATIAL PULSE LENGTH

This is the length of the pulse in millimeters and is defined as:

$$\lambda \times n$$

where *n* is the number of cycles. For a 5 MHz transducer where λ is 0.3 mm the spatial pulse length (SPL) would be 0.9 mm for a three cycle pulse (*n* = 3). The SPL has a typical range of 0.3 to 1.0 mm for diagnostic ultrasound and depends on transducer frequency as shown by the pulses in Fig. 17.10b for a low and high frequency transducer (e.g. 3.5 and 7.5 MHz). The **pulse duration** (PD), measured in µs, is given by *n/f* and varies typically between 0.4 and 1.5 µs. A range of SPL and PD values for a three-cycle pulse is given in Table 17.6.

The SPL alters during its transmission through tissue since the process of attenuation resembles a low frequency (low pass) filter removing higher frequencies. The higher frequencies of the transmitted pulse are attenuated more strongly during their travel through tissue than the lower frequencies and as a consequence the spatial pulse length increases so degrading image resolution. This filtering of higher frequencies is called **dispersion**. This has a strong influence on **spatial resolution** in the ultrasound image.

PULSE REPETITION FREQUENCY

This is the number of pulses per second and set by a master clock in the ultrasound unit. An electrical pulse generator drives the transducer which causes each resonant pulse. For a PD of about 1 µs and a pulse repetition frequency (PRF) of 1 kHz this leaves a period of approximately 999 µs between pulses so the transducer is in 'receive mode' for 99.9% of the time. Increasing the PRF increases the image information rate (echoes received) but shortens receive time so limiting the time for receiving distant echoes in the anatomical region being studied. The pulse repetition period (PRP) is the reciprocal, 1/PRF, and is a measure of time from one pulse to the next; typically from 0.1 to 0.5 ms.

IMAGE DEPTH

The time between pulses must be greater than the 'return trip' which is equivalent to image depth $D \times 2$; the maximum PRF is determined by $c/2D$. If a penetration of 150 mm is required and *c* is 1500 m s^{-1} then the PRF is about 5 kHz. A typical value in practice is 2 to 3 kHz.

17.3.5 Resonant frequency and *Q*

The pulse produced by the transducer in Fig. 17.11a is a mixture of frequencies. The shorter the pulse the greater the frequency mixture and the broader the **bandwidth**. The frequency spectrum of two signals is shown in Fig. 17.11b for both imaging and Doppler. The Doppler pulse has a greater SPL and gives a tighter frequency spectrum since increasing SPL decreases bandwidth. SPL and bandwidth are related as 1/SPL ∝ bandwidth.

BANDWIDTH

The frequency spectrum shown by curve A in Fig. 17.12a has a narrow bandwidth and curve B a broad bandwidth. This is measured between F_1 and F_2 in the graph. The frequency cut-off above and below these limits should be sharp in order to reject noise; this is the case with spectrum A. The efficiency of ultrasound production, its purity of sound (restricted frequency range) and the duration of the pulse are expressed in terms of a Q factor. A high Q transducer produces a pure single frequency with a long duration or ringing time (Doppler waveform in Fig. 17.11). A low Q transducer produces a mixed frequency sound pulse of short duration. The two signals A and B shown in Fig. 17.12a have a high and a low Q factor. Q is expressed as

$$Q = \frac{F_R}{F_2 - F_1} \qquad (17.19)$$

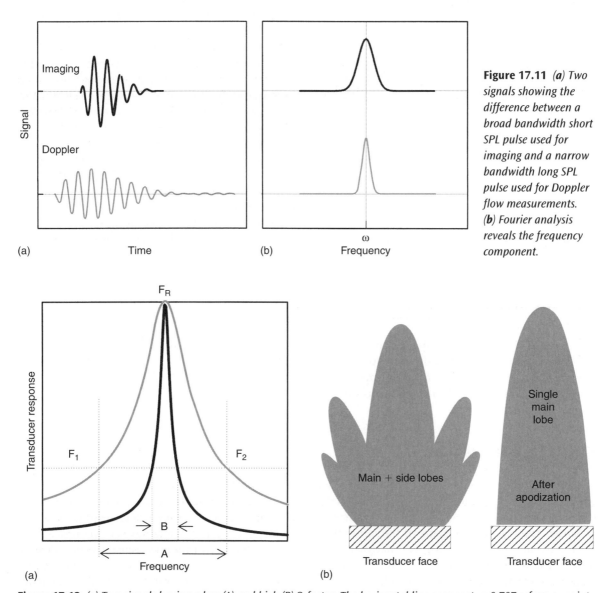

Figure 17.11 (**a**) Two signals showing the difference between a broad bandwidth short SPL pulse used for imaging and a narrow bandwidth long SPL pulse used for Doppler flow measurements. (**b**) Fourier analysis reveals the frequency component.

Figure 17.12 (**a**) Two signals having a low (A) and high (B) Q factor. The horizontal line represents a 0.707 reference point (not to scale). (**b**) The ultrasound beam projecting from the transducer face showing side lobes which can decrease main lobe power unless removed by apodization.

where F_R is the resonant or dominant frequency and F_1, F_2 are points below and above the resonance peak where the signal intensity is reduced by $1/\sqrt{2}$ or 0.707; these points are marked as dotted and dashed lines. An increased bandwidth and a decreased spatial pulse length reduces the Q factor. A high Q crystal is used for transmission when a pure ultrasound source is required (e.g. Doppler). A broader Q crystal would be used for imaging where a short SPL gives good image resolution. Transducers for medical imaging have Q factors related to the number of cycles in the pulse, typically 2 to 4.

SIDE LOBES

Ideally ultrasound pulse energy appears as a single front traveling in a forward direction from the crystal face; however, some energy travels off in different directions called grating or side lobes (Fig. 17.12b). This extraneous energy must be suppressed otherwise the transmitted energy will be dissipated in multiple lobes and degrade image quality (contrast and resolution). **Apodization** means 'removal of the feet' representing removal of subsidiary maxima in the sound pulse. Shaping the acoustic aperture changes the envelope of the transmit pulse from a square function to a Gaussian; this effectively eliminates the side lobes and markedly improves image quality.

17.4 THE ULTRASONIC FIELD

The shape of the ultrasound pulse produced by the transducer crystal determines the resolution of an imaging device. The beam dimensions change as they travel through tissue; this strongly influences image quality with depth.

17.4.1 The beam profile

The ability of the imaging device to distinguish two objects placed very close together in the plane at right angles to the direction of the beam is a measure of its **lateral resolution**. The shape of the ultrasound beam, shown in Fig. 17.13a, is at first narrow and is determined by the size of the transducer and the wavelength of the sound (which depends on the frequency). After a certain distance the beam diverges. The beam shape therefore consists of two distinct regions: the near field or **Fresnel zone** (A.J. Fresnel,

1788–1827; French physicist) and the far field or **Fraunhofer zone** (J. von Fraunhofer, 1787–1826; German physicist). The near field maintains the width of the transducer, the beam then spreads out in the far field or undergoes divergence causing a decrease in lateral resolution and intensity of the beam. The length of the near field Z_f is governed by

$$Z_f = \frac{\alpha^2}{\lambda} \qquad (17.20)$$

where α is the half the width (radius) of the transducer and λ is the wavelength of ultrasound.

As the width of the transducer is increased the length of the Fresnel zone is maintained (Fig. 17.13b) so a narrow transducer will provide high resolution over a short distance while a wider probe will maintain lower resolution for greater distances. Equation 17.20 shows that the length of the Fresnel zone is proportional to the square of the transducer radius and inversely proportional to the wavelength. Figure 17.13c and d demonstrates that length of the near field (and therefore the lateral resolution at depth) is improved as the wavelength is shortened, i.e. using a higher ultrasound frequency from 1 MHz to 5 MHz but the attenuation of ultrasound increases with frequency, so while the lateral resolution is maintained for greater depths the amplitudes of returning echo signals will be decreased and **image depth** reduced.

17.4.2 Divergence

At the end of the near field (Fresnel zone) the beam begins to spread out or diverge; this is the far field or Fraunhofer zone. The magnitude of this divergence is given by

$$\theta = \sin^{-1}\left(\frac{0.61\lambda}{\alpha}\right) \qquad (17.21)$$

where θ is the **angle of divergence**, λ is the wavelength and α is again the half width of the transducer. Field divergence decreases with increasing transducer width and with decreasing wavelength or increasing frequency; so **resolution at depth** is best with wide transducers and high frequency. Clearly, compromises are made to optimize image quality with image depth; this will be a problem as frequencies are increased. Ophthalmology requires high resolution for shallow depths and the frequency of ultrasound is

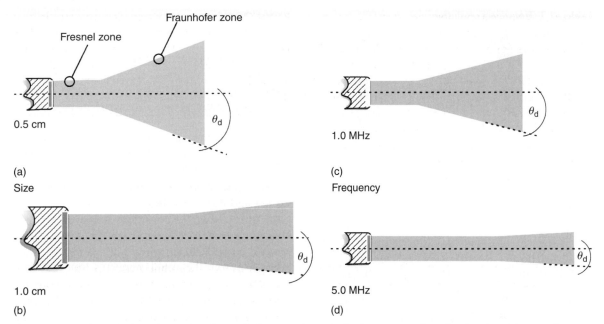

Figure 17.13 *The variation of Fresnel and Fraunhofer zones for a single element transducer having sizes (a) 0.5 and (b) 1.0 cm. The beam profile for the 0.5 cm transducer is then shown at (c) 1 MHz and (d) 5 MHz.*

generally higher than for conventional diagnostic imaging.

17.4.3 Resolution

There are two axes of resolution in an ultrasound image: **lateral** resolution which describes resolving power across the beam and **axial** in the path or parallel to the beam. Both the axial and lateral resolution is a measure of the system's ability to separate closely placed reflecting surfaces.

AXIAL RESOLUTION

Resolving two closely placed surfaces parallel to the direction of the beam is determined by the spatial pulse length (SPL) so the higher the frequency of the ultrasound the shorter the pulse length (Fig. 17.10b). Since the high frequency component of the pulse is preferentially absorbed by its passage through tissue (frequency dispersion) the SPL increases and axial resolution becomes degraded. A measure of axial resolution is given by SPL/2.

LATERAL RESOLUTION

The resolution across the beam depends on the focusing ability of the transducer as shown in Fig. 17.14.

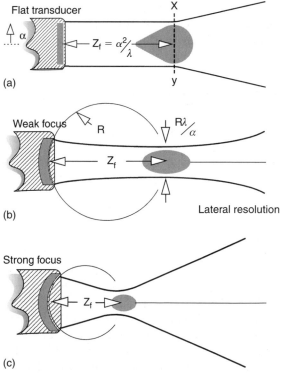

Figure 17.14 *The various focal positions for (a) flat (b) a weakly focused and (c) a strongly focused transducer showing the length of the near field (Z$_f$) and focal zone.*

Table 17.7 *Transducer resolution.*

Frequency	Image depth	Axial resolution	Lateral resolution
2.0	30	0.7	3.0
3.5	17	0.4	1.7
5.0	12	0.3	1.2
7.5	8	0.2	0.8
10.0	6	0.15	0.6

The distance to the focal zone Z_f where the beam starts to diverge is given by eqn 17.21. The lateral resolution at this point depends on the radius of curvature R determining the focal dimensions. These are usually termed weak focus ($Z_f/R < 2$), medium ($Z_f/R \approx 2$ to 3), and strong ($Z_f/R \approx 3$ to 4). In general, ultrasound transducers have better axial than lateral resolution but strongly focused beams can provide symmetrical resolution performance.

Examples of image depth and approximate axial resolution/lateral resolution are listed in Table 17.7 for selected frequencies. Examples will be given in the next chapter on ultrasound imaging.

SUMMARY

In the following relationships λ is wavelength, c the speed of sound in the medium and f the ultrasound frequency and n the number of cycles in the pulse:

- Intensity $= p/A$, where p is the power (in mW) and A is the area (in mm^2)
- In wavelength matching:
  - Crystal thickness (in mm) $= \lambda/2$
  - Matching layer (in mm) $= \lambda/4$
  - Matching layer impedance $Z_M = \sqrt{Z_T \times Z_L}$ where Z_T represents the transducer and Z_L the matching layer
- Propagation period (in μs) $= 1/f$
- Pulse wavelength (in mm) $= c/f$
- Spatial pulse length (in mm) $= n \times \lambda$
- Pulse duration (in μs) $= n/f$
- Near field length (Fresnel zone) $Z_f = \alpha^2/\lambda$ where α is the half width (or radius) of the transducer
- Diversion angle (Fraunhofer zone) $\theta = \sin^{-1}(0.61\lambda/\alpha)$
- Axial resolution $=$ SPL/2
- Lateral resolution $= R\lambda/\alpha$

KEYWORDS

acoustic absorption: the loss of sound energy by attenuation and scatter

acoustic amplitude: this is measured from the zero (cross-over) point of the sine wave to its peak in mV or μV

acoustic frequency, f: the compression and rarefaction events translated as a sine wave whose frequency range is 2.5 to 15 MHz in clinical ultrasound

acoustic impedance, Z: is the product of material density and speed of sound

acoustic intensity: the power per unit area (W cm^{-2})

acoustic parameters: pressure density, temperature, acoustic impedance

acoustic power: the sound energy per unit time J s^{-1} or watts

acoustic pressure: the pressure difference from normal pressure induced by sound wave. Units are pascals: 1 Pa $=$ 1 N m^{-2} $=$ 10 μbar. A typical range is 0.06 to 1.5 MPa

amplitude: wave peak height

anechoic: echo free

angle of incidence: angle between beam direction and the perpendicular axis

angle of reflection: equals the angle of incidence

apodization: removal of sound beam side lobes by using gaussian beam profile

continuous wave: indefinite wave not pulsed

coupling gel: soft grease provides continuous interface excluding air

cycle (Hz): complete transition of waveform measured from identical points (zero crossing or peaks)

cycles per pulse: typical pulse contains 1 to 3 cycles

decibel (dB): the logarithmic comparative measure of power, intensity, and amplitude or voltage gain

diffraction: bending of a beam at the edge of an absorbing surface into the shadow area of the surface

dispersion: pulse spreads out as it passes through medium. Pulse height decreases as pulse width increases. Depends on the property of the medium

divergent angle: the angle describing far field divergence (see Fraunhofer zone)

duty factor, DF: time fraction that the pulse is on. Typical value 5 ms, range 1 to 10 ms: DF $=$ PD/(PRP $\times$ 1000) or (PD $\times$ PRF)/1000 ms

elongation velocity: velocity of a particle about its equilibrium position. Typical value 35 mm s^{-1}

Fraunhofer zone: far-field divergence related to wavelength and transducer diameter as $\sin \theta = 0.612 \times (\lambda/r)$

frequency (Hz): cycles per second. Typical ultrasound values are 2 to 10 MHz

Fresnel zone: near zone dependent on transducer diameter d or aperture $d^2/4\lambda$

imaging depth: maximum penetration that will yield image information. Proportional to 75/PRF

impedance, Z: material density $\times$ propagation speed. Typical range 1.3×10^6 to 1.7×10^6 rayls

longitudinal wave: compression wave in parallel to wave direction

modulus of elasticity, E: a measurement of material stiffness represented by stress/strain. The inverse is compressibility or $1/E$

particle velocity: typically 3.5 cm s^{-1} displacement to and fro from the rest position

period, T: time per cycle. Range 0.1 to 0.5 μs. $T = 1/f$

piezoelectric effect: shown by a material whose dimensions change with electric charge. Mechanical deformation produces an electrical charge

power: work done per unit time J s^{-1}

propagation velocity, c: speed of displacement through the medium. Typical value 1500 m s^{-1} for soft tissue

pulse duration: a typical pulse duration is 0.5 to 3 μs. PD = cycles $\times$ period or cycles/f

pulse repetition frequency, PRF: time to repeat ultrasound pulse. Range 2 to 10 kHz

pulse repetition period, PRP: time from one pulse to the next RPR = 1/PRF range 0.1 to 0.5 ms

rayl: a measure of acoustic impedance. The units are kg m^{-2} s^{-1}

reflection (specular): reflection of ultrasound from a smooth surface

reflection (nonspecular): reflection of ultrasound from a rough surface

refraction: the bending of the transmitted beam due to change in propagation velocity. The change of beam direction when traveling from one medium to another

relaxation frequencies: frequency of maximum absorption in a medium

resolution (axial): resolving power parallel to the beam travel. Influenced by SPL/2

resolution (lateral): resolving power across the beam. Depends on focal dimensions of the beam influenced by aperture size and electronic focusing

scattering: redirection of sound beam in several directions

side lobes: minor sound beams traveling at an angle from the main beam in a single element

spatial pulse length, SPL: length of a single pulse. Typical values 0.1 to 1.0 mm

specular reflection (mirror reflection): reflection from a large smooth surface. SPL = cycles $\times$ wavelength

wavelength: (propagation speed)/frequency. Typical ultrasound range 0.1 to 0.5 mm depending on medium

18

Ultrasound imaging

18.1 ULTRASOUND IMAGING

Since the development of multi-element array technology in the early 1970s mechanical scanning methods have been gradually superseded. Electronically switched transducer arrays are now used exclusively for ultrasound imaging except for annular transducers that still use mechanical methods.

DISPLAY MODES

There are two basic display modes offered by diagnostic ultrasound: brightness modulation or B-mode which gives a gray-scale picture and M-mode which instead of a 2-D spatial image traces out a 2-D time-versus-movement graphic display, which indicates the motion of cardiac chambers or valves.

The B-mode display gives a brightness scale (gray scale) depending on echo strength. Distinct interfaces between different tissues are seen as white regions. The B-mode picture displays a section through the body anatomy whose image depth depends on transducer parameters (frequency, focusing etc.). The image display, or **frame**, is constructed from **scan lines**, the number depending on the number of individual elements in the transducer. The image is refreshed at regular intervals called the **frame rate**. If the frame rate is fast enough then a 'real-time' display can be observed. Single frames can be held in the computer memory for inspection; this is a 'freeze-frame' display.

MULTI-ELEMENT PROPAGATION

The array transducer consists of many small elements that combine to give a single ultrasound wavefront. Figure 18.1 shows the propagation of a sound front formed in front of a transducer array. The sound issuing from a multiple transducer was developed by

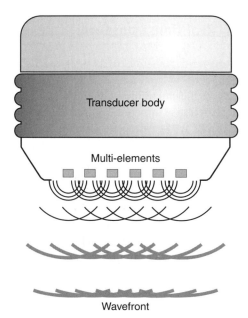

Figure 18.1 *Sound wave propagation from multiple transducers forming a wave front according to Huygen's principle.*

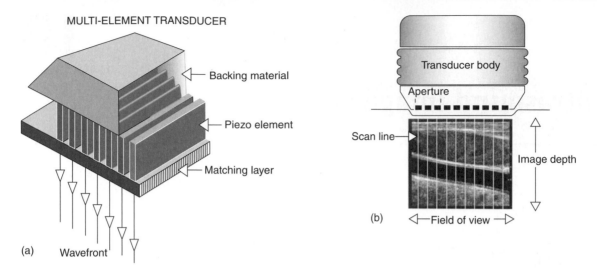

Figure 18.2 (*a*) *Three-dimensional plan of a multi-element transducer showing individual elements, the common backing material and matching layer.* (*b*) *Basic multi-element linear transducer showing scan length and field of view and image depth.*

Huygens to explain the propagation of light (C. Huygens, 1629–93; Dutch physicist). Each transducer element serves as a point sound source radially expanding until they interact with each other and produce a combined **wavefront.** The ultrasound from these **real-time** transducers travels as a wavefront through the tissue.

18.1.1 Real-time transducer

The ultrasound real-time transducer consists of a series of identical rectangular shaped piezoelectric elements, each element individually pulsed. The general construction is shown in Fig. 18.2a. The width of each element is measured in wavelengths ranging from 1λ to 4λ, the absolute dimension decided by transducer frequency (see Table 17.2).

The wavefront issuing from the multi-element transducer has the same dimensions, in the near field (Fresnel zone), as the total transducer surface. The near field converges slightly just before diverging in the far field. The near and far field dimensions are governed by transducer frequency and array dimensions (**aperture**) and electronic focusing procedures.

SCAN LINES

Figure 18.2b shows that each element of a linear transducer produces a **scan line** whose length is the **image depth**. Linear arrays produce parallel scans

lines while other array designs produce sector shapes. The image depth depends on beam penetration (sound frequency) and pulse timing. The physical size of the array head (area) is its **footprint**; linear arrays have large footprints, other array designs have smaller footprints.

APERTURE

The transducer **aperture** is determined by the group of transducer elements working in unison. Aperture size can vary during data transmission and reception giving the transducer a **dynamic aperture**. A linear transducer produces a 3-D ultrasound beam whose propagation pattern, shown in Fig. 18.3a, gives a rectilinear cover whose area depends on the number of elements in the transducer. The side dimension of the beam edge is defined by an acoustic lens which determines the **section thickness**.

18.1.2 Ultrasound pulse timing

The ultrasound signal is produced by a high voltage pulse delivered to each element in the transducer array. This produces a **critically damped** ultrasound 'ring' of two to three wavelengths. The length of this pulse (spatial pulse length (SPL)) and the frequency of pulse production (pulse repetition frequency (PRF)) defines certain important image characteristics that have been defined in Chapter 17.

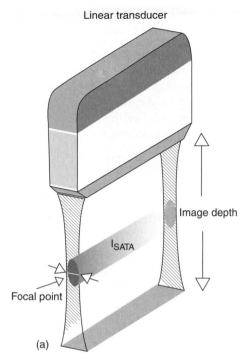

Linear transducer

Image depth

I_{SATA}

Focal point

(a)

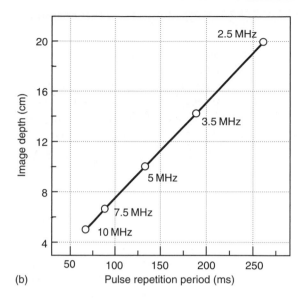

(b)

Figure 18.3 *(a) A linear transducer giving a beam shape which narrows toward the middle. This is the section thickness.* I_{SATA} *is a measure of sound intensity referred to in the section on safety. (b) The change of image depth with pulse repetition period (PRP). Transducer frequency from 2.5 to 10 MHz is also identified on the slope.*

SPATIAL PULSE LENGTH

This is related to wavelength as

$$SPL = \lambda \times \text{number of cycles} \quad (18.1)$$

Transmission pulses are damped to give two to three complete cycles. Three cycles of a higher frequency clearly have a shorter SPL than three cycles of lower frequency (see Chapter 17) but as the frequency is increased penetration of the ultrasound beam is reduced (absorption increases linearly with increasing frequency). Dimensions are typically between 0.45 and 2.25 mm for a diagnostic imaging range.

PULSE DURATION

This measures the time period of the pulse. Ultrasound imaging typically uses pulses that are two to three wavelengths long.

$$PD = \text{pulse wavelength} \times \text{number of cycles} \quad (18.2)$$

The PD is generally measured in microseconds, and is typically between 0.5 and 3 μs for current machines.

PULSE REPETITION FREQUENCY

The transducer element group is excited by an electrical signal which generates the ultrasound **transmission pulse** whose frequency depends on the transducer element dimensions. A chain of timed transmission pulses is delivered to the transducer while imaging. The timing between the transmission pulses, the **pulse repetition period** (PRP), is critical for each transducer type since this determines the rate of image formation or **frame rate** and **imaging depth** D_{max} identified in Fig. 18.3b. If a 1 μs transmission pulse is followed by a waiting period of 200 μs (receive period) this will give

$$PRF = \frac{10^6}{200} = 5000 \text{ Hz (5 kHz)}$$

Typical PRF values range from 2 to 10 kHz for diagnostic imaging. Over 99% of the timing cycle is spent listening for echoes since pulse duration is typically 1 μs compared to a pulse repetition period of 200 μs. The PRP is matched to the image depth or scan line length (SL) otherwise echo pulses may clash with transmission pulses if the PRP is too short.

Sound attenuation increases with frequency and this is the major determining factor for image depth. The graph in Fig. 18.3b plots the relationship between PRP and imaging depth for a speed of sound of $1500 \, \text{cm s}^{-1}$; transducer frequencies used at various PRP values are superimposed on the graph. Various clinical factors decide which frequency is used since higher frequency transducers give improved image resolution and owing to faster PRP are more able to give real-time displays and follow pulsatile (cardiac) movement.

DUTY FACTOR

This is also the duty cycle and is the percentage or fractional measure of the time that the pulse occupies in the transmit receive cycle. The duty factor (DF) increases with increasing PRF.

$$DF = \frac{PD}{PRP} \qquad (18.3)$$

IMAGE DEPTH

This can be calculated from the speed of sound in soft tissue $(1500 \, \text{m s}^{-1})$ and allowing for a return path (so halving this distance) then the image depth, D_{max}, is $150\,000 \times 0.5 \times PRP$ or $75\,000 \times PRP$ cm. For a PRP of $200 \, \mu s$ this would give an imaging depth of 15 cm. Alternatively, D_{max} can be calculated as $75\,000/PRF$. Similarly, for soft tissue imaging,

$$PRF = \frac{1500}{2 \times D_{max}} \qquad (18.4)$$

Higher frequency transducers have higher PRP values so give shallower image depths as demonstrated in Fig. 18.3b.

Both PD and PRP are measured in μs to give the DF as a unitless fraction. The duty factor is an important measure of ultrasound power used in ultrasound safety.

BANDWIDTH

As improvements are made to transducer materials the characteristic impedance is lowered along with degrees of mismatch. Backing material is used which does not absorb as much sound energy so transducer sensitivity is improved giving increased dynamic range and image depth. Transducer bandwidth is also increased which can be used in one of two ways:

- Operator choice of center frequency in a narrow window moved over the larger bandwidth giving multi-frequency probes and choice of image depth
- Alternatively, large bandwidth transmission which gives a wide range of echo information maintaining maximum image depth at all times

Manufacturers supply variations on these basic properties.

18.1.3 Spatial resolution

Resolution is measured as the minimum distance between objects (in mm) which can be distinguished in the image. Ultrasound transducer resolution is described in terms of:

- Axial
- Lateral
- Section thickness

AXIAL RESOLUTION

Axial resolution, R_x, is measured in the direction parallel to the beam and is illustrated in Fig. 18.4a. It is determined by the **transmission pulse width**. Ideally, this should be a single cycle duration of the particular ultrasound frequency. In practice the pulse tends to last for two to three cycles. The backing material is a mechanical damping device for reducing the SPL; electronic damping is also used to ensure a 2 to 3 cycle SPL.

Axial resolution measured as the ability to resolve reflecting surfaces along the beam path is determined by the pulse duration (spatial pulse length SPL). Axial resolution is related as:

$$R_x = \frac{\text{spatial pulse length}}{2} \qquad (18.5)$$

Axial resolution can be improved by decreasing the length of the transmission pulse. In practice this can only be achieved by increasing the pulse frequency and thereby decreasing the spatial pulse length (SPL). Figure 18.4b indicates that higher frequency transducers have higher axial resolutions but poorer imaging depth. Axial resolutions are on the second y-axis in Fig. 18.4b for the range of clinical ultrasound frequencies. Axial resolution varies due

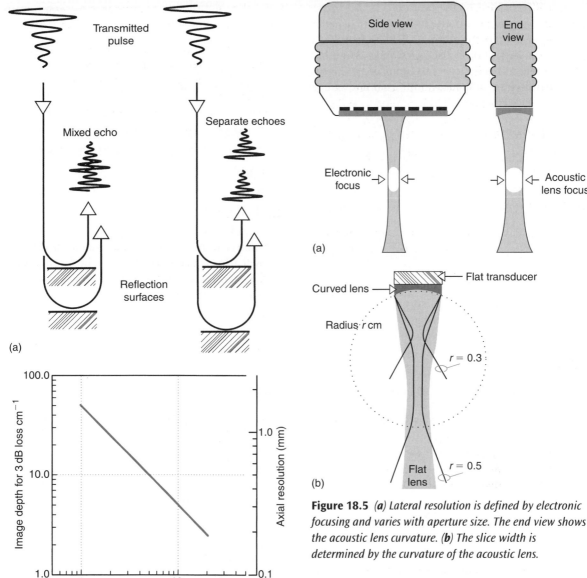

Figure 18.4 (**a**) Signal separation defining axial resolution. This depends on the spatial pulse length (SPL) so the two surfaces could be resolved by using a higher frequency and shorter SPL. (**b**) The pulse repetition period (PRP) and imaging depth for various frequency transducers identified on the slope. Image depth for 50 dB attenuation and transducer frequency with approximate axial resolution.

to high frequency loss with depth; the center frequency of the pulse decreasing with a consequent broadening of the SPL. **Contrast resolution** is determined by how effective the system is in separating

Figure 18.5 (**a**) Lateral resolution is defined by electronic focusing and varies with aperture size. The end view shows the acoustic lens curvature. (**b**) The slice width is determined by the curvature of the acoustic lens.

pulse overlap as illustrated in Fig. 18.4a; this is influenced by signal strength and system sensitivity.

LATERAL RESOLUTION

This is governed by the beam width which depends on the number of element groups (the **aperture**) of the transducer during transmission and dynamic focusing during echo reception. Lateral resolution for a linear transducer is identified in Fig. 18.5a, a deeper focal zone would be given by a larger aperture.

Dynamic focusing and dynamic aperture maintain optimum lateral resolution for all depths, which will be described later. Lateral resolution, across the beam, is determined by the beam width and shape. Beam shape is not a constant dimension and depends on the focal point of the beam. A 3.5 MHz transducer has an axial resolution between 0.6 and 0.8 mm but lateral resolution is three to five times larger. Transducer **bandwidth** influences both axial and lateral resolution (see Chapter 17).

SLICE THICKNESS

The slice width or section thickness has already been identified in Fig. 18.3a and is further defined by the end view in Fig. 18.5a. The focal planes which determine slice width are identified in Fig. 18.5b. Beam width in this dimension is achieved by shaping either the transducer crystal or matching layer (see Chapter 17 and refraction). A focused beam is produced by providing a concave crystal and/or a matching layer as a lens system. The concave shape is not ideal for obtaining good contact with the skin. A focused crystal with a convex matching layer will usually provide an adequate amount of focusing and allow good skin contact.

SUMMARY

Lateral resolution can be described as follows:

- It is a measure of minimal separation of points across the beam.
- It varies with distance from the transducer (focal region) and aperture.
- It decreases (poorer resolution) with increasing beam width. It increases with frequency.

- Axial resolution.
- It is the minimal separation of surfaces in line with the beam.
- Governed by SPL as SPL/2 and therefore decreases with increasing SPL.
- Imaging depth decreases with frequency.

18.2 IMAGE PROCESSING

The component parts of an ultrasound imaging system is shown in Fig. 18.6. The ultrasound signal processing sequences are:

- The **pulser** consisting of clock and pulse transmitter
- **Amplification** increases the amplitude of the small echo signals in increased
- **Time gain compensation** where correction is made for tissue attenuation
- **Signal compression** reducing the broad range in echo amplitude before displaying the signals as an image
- **Demodulation** or signal thresholding
- **Signal rejection** or filtering prepare the signal for digitization

THE TRANSMITTER

The heart of the system is the **clock**. This controls all the timing of the transmission pulse, the pulse frequency (PRF), and image data (echo) collection by preparing receiving and digitization circuits. It

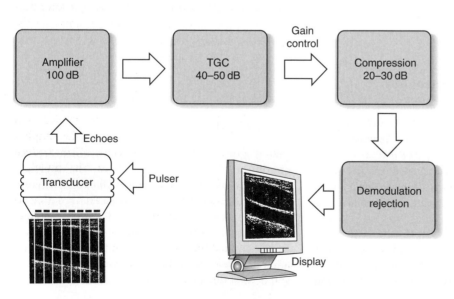

Figure 18.6 *A simplified block diagram of the transducer processing circuits. The ultrasound pulse is driven by the pulser and returning echoes received by the amplifier/processing chain. The gain control is operator adjusted for image depth.*

synchronizes dynamic focusing and controls the dynamic transducer aperture. The transmitter (combined with the clock as the pulser in the diagram) supplies the electrical pulse to the transducer array at times decided by the clock. Transmitter voltages range from about 5 V up to a few hundreds of volts; this can be operator adjusted. Piezoelectric materials can tolerate field strengths of up to 1 kV mm^{-2}.

THE RECEIVER

The simplest image involves only one reflecting object in the path of the beam but in practice, of course, there are many hundreds. A series of echoes will be received from these objects whose amplitudes will vary in size depending on the size of the echo and the depth at which the echo originates.

18.2.1 Signal pre-processing

APODIZATION

This has been referred to in Chapter 17. The main intensity of an ultrasound beam is directed perpendicular to the transducer face; this is the main lobe. High side lobe and grating lobe level must be kept to a minimum since they will reduce image contrast due to off-axis echo signals which interfere with the main axis signals. Nonlinear signal processing accentuate these off axis signals. Apodization of the acoustic aperture by shaping the electrical pulse applied to the transducer reduces side lobes in the ultrasound pulse and grating lobes in the multi-element array where the width of each element also influences the magnitude of grating lobe dimensions.

AMPLIFICATION

Small echo signals (μV) undergo linear amplification from a few microvolts to millivolts so that they can be handled by the signal processing circuits.

DYNAMIC RANGE

This describes the ratio of the smallest to the largest signals that can be handled by the amplifier. Echoes returning from tissues can have dynamic ranges of between 100 and 150 dB giving amplitude differences A of

$$20 \log \frac{A}{A_0} \text{ dB} \qquad (18.6)$$

For 100 to 150 dB this would represent a signal range of 1 μV to 316 μV. Power differences (intensity) would cover nanowatts to picowatts. Amplified signals are processed by the signal conditioning circuits before being digitized for computer storage and eventually displayed as gray-scale images. Dynamic range is decreased as the signals are processed since small signals carry mainly noise and little information so are rejected so improving the signal-to-noise ratio. The image depth D of a transducer typically represents a dynamic range limit of 50 dB and the depth of penetration based on this figure is plotted in Fig. 18.4b. This is influenced by the attenuation coefficient α in dB cm^{-1}MHz^{-1} and frequency f so that the product $\alpha \times f \times D = 50$ dB for soft tissue. As $\alpha = 1$ dB cm^{-1} MHz^{-1} the image depth is related to transducer frequency as

$$D = \frac{50}{f} \qquad (18.7)$$

A final dynamic range of 50 dB is typical of modern ultrasound systems which would give practical image depths plotted in Fig. 18.3b and Fig. 18.4b. The displayed dynamic range is operator controlled.

TIME GAIN COMPENSATION (SWEPT GAIN)

Echoes originating from greater tissue depths will have smaller amplitudes as the sound has undergone attenuation with distance traveled. In order to produce good quality images it is necessary to compensate for echo attenuation and a time varying gain control or time gain compensation (TGC) circuit amplifies the signal depending on time of arrival; later signals undergo greater amplification so correcting signal amplitude loss from tissue attenuation. The process is also known as **swept gain** or **time varied gain**.

TGC techniques amplify the signal proportional to the time delay between the transmission and detection of the ultrasound pulses. In the simplest form of TGC the amplification is linear but modern imaging systems also provide nonlinear amplification. Either analog or digital methods which use look-up tables may be used. This form of signal compensation is illustrated in Fig. 18.7a where linear amplification dependent on depth is given to echo-signals originating from 2 to 6 cm (in this example); echoes outside this range receive no amplification. The overall effect is illustrated in Fig. 18.7b.

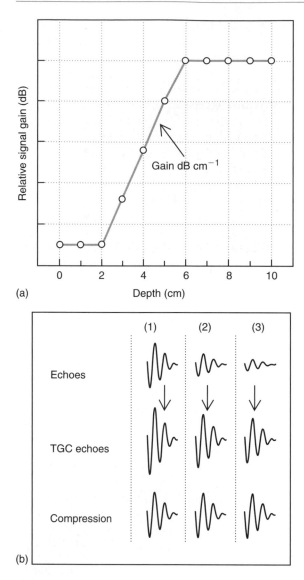

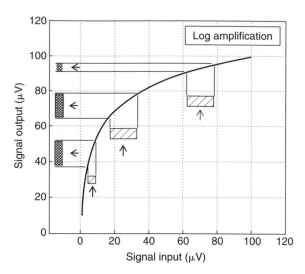

Figure 18.8 *Signal compression achieved by logarithmic amplification. Small signal amplitudes are increased, large signals are reduced.*

larger signals and gives the final signal series illustrated by the bottom line of pulses in Fig. 18.7b. Dynamic range is usually reduced to about 20 to 30 dB which can be handled more easily by the electronics.

DEMODULATION AND REJECTION

After compression the signals undergo the equivalent of full-wave rectification which defines their outline or shape (envelope). This is the **demodulated signal**. A threshold is placed on the demodulated signals to reject smaller amplitude pulses which mostly carry acoustic or electronic noise and have very little useful information. The signals above threshold are then digitized.

PHASE DECODING

The conventional ultrasound image represents changes in signal amplitude, although current developments use information derived from both **phase** and **amplitude** with a consequent improvement in signal-to-noise ratio (SNR). Both spatial and temporal resolution are improved (faster frame rates). Dynamic range is also increased to 100 dB which improves image depth.

18.2.2 Signal digitization

In current ultrasound equipment image formation is controlled by computer and the clinical image is

Figure 18.7 *(a) Time gain compensation (TGC) curve showing the slope representing dB cm^{-1} gain. (b) TGC altering the signal amplitude where late arriving signals receive more gain than earlier ones, the signals then undergo compression.*

COMPRESSION

After TGC the large dynamic range of signal amplitude cannot be displayed effectively so the signal range is compressed using logarithmic amplification represented in Fig. 18.8, where smaller input signals (10 to 20 µV) will undergo greater amplification than stronger signals (70 to 80 µV). This increases the amplitude of the smaller signals at the expense of the

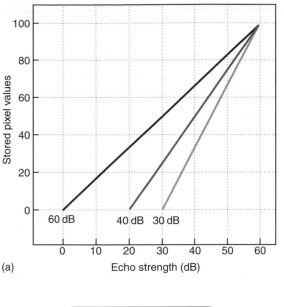

(a)

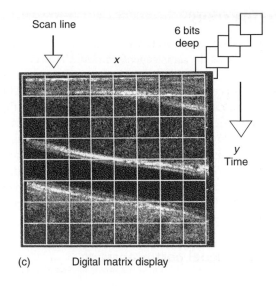

(c) Digital matrix display

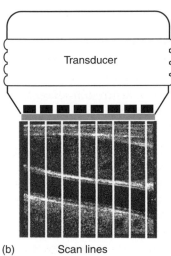

(b) Scan lines

Figure 18.9 *(a) Echoes are digitized according to time of arrival and strength. Three dynamic display ranges are shown, 30, 40, and 60 dB. (**b**) Transducer elements dividing the area of interest into scan lines. (**c**) The image matrix superimposed on the area of interest, showing image formation determined by scan line position in the x-axis and echo time of arrival in the y-axis.*

viewed on a video monitor in a continuous or real-time mode. First the echo signals undergo some processing and are then digitized according to echo strength. Figure 18.9a indicates how the stored pixel values (*y*-axis) in computer memory relate to echo signal strength (*x*-axis) for three selected dynamic ranges 30, 40, and 60 dB. Fig. 18.9b and c show scan line information from each transducer element group is located in an image matrix according to element position (matrix *x*-axis) and echo depth (matrix *y*-axis). The matrix column (*x*-axis) is **time coded** for echoes arriving at fixed depths. The matrix rows (*y-axis*) are chosen by the transducer **group position**.

The **echo strength** is stored as a 6, 7 or 8-bit number in each memory location depending on dynamic range. An imaging device, which uses a linear probe having 128 parallel beams, allocates two columns in computer memory for each beam so the 2-D image memory has a capacity of 256 × 256 storage locations.

Locations in the memory array are addressed as columns 1 to 256 and rows 1 to 256. Echoes from beam-1 occupy columns 1 and 2, those from beam-2 occupy 3 and 4 and so on until beam 128 occupies columns 255 and 256. Each location or address in the 256 × 256 memory holds a digital number representing echo strength.

SECTOR SCANS

The production of sector scans (see phased arrays later) follows the same general principle. However, in sector scans the relationship between memory location and echo position is by **polar coordinates**. The angle and radius at which the echo occurs defines the memory location. The digital memory (frame) of a modern ultrasound display is typically 512×512 pixels; each pixel 6, 7 or 8 bits deep. Several of these frames can be acquired each second. If the imaging depth is 15 cm then each of the 512 pixels in the y-axis represents $150/512 = 0.3$ mm; for a 20 cm imaging depth each pixel would represent 0.4 mm.

18.2.3 Signal post-processing

Many aspects of image presentation are under user control. Echoes emanating from deep structures experience greater signal attenuation than those from superficial structures. Diagnostic imaging equipment allows the user to vary the amplification of echoes from different depths by using variable TGC (see Fig. 18.6 and Fig. 18.7). Usually, the amplification increases with depth but the user may decide not to amplify echoes from a variety of depths depending on whether that information is useful or not.

SENSITIVITY

The simplest image involves only one reflecting surface in the path of the beam but in practice of course there is more than just one. A series of echoes will be received from these surfaces whose amplitudes will vary in size depending on the size of the echo and the depth at which the echo originates.

It may happen that echoes from diffuse structures at depth are so small as to be indistinguishable from the noise level which would also be amplified. The user may vary the depth of field of view by using zoom or expansion controls and, in sector imaging, the **field angle**. In real-time imaging the operator is depth limited, e.g. the depth that can be interrogated while still maintaining real-time or continuous effect. The continuous real-time effect may be sacrificed if extra image depth is required.

GRAY-SCALE DISPLAY

Each pixel contains a numerical value representing signal strength; stronger reflections have larger pixel values than weaker reflections. A gray-scale display represents echo signal strengths. Pixel depth influences displayed image contrast; more bits per pixel increases this contrast range. Typical pixel depths are:

- 6 bits or 2^6 giving 64 gray scales
- 7 bits or 2^7 giving 128 gray scales
- 8 bits or 2^8 giving 256 gray scales

The binary values in each pixel are converted to analog (voltage) levels for display on a video monitor for visual inspection or film recording. The digital values are fed out from the matrix in sequence into a digital-to-analog converter (DAC) and the varying analog voltage coded with a video signal to give a video raster display.

18.3 TRANSDUCERS

Mechanical scanning methods previously used in ultrasound imaging have almost entirely been replaced by electronically scanned multi-element array transducers. There are two basic types of electronically scanned transducer:

- Sequenced (switched) transducer arrays (linear or curvilinear designs)
- Phased transducer arrays (linear or annular)

These transducers give different image shapes or scan fields and are shown in Fig. 18.10. Each transducer has its own advantages and disadvantages, these are described for each transducer type and typical applications are given.

Sequenced arrays selectively pulse a group of transducer elements. The picture is constructed by moving the group sequence along the transducer. Resolution is determined by the number of scanned lines, field of view and transducer aperture already shown in Fig. 18.2b. The electronic distinction between sequenced and **phased** arrays is decided by the excitation pulse timing.

Annular array transducers differ from these designs since their separate elements form an annulus which is mechanically scanned.

18.3.1 The linear sequence array

The linear array is formed from a large number (up to 128) individual transducer **elements** arranged in groups. During each transmission/receive cycle only

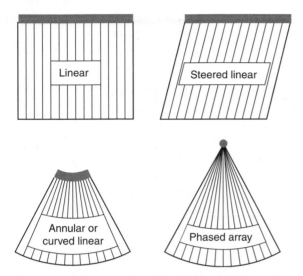

Figure 18.10 *Image scan fields delivered by different transducers commonly used in diagnostic ultrasound.*

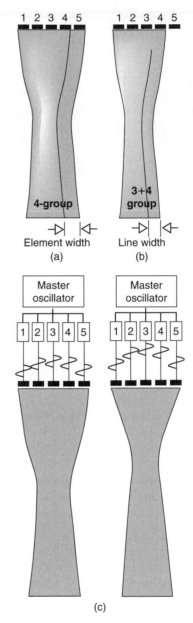

Figure 18.11 *(a) Linear array beam sequence switching where the aperture varies between three and four elements which gives (b) a scan line separation less than the width of the individual element. (c) Varying the delay times applied to each element group influences the depth of focus of the aperture.*

one transducer group (from 16 to 32 elements) is active. The information for each scan line is obtained by switching; a single element is added to the group while the last element is removed.

The transducer group or **aperture** thus advances along the length of the transducer and reconstructs the sectional image line by line defined by the individual element width. The ultrasound field from an individual small element in a multi-element linear array would be a very fine beam. Due to these narrow dimensions the beam would have a very short near field and would diverge very quickly giving poor resolution at depth. This problem can be solved by pulsing groups of transducers in unison; usually 8 to 32 elements on a 60 to 120 element array. This produces a wider beam with much improved resolution characteristics at depth. The group size defines the transducer aperture. A scanning motion is obtained by shifting an element one at a time as seen in Fig. 18.11a.

The number of scan lines can be doubled if two groups having different sizes are used. In Fig. 18.11b, where $n = 3$, if the first group consists of n elements transmitting and receiving as a unit and the second group has an extra element added, giving $n + 1$ elements then the central axis of this unit only shifts by a half-element compared with the first group. During each transmission/receive cycle only a single transducer group is active (n or $n + 1$).

Although linear arrays can operate in an unfocused mode linear sequential arrays are commonly focused

by delaying or phasing the excitation pulses (Fig. 18.11c). This produces either a short or long focal length; the delay pulses have nanosecond timing. A focused linear array is sometimes called a **phased**

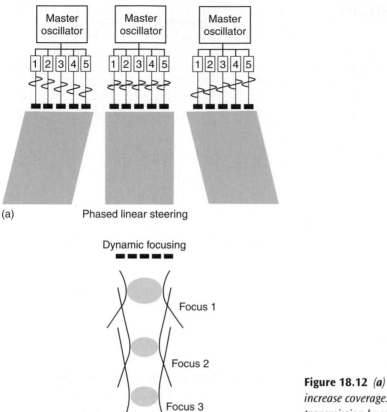

(a) Phased linear steering

Dynamic focusing

Focus 1

Focus 2

Focus 3

(c)

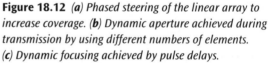

(b)

Figure 18.12 *(a) Phased steering of the linear array to increase coverage. (b) Dynamic aperture achieved during transmission by using different numbers of elements. (c) Dynamic focusing achieved by pulse delays.*

linear array. Pulse delay focuses the beam but the linear array is still operated in a **sequenced** manner.

Linear scanning uses **rectilinear coordinates**; the beam is moved in a rectangular or parallelogram pattern as demonstrated in Fig. 18.12a giving equal dimensions in the near and far fields seen in the top row of Fig. 18.10. The position of the narrow section of the beam at various depths is controlled by the **aperture size** (size of element group), therefore the focus at various depths is maintained by dynamically varying the aperture (see Fig. 18.12b) giving a **dynamic aperture** to the transducer.

MULTIPLE FOCUSING

During transmission the focusing can be altered by delaying the pulses in set patterns (focus 1, 2, and 3 in Fig. 18.12c). The echoes are then received from each focal point before the beam is switched to the next focus. The transducer frame rate is reduced as $1/F_n$ where F_n is the number of foci. **Dynamic focusing** is achieved during echo reception by switching receiver

delays so collecting accurately timed echoes from focus points 3, 2, and 1 in Fig. 18.12c.

There is no reduction in frame rate for dynamic focusing during reception. Both dynamic aperture and dynamic focusing maintain optimum image resolution over the entire image depth. The same field dimensions can also be maintained with depth by simultaneously applying **dynamic aperture**.

FRAME RATE

Several transducer elements provide a scan line (see Fig. 18.11a and b) which makes up a sectional image having a typical frame rate of between 25 and 30 frames per second. Each frame is made up from a complete set of scan lines. The action of the real-time transducer moves the scan line prior to the next transmission pulse. The rate of scan-line movement influences the frame rate which is related to the pulse repetition frequency as

$$FR = \frac{PRF}{\text{number of scan lines}} \quad (18.8)$$

Table 18.1 *Pulse repetition frequency (PRF) beam penetration and frame rate.*

Frequency (MHz)	PRF (kHz)	Penetration (cm)	Frame rate (100 lines)
3.5	3.8	20	38
5.0	5.0	15	51
7.5	7.7	10	77
10.0	15.4	5	154

The frame rate is therefore determined by the PRF and the number of scan lines. The frame time (FT) is the time taken to acquire the complete image of N scan lines and the frame rate is the inverse of this so

$$\mathrm{PRP} \times N = \mathrm{FT} \qquad (18.9)$$

The frame rate should exceed 20 fps if image flicker to be avoided. Frame rate is limited by image depth and number of multiple focuses so that:

$$\mathrm{PRF} = \text{scan lines} \times \text{number of focuses} \\ \times \text{frame rate} \qquad (18.10)$$

If extra depth is required then the frame rate may be slowed since the PRF must be reduced. Table 18.1 compares frequency, PRF, image depth, and frame rate. Each focus during dynamic focusing requires a transmission pulse. If sound velocity is $150\,000\,\mathrm{cm\,s^{-1}}$ for soft tissue and making allowances for the return path then the PRF is determined by the factor $150\,000 \times 0.5 = 75\,000$, so

$$\text{beam penetration} \times \text{focuses} \times \text{scan lines} \\ \times \text{frame rate} = 75\,000 \qquad (18.11)$$

Box 18.1 calculates the frame rate for a 5 MHz transducer having 128 elements.

LINEAR ARRAY SPECIFICATIONS

The linear array is commonly used for examining the abdomen. A typical linear transducer would have:

- 60 to 120 transducer elements
- 8 to 32 group width (aperture)
- 3.5 to 7.5 MHz frequency range.
- Element width 1 to 41
- Size of footprint from $2 \times 0.6\,\mathrm{cm}$ to $1.4 \times 10\,\mathrm{cm}$

Box 18.1 Transducer frame rate

A 5 MHz transducer having 128 elements is required to give a 12 cm image depth. What is the frame rate? The velocity of sound in soft tissue is $1500\,\mathrm{m\,s^{-1}}$. This is $\approx 13\,\mathrm{\mu s\,cm^{-1}}$ for the returning echo, so

$$\mathrm{PRP} = 12 \times 13 = 156\,\mathrm{\mu s}$$
$$\mathrm{FT} = 156 \times 128 = 20\,\mathrm{ms}$$
$$\mathrm{FR} = 50\,\mathrm{Hz}$$

Increasing PRP, image depth or scan line density will decrease frame rate.

The applications include:

- Large body areas such as abdomen
- Gynecology
- Thyroid
- Superficial vessels
- Ultrasound guided biopsy

Advantages are a rectangular field of view which gives good definition to both near and distant anatomy as seen in Fig. 18.13a and b and good image quality across the full image depth and field of view. The disadvantages are a large footprint (surface contact area) and a limited field of view with depth.

CURVED ARRAYS

These are a modification of the linear array design having a convex transducer surface. The scan is produced by sequential element switching as before but a **sector scan** is produced (Fig. 18.13c and d) having a curved top. The size of this transducer is smaller than the linear array giving it a smaller footprint (surface contact area). The beam is much wider at depth so gives a larger anatomical image. The size of the sector, which is variable, is determined by the pulse delay variation.

A linear array can give a diverging field of view; this is the **vector array** and the scan lines fan outwards. The image format is similar to the curvilinear array except that the footprint is smaller still and the display format has a flat top.

SPECIFICATIONS

A typical sequenced curved array would have:

- Radius of curvature 40 to 80 mm
- Frequency 3.5 to 5.0 MHz

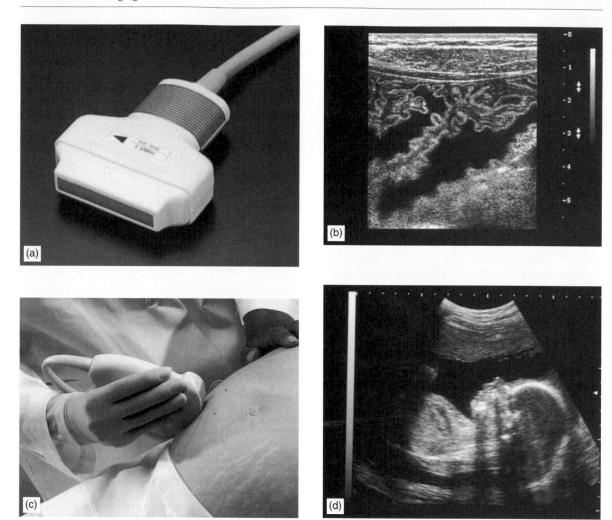

Figure 18.13 *Linear array (a) and curved linear array (c) transducers with their respective clinical images (b) and (d).*

- Elements >100
- Aperture 16 to 32 elements
- Frame rate 58 fps

18.3.2 The phased array

The principle of the phased array is shown in Fig. 18.14. The transmit pulses are applied to each element via a delay which gives a swiveled (angled) wavefront. The degree of swivel ($\pm 45°$) requires very narrow elements of about $1/2\,\lambda$ dimensions. The effective aperture A' is $A \times \cos j$ where A is the total aperture or array length without the swivel. During receive mode the same pulse delays are used.

The phased array can also produce directional and focused beams as used in the sequenced array which moves the focal point to position it shallow or deep giving electronic dynamic focusing in conjunction with beam steering. Unlike the linear sequenced array all the elements are pulsed at the same time during transmission and reception and the phased array image formation is achieved by using polar coordinates and not rectilinear.

Phased arrays use a smaller number of elements than a linear array (48 to 128) and consequently their footprint is smaller allowing inspection of more restricted anatomy (between the rib cage). Phased array probes are shown in Fig. 18.15a and c. A pie-shaped or **sector scan** is obtained which is shown in Fig. 18.15b. The phased array has demanding requirements since

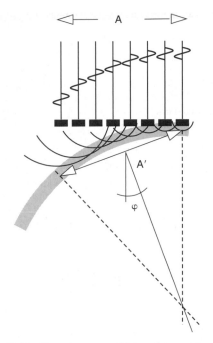

Figure 18.14 *Phased array switching giving a planar or focused beam. All the elements usually act in unison.*

separate transmit and receive delay circuits are present for each element. All elements are pulsed using various delay timings; the pulse rate determines the number of scan lines. The directional characteristic of the elements determines the swivel angle ($\pm 45°$) which is achieved with very narrow elements ($\approx 1/2\lambda = 0.22$ mm for 3.5 MHz). In the receive mode delays are introduced into the received signals which enable the transducer to be sensitive to echoes returning from specific directions. These effects produce arrays which are preferentially sensitive to echoes emanating from chosen regions which can be user selected by variation of the delay times. If delay times are changed during the receiving cycle the focal plane can be varied to give **dynamic focusing** but increasing the number of focal planes decreases the frame rate. **Dynamic apertures** are achieved by using a proportion of the total available elements, so in some circumstances not all the elements in a phased array are being used.

PHASED ARRAY PROBE

The design of the phased array lends itself to miniature probe design for internal examinations (rectum,

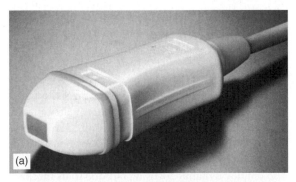

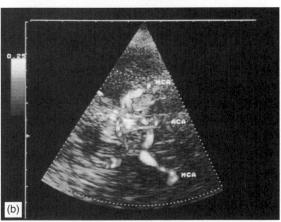

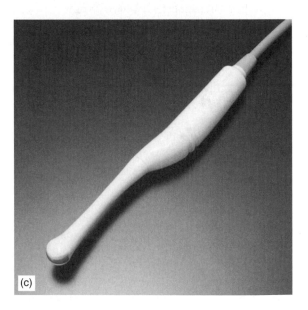

Figure 18.15 *(a) Phased array transducers. (b) Example sector display. (c) Phased array probe (courtesy Toshiba Medical Systems).*

vagina, and esophagus). Tiny catheter sized ultrasound transducers are available for intra-luminal inspection of blood vessels. This bi-planar probe allows imaging in transverse (360°) and longitudinal planes (240°); frequency range is typically 5 to 7.5 MHz. Acoustic coupling can be obtained either by close application to the epithelial mucous or by inflating an 'on-board' water balloon.

SPECIFICATIONS

Phased array transducers with small arrays (14 mm aperture) are useful for echocardiography. Larger arrays give large field of view pictures of the abdomen and special applications are found in rectal and gynecological probes.

Advantages are the large field of view relative to its footprint size and the fast frame rate. The disadvantage is that the sector scan pattern gives a poor near field of view. Typical specifications for a phased array would be:

- Frequency 2.5, 3.5, 5.0, and 7 MHz
- Frame rate up to 156 fps
- Imaging depth 25 cm
- Aperture (transducer size) 14 to 28 mm
- Swivel 40 to 45°

18.3.3 Annular transducer

Instead of individual small linear elements a series of concentric transducers operates as an annular phased array; the side and plan view are given in Fig. 18.16a. This produces a conical beam section. The concentric rings resemble an optical Fresnel lens. The signals are delayed to each ring in order to give a focused beam (Fig. 18.16b) which is mechanically moved in an arc.

Excellent image quality can be obtained from annular arrays since the lateral resolution and resolution at depth can be influenced by signal phasing giving a superior constant focus with depth. The focusing effect is achieved by pulsing the two outermost elements before the two next inner neighbors. The composite wavefront then has a focus along the mid-line. The overall depth of focus is controlled by the delay between pulsing signals. Annular arrays also provide superior slice thickness uniformity.

Annular arrays cannot be steered electronically as linear phased arrays, so a mechanical 'wobbler' method is employed. A typical design with the transducer

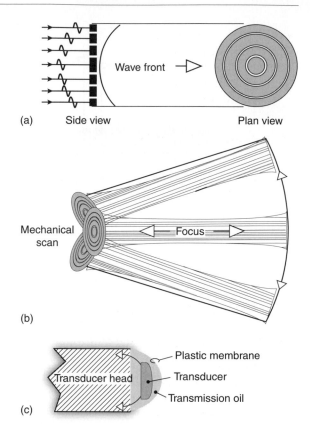

Figure 18.16 (a) Annular array transducer design and (b) the mechanical scan pattern achieved by the mechanical scan head. (c) The transducer in its oil bath.

moving within an enclosed bath of transmission oil is shown in Fig. 18.16c. Reduced scan frequency enables increased line density with better resolution. There is a free choice of sector angle and system resolution is optimized by altering scan frequency. Annular arrays also employ dynamic focusing but due to its mechanical scanning it is difficult to incorporate Doppler scan techniques since the mechanical movement would introduce interfering signals.

SPECIFICATIONS

Annular arrays are employed whenever fine detail is important such as fetal examinations. They give very good image quality over a long focal length. Their disadvantages are that they require mechanical scanning which restricts their use for Doppler/duplex imaging. A typical transducer would consist of:

- Annular array 3.5 and 5.0 MHz
- Electronic focusing

- Adjustable transmit focus
- Dynamic receive focus
- Imaging depth 25 cm (3.5 MHz)
- 17 cm (5 MHz)
- Frame rate 30 fps

18.4 IMAGE ARTIFACTS

Image artifacts are caused by a variety of technical factors which give false or misleading information in the final image. There are two main sources of artifact in diagnostic ultrasound images due to:

- Propagation
- Attenuation

18.4.1 Propagation errors

REVERBERATIONS (MULTIPLE ECHOES)

This effect may occur between the face of the transducer and a strongly reflecting surface. The echo signal from this surface returns to the transducer where it is reflected again to the structure surface back to the transducer and so on. In the image the structure is imaged as expected but it also contains 'structure' at regular intervals (successively reduced in amplitude) due to reverberation of the initial strong reflector. This occurs because the probe acts as though it has received an echo which has taken twice as long as the first. This is commonly seen in images which include bowel gas or sections of the bladder wall.

MULTIPLE PATH REFLECTION

The incident ultrasound beam may be obliquely reflected onto a second reflector. The echo returns to the transducer via the initial reflecting surface as illustrated in Fig. 18.17. There is a miscalculation based on the time taken for the pulse's round trip giving misregistration beyond the oblique reflecting surface causing a ghost or apparent image.

SECTION THICKNESS/SLICE WIDTH

The width of the beam is defined by the acoustic lens as shown in Fig. 18.5. Off-axis echoes from outside the section thickness appear in regions that should be echo free. This is commonly seen in the lumens of large blood vessels and large cysts.

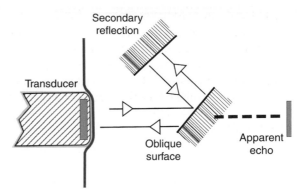

Figure 18.17 *The origin of multiple path errors from an off beam reflecting surface giving an apparent echo.*

REFRACTION

This has been described fully in Chapter 17 and is the bending of the ultrasound beam as it passes through tissues having different characteristic velocities. The refracted beam causes echoes to be misregistered. This is commonly seen in tissues having marked differences in acoustic impedance particularly the eye (lens and vitreous humor) and fatty tissues.

SPECKLE

If the scattering surfaces are spaced at distances less than the axial resolution then echo interference gives constructive and destructive interference patterns which increase image noise seen as speckle on the display.

BEAM LOBES

The weak echoes from **side** or **grating lobes** are not usually visualized but they become visible from strong reflectors outside the beam section causing misplaced artifacts within the image; commonly seen when imaging the fetal skull.

18.4.2 Attenuation errors

SHADOWING

If several objects of interest are aligned in the path of the beam and the first object in the beam's path is a very strong reflector then almost all of the sound will be reflected at the first object leaving very little to interact with the remaining objects in the path. As a result the area behind the first structure appears uniformly black indicating absence of echogenic structures. These structures are being 'shadowed' by the first strong reflector. An example of this phenomenon is found distally to bone and air structures. One solution is to change the probe's direction or angle of attack.

ENHANCEMENT

When the beam is intersected by a low attenuation object (traveling between higher attenuation and low attenuation pathways) there is a much lower attenuation for the returning echoes from the distant wall of this object. These echoes will have abnormally large amplitudes. Commonly seen in fatty cysts and other substances having a high lipid content such as bile.

18.5 DOPPLER IMAGING

Blood velocity can be measured very accurately using the **Doppler effect** which is the apparent change in frequency (pitch) when the sound source is moving with respect to the listener (or transducer). This is illustrated in Fig. 18.18a showing expansion of the wavefront; lower frequency of sound sources passing away from the receiver and compression of the wavefront with source towards the receiver. A common example of this phenomenon is the change in sound pitch from the siren on a passing ambulance or police car.

18.5.1 The Doppler shift

Figure 18.18b shows two waveforms, a transmitted signal and the returning signal, of slightly higher frequency, from a moving object (blood corpuscles). The interference signal has a much lower beat-frequency, its changing frequency giving useful qualitative information to an experienced sonographer when measuring blood velocity.

For a simple case where the transducer is in line with the flowing medium (blood) the apparent frequency f' observed is given by:

$$f' = \left(\frac{v}{v \pm S}\right) f_0 \qquad (18.12)$$

where v is velocity of sound in medium S the blood velocity (+ towards; − away) and f_0 is the transmitted

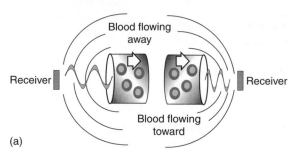

(a)

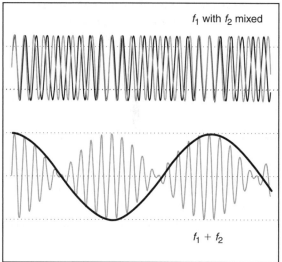

f_1 with f_2 mixed

$f_1 + f_2$

Figure 18.18 (**a**) The Doppler principle showing one sound source traveling away from the receiver and another towards the receiver showing expansion and compression of the wave front. (**b**) Two frequencies f_1 and f_2 mixed to give a beat frequency.

ultrasound frequency. When ultrasound is incident on the moving blood corpuscles there will be a change in the frequency of the returning sound energy. The detected frequency will increase if the blood is moving towards the transducer and decrease if the blood is moving away. For a transducer angle θ the Doppler frequency of the reflected ultrasound is given by

$$f_D = \frac{2 f_0 v}{c} \times \cos \theta \qquad (18.13)$$

where f_D is the Doppler shift frequency, c is the velocity of sound in the medium and θ is the angle between the direction of the sound beam and the direction of the blood flow. Box 18.2 calculates the frequency change for transducers having different angles to the skin surface using the parameters in Fig. 18.19.

Box 18.2 Examples of Doppler shift

The basic equation is

$$f_D = \frac{2 f_0 v}{c} \times \cos \theta$$

where

f_D = frequency change or Doppler shift
f_0 = frequency of ultrasound transmitted beam
c = sound velocity in medium
v = blood velocity
θ = angle between transducer and vessel

Example

If the velocity of blood is $20\ \mathrm{cm\ s^{-1}}$, the transducer frequency is 5 MHz and 60° then 45° are chosen as the angles to the vessel, what are the Doppler shifts? Using the basic equation:

$$f_D = \frac{2\left(5 \times 10^6\right) \times 20}{15.7 \times 10^4} \times 0.5 = 637\ \mathrm{Hz\ for\ 60°}$$

$$f_D = \frac{2\left(5 \times 10^6\right) \times 20}{15.7 \times 10^4} \times 0.7 = 900\ \mathrm{Hz\ for\ 45°}$$

Note that:

- Doppler shift increases as transducer is aligned with the vessel axis.
- Doppler shift has a positive or negative value depending on flow direction: +, flow toward; −, flow away from transducer. These are color coded in Doppler imaging.
- Percentage frequency change is *very* small: 637 Hz represents 0.0127% and 900 Hz represents 0.018% of the 5 MHz carrier frequency.

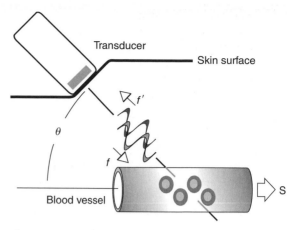

Figure 18.19 *The basic Doppler geometry referred to in the text.*

of the ultrasound. The corpuscles cause the beam to be scattered and not specularly reflected. The intensity of the scattering increases with frequency f as f^4.

Thus higher frequency ultrasound is preferred for Doppler studies. These higher frequencies provide a larger shift in frequency for a given velocity of scatterer. However, it should be remembered that the penetration of the Doppler beam would be compromised with increasing frequency.

18.5.2 Doppler transducers

CONTINUOUS WAVE DOPPLER

The simplest case is where a continuous ultrasound signal is applied to the patient's skin and the change in frequency of the reflected sound is computed; information on any movements in the beam can be determined often as an audible signal such as a fetal monitor. The transducer design is illustrated in Fig. 18.20a. The two signals are mixed electronically in a demodulator to separate the interference or beat signal having a lower frequency in the audible range.

PULSED DOPPLER

Using a source of pulsed ultrasound it is possible to select the tissue depth at which echo signals are examined for Doppler shifts. This is achieved by limiting the frequency analysis to echo pulses which are received at specific time intervals after pulse generation shown in Fig. 18.20b; pulsed wave Doppler probes have a single transmit/receive transducer. The pulse repetition

DEMODULATION

The two signals are mixed electronically in a demodulator to separate the interference or beat signal having a lower frequency, typically in the audible range, which is represented in Fig. 18.18b as the envelope. The beat frequency changes with the Doppler shift. The source of the echoes for Doppler studies is the blood corpuscles which are very much smaller than the wavelength

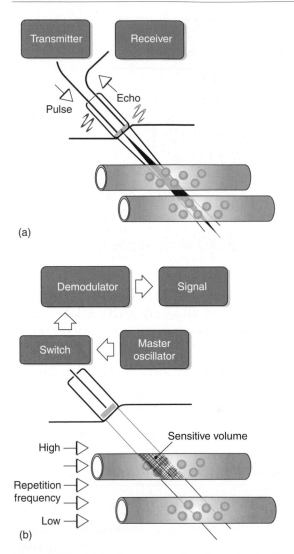

(a)

(b)

Figure 18.20 (a) Continuous wave Doppler probe showing extended depth of response. (b) Pulsed Doppler probe selecting the depth for blood velocity measurements by altering the pulse repetition frequency.

frequency determines the maximum depth of the sensitive volume.

The time at which the analysis begins and its duration determine the depth and axial length of the volume of tissue which is examined for flow information (the area from which the echoes are received). This is equivalent to opening a signal gate so the procedure is known as 'gating'. It is possible to divide the length of the ultrasound beam into a sequence of gates each having a size of one pixel which provides flow information for color coding.

There are two important limitations on the use of pulsed Doppler ultrasound measurement of blood flow. The maximum depth that can be examined and the maximum frequency shift detected is limited by the pulse repetition frequency. Increasing the repetition frequency increases the maximum frequency shift that can be detected but decreases the interrogation depth.

MAXIMUM VELOCITY

This depends on the transducer frequency and its PRF. From eqn18.13 the velocity is

$$v = \frac{\Delta f \times c}{2 f_0} \times \cos \theta \qquad (18.14)$$

For soft tissue $c = 150\,000 \text{ cm s}^{-1}$. So

$$v = \frac{\Delta f \left(7.5 \times 10^4 \right)}{f_0} \times \cos \theta \qquad (18.15)$$

If the Nyquist frequency determines the highest Doppler frequency that can be accurately resolved then this is PRF/2; from eqn 18.15 yields:

$$v_{max} = \frac{\text{PRF} \times c}{4 f_0 \times \cos \theta} \qquad (18.16)$$

Blood velocity in humans varies between 20 to 200 cm s^{-1}. Equation 18.16 indicates that high PRF values are necessary in order to measure fast flow rates, but PRF is also related to image depth, so fast flow rates can only be detected at small distances from the transducer face. The depth of response represented in Fig. 18.20b can be calculated if the speed of sound in soft tissue is taken to be 1500 m s^{-1} or ≈ 6.5 cm μs^{-1}. Transmission and reception takes about 13 μs cm^{-1} so for 6 cm tissue depth the **pulse repetition period** must be $>6 \times 13$ or 78 μs. The PRF is the inverse or 12.8 kHz. Similar relationships between PRF, PRP, and depth are given in Table 18.2. The maximum Doppler shift that can be detected is half the repetition frequency which is 6.25 kHz for a PRF of 12.5 kHz so from eqn 18.16 this gives 98 cm s^{-1}.

ALIASING

This has been discussed in Chapter 14 and concerns signal sampling rate and the Nyquist frequency.

Table 18.2 *Relationship between pulse repetition frequency (PRF), pulse repetition period (PRP), and depth.*

PRF (kHz)	PRP (μs)	Depth (cm)
5	200	15.4
8	125	9.6
12.5	80	6.0
15	66	5.0
20	50	3.8

Aliasing artifacts in pulsed Doppler give false flow direction signals. The highest Doppler shift that pulsed Doppler can measure is PRF/2; a maximum repetition frequency is related to maximum image depth (D_{max}) then maximum recorded velocity and image depth are related as

$$PRF = \frac{c}{D_{max}} \qquad (18.17)$$

High blood velocities which produce Doppler shifts greater than half the repetition frequency cause an effect known as aliasing, so the frequency shift recorded will incorrectly underestimate the value of the blood velocity.

18.5.3 Duplex and color velocity imaging

DUPLEX IMAGING

This combines Doppler information with a real-time gray-scale image. A pulsed Doppler transducer is combined in the array (linear or phased) at an angle so that it can be directed into the area of interest as shown in Fig. 18.21. The placement of the sensitive area or sample volume is operator controlled so that a particular vessel can be targeted. This technique produces a 2-D representation of the direction and velocity of blood flow on a gray-scale image. In a typical display blood flowing towards the transducer is coded as red and blood flow away from the transducer is represented as blue.

Various intermediate colors represent the different velocities of the flow. Images of blood flow are produced by examining the change in the echo pattern for each line in the image. The two patterns are examined for differences which would have been produced by movement of blood. Variations in pattern are then color-coded red or blue depending on the

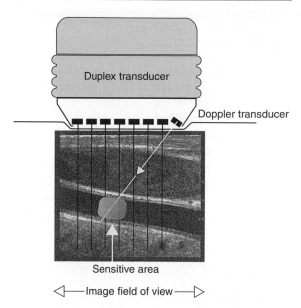

Figure 18.21 *Linear array containing a Doppler transducer used for combined color flow in duplex imaging.*

Table 18.3 *Advantages and disadvantages of duplex imaging.*

Advantages	Disadvantages
Visual display of blood flow	Low spatial resolution
Rapid localization of vessel	Low frame rates
Flow disturbances visualized	Aliasing problems
Small flow values measured	
Identification of hypo-echoic plaque	High power requirements
Surface features identified	

direction of the change. The resolution of Doppler flow images is commonly restricted to 128×128 matrices. Advantages and disadvantages of duplex imaging are given in Table 18.3.

COLOR DOPPLER DISPLAYS

Flow echoes in the display itself are assigned colors according to the color map chosen by the manufacturer. Red, orange, yellow, blue, cyan, and white typically indicate positive or negative Doppler shifts (approaching or receding flow). The phase quadrature and auto-correlation processes used in most color-Doppler imaging systems yield the sign, mean, variance, and amplitude or power of the Doppler spectrum at each of many volume-sample locations in a tissue cross section. Traditionally, in color-Doppler imaging, sign and mean Doppler shift, and sometimes, variance (usually in cardiac applications), are color-encoded and displayed. These parameters are dependent on Doppler angle and are subject to aliasing. Yellow, cyan or green is sometimes used to indicate variance (disturbed or turbulent flow).

Linear, convex, phased, and vector arrays are used to acquire the gray-scale and color-flow information. The color controls include gain, map selection, variance on/off, persistence, color/gray priority, scale (PKF), baseline shift, wall filter, and color window angle. Since Doppler color-flow instruments are pulsed they are subject to the limitations of Doppler angle dependence and aliasing.

18.5.4 Power Doppler

In the Doppler color flow image the magnitude of the frequency shift color encodes the pixel value and assigns a color depending on blood flow direction; (positive or negative). This Doppler signal processing places a restriction on motion sensitivity since the signals received must be extracted to determine velocity and direction from the Doppler and phase shifts in the returning echoes within each gated region.

Power Doppler information encodes the strength of the Doppler shifts (amplitude, intensity, power, energy) with colors based on the selected power map and ignores directional (phase) information. In power Doppler, the density of the red blood cells is depicted, as opposed to their velocity. This improves the sensitivity to motion (e.g. slow blood flow) at the expense of directional and quantitative flow information and is free of aliasing and angle dependence. It therefore exhibits increased sensitivity to slow flow rates, picking up flow in small or deep vessels which would otherwise be missed in color velocity imaging. Greater sensitivity allows detection of very subtle and slow blood flows. Since the amplitude (or power) of the Doppler shifts is determined by the concentration of moving particles (blood cells) it is independent of Doppler shift frequency. Power Doppler integrates the area under the echo signal spectrum and this information is independent of probe angle and aliasing. This uniformity of signal display is the important advantage of power Doppler, although this is accomplished with a loss in flow direction, speed, and character information.

A noticeable disadvantage of power Doppler is the susceptibility to motion artifacts, which severely limits its application to areas with considerable motion (e.g. the heart) unless substantial weighted temporal averaging is employed (i.e. high frame-to-frame averaging or high persistence). This reduces motion artifact but increases the display response time (i.e. the color map seems to lag behind the gray-scale image).

The use of the expression 'power Doppler' suggests increased transmitted ultrasound power to the patient but the power levels are about the same as those in a standard color flow procedure. The difference is in the processing of the returning signals, where the **total power information** of the signal is used in the display.

18.6 SAFETY

The two important mechanisms of potential hazard in diagnostic ultrasound that are considered relevant to present day transducers are **heating** and **cavitation**.

Heating is caused by the conversion of ultrasonic energy to heat in the tissue. The intensity I of ultrasound energy is defined as the energy flux crossing unit area in unit time or the rate of delivery of ultrasound energy per unit area of tissue. Intensity is measured in watts as $\mathrm{W\,cm^{-2}}$ or $\mathrm{mW\,cm^{-2}}$.

Cavitation or gas bubble growth is related to acoustic pressure p. Intensity and pressure are related as

$$I = \frac{p^2}{z} \qquad (18.18)$$

where z is the acoustic impedance of the tissue. A typical pulsed beam, as used in diagnostic ultrasound, has an 'on time' or **mark** and an 'off time' or **space**; the mark to space ratio ($m{:}s$) and **duty factor** $[m/(m+s)] \times 100\%$ are important measurements when considering safety factors. Ultrasound **power** is defined as the energy flux per unit time through the whole cross section of the beam.

The pulse from a diagnostic ultrasound transducer delivers an acoustic pressure in tissue that alternates between positive and negative values. The major hazards associated with these pressure events are the acoustic output measured in several ways but commonly as the **spatial time averaged intensity** I_{SPTA} in $\mathrm{W\,m^{-2}}$ and the **time averaged power** measured in milliwatts (mW).

18.6.1 Units of intensity

The beam profile from an ultrasound probe has already been shown in Chapter 17. A modified version in Fig. 18.22 is used for defining the basic and derived spatial intensity parameters:

- Spatial peak (SP): The peak beam intensity measured on the central axis
- Spatial average (SA): The mean intensity of the transducer beam

Ultrasound is delivered in a series of pulses, each giving a peak output. The number of peaks per unit time depends on the pulse repetition frequency (PRF). The pulse train shown in Fig. 18.23a describes the temporal parameters that are related to the duty factor and **mark:space** ratio which is influenced by the pulse width.

- **Pulse average** (PA) is the intensity during 'on-time' (mark).
- **Temporal peak** (TP) is the highest intensity of the pulse. Since the pulse amplitude of Doppler is constant but that of diagnostic ultrasound is varying, the **peak intensity** within each pulse of the diagnostic waveform is the temporal peak TP and the average intensity over each pulse is the pulse average PA.
- **Temporal or time average power** (TA) is the intensity of the entire pulse train averaged over time defined as

$$\frac{\text{total power per frame}}{\text{frame duration}} \quad (18.19)$$

which gives the average intensity of the pulse train.

This gives a guide to the heating effects. It is related to transducer aperture and transducer PRF. As the aperture in linear arrays is increased to access greater depths time averaged power will increase but PRF is reduced with depth so there is a balance. Time averaged power will tend to decrease with depth owing to beam attenuation, although, in practice, with the use of multiple focal zones (dynamic focusing) which give deeper focus settings, slightly higher time averaged powers will result.

If the PRF of the transducer is high then the TA will be high; if the PRF is decreased then the TA will be lower. If the ultrasound is continuous instead of

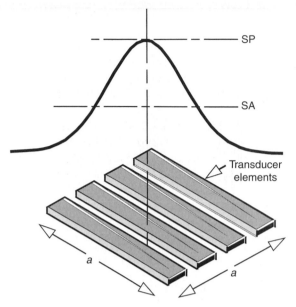

Figure 18.22 *Power levels measured in an ultrasound beam.*

pulsatile (CW Doppler) then the duty cycle is 1 and PA = TA.

18.6.2 Combined intensity units

The spatial average, SA, and the temporal average, TA, are combined to give a basic overall intensity measurement which is used for deriving other intensity parameters.

SPATIAL AVERAGE TEMPORAL AVERAGE INTENSITY, I_{SATA}

This is the temporal average divided by the area of the transducer face (referring to Fig. 18.22):

$$I_{SATA} = \frac{TA}{a^2} \quad (18.20)$$

The units are mW cm^{-2}. As a spatially and temporally averaged acoustic intensity it is usually maximum at the surface of the scan head or where the cross-sectional area of the scan profile is smallest. In a linear array I_{SATA} would be greatest at the mechanical focal point given by the acoustic lens previously identified in Fig. 18.3a. A complete family of other intensity values can be derived from I_{SATA} and some of these are illustrated in Fig. 18.23b.

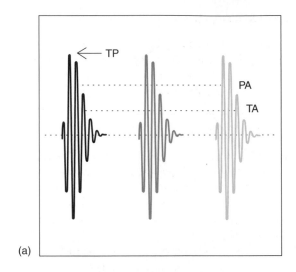

(a)

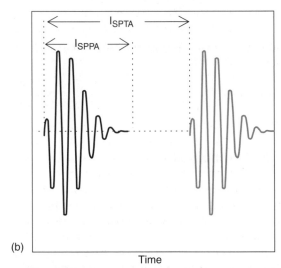

(b)

Time

Figure 18.23 *(a) Peak and average intensities of the ultrasound pressure waveform identified in the text. (b) Combination intensity units identified in the text.*

SPATIAL PEAK TEMPORAL AVERAGE INTENSITY, I_{SPTA}

This is derived as:

$$I_{SPTA} = I_{SATA} \times \frac{SP}{SA} \qquad (18.21)$$

The units are mW cm^{-2}. This is the time averaged power relating peak power to the pulse width and **duty factor**; a higher PRF will increase the I_{SPTA} value. For a peak power of 1 W cm^{-2} and a duty factor of 0.1 the SPTA would be 100 mW cm^{-2}, increasing the pulse width or PRF increases this value.

Table 18.4 *Intensity range in practice.*

Display mode	Time average power (mW)	I_{SPTA} (mW cm^{-2})
B-mode	0.5 to 350	1 to 1000
M-mode	0.5 to 350	5 to >1000
Duplex/pulsed Doppler	10 to >400	20 to >1000
CW Doppler		
Obstetric	16 to 25	10 to 20
Vascular	2 to 90	20 to 600

Likely manufacturer's limits.

Mode	I_{SPTA}, B-mode	I_{SPTA}, M-mode	I_{SPTA}, Doppler
Linear array	3.1	118	
Phased array	117	243	1266
Annular array	42	321	

I_{SPTA}, spatial time average intensity; CW Doppler, continuous wave Doppler.

This intensity measurement is a good indicator for heating effects and this, together with the time averaged power figures for various investigations, is given in Table 18.4. Absolute maximum values in milliwatts per cm^2 that various manufacturers quote are also appended.

SPATIAL PEAK PULSE AVERAGE INTENSITY, I_{SPPA}

This is a measurement of the maximum mean intensity that occurs within the ultrasound beam at any instant as shown in Fig. 18.23b. It is a good indicator for **cavitation** and other mechanical bio-effects.

SPATIAL PEAK TEMPORAL PEAK INTENSITY, I_{SPTP}

This is also shown in Fig. 18.23b and is derived as:

$$\frac{I_{SPTA}}{\text{duty cycle}} \qquad (18.22)$$

The units are W cm^{-2}. This value may be a useful indication for cavitation effects. The **spatial peak temporal peak pressure** measured in MPa is similar to I_{SPPA} but refers to the peak pressure.

Table 18.5 *Acoustic output limits, as given by the US Food & Drug Administration.*

Value	Heart	PV	Op	Abdomen (fetus)
I_{SPPA} (W cm^{-2})	190	190	28	190
I_{SPTP} (W cm^{-2})	310	310	50	310
I_{SPTA} (mW cm^{-2})	430	720	17	94
I_{SATA} (mW cm^{-2})	430	720	17	94

SPATIAL AVERAGE PULSE AVERAGE INTENSITY, I_{SAPA}

Since PA = TA/duty cycle then

$$I_{SAPA} = \frac{I_{SATA}}{\text{duty cycle}} \quad (18.23)$$

The units are mW cm^{-2}.

INTENSITY MAGNITUDES

The magnitude of these intensity values follows the sequence:

$$I_{SPTP} > I_{SPPA} > I_{SPTA} > I_{SAPA} > I_{SATA}$$

The commonly used intensity measures are I_{SPPA} (the maximum transducer pulse intensity) and I_{SPTA}. Both are used in specifying maximum levels by the various national licensing authorities (FDA in USA).

The absolute values will be influenced by focal dimensions. Transducers which have a tight focus in the near field will produce a higher I_{SPTA} value than those which are focused in the far field. Recommended maximum levels quoted by the FDA in the USA for cardiac, peripheral vascular, ophthalmology, and obstetrics are listed in Table 18.5.

Most machines provide an output control which adjusts the amplitude of the transmitted pulse but at 'switch-on' the power setting is often at maximum.

SCANNED MODE IMAGES

(B-mode and color flow imaging) There will be a maximum energy when the axis of the scanning beam passes over a particular point. Beam overlapping will also increase this axial power level. Using linear arrays can increase beam overlap in the proximal image field. For sector scanners the considerable beam-overlap close to the transducer face means the I_{SPTA} value will always be proximal to the focus.

UNSCANNED MODES

In unscanned modes (pulsed Doppler and CW Doppler) the highest values of I_{SPTA} are seen since tissue points on the beam axis will receive the maximum beam strength repeatedly.

HEATING EFFECTS

The rate of local heat production is related to the average intensity and the tissue absorption. In the absence of any heat losses the temperature rise depends on the time exposed. There is not a great deal of difference in heat gain for most soft tissues; the important exception is bone.

Thermal effects depend on energy deposited and heat removal (organ blood flow). Both tissue attenuation and transducer frequencies influence heat production; higher frequencies are more attenuated and thus higher energy absorbed. Bone/tissue interface can cause heat build-up. Doppler power outputs can approach hazard levels and also ultrasound probes (rectal, vaginal). A Doppler probe operating in air has given a temperature approaching 80°C. A skin temperature of over 41°C was measured using a 5 MHz phased array in pulsed Doppler mode for 30 s and a skin temperature elevation of 10°C has been reported at a depth 2 mm below the skin surface.

Probe temperature increases are particularly important in intra-vaginal examinations where the probe face may be in close contact to the conceptus. Temperature rise is of most significance during organo-genesis so the embryo is most vulnerable during the first 8 weeks of development. Some proliferating adult tissues (testes, bone marrow) are at risk.

A statement from the American Institute of Ultrasound in Medicine (AIUM) October 1992 states that in the low MHz range there have been no deleterious thermal effects to mammalian tissue due to exposure from:

- Unfocused beam intensities < 10 mW cm^{-2}
- Focused beam intensities < 1 W cm^{-2}

CAVITATION

At high intensities used in therapy, cavitation (bubble precipitation in liquid) has been demonstrated but it has not been reported at diagnostic intensities. The AUIM and the FDA have introduced a mechanical index (MI) derived from peak negative pressure giving an index for cavitation values for diagnostic ultrasound between 0.2 and 1.9.

18.6.3 Bioeffects

CHROMOSOME DAMAGE

Single-strand DNA breaks have been seen in hymen leukocytes. Various continuous and pulsed frequencies were used but $94\,W\,cm^{-2}$ spatial peak-temporal average (SPTA) at $8\,MHz$ continuous wave (CW) yielded consistent breaks associated with cavitation effects. This is much higher power than would be available from diagnostic equipment.

SISTER CHROMATID EXCHANGE

The most extensive literature deals with sister chromatid exchange *in vitro*. The occurrence is small but statistically significant. Because *in vitro* and *in vivo* effects are different, extrapolation should be attempted with caution. The statement from the AIUM is:

> It is difficult to evaluate reports of ultrasonically induced in-vitro biological effects with respect to their clinical significance. The predominant physical and biological interactions and mechanisms involved in an in-vitro effect may not pertain to the in-vivo situation. Nevertheless an in-vitro effect must be regarded as a real biological effect. While it is valid for authors to place their results in context and to suggest further relevant investigations reports of in-vitro studies which claim direct clinical significance should be viewed with caution.

18.6.4 Safety levels

The boundary of accepted safety levels in the USA is given in Fig. 18.24. In the low MHz range there have been no confirmed biological effects in mammalian tissue exposed *in vivo* to unfocused ultrasound with I_{SPTA} values below $100\,mW\,cm^{-2}$ for less than $500\,s$ or for focused ultrasound with I_{SPTA} below $1\,W\,cm^{-2}$ for less than $50\,s$. Furthermore, for exposure times more than $1\,s$ and less than $500\,s$ (unfocused) or $50\,s$ focused such effects have not been demonstrated at even higher intensities. The power of current machines, however, is able to penetrate the harmful

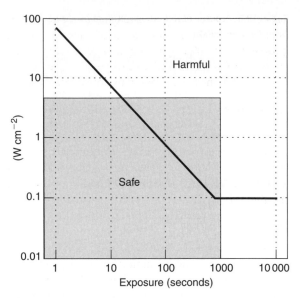

Figure 18.24 *The boundary of safe intensity levels for time spent in the examination.*

region as indicated by the hatched area on the graph. Biologically sensitive areas would be:

- 1st trimester embryo
- Fetus skeletal heating
- Transcranial Doppler
- Eye
- Intracavitary

FETAL EXPOSURE

The calcium channels appear to be the first to develop in the cell membranes of embryos and prolonged ultrasound intensities could have undesirable side-effects not only on embryo-genesis but on late prenatal and postnatal development. There is a growing realization of the potential importance of nonthermal effects and increasing evidence that the temporal peak intensity is potentially related to the production of some effects (cavitation). Doppler flow studies of the fetus are of major concern since this can induce heating in mineralized bone.

A recent safety statement from the Ultrasound Safety Committee states that routine Doppler investigations of the first trimester embryo are inadvisable and that exposure time should be minimized in any pulsed Doppler examination of the fetus particularly if fetal bone is within the Doppler beam. A study of 10 000 pregnancies exposed to ultrasound is currently being carried out in Canada. A preliminary report from this group on 2428 children showed no increase in malformation or other developmental problems. No difference was found between matched pairs of siblings followed up to 6 years of age, one of each pair having been exposed to ultrasound *in utero*.

SUMMARY

There seem to be no limits on acoustic output in most European countries (including the UK and Ireland) but there are limits imposed in the USA and Japan where most manufacturers of ultrasound equipment are located.

The USA requires I_{SPTA} and I_{SPPA} levels to be lower than the values in Table 18.3 and under defined operating procedures (nonfetal Doppler) requires AIUM thermal and mechanical indices to be displayed on-screen. Japan requires an I_{SATA} limit of $10\,\mathrm{mW\,cm^{-2}}$ for B-mode and fetal Doppler, $40\,\mathrm{mW\,cm^{-2}}$ for M-mode and $100\,\mathrm{mW\,cm^{-2}}$ for A mode. A European standard is being prepared which will require an $I_{SPTA} < 100\,\mathrm{mW\,cm^{-2}}$.

MINIMIZING RISKS

Practical general measures to minimize risks in ultrasound scanning would be:

- Do not scan unless there is a clear clinical objective.
- Make sure equipment is checked regularly.
- Discover if the sound output is disabled during freeze frame. If not, remove the probe.
- Use the output attenuator to reduce the output to the lowest levels consistent with giving the required quality of image.
- If the output of the equipment exceeds $100\,\mathrm{mW\,cm^{-2}}$ calculate the time you can safely dwell at one point before the $50\,\mathrm{J\,cm^{-2}}$ limit is exceeded.
- Take special care when scanning sensitive organs (early pregnancy, eye, gonads).
- Keep up to date on scanning techniques to minimize exposure.
- Ensure that trainee radiographers do not spend an undue amount of time on any one patient.
- Keep well informed of the experimental findings on the safety of ultrasound.

FURTHER READING

Fish P (1990) *Physics and Instrumentations of Diagnostic Medical Ultrasound*. John Wiley, Chichester, UK.

Kremkau F (1998) *Diagnostic Ultrasound*, fifth edition. Saunders Company, Philadelphia.

KEYWORDS

annular array: transducers arranged in concentric circles

aperture: the size of the transducer or size of a number of transducer elements

aperture (dynamic): change in aperture size during transmission to maintain focus with depth

auto-correlation: a rapid technique, used in most color-flow instruments, for obtaining mean Doppler shift frequency

beat frequency: a low frequency interference between two waveforms having a different frequency

cavitation: gas bubble production due to rarefaction events in a liquid

clutter: noise in the Doppler signal that is generally caused by high-amplitude, Doppler-shifted echoes from the heart or vessel walls

color flow display: the presentation of two-dimensional, real-time Doppler shift or time shift information superimposed on a real-time, gray-scale, anatomic, cross-sectional image. Flow directions toward and away from the transducer (i.e., positive and negative Doppler or time shifts) are presented as different colors on the display

cross-correlation: a rapid technique for determining time shifts in echo arrival; a technique used to determine flow speeds without using the Doppler effect

curvilinear array: a linear sequence array with a curved outline

demodulator: an electronic circuit which separates a single signal from a mixed signal

depth of response: the point from the transducer face where echoes are $-50\,\mathrm{dB}$

Doppler (continuous): measuring the Doppler frequency by continuous transmission reception. Separate crystals necessary

Doppler (pulsed): measuring the Doppler frequency by pulsing the ultrasound beam. A single crystal is used

Doppler effect: change of reflected frequency with movement

duplex imaging: combining a gray-scale image with a color Doppler image

duty cycle (factor): the percentage of time the pulse occupies in the operational cycle

dynamic range: the range of echo intensities. This can be up to 100 dB at the input amplifier, 60 to 80 dB at the TGC and 50 dB after compression

ensemble length: number of pulses used to generate one color-flow image scan line

focus: determines the slice thickness by shaping the crystal or matching layer or an electronic focus can influence lateral resolution

footprint: area of transducer in contact with the patient

frame rate: number of complete scanned images per second, or number of frames displayed per second

grating lobes: side lobes produced by a multi-element transducer

imaging depth: visible distance from transducer face determined by the PRP and transducer frequency

linear array: a transducer whose elements are pulsed in a sequence to give a rectilinear shaped image or curvilinear for a curved face

phased array: a transducer where the elements are pulsed together using signal delays to steer the beam in a sector scan

polar coordinates: the positional geometry used by a phased array transducer producing a sector scan

power Doppler: color-flow display in which colors are assigned according to the strength (amplitude, power, intensity, energy) of the Doppler-shifted echoes

pulse average intensity (PA): average intensity over repetition period

pulse duration (period) (PD): the time for 2 to 3 wavelengths; typically 0.5 to 3 μs

pulse repetition frequency (PRF): 1/PRP, typically 2 to 10 kHz

pulse repetition period (PRP): the time between pulses or waiting time for echo collection, typically 200 μs

rectilinear coordinates: position geometry used by a linear sequenced array

scan line: produced by a transducer element whose length defines image depth

section thickness: the narrowest or focal point of a section or slice

sector scan: produced by a phased or annular array

spatial average intensity (SA): average intensity over transducer area

spatial peak intensity (SP): highest intensity in beam

spatial pulse length (SPL): the wavelength × number of cycles. Typically 0.45 to 2.25 mm

swept gain: (see time gain compensation)

temporal average intensity (TA): time averaged intensity for the time transducer is used

temporal peak intensity (TP): highest intensity at any time within beam

time-gain compensation (TGC): signal post-processing amplification for correcting attenuation loss

variance: square of standard deviation; one of the outputs of the auto-correlation process; a measure of spectral broadening (i.e. spread around the mean)

wall filter: an electric filter that passes frequencies above a set level and eliminates strong, low-frequency Doppler shifts from pulsating heart or vessel walls

19

Magnetic resonance: principles

19.1 INTRODUCTION

Medical diagnostic imaging uses the upper end of the electromagnetic spectrum almost exclusively for investigating the living body, commanding the shorter wavelengths of X- and gamma radiation. The longer wavelength region embracing the radio-band wavelength 150 cm to 150 m (200 MHz to 2 MHz) has only recently been used by diagnostic imaging due to the application of nuclear magnetic resonance (NMR).

Nuclear magnetic resonance does not rely on ionizing radiation (as conventional radiography, CT and nuclear medicine do), nor does it depend on the transmission of energy through tissue like ultrasound. It utilizes an entirely different principle, involving the interaction of atomic nuclei with imposed magnetic fields which cause radio frequency NMR signals. The nuclei studied in NMR all have odd numbers of protons, the most common nucleus being hydrogen, which is a single proton.

NMR generates very small signals and their strengths and frequencies give unique information about tissue chemistry. Methods for measuring nuclear resonance in organic materials were simultaneously developed in 1946 by E.M. Purcell and co-workers at Harvard and F. Bloch and his team at Stanford. Both physicists received the Nobel Prize for this work. Since then nuclear magnetic resonance has rapidly become a valuable non-destructive laboratory technique for showing molecular differences in biological materials.

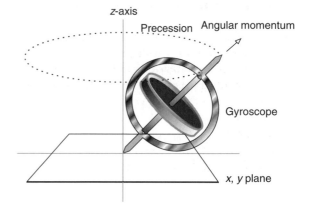

Figure 19.1 *Spinning gyroscope showing an off center wobble or precession representing a very simple model of the precessing proton.*

The NMR signal given by a spinning nucleus can be likened to a spinning top, shown in Fig. 19.1, which normally spins around its own central axis but when disturbed traces out, or **precesses**, at an angle to the vertical axis. This is also shown by a nucleus in a strong magnetic field: when it is disturbed by an opposing magnetic field it will also precess.

IMAGE FORMATION

Magnetic resonance imaging (MRI), introduced commercially in the early 1980s employs these same NMR signals but in addition provides spatial information that yields tomographic sectional images of the human body in the axial plane (as CT), and also in the coronal and sagittal planes as well as any chosen oblique plane.

The images obtained from MRI convey information that is entirely different from the transmission tomographic images of CT and ultrasound. Magnetic resonance images reflect NMR signal changes that are altered by the chemistry of hydrogen and the configuration of hydrogen atoms within molecules, e.g. water, fats, proteins, and carbohydrates. Bone, which has a relatively poor hydrogen concentration, is poorly displayed and any bony anatomy that is seen is due to fatty marrow or pathological changes that involve invasion by soft tissue.

Before describing magnetic resonance imaging it is necessary to understand the fundamental principles of nuclear magnetic resonance and the basic signals. The principles of nuclear magnetic resonance can be very complex but in order to understand their application to imaging many of the complexities can be stripped away and the basics much simplified. This chapter is therefore an abridged version of the true process. More detailed descriptions are given in the books listed at the end of this chapter.

19.2 THE PROTON IN A MAGNETIC FIELD

The phenomenon of nuclear magnetic resonance is not shown by all nuclei; they must contain an odd number of nucleons (protons plus neutrons) and so have a magnetic component or **moment**. The most common is the hydrogen nucleus ^1H, which is a single proton. Other physiologically important atoms are ^{13}C and ^{31}P.

Since the diagnostic imaging applications of NMR almost exclusively involve the hydrogen proton, the following descriptions will use this simple nucleus as a model. The hydrogen proton can be compared to a bar magnet as shown in Fig. 19.2a. It behaves as a dipole having a magnetic dipole moment μ, which is analogous to a pole of a bar magnet. Unlike the bar magnet the proton has spin giving it angular momentum. The proton, in the absence of an external magnetic field can take up any orientation in free space; three protons are shown in Fig. 19.2b freely spinning at different angles on their axes.

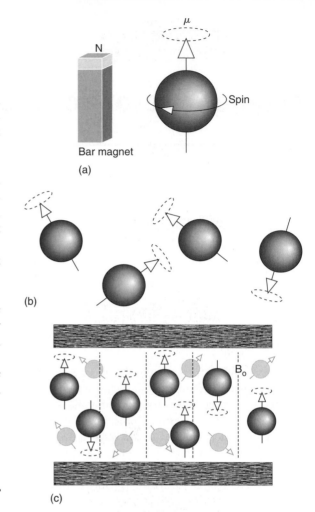

Figure 19.2 (*a*) *The hydrogen proton compared to a bar magnet showing the proton spin creating a magnetic dipole* μ *analogous to the magnetic pole of the bar magnet.* (*b*) *A group of three protons showing various orientations of their axis in free space.* (*c*) *The proton axis aligned in a strong magnetic field* B_0. *A smaller proportion take up opposing direction.*

When the protons are placed in a strong magnetic field B_0, as shown in Fig. 19.2c, the proton axes line up with the magnetic flux lines. In reality, protons can adopt two alignment modes: parallel (with the magnetic flux) and anti-parallel (inverted or opposing the flux) although slightly more align with the magnetic field. The proportion that is in alignment varies with the magnetic field strength. In order to simplify the following descriptions only the majority nuclei, parallel to the magnetic field, will be illustrated.

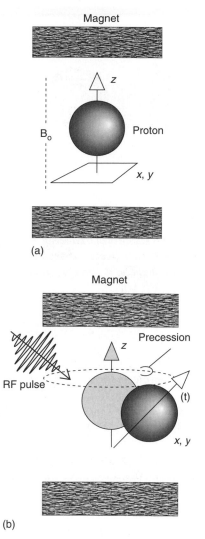

Magnet

z

B_0 Proton

x, y

(a)

Magnet

Precession

RF pulse

z

(t)

x, y

(b)

Figure 19.3 *(**a**) The proton in a magnetic field aligned with the longitudinal z-axis, the transverse* x, y *plane is empty. (**b**) The RF pulse displaces the proton axis into the transverse plane.*

Table 19.1 *Definition of parameters.*

Symbol	Definition
B_0	Static magnetic field
z	Longitudinal plane
x,y	Transverse plane
M	Sum magnetization vector
M_z	Proportion of M in z
	Longitudinal magnetization
M_{xy}	Proportion of M in x,y
	Transverse magnetization
$M(t)$	M at time t after the RF pulse
	Magnitude $\propto$ spin density

part of the transverse plane. The proton loses this excess energy by precessing (the precession frequency determined by the magnetic field strength) until it regains equilibrium in the longitudinal axis once again. Location(t) denotes position of the proton axis at time t after the RF pulse. There are many protons undergoing this transition in a tissue sample so the sum behavior is best described by using **vectors**.

19.2.2 The NMR signal

The following descriptions are simplified so that the overall picture can be grasped. The full story involves the complexities of quantum mechanics described in more specialist literature. In order to describe the source of the NMR signal certain parameters must be identified; these are given in Table 19.1 and identified in the vector diagrams of Fig. 19.4.

The static magnetic field B_0 represents the machine's magnetic field, typically 1 tesla (1 T). The **longitudinal** magnetic plane is z and the **transverse** magnetic plane (at 90°) is x, y.

The simple diagrams in Fig. 19.4 use a magnetization vector M to represent the net magnetic moment or the 'sum behavior' of all the protons in the sample. The magnitude of this signal depends on the proton numbers or more correctly the **spin density**. When this aligns with the z-axis the **longitudinal magnetization** is 100% (M_z). If this stable configuration is now disturbed by injecting an RF pulse M is displaced $M(t)$. The total displacement is proportional to the RF pulse energy; a 90° RF pulse will displace M from the z-axis into the **transverse** x,y plane ($\alpha = 90°$); the longitudinal magnetization will be 0% and the transverse magnetization will be 100% (M_{xy}).

19.2.1 Precession

The three-dimensional geometry is represented by three axes, $z, x,$ and y in Fig. 19.3a which shows a proton at equilibrium in a strong magnetic field. The longitudinal z-axis is parallel to the flux lines of the magnetic field and the x and y axes are at right angles to the z-axis in the **transverse plane**. Figure 19.3b shows that energy from an RF pulse has disturbed the equilibrium, displacing the proton axis so that it now occupies

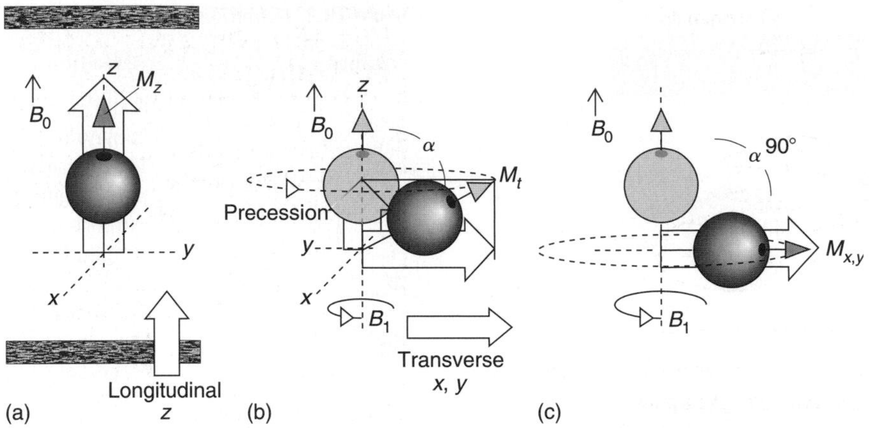

Figure 19.4 *(a) The proton in a magnetic field* B$_0$*. The total proton contribution is represented by a vector* M$_z$ *at equilibrium in the z-plane (z-component maximum, x, y component zero). (b) An RF pulse creates the opposed field B$_1$ displacing M by α°; the x, y transverse component has grown. (c) A large RF pulse displaces M into x, y (z-component zero, x, y component maximum). Longitudinal recovery now takes place.*

The intermediate vector position $M(t)$ contains a proportion of longitudinal and transverse magnetization depending on the RF pulse energy; this decides $α$ the **flip angle**. The speed of relaxation or the time to lose transverse magnetization M_x and regain equilibrium is the **longitudinal relaxation time**. This is an exponential event and is represented by a time constant: T1.

The shape and frequency of the RF pulse is also critical. It is commonly bell-shaped containing a short burst (3 to 4$λ$) of a frequency matching the proton's precessional frequency. The various stages of proton interactions within a magnetic field can be described by reference to Fig. 19.4.

STAGE 1

(Fig. 19.4a) With the proton axis at **equilibrium** magnetic vector M_z is aligned with B_0. The component of M in the longitudinal plane z is M_z (maximum at this stage); likewise the component of M in the transverse plane x, y is M_{xy} (zero at this stage).

STAGE 2

(Fig. 19.4b) When an external force in the form of an RF pulse imposes a field B_1 on the system perpendicular to B_0 then M acquires energy and moves away from its equilibrium taking up some point $M(t)$. The representative magnitudes of M_z and M_{xy} change as indicated by the white arrows.

STAGE 3

(Fig. 19.4c) If the RF pulse has sufficient energy (90° RF) then M is projected into the transverse plane x, y and $M(t) = M_{xy}$ having undergone full saturation. A sufficiently powerful RF pulse will invert the proton axis entirely into $-z$ (180° RF); the magnetic vector will then occupy $-M_z$.

On return of M to its equilibrium value M_z the magnetic vector $M(t)$ undergoes longitudinal relaxation and traces a spiral motion described by the Bloch equations:

$$M_x = e^{-\frac{t}{T2}} \cos \omega_L t$$
$$M_y = e^{-\frac{t}{T2}} \sin \omega_L t \qquad (19.1)$$
$$M_z = M_0 \left(1 - e^{-\frac{t}{T2}} \right)$$

These equations were derived by F. Bloch in 1946 to explain the basic properties of NMR and predicted that the motion of $M(t)$ would be a simple precession (already sketched in Fig. 19.4b) with a frequency $ω$ dependent on the magnetic field. If proton spins interfere with each other's value of $M(t)$ precession will lose energy and return to its equilibrium position M_0; this energy loss is the relaxation process.

Two time constants T1 and T2 are introduced to describe this: T1 the growth in M_z and T2 the decay of the transverse component M_{xy}; both T1 and T2

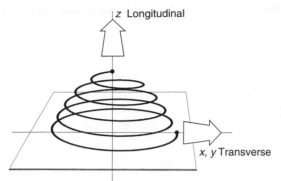

Figure 19.5 *The magnetic vector tracing out a spiral path as it regains equilibrium with the z plane.*

follow exponential decay patterns. The Bloch equations have been used to give the tracing in Fig. 19.5 showing the spiral pathway during **free induction decay** (FID). The sum magnetization vector M_{xy} contributes to the transverse relaxation time. From these equations it will be seen that the longitudinal relaxation time T1 represents the time taken for $M(t)$ to reach the position on the curve $1 - e^{-1}$ or 63% of M_0. The **transverse relaxation time** is the time taken for the FID to decay to e^{-1} or 37% of the M_{xy} value. The overall signal strength S obtained from $M(t)$ during longitudinal and transverse relaxation depends on three parameters: spin density ρ, T1 and T2 relaxation times, so:

$$S = \rho \times \exp\left(-\frac{TE}{T2}\right) \times \left[1 - \exp\left(-\frac{TR}{T1}\right)\right] \qquad (19.2)$$

where TE and TR are pulse sequence parameters described later.

FLIP ANGLES

The angle of precession α or the flip angle, shown in Fig. 19.4b, depends on the RF pulse energy. If the RF pulse is less energetic than 90° then intermediate angles of rotation can be induced. If the rotating magnetic field of the RF pulse is B_1 then the angle of rotation (the flip angle) is

$$\alpha = \gamma B_1 t \qquad (19.3)$$

where t represents the RF pulse duration. The flip angle can therefore be controlled by varying the pulse time or amplitude. After time t the magnetic vector M is orientated at an angle α in the diagram.

Box 19.1 The gyromagnetic ratio γ for hydrogen

The proton magnetic moment is 1.41031×10^{-26} J T^{-1} and the proton spin angular momentum is 0.527×10^{-34} J s^{-1}. Hence,

$$\gamma = \frac{\mu}{2\pi L} = \frac{1.41 \times 10^{-26}}{2\pi \times 0.527 \times 10^{-34}}$$
$$= 42\,582\,252\,\text{Hz}$$

or 42.58... MHz T^{-1}.

Clinical magnet strengths

The precession frequencies of ^{1}H (proton) for high, medium, and low strength magnets are as follows:

High 1.5 T	$f = 42.58 \times 1.5$	63.87 MHz
Medium 0.3 T	$f = 42.58 \times 0.3$	12.77 MHz
Low 0.064 T	$f = 42.58 \times 0.064$	2.72 MHz

19.2.3 The Larmor frequency

The **precessional frequency** f of the nucleus can be calculated as

$$f = \frac{\mu B_0}{2\pi L} \qquad (19.4)$$

where μ is the proton magnetic moment shown in Fig. 19.2, L is the proton spin angular momentum and B_0 the magnetic field strength in tesla. In order to simplify matters μ and $2\pi L$ can be treated as constants since they are fixed for any particular nucleus (in this case a hydrogen proton). Together they describe the gyromagnetic ratio γ:

$$\gamma = \frac{\mu}{2\pi L} \qquad (19.5)$$

This is a constant specific to the nucleus in question. The gyromagnetic ratio for the hydrogen proton is calculated in Box 19.1 Simplifying Equation 19.4 by substituting γ:

$$\omega_L = \gamma B_0 \qquad (19.6)$$

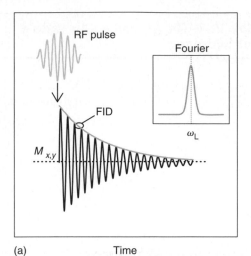

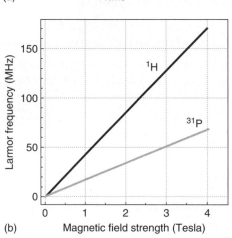

(a)   Time

(b)   Magnetic field strength (Tesla)

Figure 19.6 *(a) Free induction decay (FID). After the RF pulse the proton precession at the Larmor frequency decays yielding the FID. The envelope of this decay measures T2*. The frequency of the FID is measured from its Fourier spectrum. (b) Influence of magnetic field strength on Larmor frequency for ^{1}H and ^{31}P nuclei.*

This is an important basic equation since it relates the precession frequency to magnetic field strength B_0 and is the **Larmor equation**; ω_L is the **Larmor frequency** (J. Larmor, 1857–1942; Irish mathematician) where ω represents the angular frequency of precession.

In Figure 19.4b B_1 will influence M only if it rotates at the Larmor precession frequency ω_L. At 1 T ω_L is ≈ 42 MHz. When the RF pulse is switched off M regains its equilibrium state M_0 by precessing as depicted in the figure. Box 19.1 shows how the Larmor frequency varies with the magnetic field strength. Figure 19.6a illustrates that after an RF pulse the NMR precessional

signal undergoes **free induction decay** (FID) and M_{xy} regains equilibrium M_z. This is the **transverse** or **spin–spin relaxation time** where individual protons lose energy to the surrounding tissue. The frequency components of the FID can be identified by Fourier analysis. Figure 19.6b shows the linear relationship between Larmor frequency (in MHz) and magnetic field strength (in tesla) for two nuclei: ^{1}H and ^{31}P.

19.2.4 Signal measurement

Simple equipment for measuring the exact Larmor frequency for any particular substance can be seen in Fig. 19.7a. The sample is positioned in a strong magnetic field B_0 surrounded by a signal coil, which acts as a transmitting and receiving antenna. The coil is connected to a variable radio frequency (RF) oscillator which transmits a series of RF pulses changing in

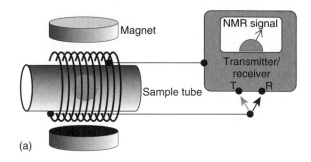

(a)

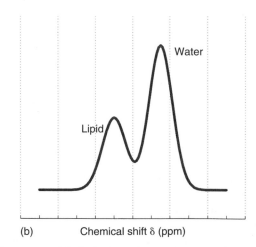

(b)   Chemical shift δ (ppm)

Figure 19.7 *(a) The basic equipment for generating and detecting the NMR signal from a sample placed in a magnetic field. T/R is the transmit/receive switch. (b) Chemical shift between water and lipid measured in parts per million of ω_L.*

Table 19.2 *Useful nuclei in nuclear magnetic resonance.*

Isotope	Natural abundance (%)	Gamma (MHz)	Signal intensity
^1H (proton)	99.98	42.58	1.0000
^{19}F	100	40.05	0.8300
^{23}Na	100	11.26	0.0930
^{31}P	100	17.24	0.0660
^{17}O	0.037	5.77	0.0290
^{13}C	1.11	10.71	0.0160
^{35}Cl	75.5	4.17	0.0084
^{15}N	0.37	4.30	0.0010
^{39}K	93.1	1.99	0.0005

frequency until resonance is achieved. The weak NMR signals received from the precessing protons are amplified and passed on to a sensitive RF receiver which measures the strength of the NMR frequency. This is highest when the RF pulse frequency is at **resonance** with the Larmor frequency.

The NMR signal strength (amplitude) at resonance depends on hydrogen atom concentration. The Larmor frequency for the same magnetic field strength differs for each nucleus.

Table 19.2 lists important physiological elements, their abundance, γ, and NMR signal strength relative to hydrogen.

SPIN DENSITY

The density of the excited spins in a region is one of the major factors influencing MR signal intensity (spin density ρ, see eqn 19.2). This influences tissue contrast and depends on the number of hydrogen nuclei and not all the protons as the equation would imply; it is therefore more appropriate to use the term spin density or intermediate scans. The simple equipment illustrated in Fig. 19.7a measures the signal from the FID at resonance obtained from a 90° RF pulse. The signal strength is directly proportional to the number of hydrogen protons. Magnetic resonance imaging, however, does not measure the proton density directly but image characteristics heavily dependent on T1 and T2. This will be described in the next chapter.

This simple equipment contains all the basic components found in larger magnetic resonance imaging machines. They are:

- A strong magnetic field B_0
- A transmitting/receiving signal coil

- An RF transmitter
- A sensitive RF receiver
- A display device

19.2.5 Chemical shift

A typical NMR spectrum is shown in Fig. 19.7b. The precise resonance frequency of a proton is determined by its local magnetic field comprising the static field and its position on the molecule. Therefore all hydrogen protons within a certain tissue do not have exactly the same Larmor frequency. Proton position can be influenced by the magnetic shielding effects of electron orbitals which induce secondary magnetic fields. This effect can either diminish the local field so shielding the proton or enhance the local field so deshielding the proton. The small changes in Larmor frequency or shifts can be represented as a spectrum, the spectrum peak positions proportional to local magnetic field strength differences specified in parts per million (ppm) of the resonance frequency relative to a standard. The chemical shift reference is a compound whose proton Larmor frequency is used as a standard. The reference material is commonly tetramethylsilane $Si(CH_3)_4$ since it exhibits one of the greatest proton shielding, exceeding tissue molecules, so any chemical shift measured would all be moved in the same direction away from this reference peak. By referring to this standard the chemical shift has a constant value independent of machine characteristics (magnetic field strength or radio frequency).

Most molecules of physiological importance have shifts (δ) between 0 and 10 ppm. Water has $\delta = 4.7$ ppm so for a 1 T magnet with a ω_L of 42.58 MHz this will give a frequency difference of $(42.58 \times 10^6) \times (4.7 \times 10^{-6}) = 200$ Hz. Figure 19.7b is an NMR spectrum for a mixture of fat and water showing the small separation of about 3.5 ppm. For lower magnetic field strengths the frequency difference, and consequently resolution, is less.

SUMMARY

These sections can be summarized as follows:

- The proton spin induces a magnetic dipole and the proton axis aligns with the magnetic field.
- Protons align parallel and anti-parallel but more align parallel.

- The proton magnetic vector is represented by M. At equilibrium this aligns with z the longitudinal axis. The x and y axes are at 90° in the transverse axis.
- Protons precess by an RF pulse at resonance with the proton's precessional frequency.
- The resonant frequency is related to the magnetic field strength (in tesla) by the Larmor equation: $\omega_L = \gamma B_0$.
- The magnetic vector M is displaced from z into x, y.
- The angular displacement of the M vector is measured as a flip angle, α.
- The gyromagnetic ratio γ is 42.58 MHz T^{-1}.

19.3 RELAXATION TIME CONSTANTS

Two signals are obtained from the proton's realignment with the static magnetic field; these are measured as time constants:

- The longitudinal time constant **T1**
- The transverse time constant **T2**

T1 and T2 signals are affected by the tissue molecular structure and chemistry. Small changes in tissue chemistry and differences between normal and abnormal tissue can alter the values of T1 and T2.

19.3.1 Longitudinal time constant: T1

The return of longitudinal magnetization M_z to its equilibrium value M_0 requires exchange of energy between the nuclear spins and the material lattice. Following excitation by a 90° RF pulse M_z will return from the transverse plane (M_{xy}) approaching M_0 with a characteristic time constant (Fig. 19.8a). This spin lattice or longitudinal relaxation time is measured as T1.

The speed of relaxation or the time to lose transverse magnetization M_{xy} and to regain equilibrium is the **longitudinal relaxation time** but since this is an exponential event the time constant itself is measured when the longitudinal magnetization reaches 63% of its original value. Figure 19.8b plots this exponential realignment of M with the z-axis and shows that T1 is measured at a point marking 63% of maximum recovery; this is explained in Box 19.2. Both short and long T1 times are shown in the figure.

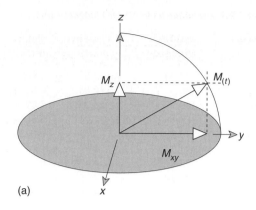

(a)

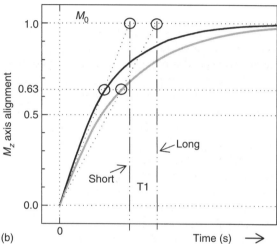

(b)

Figure 19.8 (*a*) *The vector diagram identifying the proportion of* M_z *and* M_{xy} *in the proton magnetic vector* M *at time* t. (*b*) M *traces out an exponential decay as it regains equilibrium (*M_z = 1*). The T1 time is measured at 63% recovery. Both short and long T1 examples are shown.*

Box 19.2 The measurement of T1

After a 90° RF pulse the M_z curve $= 1 - \exp(-t/T1)$. By setting t at various values of T1, the calculation of M_z is as follows. When

$$t = T1, \quad M_z \text{ is } (1 - e^{-1}) = 63$$
$$t = 2 \times T1, M_z \text{ is } (1 - e^{-2}) = 86$$
$$t = 3 \times T1, M_z \text{ is } (1 - e^{-3}) = 95$$
$$t = 4 \times T1, M_z \text{ is } (1 - e^{-4}) = 98$$
$$t = 5 \times T1, M_z \text{ is } (1 - e^{-5}) = 99.3$$

Measurement of T1 time is made when M_z reaches 63% maximum.

Table 19.3 *The variation of T1 with magnet field.*

Tissue	T1			T2
	0.5 T	1.0 T	1.5 T	
Fat	210	240	260	80
Liver	350	420	500	40
Kidney	430	590	690	58
Muscle	550	730	870	45
Heart	570	750	880	57
White matter	500	680	780	90
Gray matter	650	810	900	100
CSF	1800	2160	2400	160

During longitudinal relaxation the protons lose energy to the surrounding tissue. The rate of proton energy loss depends on the material or tissue composition. Protons lose energy more rapidly to those tissues with greater complexity (T1 time is short). With simple molecular structures (water), the energy loss is slower and T1 is long. The exception to this rule is fat which, in spite of being a simple compound, has chemical bonds at the ends of its fatty acid molecules which have frequencies near the Larmor frequency of hydrogen. These allow fast energy transfer and consequently T1 times are short for fatty tissue. More complex or solid tissue (muscle protein) absorbs proton energy quickly so T1 is shorter for solid tissues. T1 is strongly related to tissue water content; time periods range between 300 and 2000 ms. T1 varies with magnetic field strengths since precessional frequencies increase with B_0 (see Larmor equation) which tends to slow the loss of energy to the surrounding tissues, consequently T1 times increase, approximately as $B_0^{0.3}$. The broad range of T1 values versus field strength is also plotted in Fig. 18.8a. Table 19.3 gives the values of various tissues for 0.5, 1.0, and 1.5 T magnets; the T2 time remains virtually unchanged.

19.3.2 Transverse time constant: T2, T2*

The transverse magnetization M_{xy} is the component of the macroscopic magnetization vector M at right angles to the static magnetic field B_0. During equilibrium recovery precession of the transverse magnetization occurs at the Larmor frequency which is the detected MR signal. After the RF pulse the transverse magnetization M_{xy} will decay to zero with a **transverse**

or **spin–)spin** relaxation time constant T2 or T2* (already indicated by the FID envelope in Fig. 19.6a).

The overall T2 signal represents the loss of phase coherence among spins orientated at an angle to the static magnetic field. Local deviations in the microscopic magnetic fields generated by interactions between magnetic moments of atoms lead to slight differences in resonance frequencies which cause phase interference or dephasing of the spins. This is demonstrated in Fig. 19.9b where a single signal in (a) is joined by two others in (b) whose slight differences destructively interfere to yield the sum signal in (c).

The composite signals in (b) **dephase** as the phase diagrams in Fig. 19.9c for $t = 0$ (FID start), $t = 0.5$, and $t = 1$ show. The FID envelope is again shown in Fig. 19.10a identifying the T2 time constant measured at 37% of the decay curve. The simple T2 measured here suffers from distortions due to the main magnetic field inhomogeneities and is distinguished by calling it T2* (T2 star, the * denotes a distorted signal influenced by magnetic field inhomogeneities). The additional effect of these inhomogeneities causes M_{xy} to decay far more quickly than the expected T2 so T2* < T2. Image contrast is a function of T2 in spin echo images but T2* determines image contrast in fast sequences or gradient echo images. The pure T2 signal is complex and must be obtained by indirect means, to be described later.

FREE INDUCTION DECAY

From Section 19.2.3 equilibrium recovery provides a radio-frequency signal generated by the precessional movement, its decay giving a proton spin–spin relaxation time or T2*.

Figure 19.4c illustrates how a 90° RF pulse shifts the magnetization vector M into the transverse x, y plane M_{xy}. After the RF pulse the NMR precessional signal undergoes free induction decay FID and M_{xy} regains equilibrium M_z. This is the transverse or spin–spin relaxation time where individual protons lose energy to the surrounding tissue.

The FID outline or signal envelope of this decay is shown in Fig. 19.10a for two tissues with a short and long T2; it follows an exponential slope whose time constant T2* is taken at 37% maximum. Box 19.3 explains why this point is chosen. The Larmor frequency of the FID is sensitive to small magnetic field variations, consequently T2 is distorted by small

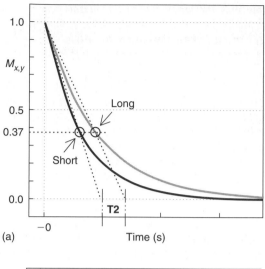

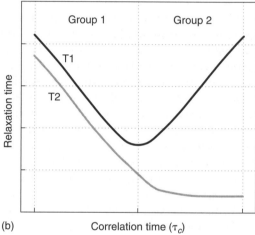

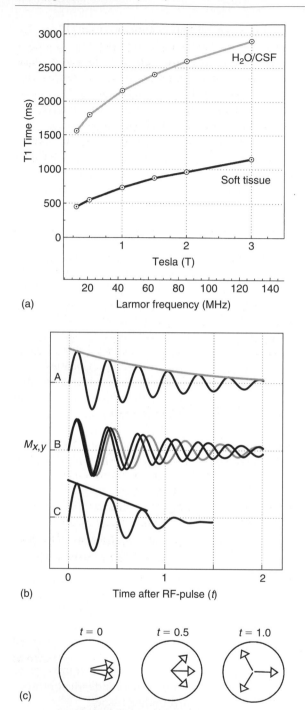

Figure 19.10 (**a**) The measurement of T2 time from the FID decay envelope. (**b**) Correlation time τ_c for T1 and T2. Group 1 consists of small molecules; group 2 consists of more complex molecules including protein and lipids.

Figure 19.9 (**a**) The variation of T1 time with magnetic field strength for liquid (water, CSF) and soft tissue, other tissues have intermediate values (Table 19.3). (**b**) A single FID (A) and signal interference amongst three FIDs (B) having slightly different frequency giving a much shorter time constant (C). (**c**) Phase diagrams for (B) at times 0, 0.5, and 1.0 s.

magnetic field inhomogeneities caused both by neighboring protons and the magnet itself. Magnet inhomogeneities obscure the true T2 tissue so the true value of T2 must be separated from magnet inhomogeneities by using a special pulse sequence (described later).

DEPHASING

The sum effect of frequency and phase differences from neighboring FIDs, demonstrated in Fig. 19.9b, cause mutual interference. Loss of phase coherence occurs exponentially due to spin–spin interference, thus the decay time of the composite FID signal is

Box 19.3 The measurement of T2 from the free induction decay

Figure 19.10a shows that free induction decay is according to the expression $e^{-t/T2}$. By setting t at various values of T2 the calculation of $M_{x,y}$ is as follows. When:

$t = $ T2,$\quad$ $M_{x,y}$ is $(e^{-1}) = 37$
$t = 2 \times $ T2, $M_{x,y}$ is $(e^{-2}) = 13$
$t = 3 \times $ T2, $M_{x,y}$ is $(e^{-3}) = 5$
$t = 4 \times $ T2, $M_{x,y}$ is $(e^{-4}) = 2$

Measurement of T2 time is therefore made when the $M_{x,y}$ falls to 37% maximum.

shortened. T2 signal differences in a perfectly homogeneous magnetic field would reflect tissue chemistry.

The FIDs undergo less proton **spin–spin interference** in simple compounds (liquids such as CSF) and maintain in-phase conditions for a longer time, so T2 times are longer. T2 for solid material is shorter as protons are in close proximity and the FIDs lose phase relationships more rapidly. The loss of transverse magnetization M_{xy}, given by T2, occurs relatively quickly whereas longitudinal recovery M_z, given by T1, takes longer. In order of time span therefore T1 is longer than T2 which is longer than T2* (T1 > T2 > T2*). Examples of T1 and T2 times for three main field strengths have been listed in Table 19.3.

Although the Larmor frequency is very sensitive to changes in magnetic field strength the transverse relaxation time (T2) is not much influenced (unlike T1), indeed spin–spin interactions at higher field strengths may be more efficient and T2 could shorten.

CORRELATION TIME

The local magnetic fields produced by various protons are produced by molecular movements or 'tumbling'. Movements at or near the Larmor frequency have the most effect.

Figure 19.10b plots the tumbling or correlation time τ_c for a variety of molecular types showing the separation of T1 and T2 times. These can be broadly divided into two groups. Group 1 represents small molecules such as water and CSF with a short τ_c and a long T1. As the molecular structure becomes more complex τ_c slows to a rate near the Larmor frequency.

Hydrogen protons incorporated into large macromolecules such as proteins and lipids have longer τ_c times (group 2 in graph) and much shorter T1 times. Molecules with correlation times less than about 500 kHz are relatively static in an environment where spins are typically 30 to 60 MHz. All molecules in group 2 give short T2 values. Extremely short T2 values of <10 µs are too rapid to be visualized in MRI; these are associated with membrane surfaces and structures having large protein molecules.

19.4 PULSE SEQUENCES

The subtle differences in tissue chemistry can be thoroughly explored by exposing them to a series of 90° and 180° RF pulses of different sequences, altering their strength and time interval. The tissue's response to these pulse sequences, shown by the T1 and T2 signals, can uncover small differences in composition not only between tissue types but within the same tissue, perhaps revealing early pathology.

19.4.1 Saturation recovery

Figure 19.4c shows the movement of the M vector into the x, y transverse plane ($\alpha = 90°$); this is the saturation point and the 90° RF pulse is the **saturation pulse**. After the 90° RF pulse the proton loses energy and recovers equilibrium. The process shown in Fig. 19.4c is reversed: the M vector regaining longitudinal magnetization and undergoing **saturation recovery**. The basic NMR signals given during saturation recovery are:

- The rate of realignment of M with z. This is **equilibrium recovery**, relaxation time or loss of transverse magnetization and is known as the T1 signal.
- During saturation recovery the proton loses energy by emitting an NMR radio-frequency signal. The decay rate of this NMR signal is known as the T2 signal.

SATURATION RECOVERY SEQUENCE

It can be seen that after a 90° RF pulse the proton undergoes relaxation, to gain equilibrium, moving from the x, y transverse plane towards the z-axis. A simple pulse sequence of 90° RF pulses at fixed TR times in Fig. 19.11a and b show the signal strengths. For long TR times, as in (a), protons recover full equilibrium between RF pulses so each FID is maximum. For faster TR times, as in (b), protons do not recover full equilibrium and the succeeding 90° pulses appear during incomplete recovery ($M(t)$ between transverse and longitudinal planes); the resultant FIDs therefore get successively smaller, shown by the sloping line for each sequence in the diagram. These are **partial saturation** pulse sequences.

19.4.2 The spin echo sequence

SPIN ECHO SIGNAL

At saturation the protons are precessing in-phase (M_{xy} is maximum) but during saturation recovery

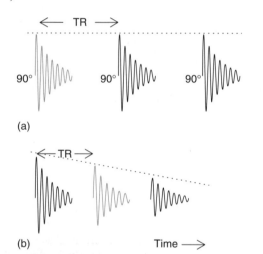

(a)

(b)

Figure 19.11 *Saturation recovery sequence for a sequence of 90° pulses at different repeat times: (a) long TR and (b) short TR times.*

($M(t)$ attaining equilibrium) protons dephase. This is shown again as the phase diagram at the end of the FID in Fig. 19.12.

Applying a 180° RF pulse will achieve proton inversion, shifting the M vector so that it is anti-parallel to the z-axis ($-M_z$). This has a most valuable property: the phase relationships lost during the saturation recovery process at (B) are regained by reversing the precession, the destructive interference is also reversed. The protons dephased at (B) are inverted by the 180° pulse thus rephasing the signals (C) and so refocusing the protons' precession (D). This gives a strong **spin echo** signal, which again decays due to dephasing (E). Due to the re-phasing of saturation recovery signals after a 180° inversion pulse, the NMR signals give a spin echo signal. This echo signal is used in a **spin echo pulse sequence** (Fig. 19.13a) which consists of a 90° RF pulse followed by a 180° RF pulse; TR time determines the T1 contribution. The time from the 90° pulse to the received echo signal is the **TE** time (time to echo). The larger the TE time the greater the T2 information. The 180° pulse is placed at ½TE, which fixes the time of signal measurement at TE. The spin echo pulse sequence is a fundamental imaging sequence, TR and TE times determining the proportion of T1 and T2 information (weighting) in the image.

19.4.3 Gradient echo

The spin echo signal can be produced by reversing the direction of the magnetic field, as shown in Fig. 19.13b. This is a much faster technique for obtaining the spin echo signal and is the technique used for fast

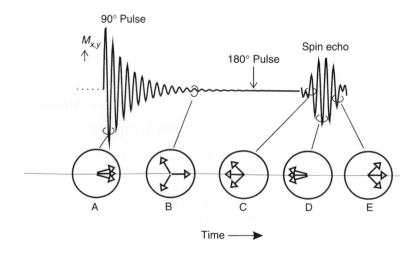

Figure 19.12 *The rephasing of the free induction decay (FID) by applying a 180° pulse at a predetermined time after the initial saturation 90° RF pulse. The phase diagrams show the phase loss by the FID (A and B) reversed by the 180° pulse (C and D) rephasing in (D) to give the spin echo signal and again loss of phase (E) as saturation recovery occurs once again.*

imaging sequences. The gradient coils are part of the imaging system of a magnetic resonance machine (described in the next chapter).

19.4.4 Inversion recovery

The inversion recovery process, shown in Fig. 19.14a, resembles saturation recovery but now a 180° RF pulse places M in the $-z$ axis. During inversion recovery $-M_z$ travels from $-z$, through the transverse x, y plane, reaching equilibrium at the $+z$ axis (M_z). The $-M_z$ realignment is compared in this graph with the 90° RF pulse saturation recovery. For the 180° recovery the T1 passes through the x,y transverse plane

when time t equals $0.693 \times$ T1, completing its recovery when t reaches $4 \times$ T1.

INVERSION RECOVERY SEQUENCE

Inversion recovery produces a signal that contains more T1 information than the saturation recovery sequence. The pulse sequence shown in Fig. 19.14b consists of a 180° pulse followed by a spin echo sequence, when the signal strength is measured. The time period TI between the initial 180° RF pulse and the 90° pulse is the **inversion time** or τ. Since different tissues will show different T1 times the proton M vector will be at varying intermediate stages of equilibrium depending on the length of TI. The inversion

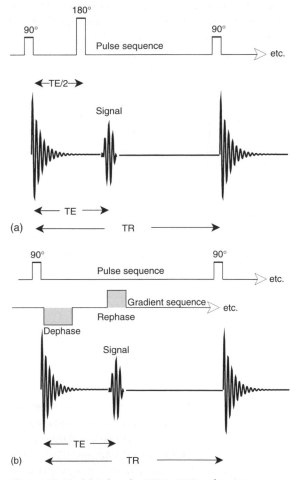

Figure 19.13 *(a) Spin echo 90° to 180° pulse sequence. The spin echo signal is measured at time TE which is chosen by the operator. (b) Gradient echo sequence which can replace the spin echo sequence; the reversed gradient performing the same function as a 180° RF pulse.*

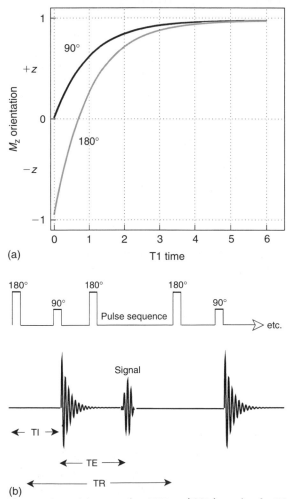

Figure 19.14 *(a) Comparing 180° and 90° inversion for T1 measurement. (b) Inversion recovery pulse sequence of 180° followed by 90° after inversion time TI.*

time between the 180° and 90° pulses and therefore determines how much T1 information the signal will contain.

19.5 T1 AND T2 SIGNAL MEASUREMENT

For non-imaging chemical analysis exact values of T1 and T2 are routinely obtained. In an imaging system, where short acquisition times are most important, exact measurement is never attempted. A rapid estimate of T1 and T2 is made for image display. A description of the full T1 and T2 measurement is included here for reference.

19.5.1 T1 measurement

The standard indirect technique for measuring T1 uses a series of 90° pulses at specific intervals (TR: time to repeat). If TR is shorter than the T1 recovery time then the resulting peak value of the FID curve will become successively smaller due to incomplete equilibrium recovery. The peak value of the FID signal will follow the T1 saturation recovery curve. Interfering processes will not influence these first peak values. The peak FID values at various TR times provide the signal outline or envelope for accurate T1 measurement. The effect of different TR times is shown in Fig. 19.15a.

The accuracy of T1 measurement depends on the number of points along the curve, only two readings are taken to obtain an estimated value when imaging. Measurements are repeated a number of times to improve accuracy: this is signal **averaging**.

19.5.2 Pure T2 measurement

The simple free induction decay (FID) will be influenced by both proton spin–spin interactions (a property of the tissue) and magnetic field inhomogeneities to give the T2* value. Spin–spin interactions cause nonreversible signal dephasing which is retained for some time, consequently repeated 90° RF pulses do not reveal the original signal peak since remnant interference from previous RF pulses will remain.

If a 180° RF pulse is applied then this remnant dephasing can be reversed and the signals will rephase to give a full peak signal: this is the spin echo signal appearing at TE (Fig. 19.12 and Fig. 19.13). The 90° pulse followed by a series of 180° pulses at time interval TE/2 is the Carr–Purcell sequence. Slight

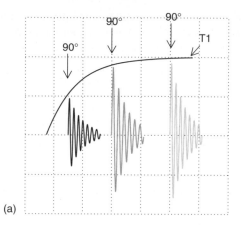

(a)

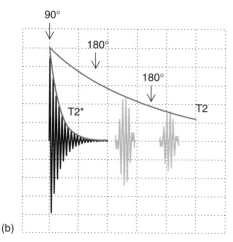

(b)

Figure 19.15 *(a) Accurate T1 measurement achieved by using different TR times. TR = 1 is short, TR = 3 is a longer 90° pulse interval. (b) Pure T2 measured by a 90° to 180° to 180° pulse sequence is much longer than T2* measured from the free induction decay.*

variations in this sequence are sometimes used to overcome inhomogeneities in the signal coils. The envelope of signal decay is now the pure T2 signal, unaffected by remnant phase differences and magnetic field non-uniformities (unlike T2*) reflecting the T2 effects of the tissue itself. Figure 19.15b shows this pulse sequence and signal averaging again improves the accuracy of these readings.

SUMMARY

Sections 19.3 to 19.5 can be summarized as follows:

- The 90° RF pulse is called the saturation pulse. The precessing proton recovers equilibrium and undergoes saturation recovery.

- A faster 90° pulse sequence will prevent complete recovery and give smaller T1 signals. Partial saturation pulse sequences result when 90° pulse timing shorter than T1.
- The spin echo sequence is a 90° RF pulse followed by a 180° pulse.
- After the 90° RF pulse photons lose phase (are dephased) and phase differences interfere with individual FIDs, shortening T2.
- The 180° inverting RF pulse rephases the dephased protons producing a spin echo pulse.
- The time between 90° pulses is the pulse repetition frequency TR time.
- After the second 90° the strength of the T1 signal depends on the longitudinal magnetization recovery. Total recovery will be given by tissues with a short T1.
- In a 90° to 180° sequence the time from the 90° pulse to reception of the spin echo signal is the TE time.
- By increasing the TE times (after the 90° RF pulse) the signals can become increasingly T2 weighted.
- T1 weighting is achieved by using a short TR time.
- A TR <0.5 s is considered short. A TR > 1.5 s is long.
- A long TE is about three times longer than a short TE (30 ms).

FURTHER READING

RSNA Syllabus. Categorical Course in Physics: the Basic Physics of MR Imaging.

Elster AD (1994) *Questions and Answers in Magnetic Resonance Imaging.* Mosby.

KEYWORDS

angular momentum: a vector quantity given by the vector product of momentum and position. This remains constant until an external force changes the direction of rotation causing precession. Atomic nuclei possess intrinsic angular momentum called spin

B_0: the magnetic field, measured in tesla

B_1: the radio frequency magnetic induction field opposed to B_0

bandwidth: a general term describing the range of frequencies in a signal

Bloch equations: describe motion of the magnetization vector. They include precession effects and T1, T2 relaxation times

chemical shift: change in Larmor frequency caused by chemical binding

diamagnetic: a material with a small negative magnetic susceptibility which will decrease a magnetic field. Water- and oxygen-rich compounds

dipole: magnetic dipole

dipole interaction: interaction between a nuclear spin and its neighbors due to magnetic dipole moments, contributing to relaxation times

ferromagnetic: a substance that has a large positive magnetic susceptibility, e.g. iron

free induction decay: when transverse magnetization M_{xy} is produced a signal will be produced decaying toward equilibrium M_0 with a characteristic time constant T2 or T2*

gauss, G: unit of magnetic flux in the c.g.s. system (1 T = 10,000 G)

gyromagnetic ratio, γ: the ratio of the magnetic moment to the angular momentum. A constant for a given nucleus

homogeneity: magnetic field uniformity measured in parts per million of the main field

inversion: the magnetization vector orientated opposite to the magnetic field produced by 180° pulse or gradient switching

inversion recovery: a pulse sequence where the nuclear magnetization is inverted prior to a spin echo pulse sequence. The time between the 180° pulse and the SE sequence is the inversion time TI

Larmor equation: this describes the frequency of precession of the nuclear magnetic moment being proportional to the magnetic field: $f = \gamma B_0/2\pi$ Hz

Larmor frequency: the frequency at which magnetic resonance can be excited; given by the Larmor equation. For H+ the Larmor frequency is 42.58 MHz T^{-1}

longitudinal magnetization: M_z the component of the magnetization vector along the static magnetic field. Following the RF pulse M_z will approach the equilibrium value M_0 with time constant T1

longitudinal relaxation: return of M_z to M_0 after excitation. Requires an exchange of energy between the proton spin and the molecular lattice. Measured by the time constant T1

magnetic moment, μ: given by a nucleus (proton) with spin. The associated magnetic dipole moment will interact with an external magnetic field mimicking a tiny bar magnet

magnetic susceptibility, c: a measure of the ability of a material to become magnetized

$M(t)$: The M value dependant on flip angle. The magnitude is proportional to spin density

MR signal: radio frequency electromagnetic signal produced by the precession of the transverse magnetization of the nuclear spins

M_{xy}: transverse magnetization

M_z: longitudinal magnetization

paramagnetic: a material with a small but positive magnetic susceptibility. Paramagnetic substances reduce relaxation times. Gadolinium and manganese are examples

partial saturation: applying repeated RF pulses at times shorter than T1. Can be used for calculating T1 for the region

permanent magnet: one whose field originates from a permanently magnetized material

permeability: tendency of a substance to concentrate a magnetic field. μ-metal has a high permeability

precession: the movement of a spinning body which traces out a conical shape. The magnetic moment of a proton with spin will precess at an angle to the magnetic field, precessing at the Larmor frequency

pulse 180° (π pulse): RF pulse which inverts the magnetization vector as $-M_z$

pulse 90°: ($\pi/2$ pulse) an RF pulse which rotates M_z into the transverse plane M_{xy}

pulse length: time duration of an RF pulse. The longer the pulse length the narrower the bandwidth

pulse sequence: a set of RF pulses, with or without gradient reversal to give an MR signal

receiver coil: a coil or antenna which picks up the MR signal

relaxation times: after excitation nuclear spins will return to their equilibrium state where M_{xy} is zero and M_z is maximum. Transverse magnetization returns to zero with a characteristic time constant T2 and longitudinal magnetization returns toward M_0 with time constant T2

resistive magnet: an electromagnet whose magnetic field is due to an electric current which consumes power (unlike superconducting magnet)

saturation: a non-equilibrium state where equal numbers of spins are aligned against and with the main magnetic field; zero net magnetization. Produced by repeated short interval RF pulses compared to T1

saturation recovery: pulse sequence that achieves partial saturation allowing recovery before next pulse

sensitive volume: the region from which the MR signal originates. Influenced by shape and bandwidth of RF pulse

Table 19.4 *Summary of the properties of T1 and T2.*

T1	T2
Longitudinal relaxation	Transverse relaxation
Spin lattice	Spin–spin
Water has long T1	Water has long T2
Fat and solids short T1	
Times between 300 and 2000 ms	Times between 30 and 150 ms
Varies with field strength	Only slight variation with field strength
Related to water content	Variation linked to water lipid and magnet inhomogeneities
Malignant tissue typically has higher T1	
Measured at 63% of maximum	Measured at 37% decay point

sequence time: or repetition time TR. The period between repeating an identical pulse sequence

spin: intrinsic angular momentum of a nucleus. Responsible for the magnetic moment

spin density, N: the density of resonating spins in a given volume, determined by the MR signal strength. Measured as moles m^{-3}. For water this is 1.1×10^5 moles H per m^3

spin echo: reappearance of an MR signal by reversing the dephasing of the spins

superconducting magnet: a magnet whose magnetic field is obtained from an electromagnet constructed from superconducting materials enclosed in a cryostat (bath of liquid helium). No electrical energy is consumed unlike a resistive magnet

T1: longitudinal relaxation time

T2: spin–spin or transverse relaxation time. (A summary of the properties of T1 and T2 is given in Table 19.4)

T2*: the time constant of the FID which is influenced by a combination of magnetic field inhomogeneities and spin–spin relaxation

TE: echo time between middle of 90° pulse and middle of spin echo signal

tesla: the SI unit of magnetic flux density $1\,T = 10{,}000\,G$. The fringe field of 0.5 mT is equivalent to 5 G

TR: repetition time (see sequence time)

transverse relaxation: loss of transverse magnetization from a non-zero value in the M_{xy} plane

voxel: volume element, representing matrix resolution and slice depth

20

Magnetic resonance imaging

20.1 THE MAIN MAGNET

The phenomenon of nuclear magnetic resonance was developed as an imaging technique in the early 1970s. Its non-ionizing characteristic makes it ideal for detailed study of anatomical structures.

Present techniques in magnetic resonance imaging (MRI) can display:

- **Chemical differences** between tissues as changes in a gray-scale image (tumor pathology)
- **Blood flow** as a high intensity image of vessels either in thin slices or 3-D images
- **Axial**, **coronal**, **saggital**, and **oblique** images from a complete 3-D voxel data set (head)
- **Long slices**, particularly in saggital view (spine)

Fast imaging techniques have been developed so that organ movement (cardiac, respiration) can be effectively frozen giving sharp pictures of the heart and abdomen. Fast data collection has enabled clinically routine 3-D imaging for investigating cranial anatomy and vascular pathways (magnetic resonance angiography (MRA)).

MRI does not offer the same clinical information as CT: the latter still provides faster imaging and higher resolution but the non-ionizing properties of MRI are a distinct advantage for imaging sensitive areas (breast).

Signal data is related to physiological properties of the tissue, unlike X-ray transmission properties shown by CT. Blood flow can be demonstrated by MRI and further refinements to sensitivity enable micro-circulation pathways in the brain to be seen.

A complete magnetic resonance imaging system consists of:

- A large bore **magnet** (resistive, permanent or superconducting)
- Very stable **power supplies** for precise magnet control
- **Transmitter/receiver** electronics for RF
- Small field of view receiving **coils** for specific anatomy
- Imaging **computer** and **array processor** with fast Fourier transform (FFT) hardwired for rapid computation of reconstructed images

20.1.1 Magnet strength

Magnetic flux density is measured in either gauss (G) or tesla (T), the conversion being: $10\,000\,G$ equals $1\,T$, so $1\,G$ equals $0.1\,mT$. Tesla is commonly used for describing MRI magnet strengths. Fractions of a tesla are expressed as millitesla (mT) or microtesla (μT).

MRI magnets have field strengths between 0.2 and 2.0 T, the outer interference boundary is 5 mT compared to Earth's magnetic field of about 50 μT. The choice of magnet strength depends exclusively on the clinical application. This is discussed in Section 20.7.

LOW TO MEDIUM FIELD

These have strengths from <0.1 to 0.2 T and are mostly **permanent** or **resistive magnets** suitable for private clinics or hospital installations where space is limited.

MEDIUM FIELD

These have fields of 0.2 to 0.3 T and include the largest practical **resistive** and **permanent magnets**. The latter are useful for mobile MRI units where energy consumption is a prime consideration.

MEDIUM TO HIGH FIELD

The common field strengths are 0.5 T, 1.0 T, 1.5 T, and 2.0 T and are exclusively **superconducting** magnets which use liquid helium as a cryogen. Magnet strengths for clinical use can reach 4 T. Magnet field strength has limits depending on the magnet type:

- The field strength of a **permanent** magnet is restricted to about 0.3 T due to weight considerations.
- A **resistive** magnet is restricted to about 0.3 T since power consumption is limited to 100 kW which restricts a resistive magnet size and an increased volume can only be achieved by sacrificing field strength.
- **Superconducting** magnets do not suffer from restrictions of field strength or volume size.

20.1.2 Magnet types

The largest component of any MRI system is the magnet itself. Three types exist commercially:

- Permanent magnet
- Resistive electromagnet
- Superconducting electromagnet

PERMANENT MAGNET

This has considerable advantages in terms of running costs since the generation of its main magnetic field consumes no electricity. Figure 20.1 shows it has a small **fringe field** (external magnetic field) which is a

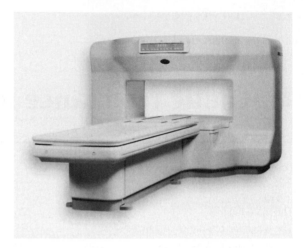

Figure 20.1 *A permanent magnet 0.2 T design showing two separate magnets, top and bottom, giving an open aspect y-axis design (courtesy of GE Medical Systems).*

considerable advantage in a small area (mobile installation). There are some major disadvantages, however:

- Weight, which can be up to 100 tonnes, needing a strengthened floor
- Continual loss of magnet field strength throughout its working life
- Comparatively poor magnetic field uniformity

In spite of these drawbacks it has become the favorite option for low field machines where the orientation of a permanent magnet MRI machine can be either along the length of the body (Z-axis) or perpendicular to the patient's body (Y-axis) shown in Fig. 20.1. The latter allows an open aspect which is more convenient for interventional work using a resistive magnet.

RESISTIVE MAGNET

This was a common design in the early MRI machines since it gave good field strengths and had a good power/weight ratio giving medium field strengths. The major disadvantage was its running costs since it can consume in excess of 30 kW. The magnet windings offer some electrical resistance so considerable heat is generated which must be removed by water cooling. Some designs use a vertical magnetic field (Fig. 20.1) which proves convenient for patient interventional studies. Magnetic field uniformity (homogeneity) is good. Emergency shut-down capabilities are important if interventional work is considered within the main magnetic field.

SUPERCONDUCTING MAGNET

The heat generated by a resistive magnet is caused by the electrical resistance at high field currents. This problem can be eliminated with a superconducting magnet using windings constructed from niobium–tantalum alloy. The windings are divided into several sets in order to create a homogeneous magnetic field and are immersed in liquid helium which causes the windings to become superconducting (zero electrical resistance). The magnet is now activated by connecting the windings to an electrical supply. The field current (up to 500 A) continues to circulate when the supply is removed; electricity costs are therefore minimal. If the magnet temperature rises above the superconducting limit (≈ 4.2 k) then heat is generated and the helium boils off, **quenching** the magnetic field (magnetic properties vanish). Helium cryogens used in a superconducting magnet can be recirculated and normally only need topping up every 6 months or so.

The construction of a typical superconducting magnet has supplementary shielding coils which significantly reduce the large magnetic fringe field (see Fig. 20.3). Figure 20.2 is a commercial MRI system showing a similar design to a CT machine although the magnet unit is considerably deeper. Table 20.1 lists the basic properties given by the three magnet types. The considerable weight (in tonnes) is a significant consideration when planning an MRI installation.

20.1.3 Magnet homogeneity

Uniformity of magnetic field throughout the imaging volume (20 to 35 cm) is essential for good image quality. As the magnet strength increases field homogeneity becomes a major problem. Magnet field inhomogeneities originate from adjacent external influences (high fields from power lines, elevators, and other electric equipment) or ferromagnetic materials (iron pipes or reinforcing rods) within the room. Inhomogeneities can also be caused by small imperfections in magnet construction. The resulting main field inhomogeneity requires careful correction by **shimming** to achieve a uniform field.

Magnetic field inhomogeneities are measured in parts per million, a relative measurement, independent of field strength using the reference proton Larmor frequency for water which is 42.58 MHz T^{-1}. Worked examples are given in Box 20.1. Magnet

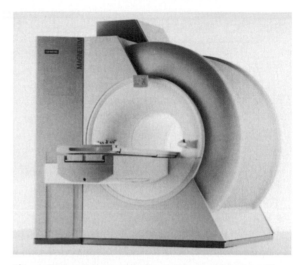

Figure 20.2 *A superconducting 1.5 T magnet system. The bulk of the cylindrical housing holds the main winding and active shim coils in a liquid helium bath. The helium vent and access can be seen on top (courtesy of Siemens Medical Systems).*

Table 20.1 *Properties of different types of magnet.*

Property	Type of magnet		
	Permanent	**Resistive**	**Super-conducting**
Strength (T)	0.064 to 0.3	0.1 to 0.3	0.5 to 4.0
Fringe field	Small	Small	Large
Orientation	z or y	z or y	z
Shut down	No	Fast	Slow
Weight (t)	up to 80	2	6
Energy use	None	Large	None
Cooling	None	Water	Helium

inhomogeneities can approach 100 ppm even without external influences so shimming the magnet is an essential requirement. It must be very carefully performed since small field inhomogeneities influence nuclei (proton) behavior (T2). Dislocations in the field homogeneity will influence readout or slice selection gradients. The influence of inherent small non-uniformity after correction can be reduced by increasing the gradient field strengths.

Manufacturers are continuously improving magnet field homogeneity. Methods have been developed for selectively suppressing the fat signal in images and emphasizing water photons. The Larmor frequency difference is 200 Hz at 1.5 T or 3.5 ppm demanding

Box 20.1 Magnetic field homogeneity

Hydrogen protons have a Larmor frequency of $42.5759\ MHz\ T^{-1}$. A 200 Hz variation would represent a variation in parts per million of $0.0002/42.5759 = 4.697 \times 10^{-6} = 4.7$ ppm. Typical magnetic field variations for large fields of view (40 cm) are:

- **Permanent and resistive magnets** 40 ppm representing a 1.7 kHz variation. Over smaller volumes homogeneity is much better.
- **Superconducting magnets** 15 ppm representing 600 Hz. This reduces to ± 3 ppm for fat suppression and better than ± 1 ppm for small volume spectroscopy.

Note. Magnet inhomogeneities are measured in parts per million since this is independent of magnetic field strength.

Table 20.2 *Magnet homogeneity for two field sizes.*

Field of view (cm)	Permanent (ppm)	Resistive (ppm)	Superconducting (ppm)
50	40	40	15
20	10	5	0.25

extremely homogeneous magnetic fields and, at the moment, is only possible with small fields of view.

Typical homogeneity values of commercial magnets for MRI are given in Table 20.2 for two fields of view (FOV) relating to body and head acquisitions. Homogeneity throughout the useful field of view is achieved by the combination of shim coils and iron sheets or foil carefully adjusted within the main winding.

SHIM COILS

Current-carrying coils are arranged cylindrically inside the magnet bore. The pattern or spectrum of the field inhomogeneities are mapped and then corrected by setting the shim-coil currents via a precision power supply. This is **active shimming**.

IRON FOIL

Carefully shaped iron plates can be placed inside or outside the magnet to give **passive shimming**. This

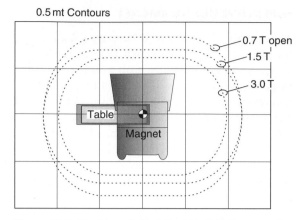

0.5 mt Contours

Figure 20.3 *The fringe field at the 0.5 mT (5 G) contour for 3 T, 1.5 T, and 0.7 T superconducting magnets. Each square has 1 m sides.*

method removes major inhomgeneities. Passive shimming is stable and is not dependent on power supply stability. It requires considerable time to fit and adjust; additional coil correction with shim coils is usually necessary.

20.1.4 Shielding

The magnetic field surrounding an MRI installation is hazardous to people and equipment; it will attract ferrous items which can act as missiles endangering staff. External flux lines (fringe field) will interfere with sensitive equipment such as gamma cameras (photomultipliers) and DSA (image intensifiers). Fringe fields are restricted by means of magnetic shielding, either passively by iron sheets or actively by a supplementary winding.

Figure 20.3 shows the 0.5 mT contour after shielding has been installed on a variety of magnet sizes. The magnet is sited within the building so that this contour does not penetrate important areas. Sensitive equipment is listed in Table 20.3 that is influenced by magnetic fields and indicates that nuclear medicine and DSA rooms should be distanced from MRI installations. **Passive or self-shielding** requires a considerable number of heavy iron plates mounted directly on the magnet. The weight of the installation is increased significantly and the room floor would require substantial strengthening. A single sheet of iron is sometimes sufficient to shield a particular area, i.e. cardiac pacemaker room. **Active shielding** uses an opposing external coil winding included within the cryostat with the main

Table 20.3 *Magnetic field limits.*

Field	Limit
Earth's magnetic field	$50\,\mu\text{T}$ ($0.05\,\text{mT}$)
Gamma camera SPECT	$50\,\mu\text{T}$
Image intensifier	$50\,\mu\text{T}$
X-ray tube	$0.2\,\text{mT}$
Cardiac pacemaker	$0.5\,\text{mT}$
Video monitors	$1.0\,\text{mT}$

winding (shown in Fig. 20.6). This increases the size and cost of the superconducting magnet but achieves effective shielding without increasing magnet weight.

RADIO-FREQUENCY SHIELDING

Efficient shielding against radio-frequency interference (radio, television signals, and power switching RF pulses) is essential owing to the high sensitivity of the receiving circuitry for the weak NMR signals. The shielding factor should be in the order of 100 dB for local radio stations. A copper or aluminum **Faraday cage** is installed which:

- Blocks radio interference from the computer and display units so they do not reach the signal coils
- Prevents RF pulses from the gradient fields interfering with other equipment

A thin (0.5 mm) copper foil should completely surround the MRI installation. Gaps in this foil should be carefully filled. Doors should be similarly shielded and cable lengths should also be enclosed so that they do not act as antenna for RF interference. A wire mesh covering the control panel window preserves the integrity of the entire RF cage.

SUMMARY

- Magnet strength is measured in tesla.
- Permanent and resistive magnets have field strengths up to 0.2 T.
- Superconducting magnets have field strengths from 0.5 to 2.0 T.
- Superconducting magnet requires liquid helium as a cryogen.
- Superconducting magnet fringe field reduced by active shielding.
- Safety contour set at 0.5 mT for pacemakers.
- Magnet homogeneity achieved by metal or coil shimming.

- Magnet homogeneity measured in parts per million; independent of field strength.
- RF shielding obtained by using wire-mesh Faraday cage.

20.2 THE MAGNETIC RESONANCE IMAGING SYSTEM

Unlike X-ray computed tomography the image forming signals in MRI are radio frequencies which convey image information by changes in:

- Frequency
- Amplitude
- Phase

The computations are performed by a dedicated fast Fourier transform (FFT) circuit which is part of an array processor. This includes a phase sensitive demodulator which gives NMR signal frequency and phase information necessary for image formation.

20.2.1 Magnetic gradients

NMR signal frequency is directly related to the magnetic field strength (as the Larmor equation explains). A carefully shimmed MRI magnet has an almost perfect homogeneous magnetic field so protons will all have the same Larmor frequency. If a magnetic field gradient G is superimposed on the main field B_0 so that there is a small linear increase over the length of the gradient then the Larmor frequency for the proton will vary along this gradient as

$$\omega = \gamma(B_0 + G) \qquad (20.1)$$

where G is the added magnetic field from the gradient. Only those protons in slice location z will resonate at frequency ω as

$$z = \frac{\omega - \gamma B_0}{\gamma G} \qquad (20.2)$$

Protons outside slice position z are unaffected and will give no signal so specific regions can be spatially located. This was first proposed by P. Lauterbur (USA) in 1973.

Specially constructed **gradient field coils** are placed within the main magnet and superimpose a linear magnetic field gradient on the main magnetic field. This gradient field is very small, typically 5 mT to

15 mT over the main field of 1 T. The main magnetic field must be perfectly uniform otherwise the small variations imposed by the gradient fields will be lost. The gradient magnetic field gives a central null point (Fig. 20.4a) with a reduced (negative) and increased (positive) magnetic gradient either side of its null

Magnetic gradients G_z G_x G_y

Positive gradient

Null

Negative gradient

(a)

(b)

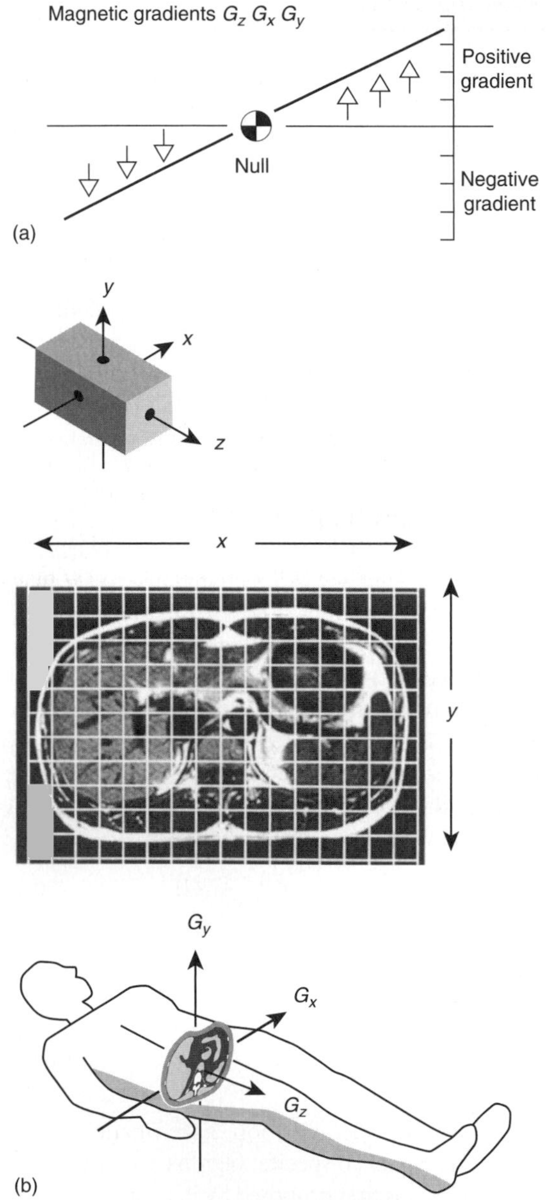

Figure 20.4 (**a**) *Superimposing a gradient field on the main magnetic field. The gradient has a central null point; to one side (left) the gradient linearly decreases in strength and to the other (right) it increases.* (**b**) *X, Y, Z image planes used for slice position and decoding the image matrix.*

point. Gradient coils serve the three axes making up the patient volume shown in Fig. 20.4b:

- A **frequency encoded** Z-axis
- A **phase encoded** Y-axis horizontally opposed to the Z-axis
- A **frequency encoded** X-axis vertically opposed to the Z-axis

These gradients are termed $\boldsymbol{G_z}$, $\boldsymbol{G_y}$, and $\boldsymbol{G_x}$, respectively, and enable spatial information to be obtained from the patient. Image data signals from these axes are produced by switching the gradient field strengths in a controlled sequence.

The gradient coils shown in Fig. 20.5a are positioned within the main magnet bore and cover the three axes. They are not active all the time (unlike the main magnetic field) but are switched on when required for signal collection. Very large gradient field switching gives the 'machine-gun' staccato

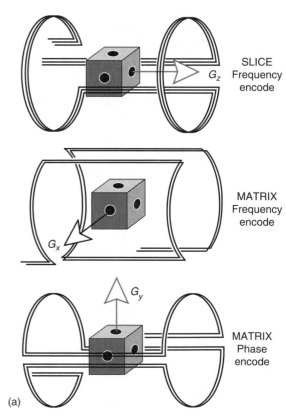

SLICE
G_z Frequency encode

MATRIX
Frequency encode

G_x

G_y

MATRIX
Phase encode

(a)

Figure 20.5 (**a**) *Gradient coil design. The Z-axis slice position is frequency encoded. The x and y gradients encode the image pixel position for frequency and phase, respectively.*

sound when an MRI machine is working. When a G_z, G_y or G_x gradient is energized the respective linear gradient field is superimposed on the main field.

Gradient field strength must be large enough to overcome magnet inhomogeneities; as the main magnet field strength increases so do the gradient field strengths. Figure 20.5b plots this relationship. Gradient strengths are measured in mT per meter ($mT\ m^{-1}$); some superconducting magnets have higher gradients in order to achieve thinner sections and better resolution.

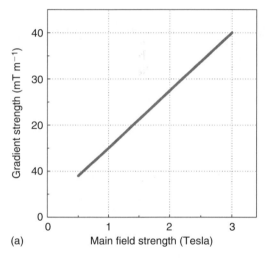

(a)

Figure 20.5 *(Contd)* *(**b**) The main field strength versus gradient strength. The slope can be steeper since large magnets (>1 T) can have gradient strengths approaching 25 mT m⁻¹.*

COMPLETE MAGNETIC RESONANCE IMAGING INDUCTORS (COILS AND WINDINGS)

The number of windings used in a complete MRI machine are shown in Fig. 20.6a. These are:

- The main **electromagnet** (resistive or superconducting coil) which is the largest winding, generating magnetic fields up to 4 T in some large machines but more commonly 0.5 to 1.5 T.
- Directly outside the main winding is a smaller winding which acts as the **active shield** in superconducting magnets, constraining the fringe field to within a narrow contour.
- Inside the main winding are various **shim coils** which, together with carefully placed iron sheets, finely adjust the uniformity of the main magnetic field.
- The **gradient coils** then form the complete coil assembly which is fixed within the gantry. The gradient coils are very thick windings since they must carry a current of up to 100 A.
- The moveable **signal coils** act as transmitter and receiver antenna; these are the body and surface coils, respectively.

The receiver coils are placed near the anatomical region of interest in order to improve signal strength.

20.2.2 Eddy currents

These have been described in Chapter 2 as currents induced in a conductor by the varying magnetic field. There is always an electrical field associated with a

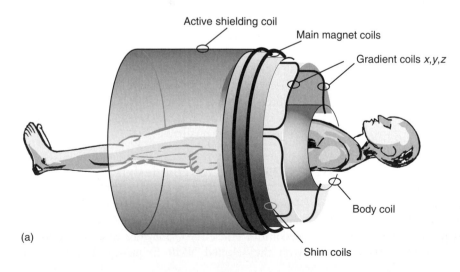

(a)

Figure 20.6 *(a) Block diagram MRI system showing the complete family of windings and coils necessary for an imaging system.*

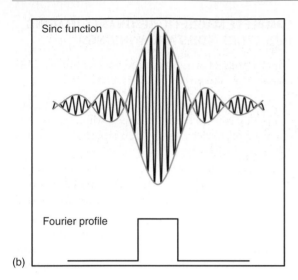

(b)

Figure 20.6 *(Contd)* *(**b**) Sinc pulse (sin x)/x transmission pulse whose shape provides a sharp rectangular frequency distribution for precise slice dimensions (lower trace).*

changing magnetic field, this induces a current to circulate in the volume of adjacent conductive material (patient tissue). These eddy currents interact against the main magnetic field causing interference and inhomogeneities. They are further undesirable because of their energy dissipation. Eddy currents are experienced in high-field superconducting magnets occurring in only a small way in smaller strength resistive and permanent magnets. They are caused by the switched gradient fields and disturb magnet field homogeneity and require compensation. Eddy currents are a particular problem in fast imaging techniques which use rapid gradient switching, they are also induced by the RF field generating an opposing field which weakens the applied RF; this skin effect causes inhomogeneities in the excitation field. At high frequencies (above 40 MHz) RF field tissue penetration also becomes a problem.

SUMMARY

- Gradient windings are in three planes: G_z (slice position and thickness) G_x and G_y (image matrix).
- The gradient has a central null point and imposes a negative and positive magnetic field on the main field either side of the null.
- G_z and G_x encode for frequency; G_y encodes for phase.

Table 20.4 *Specification for radio-frequency pulse transmitter.*

Parameter	Frequency
Nominal frequency	63.6 MHz
Tunable range	63.4 to 63.8 MHz
Bandwidth	400 kHz
Stability	4×10^{-9} Hz
Transmit power	10 kW

- Gradient field strengths are from 10 to 25 mT m^{-1}.
- Gradient windings can carry up to 100 A.

20.2.3 The radio-frequency pulse

In order to excite a sharp rectangular slice a special pulse shape is used; this is the sinc-pulse shown in Fig. 20.6b and uses the mathematical function sin x/x. The transmitter section of the MRI machine is a computer controlled RF generator whose high frequency can be tuned very accurately for frequency and bandwidth. The precisely shaped sinc-pulse is amplified to give 90° or 180° power levels or intermediate levels when smaller '**flip angles**' are being used.

The receiver section of the MRI system accepts the high frequency NMR signals which are converted (demodulated) to give low frequency signals before digitization; only frequency and phase differences are important and not the absolute frequency value. Typical specifications for a 1.5 T MRI transmitter system are shown in Table 20.4. The extremely stable frequency is necessary for accurate spatial information.

The **body coil** identified in Fig. 20.6a is used as the transmission antenna delivering precise frequencies which determine the slice position within the coil (determined by G_z). The NMR signal is picked up by either the same body coil or more commonly by specialized receiver coils designed to cover the anatomy of interest (spine, breast, knee etc.). These surface coils significantly improve the signal-to-noise ratio and hence image quality.

20.2.4 Detector coil design

The detector coil picks up the very small NMR signals from the tissue volume under investigation. For maximum efficiency Q they are tuned to resonate with the selected NMR frequency. The resonant

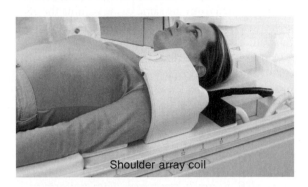

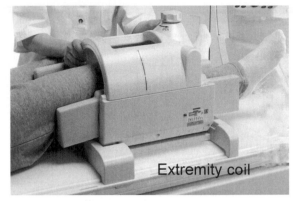

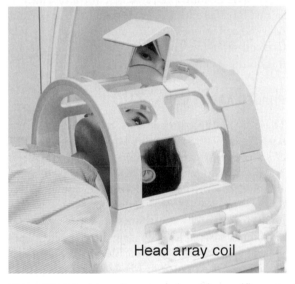

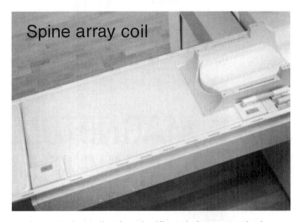

Figure 20.7 *Various coil arrays designed for specific anatomical regions. Their application significantly increases the image signal to noise ratio (courtesy of Siemens Medical Systems).*

signal is then converted to a lower frequency signal. Most detectors give phase measurement and this information is obtained by using a quadrature demodulator to extract the phase information. A selection of receiver coils is shown in Fig. 20.7.

SURFACE COILS

Surface coils are small coils placed immediately adjacent to the body region of interest (spine, neck, knee etc.). They allow the RF signals to be received with excellent signal-to-noise ratio (SNR) but cover smaller areas than obtained with the standard head or body coils. Most surface coils are used strictly as receivers with the standard body coil as the transmitter. Surface coils do not surround the body but are placed close to the organ of interest. They have a selectivity

for a tissue volume approximately subtended by the coil circumference and one radius deep from the coil center.

A simple arrangement is shown in Fig. 20.8a. In its simplest arrangement it is a simple ring tuned to resonate at the particular NMR frequency. The sensitivity along the coil axis decreases rapidly with increasing distance from the coil plane. Effective penetration depth is roughly equal to the coil radius. Surface coils are used primarily as detectors, the pulse transmission can be obtained by using the body coil.

QUADRATURE DETECTORS

By joining a pair of coils at 90° to one another and driving them during the transmit cycle through a power divider and phase shifter a rotating field can

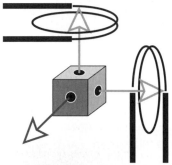

(a)   Surface coil

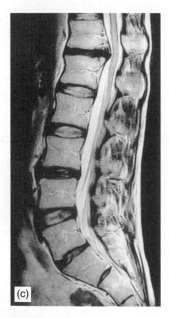

(b)   Quadrature detector

Figure 20.8 *Signal coil design showing (**a**) the smaller flat loop and (**b**) the basic quadrature coil design. (**c**) Longitudinal image of the spine using surface coils showing improved definition in the specific coil array (courtesy Siemens Medical and MRT Hoheluft, Germany).*

be produced that only requires half the RF power (Fig. 20.8b). In a similar fashion the same principle gives a quadrature detector which is phase sensitive. It is sensitive to the components of the signal which

is phase shifted by 90°. Since two separate signals are being obtained from the same tissue volume the SNR is improved by $\sqrt{2}$ or ≈ 1.4. Patient motion reduces this value, however.

Surface coils generally improve images of superficial structures. Figure 20.8c gives examples of clinical images taken with anatomically specific coils. Signal reception is increased by proximity of the organ to the receiver antenna and noise and reflections are decreased because signals outside the region of interest are very weak. Reducing the field of view also improves resolution since there is smaller voxel volume. SNR is much improved. Non-uniformity is caused by difference in signal strengths from organs near the coil to ones that are more distant. The surface coil should be chosen for the region of interest; this optimizes the image SNR.

PHASED ARRAY COILS

These are multiple surface coils, each coil served by a separate detector/receiver. A typical design consists of six coils that can be combined to give surface or 3-D configurations. A large field of view is obtained at high SNR since each coil is an independent detector. Interference between coils is prevented by low impedance receiver matching. They cover a wider anatomical area reducing imaging time for larger fields of view. Surface coils are available that use a 'ladder' configuration where individual coils are switched through to a common receiver. These are not true phased array coils.

SUMMARY

- Body coil solenoid coils act as transmitting antennae for the RF pulses.
- Specialized surface coils matched to the anatomy act as receiver antennae.
- The signal-to-noise ratio is improved by surface coils.
- Phased array coils cover larger areas.

20.2.5 Spatial encoding

The three orthogonal axes, which are used for spatially encoding, are shown as a small sketch in Fig. 20.4b. The three gradient fields G_z, G_x, and G_y are switched in a defined sequence, firstly to encode slice position and thickness G_z then to encode the x and y positions in

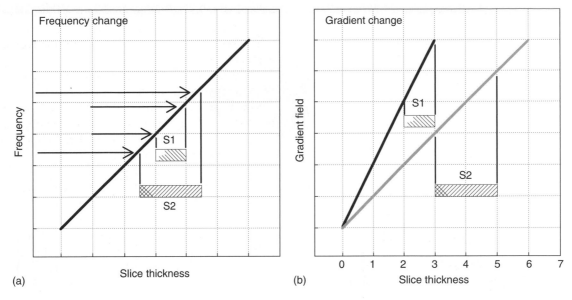

(a)

(b)

Figure 20.9 *Slice thickness can be selected by increasing frequency bandwidth or altering the slope of the gradient field.*

the image matrix. The size of the image matrix has increased with improved accuracy of location from 128 to 256 to 512. The eventual image matrix can be interpolated to a larger size (1024^2) if necessary.

THE SLICE AXIS G_z (FREQUENCY ENCODED)

The protons exposed to the G_z gradient will show differing Larmor frequencies depending on their position along it. The precise frequency of the RF pulse (transmitted via the body coil) will select a specific slice position (see eqn 20.1) described by $\omega = \gamma(B_0 + G_z)$. Slice thickness can be altered by:

- Increasing the range of frequencies in the RF pulse; the wider the frequency range the thicker the slice
- Keeping the bandwidth constant and altering the gradient slope to modify the slice thickness

These are shown graphically in Fig. 20.9, and Box 20.2 calculates the frequency difference necessary for defining a 5 mm slice. The change is very small and so the magnetic field must be uniform in order to localize the slice position precisely. The transmission pulse should have a narrow frequency range for accurate slice location and thickness and for good SNR. A wide frequency range will excite regions outside the slice of interest causing **cross-talk**. For this reason gaps between slices are maintained, usually between 30 and 50% of the slice width.

Box 20.2 Slice position and thickness

The Larmor frequency for a 1 T magnet is 42.58 MHz T^{-1}. The gradient strength for:

- a 0.5 T magnet is 10 mT m^{-1} (0.1 mT cm^{-1})
- a 1.0 T magnet is 15 mT m^{-1} (0.15 mT cm^{-1})

What is the frequency range necessary for a slice thickness of 5 mm (0.5 cm)?

For a 0.5 T magnet (Larmor frequency 21.29 MHz), 0.005 mT for 0.5 cm is

$$21.29 \times 1.00005 = 21.2910645 \text{ MHz}$$

$$\Delta f = 0.00106 \text{ MHz} \quad \text{or} \quad \approx 1 \text{ kHz}$$

So the central frequency for slice location is chosen with ± 500 Hz to give a 5 mm thickness. For a 1.0 T magnet, 0.075 mT per 0.5 cm is

$$42.58 \times 1.000075 = 42.5831935 \text{ MHz}$$

$$\Delta f = 3.2 \text{ kHz}$$

So a central frequency ± 1.6 kHz would give a 5 mm thickness.

Slice thickness is determined by the gradient strength and the bandwidth of the radio-frequency pulse. The strength of the gradient must be large enough to overcome slight inhomogeneities that are present in the main magnetic field.

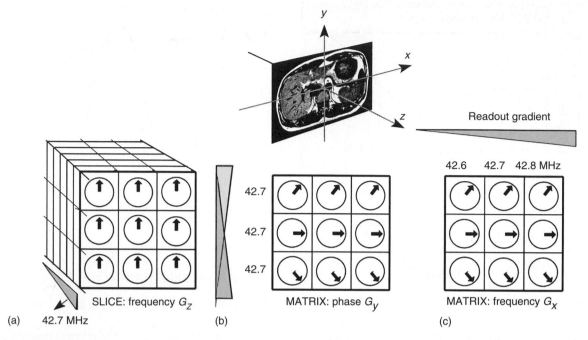

Figure 20.10 *Selecting Z, X, and Y planes by frequency ω and phase encoding φ. For this example a 42.7 MHz frequency selects the slice position in (a). The Y-gradient (b) is switched during acquisition depending on matrix size (three steps for this simplified example). (c) Larmor frequencies of 42.6 to 42.8 MHz determine the X-plane.*

IMAGE MATRIX (G_x, G_y PHASE/FREQUENCY ENCODED)

Figure 20.10a, b, and c shows how a combination of G_z, G_y, and G_x gradients can encode an image matrix. The slice position has already been identified in this example by selecting a hypothetical slice frequency G_z of 42.7 MHz. The G_y gradient is switched on for a short time which causes another frequency change in the proton signal (after G_z) depending on their position along the vertical Y-axis. When G_y is switched off the protons resume their original frequency but they have now lost their phase uniformity; they are now phase shifted according to their position on the Y-axis since the momentary change in frequency caused by G_y, caused them to be dephased. The phase differences are retained when G_y is switched off and are proportional to the strength of G_y; larger phase differences occur at either end of this gradient. Unlike the other gradients (G_z and G_x), the G_y field is switched in a series of steps in order to decode the full matrix. Step numbers are typically 128, 256 or 512. A 256 matrix having 256 phase encoding steps would mean that each step will cause a phase shift of 360°/256 or 1.4° with respect to its column neighbor.

Stepped gradients are represented as a 'ladder' symbol in MRI pulse sequence diagrams.

In the same way that the G_z gradient encodes according to position on the Z-axis, the G_x gradient encodes proton frequencies depending on their X-axis position, fixing their matrix row position by frequency encoding. The G_x gradient remains switched on while NMR signal frequency measurements are recorded. The frequency changes necessary to separate each pixel are calculated in Box 20.3 and considerable uniformity in the main magnetic field is necessary to achieve good image definition in large matrix sizes. Changes in the phase and frequency of NMR signals are measured by reference to a standard signal. This is usually the pure signal for hydrogen protons at the main magnet field strength (21.29 MHz for 0.5 T; 42.58 MHz for 1 T and 63.87 for 1.5 T). The calculations are carried out by a fast Fourier transform (FFT) in a demodulator circuit.

SUMMARY

Three gradients select z-axis (slice position) and x- and y-axes for the image matrix. These are G_z, G_x and G_y.

- G_z uses frequency encoding.
- G_y uses phase encoding.

Box 20.3 Pixel bandwidth

Pixel selection for 0.5 and 1.0 T magnets with 15 cm field of view (FOV) head coil.

For the 0.5 T magnet $(0.1\,\mathrm{mT\,cm^{-1}})$

$$0.1\,\mathrm{mT\,cm^{-1}} \times 15 = 1.5\,\mathrm{mT\ variation}$$
$$\text{over 15 cm}$$

$$21.29 \times 1.0015 = 21.3321935$$

$\Delta f = 32\,\mathrm{kHz} = 120\,\mathrm{Hz\ pixel^{-1}}$ for a 256^2 matrix.

For the 1.0 T magnet $(0.15\,\mathrm{mT\,cm^{-1}})$

$$0.15\,\mathrm{mT\,cm^{-1}} \times 15 = 2.25\,\mathrm{mT\ variation}$$
$$\text{over 15 cm}$$

$$42.58 \times 1.00225 = 42.6758$$

$\Delta f = 95\,\mathrm{kHz} = 374\,\mathrm{Hz\ pixel^{-1}}$ for a 256^2 matrix
$= 190\,\mathrm{Hz\ pixel^{-1}}$ for a 512^2 matrix.

- G_x uses frequency encoding and identifies the signal. This is the readout gradient.

Pulse and signal timing can be varied. Gradient fields impose a negative and positive field change with a middle null point where the overall magnetic field is unaltered. Gradient coils switch up to 100 A.

20.3 THE DATA MATRIX: *K*-SPACE

The concept of rotational motion has been discussed in Chapter 2, Section 2.4. If P rotates about O with a uniform speed then this describes simple harmonic oscillation. Figure 20.11 reiterates the various parameters.

As previously seen, the oscillating displacement of point P is

$$y = A\cos\frac{2\pi t}{T}$$
$$= A\cos 2\pi\nu t$$
$$= A\cos\omega t$$

where A is the amplitude of oscillation, T the period of oscillation (seconds), ν the frequency of oscillation (oscillations $\mathrm{s^{-1}}$), ω the angular frequency (rad $\mathrm{s^{-1}}$) and t is time in seconds. The equation for the transmitted wave motion may then be written as

$$y = A\cos\left(\omega t\,\frac{2\pi x}{\lambda}\right)$$

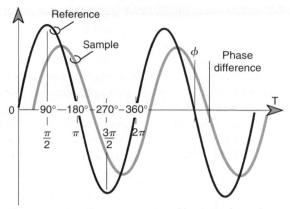

Figure 20.11 *A sine wave generated by a rotating point as seen previously in Fig. 2.1.*

20.3.1 Introduction to *k*: the wave number

The wave motion moves a distance of one wavelength (λ) for each oscillation. Wave velocity (v) is therefore $v = \lambda/T$ usually expressed as $v = \lambda\nu$. This can now be used in an alternative expression where the wave is travelling in direction x:

$$y = A\cos(\omega t - kx)$$

where 'k' is known as the wave number, and is commonly used in optics. The term wave number refers to the number of complete wave cycles that exist in 1 m of linear space (so k is in units of rad $\mathrm{m^{-1}}$). The wave number is traditionally denoted by the letter k. We define

$$k = \frac{2\pi}{\lambda}$$

A wave of wavelength 0.5 m will have $k = 4\pi_1$, in other words its phase will evolve by 4π in 1 m. This is the physical meaning of k; the phase evolved per meter. It is also a vector quantity, as the wave has direction.

20.3.2 Data collection and the gradient sequences

In its simple form *k*-space used in MRI is obtained by gradient switching the MR signals so that they undergo Fourier transformation and provide a 2-D plot of all possible wave numbers. The *k*-space data set is two-dimensional for a 2-D image containing full information on received signal frequency and phase. Application of varying gradient strengths in MRI can be used to move around in k-space.

Plane waves with identical wave numbers (same frequency) may still differ with regard to their phase, and the data on k-space is a complex data set (see above), so that the phase information is included.

The switching sequence of the gradient magnetic fields is controlled and timed by the main system computer. For basic imaging routines a typical sequence could be:

- G_z identifies the slice position; the slice encode gradient (Fig. 20.10a).
- G_y is now switched on for a short period, causing the protons in the vertical axis to alter frequency momentarily according to their position along the y-gradient. This is the phase encode gradient. The protons resume their pre-G_y Larmor frequency when G_y is switched off but retain a phase difference, depending on their position in the matrix columns (Fig. 20.10b).
- G_x is switched on causing a frequency difference in the rows, the NMR signal is now measured and the phase/frequency information stored. G_x is therefore the frequency encode or readout gradient (Fig. 20.10c).

SIGNAL STORAGE

Magnetic resonance echoes are measured as a combination of plane waves of certain frequencies (or wave numbers), and phases. Different spatial positions within the object (i.e. patient) are represented as different magnetic resonance frequencies (frequency encoding, phase encoding). Rather than recording and storing individual resonance frequencies, the time dependent radio-frequency bursts are stored which are related to the frequency domain data by an inverse Fourier transformation.

Conceptually, k-space is infinite, but practically it is limited to the frequencies which have been used in the spatial encoding of the data. Figure 20.12 shows how a simple square wave can be represented by its Fourier transform (see Chapter 1, Section 1.12.2). As the high frequency component of the Fourier transform is restricted the square wave becomes less square and the sharp edges become slopes. Describing a square wave function by a Fourier series needs high frequency harmonics of the base frequency to define the edges, but there is a practical limit to the highest frequency that can be measured (bandwidth of the electronics) so the

signals undergo some form of truncation. Typically, the bulk of the signal in an object corresponds to low spatial frequencies and the edges in the object correspond to high spatial frequencies; therefore truncation will affect the fine image detail.

20.3.3 The wave number domain: k-space

The complex information measured in MRI combine signals from all over the object being imaged. These signals are composed of a series of sine waves, each with an individual frequency and amplitude. The wave number domain or k-space describes a 2-D matrix of positive and negative spatial frequency values, encoded as complex numbers (e.g. $a + bj$, where $j = v^{-1}$, see Chapter 1, Sections 1.2.4 and 1.12.2). Euler's formula enables the **Fourier transform** to be expressed in complex form, extracting 'real' and 'imaginary' roots (phase and amplitude) where

$$e^{-j\omega x} = \cos(\omega x) - j\sin(\omega x)$$

where j is v^{-1} (sometimes represented by i) and ω is $2\pi f$ (where f is the frequency). In magnetic resonance imaging the 'real' and 'imaginary' cosine and sine wave functions describe phase and amplitude characteristics of the composite resonance signal.

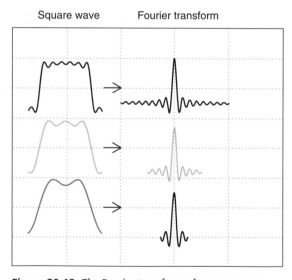

Figure 20.12 *The Fourier transform of a square wave signal yields a pulse whose waveform extends to infinity (high frequency component). In practice therefore the frequency is limited (truncation), consequently this degrades the square wave and gives it sloping sides.*

The Fourier transform describes these in terms of frequencies and amplitudes converting the signals from their time domain into frequency domain.

MR Signal: Time domain (*t* seconds)
↓
Fourier transform: Frequency domain (Hz s^{-1})

Figure 20.13 shows how the first signal is positioned in the data set representing *k*-space at the start of 2-D matrix construction (the *z*-value is stored for phase and frequency).

Further *k*-frequency signals are added to the data set as shown in Fig. 20.14 where three echoes have been collected along the *k*-frequency axis and the phase information can now be seen to gradually build up. The *k*-space matrix varies in the phase encoding direction first (from one acquired line to the next). Filling a line in the frequency encoding direction takes milliseconds whereas the full data set, which includes the phase information, can take minutes. Figure 20.15 illustrates the line-by-line acquisition. The central line of *k*-space is acquired when there is no phase encoding applied and very near the center there is only a small amount of phase encoding.

In Fourier space the image data is represented as its frequency components. Each point in the Fourier domain represents a periodic component of the image with the discrete wave numbers in *x* and *y* directions. These complex numbers carry information about the amplitude and the phase, giving the relative position of a periodic structure.

The phase encoding gradient, as well as encoding the signal, also causes dephasing, which reduces signal strength (*z*-axis). This means that at the top and bottom edges of *k*-space, where there is 'stronger' phase encoding, the amplitudes of the signals are smaller than at the center The entire data set is seen in Fig. 20.16 and in simple form represents a 'Mexican hat' distribution with strong central signal and smaller signal amplitude in the periphery.

The important part of *k*-space is the center, which contains low frequency information which determines image contrast. The matrix is divided into four quadrants, with the origin at the center representing frequency = 0. Frequency domain data are encoded in the *k x*-direction by the frequency encode gradient, and in the *k y*-direction by the phase encode gradient in most image sequences (Fig. 20.15).

The Fourier transform decomposes the spatial information of an image into periodic structures. This is an extremely helpful tool for understanding image formation, digitization, and processing. Chapter 1, Section 1.12.2 has already described the fundamentals of waveform analysis using the Fourier transform, which can be regarded as a coordinate transformation in a finite-dimensional vector space. Therefore, the image information is completely preserved. We can perform the **inverse Fourier transform** to obtain the original image. An axial image is in 2-D space so, in

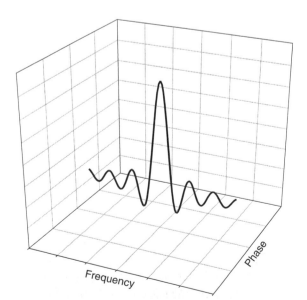

Figure 20.13 *The first signal positioned in the* k-space *matrix along the* y-axis.

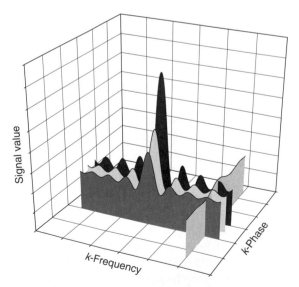

Figure 20.14 *Subsequent* k-frequency signals stored line by line gradually yielding k-phase information in the x-axis.

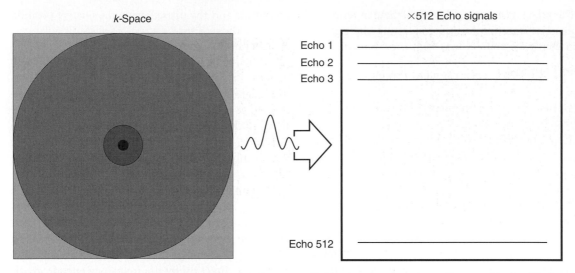

k-Space

×512 Echo signals

Echo 1
Echo 2
Echo 3

Echo 512

Figure 20.15 *The k-space is constructed a line at a time controlled by the phase encode gradient. In this simplified example the k-space represents 512 echo signals. It can be viewed as a 2-D distribution of frequency and phase information having a central peak.*

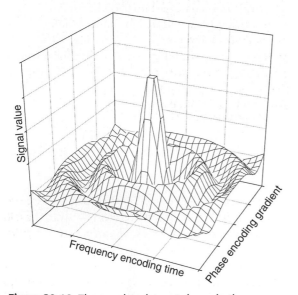

Signal value

Frequency encoding time

Phase encoding gradient

Figure 20.16 *The complete data set shown in three dimensions: holding information about frequency, phase, and amplitude. The data yields a 'Mexican-hat' shape with largest central values and smaller values on the periphery.*

Frequency ω

Phase φ

$\omega_1\,\phi_1$	$\omega_2\,\phi_1$	$\omega_3\,\phi_1$	$\omega_4\,\phi_1$	$\omega_5\,\phi_1$
$\omega_1\,\phi_2$	$\omega_2\,\phi_2$	$\omega_3\,\phi_2$	$\omega_4\,\phi_2$	$\omega_5\,\phi_2$
$\omega_1\,\phi_3$	$\omega_2\,\phi_3$	$\omega_3\,\phi_3$	$\omega_4\,\phi_3$	$\omega_5\,\phi_3$
$\omega_1\,\phi_4$	$\omega_2\,\phi_4$	$\omega_3\,\phi_4$	$\omega_4\,\phi_4$	$\omega_5\,\phi_4$
$\omega_1\,\phi_5$	$\omega_2\,\phi_5$	$\omega_3\,\phi_5$	$\omega_4\,\phi_5$	$\omega_5\,\phi_5$

Figure 20.17 *The fully encoded matrix where each voxel separates the NMR signal according to phase ϕ and frequency ω. This matrix is in k-space. An inverse Fourier transform forms the display pixel-matrix.*

this case, the *k*-space map represents a plane for the 2-D MR image, but *k*-space can represent 3-D space for 3-D volume imaging.

The axes between *k*-space and image space differ, but since the MR signals are encoded with magnetic field gradients both frequency and (rate of change of) phase carry spatial information. In *k*-space axes can be asymmetric since the axes of *k*-space are time. Acquiring one phase encoding step (filling a line in the frequency encoding direction) takes milliseconds, whereas filling *k*-space to have a full data set in the phase encoding direction can take minutes.

A simplified encoded matrix is shown in Fig. 20.17. Each voxel presents a different frequency and phase

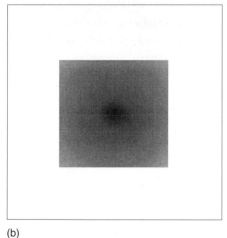

(a)

Full data set

(b)

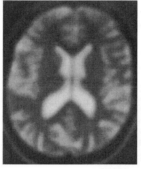

Figure 20.18 *(a) The full data set in* k-*space having undergone an inverse Fourier transform yields a gray-scale image. (**b**) Transforming only the central regions also yields a full image retaining contrast but having lost all fine detail (spatial resolution).*

as encoded by G_x and G_y. This matrix is not the displayed matrix since it carries only frequency and phase information in *k*-space. N_x and N_y are often used to signify the number of phase and frequency coded steps; these decide the final dimension of the matrix (256^2, 512^2, 1024^2).

The two-dimensional Fourier transform (2-D.FT) is able to separate the signal into its respective frequency and phase components and using these two components it is possible to identify the two spatial dimensions in the image matrix and so separate the individual voxels in the slice. *k*-space is a 2-D plot of spatial frequencies, and so there is no positional information between points in *k*-space and relevant points on the displayed image.

Every single point in *k*-space contributes to the entire image. The data in the *k*-space array are spatial frequencies, not intensity values with (x, y) coordinates

in real space. After separating the NMR signal according to its frequency and phase characteristics it again undergoes an **inverse Fourier transform** which yields signal strength information (amplitude) which is stored as a gray-scale value in a pixel display matrix (Fig. 20.18a). The contrast of an image is mapped into the center of *k*-space while high resolution fine detail structures are represented in its peripheral regions. Hence the full frequency information has to be mapped extensively in *k*-space to reconstruct a high resolution image. Removing or altering the peripheral data in *k*-space will affect image spatial resolution (Fig. 20.18b).

Phase and frequency information in *k*-space can be sampled line by line and a Fourier transform of it will then result in the desired image. Many programs have been devised to sample data points in *k*-space. Data points on each *k*-space line can be spaced at equal distances (linear sampling) or at variable distances (nonlinear sampling). More frequent sampling of the central k-space region than the periphery will provide rapid update of contrast changes in an image, i.e. after injection of contrast media, but less frequent updates of subtle high resolution changes in an image.

VOXEL SIZE

The matrix dimension m, assuming equal number of phase and frequency encoding steps N_x and N_y and the field of view (FOV) with the slice thickness determine the individual voxel size. For a 50 cm FOV, which is the typical value, occupying a 512^2 matrix and a 2 mm slice thickness the voxel size would be FOV/m or approximately 1 mm^2 by 2 mm deep.

20.4 IMAGING PULSE SEQUENCES

The gradient field switching is synchronized with 90° and 180° RF pulses transmitted by the body coil. These switching and pulse sequences yield an NMR signal along with its spatial information.

20.4.1 Spin echo sequence and two-dimensional Fourier transform

Unlike CT where image reconstruction depends on successively rotated projections (polar coordinates), MR image reconstruction utilizes Cartesian coordinates (x, y, and z) which allows direct reconstruction by means of a 2-D fast Fourier transform.

The basic spin echo pulse sequence described in Chapter 19 is shown again in Fig. 20.19a. This imaging sequence consists of a series of 90° and 180° pulses; the time between the 90° pulses is the time-to-repeat (TR) time. After the 90° pulse the proton transverse signal (T2*) will decay at a rate decided by tissue characteristics. The 180° pulse rephases the NMR signals so correcting for external magnet inhomogeneities. The NMR signal appears at TE (time-to-echo). The 180° pulse is positioned at half TE: TE/2 time.

Figure 20.19b shows the gradient switching G_z, G_x, and G_y pulse sequences necessary for image signal collection using a 90° to 180° spin echo sequence:

- G_z is applied only when 90° or 180° RF pulses are transmitted. Gradient strength remains constant during data acquisition but changes to select other slices and slice thicknesses.

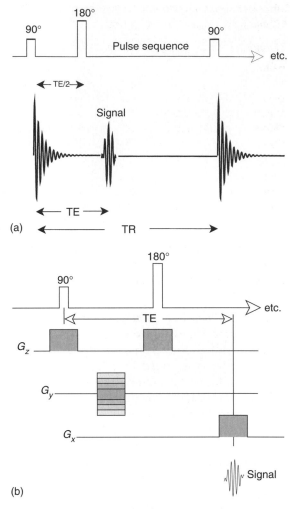

Figure 20.19 (a) The basic spin echo pulse sequence identifying TR and TE together with τ which is TE/2. (b) The spin echo sequence with gradient switching G_z, G_y, G_x and echo signal timing which yields the 2-D image.

- G_y is applied after the RF pulses but before the NMR echo is received. It is a stepped gradient, the number of steps depending on matrix size.
- G_x is applied only when receiving signals. This is a constant strength gradient.

Since G_y is a varying magnetic field, this is depicted as a stepped pulse in the diagrams. The time of TR and TE in Fig. 20.19a are termed short and long. TR is chosen to match the time constant T1 of the tissue of interest. A TR less than 500 ms is termed 'short' and >1500 ms is termed 'long'. A TE of <30 ms is short and >80 ms is long. Table 20.5 lists some T1 and T2 times for various tissue types using field strengths of 0.5, 1.0, and 1.5 T.

Table 20.5 *T1, in milliseconds, for three magnet sizes: 0.5, 1.0, and 1.5 T. T2 time does not change.*

Tissue	T1 (0.5)	T1 (1.0)	T1 (1.5)	T2
Body				
Fat	210	240	260	80
Liver	350	420	500	40
Muscle	550	730	870	45
Kidney	440	590	700	58
Heart	560	750	890	57
Brain				
White matter	500	680	780	90
Gray matter	650	810	900	100
CSF	1800	2160	2400	160

After the protons have been rephased by a 180° inversion pulse an x-gradient G_x is superimposed on the main field and the signal echo is collected. The complete 2-D.FT sequence from Fig. 20.19b is:

- A 90° RF pulse at a predetermined frequency is transmitted while G_z is switched on.
- The center frequency of this pulse selects the position on the z-axis. Its band width determines slice thickness for a given gradient strength.
- G_y is now switched on, changing the proton Larmor frequency. When the y-gradient is switched off the protons revert to their original Larmor frequency but they are dephased so giving a phase difference. A single phase gradient is not sufficient to encode the entire y-axis so it is applied in carefully scaled steps.
- A rephasing 180° signal after time TE/2 reestablishes phase relationships and the photons again have phase coherence.
- Just before TE time the G_x is switched on which distributes the Larmor frequencies depending on proton position along the x-gradient.
- Echo signals are received and digitized (fast ADC) and stored in a voxel matrix according to their position determined by their phase and frequency in a k-space (frequency and phase matrix).

This total process is repeated a number of times with further 90° to 180° pulse sequences. The following points should be noted about the data stored as phase/frequency information:

- The central voxel represents zero frequency and zero phase shift differences.
- The k-space matrix is converted to the conventional display matrix 256^2 or 512^2 which carries gray-scale information depending on signal strength.
- A Fourier transform converts the k-space into an x and y pixel matrix, each pixel carrying a gray-scale value (8 bits: 256 gray scales).

IMAGING TIME

The time taken to acquire images using the spin echo sequence depends on the number of phase encoding steps, signal averaging and 'time-to-repeat'. Acquisition time is therefore:

$$M \times N \times \text{TR} \quad (20.3)$$

where M the number of phase encode steps which matches the matrix size. N is the number of averaging (excitation) times; usually 2 but can be greater. TR is the time to repeat. For a 256^2 matrix M equals 256 so for a signal averaging of 2 and a TR time of 500 ms acquisition time is: $256 \times 2 \times 0.5 = 4.2$ min. For longer TR values this can increase to over 12 min.

INVERSION RECOVERY

This has been described in Chapter 19. The spin echo 90–180° pulse sequence is preceded by a 180° pulse. The proportion of M_z can only be measured by using the conventional spin echo sequence. The timing of the 180° pulse and tissue type influences the magnitude of M_z recovery. The negative value of M_z must pass through zero, continuing until equilibrium M_0 is reached. Owing to this increase in recovery time a longer TR period is necessary so the inversion recovery spin echo sequence (IRSE) is a slow imaging process. A modified version is described later called STIR; 'short T1 inversion recovery'.

20.4.2 Multi-image techniques

MULTISLICE IMAGING

During a simple spin echo sequence there is a delay between successive 90° pulses (TR time) which can be as long as 1.5 s. This represents an inefficient duty cycle which can be improved if data from other slices are collected by using different transmission frequencies; more than one slice can then be decoded from the Z, X, and Y image data. Multiple slices can be obtained in a single pulse sequence. Figure 20.20a shows a spin echo multislice signal train which allows multiple slices to be collected and the duty cycle efficiency improves considerably. During each

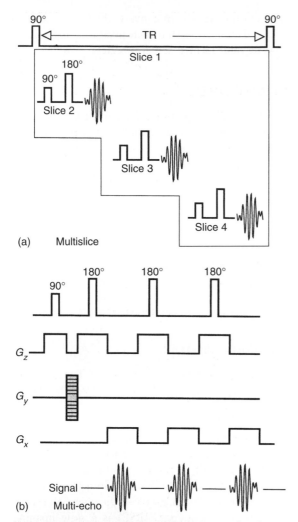

Figure 20.20 *(a) Spin echo multislice sequence showing five separate slices collected during a single TR time. (b) Multi-echo sequence giving different T2 weighted images.*

TR period other 90–180° pulse sequences can be interspersed depending on the relationship:

$$\frac{TR}{TE \times m} \qquad (20.4)$$

where m is a constant depending on machine type. For $m = 2$; TR = 1500 ms and TE = 30 ms. A theoretical 25 slices can be obtained using a multislice sequence.

CROSS-TALK

It was seen in Chapter 14 that it was not possible to obtain ideal rectangular slice profiles since the RF sinc-pulse is fore-shortened and not perfect. In MRI

the overlap of the slice profiles influences the signals in the adjacent slices. This is slice cross-talk and modifies T1 contrast. The cross-talk can be minimized by increasing the slice gap.

MULTI-ECHO SEQUENCE

A single slice will contain fixed T1 and T2 contributions. Differentiating the T1 and T2 contribution can be achieved by using a 180° pulse train (Fig. 20.20b). The successive 180° echoes have approximately the same T1 content but will reflect different T2 weighting in the image. Multi-echo techniques can be run with multislice routines and will only marginally decrease multiple-slice number.

SUMMARY

The slice can be selected with a G_z field superimposed on the main field. The slice thickness can be altered by either:

- Changing the frequency of excitation
- Altering the gradient field slope

The selected slice image matrix uses two other gradient fields:

- x-gradient frequency encoding G_x
- y-gradient phase encoding G_y.

The frequency encoding gradients give different Larmor frequencies. The phase encoding gradient is applied for a specific time by G_y. The gradient is switched off and the protons resume at the original frequency but now have different phase relationships. The fast Fourier transform gives the signal intensities for frequency and phase.

20.4.3 Image contrast

Magnetic resonance signals are influenced by three major parameters:

- The nuclear density (number of protons per unit volume)
- The vertical relaxation time T1
- The transverse relaxation time T2

These three qualities are dependent on the tissue type and with a spin echo sequence the NMR signal S is proportional to

$$S \propto \rho \times \left[1 - \exp\left(-\frac{TR}{T1}\right)\right] \times \exp\left(-\frac{TE}{T2}\right) \quad (20.5)$$

Table 20.6 *Different combinations of time-to-repeat (TR) and time-to-echo (TE).*

	Short TR	Long TR
Short TE	T1 weighted	Proton density
	TR 500 ms	TR 2000 ms
	TE 20 ms	TE 20 ms
Long TE	Not valid	T2 weighted
		TR 2000 ms
		TE 80 ms

where TR and TE are the repetition and echo time respectively and ρ is the spin density. The formula indicates that TR and TE settings significantly influence image contrast, controlling the part played by T1 and T2 times and producing T1 or T2 weighted images. Optimum image contrast depends on TR and TE timing in order to match the tissue of interest and/or pathology. Image contrast is determined by the variation of these parameters to yield **T1 or T2 weighted images** or a simple proton density image; the relevant time durations are summarized in Table 20.6. A long TR would be >1500 ms whilst a long TE would be >40 ms.

REPETITION TIME TR

This is the time interval between consecutive pulse sequences. In the case of the spin echo sequence it is the time between the 90° pulses as shown in Fig. 20.19a. T1 contrast is largely influenced by TR. Two T1 curves (A and B) are shown in Fig. 20.21a. A **short TR** time will yield a larger difference between these curves and an image will be T1 weighted for a short TR time although signal intensity will be smaller due to saturation. The minimal TR time depends on the chosen pulse sequence.

ECHO TIME

This is the time between the center of the excitation pulse and the center of the spin echo or gradient echo. This has also been identified in the spin echo sequence of Fig. 20.19a. The T2 contrast is influenced by the length of TE. Two tissue types (soft tissue and liquid) are shown in Fig. 20.21b. They have different decay times. Differences will be maximum at longer TE times. The TE times can be chosen by the operator but there is a trade-off since T2 signals rapidly decay, so losing signal strength; there is a practical limit for optimum SNR; a long T2 of 80 ms will increase T2

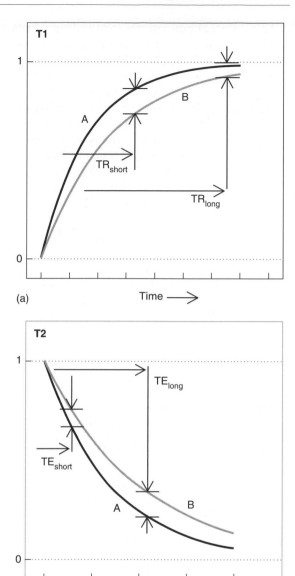

(a)

(b)

Figure 20.21 *(a) Two curves describing longitudinal relaxation with different time constants T1. Tissue A has a shorter T1 than tissue B. Their differences are greatest for short TR; the image will be T1 weighted. (b) Two curves describing transverse relaxation with different T2 times; a longer TE differentiates between tissue A and tissue B; the image will be T2 weighted.*

weighting and it will also increase image noise. T2 signals are always shorter than the corresponding T1 signals for any given substance. T2 is a measure of how long the substance holds the transverse magnetization and is influenced by the interaction of molecular fields reflecting changes in tissue chemistry. In a liquid the local magnetic fields respond rapidly, their spin–spin interferences are less and dephasing is relatively slow. Consequently, their T2 times are longer.

Solids have a fixed molecular structure and neighboring protons strongly influence FID phase relationships. After RF excitation protons in solids show spin–spin interference, their FIDs rapidly lose phase and produce a shorter T2. Since solids and tissues with low water content have protons that are influenced by their neighbor's small magnetic fields they

induce small inhomogeneities in the overall magnetic field so the individual FIDs vary slightly, behaving similarly to out-of-phase signals and giving the same result: shorter T2 times.

T1 AND T2 WEIGHTED IMAGES

An idea of signal intensity by altering TR and TE values can be obtained by superimposing the T1 and T2 curves shown in Fig. 20.22a. The TR value determines T1 signal strength as previously seen in Fig. 20.21 and the superimposed T2 curve seen in Fig. 20.22b

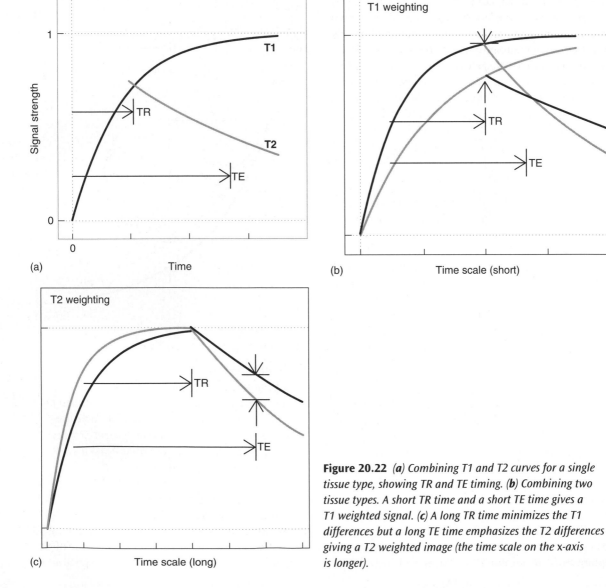

Figure 20.22 (*a*) Combining T1 and T2 curves for a single tissue type, showing TR and TE timing. (*b*) Combining two tissue types. A short TR time and a short TE time gives a T1 weighted signal. (*c*) A long TR time minimizes the T1 differences but a long TE time emphasizes the T2 differences giving a T2 weighted image (the time scale on the x-axis is longer).

gives the magnitude of the FID signal at this TR time. The TR timing determines the end point of the T1 curve which consequently fixes the start of the T2 signal. The TE period governs the magnitude of the T2 signal (Fig. 20.22c). Tissue difference (contrast) can therefore be emphasized by using different TR and TE timing.

The simulated MR brain images in Fig. 20.23a and b (exaggerated anatomy) show varying TR and TE times altering signal strengths for either T1 or T2 characteristics. Figure 20.23 illustrates proton density.

T1 and T2 weighted MR images are shown in Fig. 20.24a and b. The T1 weighted image shows dark CSF and the gray matter darker than the white matter. A proton density image would be very similar except contrast between gray and white matter would be reversed since there are more protons (water) in the gray matter, the CSF becomes lighter. Proton density images are not very sensitive to tissue pathology. Figure 20.24b is a T2 weighted image where the CSF has a higher signal than the gray or white matter as is ideal for visualizing CSF or edema.

CONTRAST AGENTS

T1 time can be deliberately altered by using specific paramagnetic contrast agents (gadolinium or manganese compounds). Paramagnetic substances have unpaired electrons causing their magnetic moments to increase by about ×1000, T1 and T2 relaxation times will shorten. Figure 20.21a, curve A, would represent the effect of a contrast agent on T1 timing and T2 timing respectively (Fig. 20.21).

The decrease in T1 and T2 is directly proportional to the concentration of the contrast agent. The effect of contrast agent on T1 times is small for short T1 tissues; their effect on T2 is smaller than T1. At small

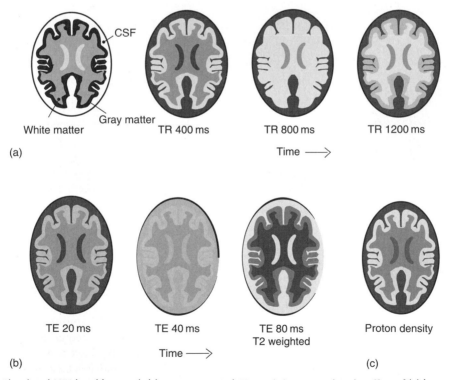

Figure 20.23 *Simulated MRI head images (with an exaggerated CSF gap) demonstrating the effect of (**a**) increasing the TR period which increases T1 information in the image. The gray/white matter contrast alters but CSF remains dark (small signal intensity). (**b**) Short TE where the CSF has a small signal (dark image), for intermediate TE periods overall contrast is poor but at longer TE there is a large signal for the CSF which is now seen as a bright area on the image. (**c**) Precise TR/TE timing to give proton density.*

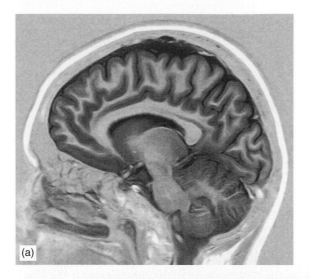

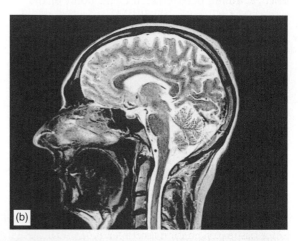

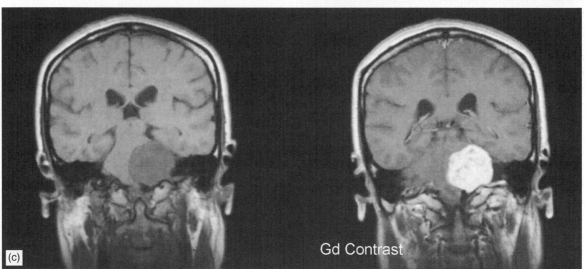

Gd Contrast

Figure 20.24 *(a) T1 weighted head image. (b) T2 weighted head image . (c) A positive contrast agent (Gd-DTPA) emphasizes this cerebral neoplasm by increasing the T1 effect.*

or intermediate concentrations T1 predominates and faster recovery gives an increased signal strength in T1 weighted images (Fig. 20.24c). At high concentrations of contrast agent T2 shortening predominates.

FUNCTIONAL MAGNETIC RESONANCE IMAGING (fMRI)

This was first attempted by using bolus contrast agents (Gd-DTPA) to study transit through the brain in real time using echo planar imaging (EPI) and mapping blood volume during brain activity (visual cortex) at rest and activity (visual stimulus). This technique bears similarities to PET studies requiring elimination of the agent between acquisitions. PET, however, operates using agent concentrations many orders of magnitude less than that achievable with fMRI.

Current interest concerns blood oxygen levels. Oxygen is a diamagnetic element (negative suscepti-bility) so fully oxygenated blood (oxyhemoglobin) is diamagnetic. Deoxyhemoglobin (reduced hemoglo-bin), however, is paramagnetic due to its unpaired electrons and can be used as an *in vivo* positive contrast agent:

$$\left\{\begin{matrix} \text{Hb}^- \\ \text{deoxyhemoglobin} \\ \text{PARAMAGNETIC} \end{matrix}\right\} \rightarrow \text{O}_2 \left\{\begin{matrix} \text{HbO}_2 \\ \text{oxyhemoglobin} \\ \text{DIAMAGNETIC} \end{matrix}\right\}$$

Its concentration is influenced by variations in oxygenation and tissue metabolism so the acronym BOLD has been given to this technique (blood oxygen level dependent). As with other paramagnetic substances deoxyhemoglobin causes a local increase in magnetic susceptibility and consequent T1, T2 shortening. Blood oxygenation reverses this action. Since tissue oxygenation levels depend on changes in perfusion fMRI can only show relatively slow events which is an unfortunate limitation.

fMRI is restricted to high field strengths. The changes being measured are tiny so it is important to maximize the signal at low noise levels; magnetic susceptibility effects increase with field strength. Most artifacts are due to patient motion since very precise image subtraction is required to reveal the small differences. Shifting the head by a fraction will give false signals.

Both spatial and temporal resolutions are critical. Using conventional gradient recalled echo (GRE) sequences about 1 mm spatial resolution can be obtained but temporal resolution is poor so the study is limited to only a few slices. Faster pulse sequences such as EPI achieve poorer spatial resolution but many more slices can be obtained.

20.4.4 Diffusion weighted imaging

In standard MR imaging, most of the signal arises from water in normal and diseased tissue. Diffusion effects contribute relatively little to overall signal intensity, causing only slight signal attenuation. However, it is possible to design MRI pulse sequences that are highly sensitive to diffusion effects. Diffusion-sensitized images generally appear 'T2 weighted' but with lower signal intensity from regions where diffusion is greatest. Including changes in the diffusion properties of tissue-water into the image has enabled the characterization of tissue structure and so the ability to identify and differentiate disease processes.

BROWNIAN MOTION

In pure liquids such as water and other small molecular compounds, the individual molecules are in constant motion in every possible direction, due to random motion initiated by thermal energy. This phenomenon is referred to as 'Brownian motion'. In tissues, however, the presence of various tissue components (larger molecules, intracellular organs, membranes, cell walls) has the effect of damping this motion.

THE DIFFUSION IMAGE

In many tissues, when averaged over the macroscopic scale of image voxels, the restriction of molecular movement is identical in every direction – the diffusion is **isotropic**. However, in some structured tissues, such as muscle or cerebral white/gray matter, the cellular arrangement creates a preferred direction of water diffusion causing **anisotropic** diffusion. This estimated diffusion coefficient gives a measure of molecular (water) motion, and it can be determined with MR imaging techniques. The motion of water molecules by diffusion through a non-uniform magnetic gradient (G) results in an irreversible signal loss through intra-voxel dephasing. This increased signal attenuation resulting from diffusion can be represented as a functional image but its quality depends heavily on the pulse sequence details.

DIFFUSION WEIGHTED PULSE SEQUENCING

The development of diffusion-sensitive pulse sequences follows two directions:

- Echo planar imaging which acquires a complete image within a single shot
- Navigator methods, which acquire images in multiple shots by employing so called navigator MR signals for each shot to detect and correct the bulk motion

Single-shot methods are simply applied but they are sensitive to magnetic field inhomogeneities leading to image distortion artifacts in areas where large variations in magnetic susceptibility exist, particularly interfaces between air, bone, and soft tissue. Single-shot methods are noisy and spatial resolution is limited so signal averaging is necessary in order to improve image quality.

Navigator pulse sequences permit much improved spatial resolution with minimal image distortion artifacts and high SNR, but they are not as straightforward and require acquisition times of 10 min or more. For cardiac studies ECG gating must be used. These pulse sequences are less prone to ghosting artifacts due to patient motion.

The use of specific pulse sequences yields diffusion-weighted images distinguishing areas of rapid proton diffusion from areas with slow diffusion. Volumes in which the protons are more mobile (less restriction to diffusion) will show increased signal when the echo is measured, compared to volumes in which diffusion is restricted. Neurology was quick to recognize this as a valuable diagnostic tool in stroke patients.

GRADIENT FIELD STRENGTH

Magnetic resonance diffusion imaging makes use of the strongest possible magnetic field gradients, which are of the order of 20 to 40 mT m^{-1} (Table 20.7). Current MRI systems can now exceed these values. The magnetic field gradient is applied to identify spins according to their location in space. A second gradient applied later then serves to probe how far, on average, the individual spins have moved between the time of the first and second gradient application. The strength of these two balanced gradients increases in one direction. Therefore, if a voxel of tissue contains water that has no net movement in this direction, the two balanced gradients cancel and the signal intensity is unchanged. However, if water molecules have undergone diffusion and have a net movement they are subjected to the first gradient pulse at one location and the second pulse at a different voxel location. The two gradients are no longer equal in magnitude and therefore no longer cancel.

The difference signal is proportional to the net displacement of molecules that has occurred between the two gradient pulses; faster-moving water protons undergo a larger net dephasing. As dephasing is proportional to time-period squared during which the gradients are switched on and also the strength of the applied gradient field, the use of high strength gradients is essential.

b-NUMBERS

In addition to the directionality of diffusion, the amount of diffusion weighting generated by the probing gradients (denoted with the *b*-value) is a

Table 20.7 *The change in* b-*value with gradient performance.*

Gradient field (mT m^{-1})	Rise time (μs)	Slew rate (T m^{-1}s^{-1})	*b*-value (s mm^{-2})
23	460	50	2500
33	430	77	4000
40	275	120	7000

potential diagnostic measure. For routine clinical scans, *b*-values between 500 and 1000 s mm^{-2} are commonly used. Increasing the *b*-value increases the contrast between tissues with different diffusion constants. With a *b*-value of 200 s mm^{-2}, for example, a fresh stroke lesion may be barely distinguishable from normal tissue, whereas at a *b*-value of 1000 s mm^{-2}, the contrast between lesion and normal tissue may reach a ratio of 2:1 or higher. Table 20.7 shows how the *b*-value improves significantly with stronger gradient fields. Higher magnet field strengths from 1 T to 3 T and above will give improved diffusion weighted images.

DIFFUSION COEFFICIENT

Each gradient is typically applied for 0.1 to 0.5 ms, during which time the average water molecule in brain tissues may migrate >10 μm in a random direction. The irregularity of the motion entails a signal loss that is used for measuring a diffusion constant.

This diffusion constant is a relative measure since the magnetic resonance measurement fails to differentiate diffusion-related motion from blood flow, perfusion, bulk tissue or tissue pulsation-related motion. Thus, the diffusion value obtained with this technique is not the real diffusion coefficient, only an **apparent diffusion coefficient** (ADC). Because of the long gradient time diffusion-weighted images are contaminated with T2 information.

In acute stroke, the ADC value within the affected area is significantly reduced within minutes of the onset of cerebral ischemia. As a result the diffusion-related signal attenuation is diminished and the lesion appears bright (Fig. 20.25).

According to Fick's law of diffusion, the net movement of molecules depends on the concentration gradient. With magnetic resonance diffusion imaging the molecular motion due to concentration gradients cannot be distinguished from molecular motion due to

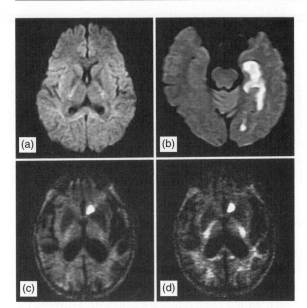

Figure 20.25 *Diffusion weighted images. (a) Image obtained with a high b-value and optimized TE. (b) Image acquired in 36 s with a b-value of 1200 s mm⁻². (c) High resolution diffusion image obtained with a b-value of 2000 s mm⁻² and (d) a b-value of 4000 s mm⁻². (Images courtesy GE Medical Systems.)*

pressure gradients, thermal gradients or ionic attraction. Therefore, when measuring molecular motion with diffusion weighted imaging, only the ADC can be calculated, so

$$SI = SI_0 \times \exp(-b \times ADC)$$

where SI_0 is the signal intensity when $b = 0 \, s \, mm^{-2}$ and ADC is the apparent diffusion coefficient. The signal intensity (SI) is more accentuated with higher b-values.

Diffusion weighted gradient pulses are applied in one direction at a time. The resultant image has information about both the direction and the magnitude of the ADC. To create an image that is related only to the magnitude of the ADC, at least three of these images must be combined. The simplest method is to multiply the three images created with the gradient pulses applied in three orthogonal directions.

DIFFUSION IMAGE ARTIFACTS

Several factors can distort the diffusion image. The most important one is motion sensitivity, which causes significant ghosting artifacts or even complete signal loss. Since molecular displacement involves molecular movement of a few micrometers, then any physical motion (patient movement) or blood flow related pulsations of the brain tissue will interfere with these precise diffusion measurements. The patient should therefore be held firmly by straps during the image acquisition.

20.5 FAST IMAGING TECHNIQUES

Producing a good quality magnetic resonance image with diagnostic quality resolution and contrast, using conventional T2 weighted spin echo sequences with long TR (Table 20.8), takes many minutes; this precludes abdominal imaging which carries respiratory and cardiac movements, particularly those involving 512^2 image matrices. Clinical applications have stimulated the need for fast data acquisition, reducing patient movement in thorax and abdomen images. Time/slice must also be reduced for three-dimensional imaging (3-D.FFT).

These original imaging pulse sequences suffered from one important drawback: imaging time which is typically between 10 and 20 min for a T2 spin echo sequence (SE T2, Table 20.8). Spin echo contrast is the 'benchmark' by which other image sequence techniques are judged, giving reference quality for T1, proton density and T2 weighted images. T2 weighted images use a long TR and long TE (Table 20.8) and to give acceptable contrast TR cannot be

Table 20.8 *Imaging times for some common magnetic resonance imaging procedures.*

Image time	Pulse sequence
1000 s	SE T2
	3-D RAGE
	3-D FLASH
	SE T1
100 s	T2 TURBO SE
	TURBO GSE
	GRASS FISP
10 s	2-D FLASH
	SPOILED GRE
1 s	FAST GRASS
	TURBO FLASH
10 ms to 100 ms	EPI

made much shorter than 300 to 400 ms giving an image time of $0.4 \times 512 \times 4$ or nearly 14 min. Conventional SE sequences cannot be used for fast imaging.

Fast imaging techniques all have a common disadvantage: reduced SNR since in approximate terms:

$$\text{SNR} \propto \sqrt{\text{imaging time}} \qquad (20.6)$$

Contrast to noise ratio (CNR) is reduced; low contrast detail is therefore poor (see Section 20.5.2).

20.5.1 Spin echo sequences

Faster spin echo sequences can be obtained by simply using additional 180° pulses following the 90° to 180° SE sequence previously shown in Fig. 20.9a; each additional 180° provides an image. An alternative more complex procedure phase encodes these echoes individually; this is RARE (rapid acquisition relaxation enhancement) and has been marketed as the so-called 'turbo spin echo'.

Scan data can be shortened by acquiring only part of the data and obtaining the remainder by interpolation since data sets are symmetrical. This is the half-Fourier method. Scan time is reduced by nearly half but there is also a concomitant reduction in SNR by 40%.

20.5.2 Gradient echo sequences

A gradient echo has been described in Chapter 19 where, by applying a pair of balanced gradients of opposite sign, a gradient or field echo can be obtained. It uses a single RF pulse usually with a flip angle of less than 90°. A major advantage of GRE is the good image quality with very short TR.

Shortening TR below about 0.3 s produces problems of rephasing with the 180° pulse and other methods of rephasing must be used. The most common is gradient reversal, echo times are considerably shortened but the disadvantage is that magnetic field inhomogeneities are not compensated. The use of a 180° pulse in the spin echo sequence corrects for inhomogeneities in the magnet field so a true T2 signal

is measured. As the fast pulse sequences do not use a 180° pulse these inhomogeneities are not corrected so the FID loses phase faster; the signal is T2*.

FLIP ANGLES

When applying a 90° pulse a comparatively long time period must elapse before repeating the pulse train. If a reduced flip angle is used with a GRE sequence then saturation effects are less and the TR can be shortened. Since much shorter flip angles are now used a thick volume of tissue can be interrogated to give a 3-D acquisition. The signal strength depends on TR/T1 timing and also the magnitude of the flip angle. Figure 20.26a shows the NMR signal strength for a 90° and a 30° flip angle. At shorter TR times the shorter flip angle produces the highest signal strength. Figure 20.26b indicates the overall loss of signal strength when the flip angle is reduced below 90°; however, the 45° pulse takes half the time of the 90° but returns 70% of the signal strength. There is a practical limit to shortening when the returning signal is too weak, as the graph illustrates.

A FLASH (fast low angle shot) pulse sequence is shown in Fig. 20.27a where gradient reversal in G_x replaces the 180° rephasing RF pulse, yielding the signal. G_y behaves the same and spoiler pulses in G_z remove residual transverse magnetization. The faster image acquisition sequences use gradient switching and flip angles less than 90°, these are indicated as 'a' in the diagram. This fast pulse sequence allows breath holding and so makes abdominal studies practical.

Echo planar imaging (EPI in Fig. 20.27b) and turbo-FLASH increase speed still further to fractions of a second per image but require very fast gradient switching. Image gating (respiration, ECG) improves image quality further at the expense of increased acquisition time.

SPOILED GRADIENT PULSES

There is also residual transverse magnetization with short TR intervals so a **spoiler pulse** is introduced into the gradient switching in order to disperse this (Fig. 20.27a). The standard 90° flip angle saturation RF pulse power is reduced to give smaller flip angles ($\alpha = 30°$) and the rephasing 180° is replaced with gradient switching since they would

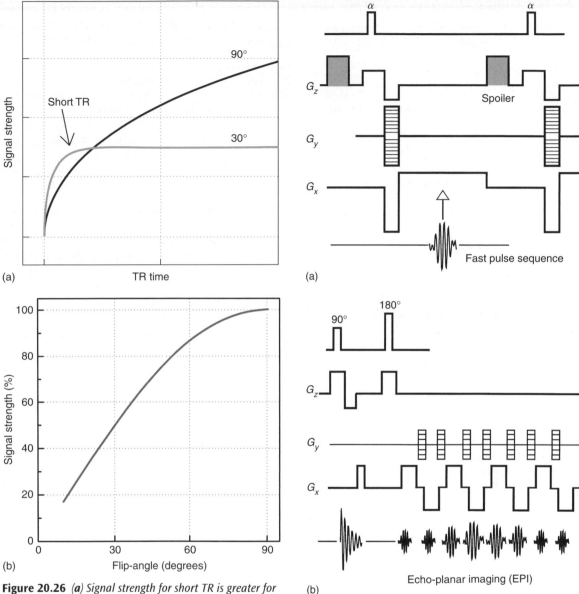

(a)

(b)

Figure 20.26 (a) Signal strength for short TR is greater for a 30° flip angle than for the conventional 90° saturation pulse. (b) Flip angle and signal strength.

Figure 20.27 (a) Fast pulse sequence (FLASH) showing the spoiler pulse which reduces residual transverse magnetization. The flip angle between 15° and 70°. (b) An echo planar (EPI) pulse sequence using 90° to 180° flip angles but collecting multiple signal echoes.

not have the previous rephasing effect. This technique removes residual signals which may persist from cycle to cycle in that before each RF pulse the transverse components of tissue signals have been neutralized ensuring maximum z component before excitation.

Spoiling is achieved by randomly changing the phase of the RF pulse which has advantages since

it does not produce eddy currents. Reversing the polarity of the phase encoding steps uses **rewinding gradients** and is applied at the end of each pulse cycle shown in Fig. 20.27a. They ensure the phase stability

Table 20.9 *A selection of commonly used fast pulse sequences.*

Generic	Commercial acronym	Acquisition (s)	Flip angle (degrees)	Use
T1 spin echo		200	90 to 180°	T1, proton density
T2 spin echo		1000	90 to 180°	T2 weighted imaging
Fast spin echo	Turbo-SE RARE	100 to 300	90 to 180°	
Gradient echo	PSIF True-FISP T2-FFE	50 to 60	15 to 70°	Enhanced intensity where T1 ≈ T2 (e.g. CSF)
Spoiled-GRE	FLASH SPGR Spoiled-FAST T1-FFE	10 to 50	15 to 70°	T1 weighted contrast, CSF imaging, myolograms, angiography
Fast-GRE	turbo-FLASH fast-GRASS (FSP-GR)	0.6	6 to 15°	Dynamic perfusion studies of various organs. T1 weighted abdominal images without breath holding
EPI	Single shot Multi-shot	0.068	90 to 180°	Ultra-fast imaging, dynamic motion studies
FAT saturation	FATSAT STIR		90 to 180°	Fat suppression
MRS	STEAM ISIS CSI DRESS			Spectroscopy

of the magnetic resonance signal. Some commonly available pulse sequences and their uses are listed in Table 20.9.

20.5.3 Fat suppression

The mixed water/lipid spectrum has already been shown in Fig. 19.7b demonstrating that separation is only 3 to 4 ppm. The chemical shift artifact occurs due to the differing resonance of protons depending on their chemical environment. Using the spin echo pulse sequence the 180° pulse causes fat and water to be in phase during each echo signal. Gradient echo pulse sequences which lack this 180° pulse cause fat and water to resonate in and out of phase. This oscillation occurs approximately every 6.6 ms for a 1 T magnet so this signal cancellation in pixels containing both water and fat is seen as a black border; an example would be the muscle sheath.

Since fat and water spectral peaks can be identified a very narrow bandwidth RF pulse can selectively saturate the fat peak so removing its influence from the image. Careful calibration is necessary in order to select the center frequency of the fat signal. Magnet field homogeneity must be high in order to ensure uniformity of the fat signal and its saturation. For less uniform homogeneity values an inversion recovery procedure is used for nulling the fat signal. Special pre-saturation pulse sequences are used to reduce the magnetic resonance signal from fat. The pulse sequence STIR is a short TI inversion recovery and is

a method for fat suppression using the inversion recovery time previously shown in Fig. 19.22b. Fat has a short TI value of about 250 ms and its null point will occur when $t = $ TI or approximately 175 ms. An inversion recovery sequence with a TI of this value is the STIR sequence. It has an added property of emphasizing tissues with long TI times so liquids (blood, CSF) appear as bright areas.

20.5.4 Multi-planar imaging (3-D.FFT)

The 3-D data set uses a very broad Z gradient representing the tissue volume to be covered but it differs from the 2-D.FFT because both G_y and G_z are now phase encoded. Image data is obtained using gradient echo techniques with TR values of about 50 ms. The 3-D volume can be acquired in isotropic or anisotropic mode (shown in Fig. 20.28a). Isotropic volumes have all dimensions identical which gives optimum resolution in all axes and 2-D slices can be extracted without distortion. Anisotropic volumes have one dimension larger than the other. This reduces the number of phase encode steps which reduces acquisition time significantly but resolution is degraded in this dimension.

It is possible to generate high-resolution 3-D data sets with a voxel size of about 1 mm (Fig. 20.28b). From a volume data set any slice orientation can be reconstructed: axial, coronal, saggital or oblique slices. The complete 3-D volume can also be displayed and rotated. Three-dimensional data sets require

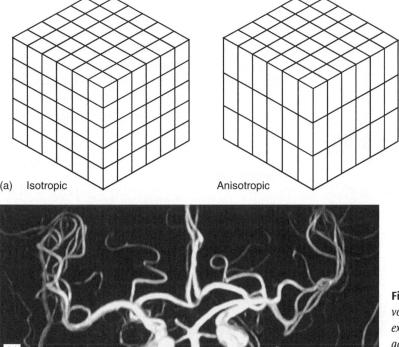

(a) Isotropic   Anisotropic

(b)

Figure 20.28 *(a) Isotropic/anisotropic volume data sets. (b) 3-D image example produced from a 1024² acquisition matrix using a 3 T machine (courtesy of Philips Medical).*

a 3-D.FFT for their reconstruction. Image acquisition is calculated as:

$$TR \times G_z \text{ phase encode steps} \\ \times G_y \text{ phase encode steps} \\ \times \text{ signal averaging} \qquad (20.7)$$

For a 256 volume and a 20 ms TR this would require $256 \times 256 \times 0.02 \times 2 = 43$ min. Smaller volumes (128) reduce this time to 27 min using a TR of 50 ms.

20.5.5 Blood flow measurement

The effect of blood moving in and out of slices that are being imaged influences the image in two ways:

- Blood entering the slice brings unsaturated protons.
- Blood leaving the slice removes spins in different saturation conditions.

Flow influences the NMR signal so that blood movement in vessels can be identified. After a 90° pulse in the spin echo sequence all the protons within the field are influenced but the original blood has left the region before the following 180° pulse or gradient reversal. The blood receiving the 180° will not yield a signal so the image will be black in the vessel region; this is the **flow-void** phenomenon. Figure 20.29a shows blood flowing into a series of slices, both ends having high signal intensity since spins are fully unsaturated and give the highest signal. Spins within the slice are saturated to various levels and give a lower intensity. The cross-sectional diagram illustrates the entrance enhancement along with a ghosting artifact. Because slice selection and frequency encoding gradients are applied for relatively long time periods any motion (blood flow) during G_z and G_x will produce these phase artifacts (in the direction of G_y phase gradient).

If blood enters the excited slice under examination the magnetic resonance signal is seen to increase at low velocities then decrease rapidly at higher velocities (Fig. 20.29c). The initial signal increase is called **paradoxical enhancement** and is due to unsaturated nuclear spins flowing into an already excited slice region. At higher velocities excited nuclear spins flow out of the slice region so depleting the overall signal strength.

Pre-saturation (shown in Fig. 20.29b) suppresses the ghost artifacts by exciting thick slice areas either side of the area of interest. Blood within these regions will be 'pre-saturated' and will give a low signal in the

imaged section. The cross section diagrams show this as a void (low signal). Two techniques are used for vessel imaging: blood flow direction can be differentiated by pre-saturating either one side or the other of the imaged slice (superior or inferior aspect); pre-saturation differentiates the blood prior to it entering the imaged slice giving information on flow direction (venous or arterial). Pre-saturation pulses can be applied outside the imaging volume in which case the in-flowing blood will show a signal loss.

PHASE SHIFT

Where gradient changes are applied moving spins will show a phase shift while static spins will not. This allows separation of vessels from surrounding tissue giving isolated vessel detail in a 3-D image and also supplies quantitative information about blood velocity depending on the degree of proton saturation.

MAGNETIC RESONANCE ANGIOGRAPHY

Phase shift imaging using low flip angles allows thin slices (1 to 2 mm) combined with short echo time imaging. These have been combined to give 3-D angiograms (Fig. 20.30). The signal intensity of the stationary tissue remains unchanged so performing a subtraction of two images leaves an isolated image of

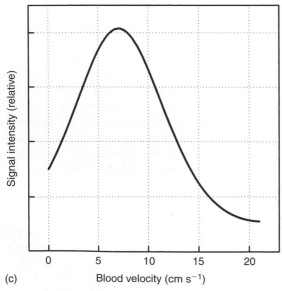

(a)

(b)

(c)

Figure 20.29 (*a*) *A series of slices containing two blood vessels flowing left to right and right to left. Phasing artifacts cause ghosting and vessels are shown as either darker or whiter than the surrounding tissues.* (*b*) *Pre-saturation (shaded slice areas) removes ghosting and gives darker vessels.* (*c*) *Flow signal strength varying with blood velocity.*

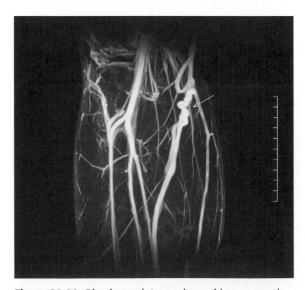

Figure 20.30 *Blood vasculature enhanced in a magnetic resonance angiography image.*

the blood vessels. Magnetic resonance angiography (MRA) is non-invasive and images can be obtained in 6 to 7 min.

SUMMARY

For fast imaging pulse sequences reducing the TR time has drawbacks. A spin echo sequence requires a 180° pulse for re-phasing the spins and with very short TR times the time taken to deliver this pulse is a limiting factor (Fig. 20.19 revises the spin echo sequence). With decreasing TR longitudinal magnetization (T1) will have very little recovery so the next pulse will influence it marginally so yielding a poor signal.

These limitations can be overcome by instead of using a 180° pulse a field gradient is superimposed as a pulse giving increased field inhomogeneities in the slice. This causes the transverse magnetization (T2) to decay faster. The gradient is switched off and then switched on again with opposite polarity and the protons rephase in a similar way to a 180° pulse: this gives the gradient echo. The poor signal strength can be improved by using flip angles of less than 90° in the range 10 to 35°. There is then sufficient remaining T1 signal which can be altered by the next pulse, even after very short TR. These are gradient echo sequences. Also:

- Missing 180° pulse allows much shorter TE but signal depends on T2*.
- Shorter flip angles give less T1 weighting.
- RF pulse bandwidth/pixel bandwidth.
- T2 weighting is not possible; this is replaced by T2* weighting.
- Fast pulse techniques enhance blood flow signals (to be described later).
- Fast pulse techniques allow <1 s per image.
- Freezes patient movement allowing abdominal and cardiac images.
- Multi-slice techniques are not available.

Blood flow imaging can be summarized as:

- Blood brings in unsaturated protons or removes saturated protons from the slice of interest depending on velocity.
- Time of flight uses pre-saturation of blood spins giving it a signal loss. Blood direction can be displayed.
- Phase shift differentiates moving and static spins allowing vessel isolation in 3-D images.

20.6 IMAGE QUALITY

The x, y, and z information during image acquisition must be obtained at the highest signal strength to ensure a good SNR, resolution, and low contrast differences. In some instances some contrast is sacrificed for fast data acquisition. Signal to noise is a very complex problem since so many factors play a part so the following assessments and summary are necessarily simplified.

20.6.1 Signal-to-noise ratio

Signal data is always accompanied by noise. The signal-to-noise ratio (SNR), which should have a high value, influences both resolution and contrast since any RF noise prevents accurate measurement of small frequency/phase differences. The fundamental limit of SNR is influenced by thermal motion of electrons in the detection coil and Brownian molecular motion of the tissue producing a noise voltage superimposed on the NMR signal. Basic small sample analytical NMR which does not have the added complexity of gradient fields shows an improvement (increase) in SNR with magnet field strength. Many extra factors, however, are associated with image signal to noise; amongst the most important are: signal frequency (and therefore field strength B_0 and bandwidth), signal coil efficiency, the pulse sequence, tissue characteristics (T1, T2, spin density) and gradient field strength.

GRADIENT FIELD STRENGTH

As we have seen, by applying a linear gradient each voxel in a slice will have a frequency distribution that depends on the magnitude and steepness of the gradient. When the spin echo is frequency decoded signals from a certain bandwidth can be assigned to each specific voxel. The gradients employed must be large enough to compensate for the main field inhomogeneity and chemical shift artifacts (3.5 ppm between fat and water). The inhomogeneity and chemical shift increase with field strength, therefore increased gradient strength (slopes) are necessary to overcome these disadvantages.

RF PULSE BANDWIDTH

Pulse bandwidth describes the range of frequencies in the RF pulse. The center frequency selects slice position and the bandwidth determines slice thickness as shown in Fig. 20.9. RF pulse bandwidth is dependent on:

$$\text{bandwidth} = \gamma \times G_z \times \text{slice thickness.} \quad (20.8)$$

Increasing gradient strength G_z will therefore increase bandwidth and so decrease the SNR.

FIELD STRENGTHS

Figure 20.31 shows the improvement in SNR, for a selection of tissue types, with increasing main magnet field strength. Larmor frequency (and hence main magnet strength) influences signal to noise as:

$$\text{SNR} \propto \sqrt{\text{frequency}} \quad (20.9)$$

The square root function causes the curves to flatten with increasing field strength. From Fig. 20.31 SNR gains above 1.0 T are slight.

Increasing the magnet field strength increases T1 time and as tissue T1 increases the full SNR cannot be attained without TR increase so patient throughput goes down, although for the same SNR value high field magnets offer a faster patient throughput since signal averaging can be kept to a minimum. Combining the advantage of detection coil efficiency with the disadvantages of signal losses due to the greater absorption of higher frequency signals, the overall improvement in image quality is minimal above 1 T.

RECEIVER BANDWIDTH

The display bandwidth describes the frequency content of the pixel and the pixel bandwidth depends on the number of phase/frequency encoding steps N_{ex} which decides the matrix dimensions and the signal sampling time T_s:

$$\text{bandwidth} = \frac{N_{ex}}{T_S} \quad (20.10)$$

Image noise approximates to $1/\sqrt{T_s}$ so shorter sampling times increase noise. Signal-to-noise ratio is dependent on:

$$\text{SNR} \propto \frac{1}{\sqrt{\text{bandwidth}}} \quad (20.11)$$

If the receiver circuits are tuned to receive signals having a narrow frequency range (bandwidth) then noise frequencies can be rejected. SNR degrades with increasing pixel bandwidth. Halving the bandwidth (for example from 4 to 2 in eqn 20.11) improves SNR by 1.4 or 40%.

RECEIVER COIL QUALITY

For small samples and low Q (efficiency) detector coils the SNR is proportional to (frequency)[1.5]; for high Q coils the SNR figure improves and becomes proportional to frequency. The fixed sample volume seen by the coil influences noise but since this volume is usually large any noise given by the RF coil is dominated by noise from the patient. The receiver Q is improved by choosing a coil to match the anatomy being imaged (matched surface coil).

SIGNAL AVERAGING (N)

The SNR can be improved by multiple measurements at the expense of examination time. Signal strength increases with n but the noise increases by EQ so SNR improves. Gradient signals are repeated a great number of times and the image signals are collected and the average signal strength used for image formation. The signal noise is decreased but imaging time is increased.

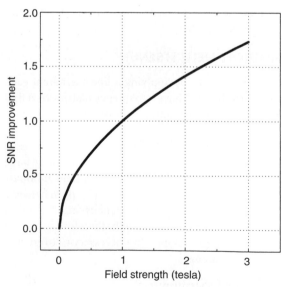

Figure 20.31 *The square root function of field strength versus image signal to noise ratio. Above 1 T only a small improvement is seen.*

VOXEL SIZE

The SNR is proportional to voxel size; determined by field of view FOV, matrix size m, and slice thickness seen in Section 20.2.5. The number of measurements performed to obtain a 2-D.FT slice ($M_{2\text{-D}}$) depends on the number of phase/frequency encoding steps in the $x \times y$ matrix which is $N_x \times N_y$. These measurements (excitations or N_{ex}) are repeated in order to reduce noise. The total number of measurements $M_{2\text{-D}} = N_x \times N_y \times N_{ex}$. The signal strength is proportional to $M_{2\text{-D}}$ and the noise proportional to $\sqrt{M_{2\text{-D}}}$ so

$$\text{SNR}_{2\text{-D}} = \frac{M_{2\text{-D}}}{\sqrt{M_{2\text{-D}}}} = \sqrt{M_{2\text{-D}}} \quad (20.12)$$

Three-dimensional data sets (3-D.FT) use a number of slices (N_z) so voxel size is

$$\frac{\text{FOV}}{m} \times \frac{\text{FOV}}{N_z}$$

3-D.FT imaging is less noisy than 2-D.FT since the number of slices comprising the 3-D volume set N_z decreases the $\text{SNR}_{2\text{-D}}$ in eqn 20.9 so $\text{SNR}_{3\text{-D}}$ is $\sqrt{N_z} \times \text{SNR}$. However, the imaging time is increased by N_z, which is significant.

IMAGING TIME (*T*)

The components of image quality are related to the time taken for accumulating two-dimensional image signals (2-D.FFT) by $t = M \times \text{TR} \times N_{ex}$ where M is the data matrix size (128^2 or 256^2), TR the repetition time between pulse sequences. Images having large TR values have better low contrast definition (more sensitive to pathological changes) where N_{ex} is the number of measurements made per voxel. SNR increases with N_{ex} so less measurements taken with faster imaging sequences give more noise tending to diminish low contrast detail.

SLICE SELECTION

By referring to Fig. 20.9 it can be seen that slice selection can be either narrow bandwidth/low gradient slope or wide bandwidth using a steeper gradient to give the same slice thickness.

Pixel bandwidth influences noise, as shown by eqn 20.8, so choosing a steeper gradient with a narrow bandwidth is preferable. Slice cross-talk has already been mentioned in Section 20.2.5. Signal strength will be influenced by the slice thickness; thicker slices give stronger signals so less noise.

OVERALL SNR

The overall image SNR is influenced by the above factors as:

$$\text{SNR} = \frac{k \times \text{voxel size} \times \sqrt{\text{Fourier terms}} \times \sqrt{N_{ex}}}{\sqrt{\text{bandwidth}}}$$

$$(20.13)$$

The constant k contains numerous terms related to the physical parameters of the MRI system (magnet strength, pulse sequence etc.) but as a rough guide $k \propto$ magnet strength so SNR tends to improve with increasing magnet field strength. Voxel size determines the volume of tissue from which the signal is derived so larger volumes improve SNR. Fourier terms refer to the complexity of the Fourier reconstruction calculation. Partial Fourier imaging where a restricted data set is used will increase noise. Bandwidth influences SNR adversely. A narrow receiver bandwidth will encompass less noise than a broadband receiver characteristic. N_{ex} refers to the number of excitations or number of signals averaged for each phase encoding step.

IMAGE RECONSTRUCTION ALGORITHMS

These have a significant effect on SNR mainly by controlling the eventual voxel size and whether isotropic or anisotropic image matrices are to be used. Reconstruction filters are designed to reduce SNR.

SUMMARY

The SNR is reduced if:

- Magnet field strength increased
- Voxel size increased
- Slice thickness increased
- Smaller matrix size
- Increased signal averaging (increase N_{ex})
- Narrow bandwidth
- Increased inter-slice gap

20.6.2 Resolution and contrast quality

This is determined by field homogeneity and steepness of the gradient fields. High resolution magnetic resonance used for spectroscopy uses steep gradients so the SNR decreases so more averaging is needed. The gradient power supply should have a high current (100 A) and high speed (sub-millisecond) for 1 mm resolution.

The high frequency signals are converted by **quadrature demodulation** into a low frequency signal before digitization and frequency and phase differences measured prior to image reconstruction. Resolution is dependent on:

- Gradient field strength (slice thickness)
- Receiver coil design
- Signal bandwidth
- Matrix size

The best resolution for general use is 0.5 mm to 1.0 mm but small FOV and high gradient field strengths can reduce this figure.

CONTRAST

This can be selected by TR and TE timing to influence T1 and T2 differences and blood flow. High field magnets increase T1 time (see Fig. 19.19a) which tends to decrease image contrast because of increased saturation of short T1 tissues relative to longer T1 tissues which then reduces the contrast between these tissues. Differences between tissue signals can be treated as a **contrast to noise ratio** (CNR); this improves only slightly beyond 1.0 T. Figure 20.32b shows the contrast for white/gray matter and muscle/ fat versus magnetic strength.

A high SNR on its own does not guarantee good image quality. The differentiation of two tissue types or the contrast between two tissue types depends on the separate SNR shown by the two tissues which gives the CNR. The first tissue may yield a strong signal but the second tissue may give a weaker signal in a poorer noise background. Figure 20.32a shows two lesions with different signal-to-noise values. Their contrasts would be given by $C = (S_1 - S_2)/S_2$. However, their contrast to noise value is given as:

$$CNR = SNR_1 - SNR_2 \qquad (20.14)$$

Worked examples in Box 20.4 show that SNR plays a more important role than measured contrast differences in making a lesion visible.

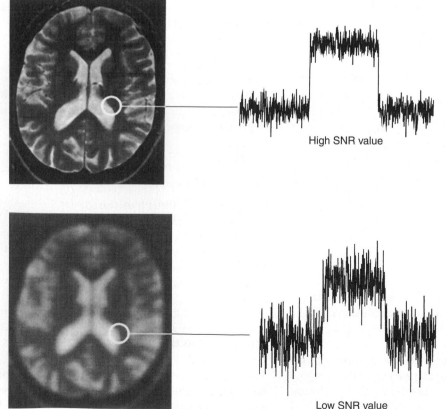

High SNR value

Low SNR value

(a)

Figure 20.32 *(a) Two profiles showing different SNR values referred to in the text.*

TRIGGERING

Data collected from a particular slice at identical points in the lung/heart cycle can be achieved by respiratory and cardiac triggering. Multiple slices combined with triggering causes different slices to hold images of different phases of the cardiac cycle. The R–R interval of the ECG decides the repetition time. Respiratory gating removes organ movement in upper abdomen slices. Fast pulse sequences have reduced the requirement for gating.

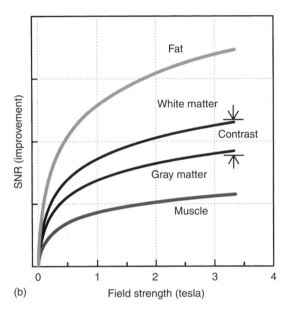

Figure 20.32 (*Contd*) (*b*) *Graph field strength tissue contrast between fat and muscle; white matter and gray matter.*

Box 20.4 Contrast to noise ratio

From the values derived from Fig. 20.32, the contrast in the top section is

$$\frac{120 - 100}{100} = 20\%$$

The contrast in the bottom section is

$$\frac{140 - 100}{100} = 40\%$$

Using eqn 20.14 the first section has a 5% noise figure giving an SNR_2 of 20 and SNR_1 of 16.6, so the CNR = 3.4.

The second section has a 10% noise figure giving an SNR_2 of 10 and SNR_1 of 7.2, so the CNR = 2.8.

SUMMARY

Noise is influenced by:

- Main magnet field strength. SNR versus field strength (Fig. 20.31)
- Gradient field strength
- Signal coil type and antenna size
- Imaging sequence
- Patient size and composition
- Spatial resolution
- Scan time
- Slice thickness

20.7 CHOICE OF MRI SYSTEM

The parameters involved with the performance of superconducting, resistive and permanent-magnet MRI systems are listed in Table 20.10. The choice of MRI system will depend on:

- Clinical application (neurological, vascular, pediatric, spectroscopy etc.)
- Image resolution and contrast required (slice thickness)
- Patient throughput/imaging time
- Costs

Other features that would influence choice would be system cooling (water supply), power consumption, degree of field homogeneity and available room size. Some arguments for and against low/high field systems are summarized in Table 20.11.

Since SNR increases with frequency the gain in SNR is roughly doubled by doubling the field strength (Fig. 20.31); good thin slice acquisition improves with magnet field strength.

To maintain the same contrast behavior at lower field strengths it might be necessary to increase TR at higher field strengths so lengthening examination time but signal averaging is less.

Faster patient throughput and shorter examination times favor higher field strengths. In regions where both water and fat are present the slope of the gradient

Table 20.10 *Choice of magnet.*

Property	Superconducting	Resistive	Permanent
Field strength (T)	0.5 to 4.0 T	0.2 T	<0.1 to 0.2 T
Gradient (mT m^{-1})	10 to 25	10	<10
Fringe field (0.5 mT)	2.5 to 4 m	–	1.5 to 2 m
Power (kW)	28	Up to 60	4
Inhomogeneity	<0.5 ppm	–	7 ppm
Magnet stability	0.1 ppm h^{-1}	–	6 ppm h^{-1}
Gradient cooling	900 m^3 h^{-1}	–	None

Table 20.11 *Comparison of low and high field magnet characteristics.*

Low field	High field
Cheap	Expensive
Short T1	Long T1
Good contrast	Poorer contrast (poor T1 separation)
T2 unchanged	T2 unchanged
No spectroscopy	Spectroscopy
Low SNR	High SNR
Low Larmor frequency	High Larmor frequency
Lower SNR	High SNR (better resolution)

fields used for encoding X, Y, and Z spatial information needs to be doubled to eliminate the chemical shift artifact. Increasing gradient field strength gives:

- Improved SNR
- Shorter TE time
- More slices per TR time
- Smaller FOV with larger matrix sizes
- Faster 3-D FLASH sequences

20.7.1 Low field system

Magnet field strengths from 0.1 to 0.2 T have certain advantages, perhaps the most important one being capital cost; they also require less room so can be installed safely in a small clinic. These magnets can be designed to have an open aspect y-axis orientation as shown in Fig. 20.1 which lends greater accessibility to the patient. The open aspect of this design is popular for interventional work.

Longitudinal relaxation time T1 is proportional to field strength (see Fig. 19.9) so low field systems require shorter TR and potentially a shorter imaging time T as

$$T = M \times TR \times N_{ex} \quad (20.15)$$

where M is the matrix size which determines the phase encoding steps (e.g. 128, 256 or 512), TR the repetition time and N_{ex} the data averaging or number of excitations. Image SNR, however, is proportional to field strength so for the same image quality in low field systems more signal averages are necessary so image time must be increased.

Low field magnets require smaller gradient strengths allowing narrower bandwidths with improvement in SNR (eqn 20.8). The advantages are:

- Cheap to run
- Simplified housing (very small fringe field)
- Short T1 time

The disadvantages are:

- Long patient imaging time (small patient numbers)
- Poor resolution

20.7.2 A medium field system (0.3 to 0.5 T)

Patient throughput is potentially improved by increasing field sizes up to 0.5 T. Permanent magnets are commonly used for some mid-field designs having field strengths of 0.2 to 0.3 T. They offer considerable advantages for mobile MRI systems since their power consumption is minimal (gradient coils). Permanent magnets are very heavy, however.

Open aspect resistive magnets are also used for interventional work; these have field strengths of about 0.3 T. They have high power consumption but resistive magnets have the important ability to be shut down instantly if required. This considerable advantage is not available for permanent or superconducting designs. The gradient field in these systems must be steep enough to compensate for magnet inhomogeneity and chemical shift artifacts, but gradient steepness is proportional to pixel bandwidth so image noise increases as $\sqrt{\text{gradient}}$. With an increase in gradient field fast imaging pulse sequences can be more widely used unlike the small field systems.

20.7.3 High field system (above 1 to 1.5T)

These machines should be considered if spectroscopy is going to be an important application since spectrum resolution improves with increased field strength. Small-bore magnets for limb or pediatric investigations are available with field strengths up to 9 T.

Their advantages can be summarized briefly as:

- Best image quality.
- High gradient field gives thin slices (3-D imaging).
- Good magnet homogeneity for fat/water separation.
- Spectroscopy.
- Fast imaging.
- Fast patient throughput.

However, they do have disadvantages:

- Superconducting magnet cannot be shut down easily.
- Cryogen replacement.
- They require a larger room because of their fringe fields.
- There are magnet hazards.

20.7.4 Harmful effects

The **specific absorption rate** (SAR) is a measure of the energy deposited by a radio-frequency field in a mass of tissue. It is analogous to the radiation absorbed dose, the gray, used for ionizing radiation. The units for the gray are joules per kilogram, the SAR for radio frequency is measured in watts per kilogram.

The energy deposited depends on the tissue radius r and electrical conductivity σ. The field strength of the magnet B_0 and the flip angle α together with the imaging sequence duty cycle d give:

$$\text{SAR} = (r^2\alpha) \times (B_0^2\alpha^2) \times d \quad (20.16)$$

The SAR value is markedly increased by:

- Increasing field strength
- Increasing the flip angle: the maximum energy being deposited by 180° RF pulses
- Increasing the duty cycle

Fast spin echo sequences with multiple 180° pulses are responsible for high SAR values while GRE sequences with low flip angles give small SAR values. Tissues with high water content have highest conductivity (CSF and blood) and the geometry of the tissue volume may increase SAR non-uniformly and double expected values. The US Food and Drug Administration (FDA) guidelines restrict SAR values to $0.4\,\text{W kg}^{-1}$ for whole-body exposure and $3.2\,\text{W kg}^{-1}$ for brain imaging.

RF PULSES

These produce warming of tissues and metallic implants since:

$$\text{heating} \sim \sqrt{\text{field strength}}$$

and

$$\text{absorbed energy} \sim \sqrt{\text{RF frequency}}$$

The acceptable limit for energy absorption was set at $0.4\,\text{W kg}^{-1}$ for whole-body imaging and $2\,\text{W kg}^{-1}$ for smaller organs.

MAGNETIC FIELD STRENGTH

The natural magnetic field of Earth is approximately $50\,\text{mT}$ and magnetic densities of about $20\,\text{mT}$ are experienced under high voltage power lines. The highest exposure experienced by humans is given by MRI where patients are exposed to between 0.15 and 2 T. This magnetic field strength has no reported ill effects on the human body. Small bore field strengths for whole-body imaging (neonates) can reach 6 T.

FAST CHANGES OF GRADIENT FIELDS

These cause Faraday currents in tissues. The most sensitive tissue seems to be the retina which causes flashing sensations. In pacemakers these cause side effects.

Large hip prostheses heat up and other smaller metal artifacts (surgical clips) suffer movement, which pose hazards. The maximum rate of change has been limited to 20 T s^{-1} (Europe); 3 T s^{-1} (USA). Contraindications for MRI examinations are:

- Pacemaker patients
- Magnetic surgical clips
- Some hip/knee metal prostheses
- Heart valve prostheses

Fatalities and injuries have been reported to patients having ferromagnetic implants (aneurysm clips); these have either been displaced *in situ* or heated.

20.8 IMAGE ARTIFACTS

These can derive from malfunction of the machine itself or be caused by the patient.

20.8.1 Machine artifacts

Eddy currents cause temporary magnet inhomogeneities and arise from gradient fields and the walls of the cryostat.

20.8.2 Patient artifacts

MOTION

Fat layers give high intensity signals and move during acquisition which disturbs frequency and phase encoding especially during long TR routines. This causes 'ghosting' on the images which are reflections of the main signal in the direction of the phase encoding gradient; the reflections are not related to the movement direction. Ghosting can be reduced by using faster image acquisition or physiological gating (respiratory or ECG) but these procedures increase acquisition time.

20.8.3 Chemical shift

This is visible as light and dark stripes on the image and is caused by the separation of lipid and water

---

Box 20.5 Chemical shift artifact

The chemical shift between water and lipids is between 3 and 3.5 ppm. In a 1 T field this represents 128 to 150 Hz (3 to 3.5 ppm of 42.576 MHz). For a read-out gradient of 0.15 mT cm^{-1} and a 256^2 matrix (see Box 20.3) the frequency/pixel is approximately 370 Hz so water and fat are displaced by 140/370 Hz or a third of a pixel width.

For lower field and gradient strengths the displacement is greater and becomes visible (see Box 20.2). For 0.5 T a 3 ppm of 21.287 MHz is 63 Hz. The frequency per pixel for this matrix is 62 Hz so there is a 100% displacement artifact.

---

components in the frequency encoded read-out gradient (usually G_x). It can cause positional displacement where fat and water are mislocated (commonly seen in head images). The degree of displacement depends on field strength and gradient strength. Box 20.5 gives an example.

20.8.4 Magnetic materials

The magnetic field is distorted by ferrous objects (iron, cobalt, nickel) which are used in the manufacture of surgical wires and clips as well as hip prostheses and stainless steel needles. Eddy currents are also induced in the implanted metal by gradient switching.

20.9 MAGNETIC RESONANCE SPECTROSCOPY

For magnetic resonance imaging the spin echo rather than the free induction decay (FID) is collected. Spectroscopy concerns itself exclusively with the FID which carries the information about the chemical nature of the material. Any NMR sensitive nucleus (H, P, C, F) will give a signal in a strong magnetic field if an RF pulse is applied at the resonant frequency for that nucleus.

Table 20.12 shows the different Larmor frequencies for each of these elements.

Table 20.12 *Elements important for clinical magnetic resonance spectroscopy.*

Element	MHz T^{-1}
^{1}H	42.58
^{19}F	40.1
^{31}P	17.2
^{23}Na	11.3
^{13}C	10.7

20.9.1 Signal origin

The local magnetic field varies slightly within the compound molecule due to chemical bonds, size of atoms and position of the atom relative to others. The hydrogen atom in a water molecule will experience a different local magnetic field to a hydrogen atom in fat for example. Since these very small differences in the local magnetic field can effect the Larmor frequency there will be frequency shifts of the NMR signal; this is the chemical shift. A plot of signal intensity versus frequency is the NMR spectrum (Fig. 20.33). The area under each peak (integral) is directly proportional to the compound concentration and the position on the frequency axis is its chemical shift measured in ppm.

The degree of shift is characteristic of the chemical bond in which the nucleus is situated. Figure 20.33 represents a mixed signal from fat and water which is resolved into its two frequencies by a fast Fourier transform. A chemical shift of about 3 ppm separates these signals.

If each separate nucleus precesses at one frequency then the Fourier analysis would yield an NMR spectrum consisting of only one line; no distinction would be observed for different compounds. The local magnetic field varies slightly within a molecule due to chemical bonds and size of various atomic groups; a hydrogen atom attached to an oxygen atom (H–O) will experience a different magnetic field to a H–C bonding (e.g. water and fat). These small differences in the local magnetic field will influence the Larmor frequency of an individual proton: this is the chemical shift.

The range of chemical shifts differs for each type of nucleus and is very small compared to the main frequency (expressed in MHz); chemical shift is given in herz and this varies with the main magnet field strength so comparison using frequency alone is difficult between two machines having slightly different magnetic field strengths. The concept of parts per

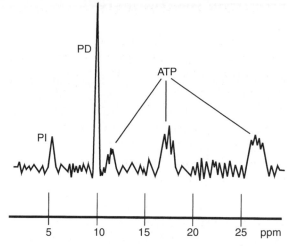

Figure 20.33 *Spectrum examples for ^{31}P compounds associated with muscle metabolism displayed using a high field (1 to 2 T) magnet.*

Box 20.6 Signal reference measurement

The frequency difference Δf between water and tetramethylsilane (a reference compound used as a standard frequency) for field strengths of 1.5 T and 2.0 T is as follows:

- For 1.5 T (where ω_0 is 63 MHz), $\Delta f = 334$ Hz
- For 2.0 T (where ω_0 is 84 MHz), $\Delta f = 445$ Hz

The chemical shift (in ppm) is:

- For 1.5 T, $334/63 \times 10^6 = 5.3 \times 10^{-6}$
  $= 5.3$ ppm
- For 2.0 T, $445/84 \times 10^6 = 5.3$ ppm

---

million or ppm is introduced in Box 20.6. Although the term parts per million is not a measure of chemical concentration, it is related because the chemical shift can be changed by chemical dilution. Chemical shift tables give chemical shift ranges for various compounds. Adjacent proton spins interact with each other as well as with the main magnetic field (T1 and T2 times). The extent of this interaction or coupling depends on the chemical bonding. Coupling causes a single line spectrum to be split, producing multiplets or groups of lines; a three line spectrum is a triplet; four lines a quartet etc.

RESOLUTION AND SENSITIVITY

The resolving power of the spectroscopy system depends on field strength, magnet homogeneity and molecular line width. Large sample volumes decrease resolution since inhomogeneity increases with volume size. Sensitivity (the ability to detect weak signals) depends on SNR which is improved by increasing field strength, concentration of material, volume size and acquisition time. There is therefore a balance between resolution and sensitivity and volume size should be chosen carefully to optimize both resolution and sensitivity.

VOLUME LOCALIZATION

Considerable improvements in acquisition accuracy are required in order to select areas for regional MRS. These include RF coil design, a very homogeneous magnetic field, stability of magnetic field after gradient switching and elimination of eddy current interference.

Special pulse sequences have been developed based on spin echo (SE) or stimulated echo (STEAM). These are able to give 'volume of interest' spectra of brain or muscle which are better resolved by high field magnets.

SUMMARY

For magnetic resonance spectroscopy:

- The FID signal gives a frequency spectrum representing chemistry.
- The frequency spectra exhibit chemical shifts (ppm).
- The degree of shift depends on the chemical bonding.
- Higher field magnets give finer resolution.
- Chemical concentration and pH can be measured.

FURTHER READING

Elster A.D. (1994) *Questions and Answers in Magnetic Resonance Imaging.* New York, Mosby.

KEYWORDS

acquisition matrix: the number of independent data samples in each direction. 2-D.FFT number of samples in-phase and frequency coded directions

aliasing: poor sampling increments. Components of the signal are at higher frequency than the Nyquist sampling frequency. In the Fourier transform this gives wrap-around image artifacts

array processor: dedicated computer for reconstructing the image matrix

Carr–Purcell (CP) sequence: spin echo sequence of 90° followed by a 180° pulse

chemical shift: the change in Larmor frequency of a nucleus due to molecular binding; caused by local alteration in the magnetic field. It is measured in parts per million relative to a reference compound

chemical shift imaging: an image of a restricted range of chemical shifts corresponding to individual line spectra

contrast agent: typically a paramagnetic substance (e.g. gadolinium) administered to a patient which shortens both T1 and T2 times

contrast to noise ratio (CNR): ratio of the difference between to regions measured by their signal-to-noise ratios (SNR)

demodulator: a component of the NMR signal receiver that converts it to a lower frequency for analysis. This is also phase sensitive (now called a quadrature demodulator) and will give phase information (detecting phase encoded RF signals)

echo-planar imaging (EPI): a complete planar image obtained from one excitation pulse. The FID is detected while switching the y-gradient magnet with a constant x-gradient. The Fourier transform of the spin echo sequence then supplies the image of the selected plane

eddy currents: electric currents induced in a conductor by a changing magnetic field (e.g. gradient fields)

Faraday shield: metal mesh between an RF transmitter and receiver to block signals such as interfering RF noise from TV, radio and power appliances

fast Fourier transform (FFT): a modified Fourier transform for computer use

flip angle: amount of magnetization vector rotation produced by RF pulse. Flip angles of 15 to 30° used in fast acquisition sequences

flow: nuclei from liquids moving into an excited slice-region can be distinguished from static tissues

flow enhancement: the increased intensity that may be seen due to flowing blood due to loss of saturated spins from the imaged slice

frequency encoding: applying a magnetic gradient causing a consequent gradient in resonance frequency

gradient coils: coils designed to produce a magnetic field gradient in the Z-axis (slice position) or X- and Y-axis (matrix dimensions) gradient echo (field echo): spin echo produced by reversing the direction of a magnetic field gradient. A substitute for the 180° pulse in the spin echo sequence

G_x G_y G_z: abbreviations used to describe the three magnetic field gradients

homogeneity: uniformity. Homogeneity of the main magnetic field defines the quality of the main magnet over a large field of view

inversion–recovery: NMR pulse sequence where nuclear magnetization is inverted before 90° pulse

multiple slice imaging: sequential plane imaging used with selective excitation techniques that do not affect adjacent slices. Adjacent slices are imaged while waiting for relaxation of the first slice toward equilibrium. Reduces imaging time for a slice set

partial saturation: excitation applying repeated RF pulses shorter than the T1 time. Causes increased contrast between similar tissue types

phase encoding: applying a pulsed magnetic field gradient to change frequency for a short time so that after this pulse the nuclei resume their original frequency but now with phase differences

quadrature detector: a demodulation circuit that detects signal phase by comparing with a reference frequency

quenching: loss of superconductivity due to temperature rise causing cryogen boil off

rephasing gradient: magnetic field gradient applied for a brief period after a selective excitation pulse. The gradient reversal rephases the spins forming a gradient echo

shimming: correction of magnet inhomogeneity; 'active' using shim coils, 'passive' using iron sheets

signal averaging: combining signals from identical acquisition procedures to reduce signal noise

spin density: the density of resonating spins which determines the strength of the NMR signal

spin echo sequence: an RF pulse series having 90° followed by 180° gives the Carr–Purcell sequence; depends strongly on T2

spoiling pulse: use of a reverse magnetic field gradient to eliminate residual magnetization in the nucleus

surface coil: a surface coil placed over a region of interest will have a selectivity for a volume approximately subtended by the coil circumference and one radius deep. Improves signal-to-noise ratio

21

Radiation protection: radiobiology and risk estimation

21.1 INTERACTION OF RADIATION WITH TISSUE

The use of ionizing radiation for diagnostic imaging requires careful thought and handling so that maximum benefit can be obtained for minimum risk. Its use has increased dramatically over the last decade; more and more people are being exposed to medical X- and gamma radiation. Figure 21.1 shows the rapid increase in their use over the past 100 years. Increased machine sensitivity has lowered the dose in diagnostic imaging but exposure even from low levels of radiation is still an unknown risk especially when applied to larger and larger numbers in the population. Although a great deal of knowledge exists about the risks of high radiation levels, extrapolation to low doses is fraught with complications.

21.1.1 Radiation type and interactions

The degree of radiation damage depends on the density of ionizing events along the radiation pathway in tissue. Figure 21.2 represents these ionization events in tissue; the degree of tissue damage depending on radiation type, which is either particulate or electromagnetic. Particulate radiation is rarely a feature in diagnostic radiology (see Chapter 15), alpha radiation is almost never encountered and beta radiation only occasionally, either in the form of therapy (^{32}P) or with a non-ideal imaging nuclide (e.g. ^{133}Xe).

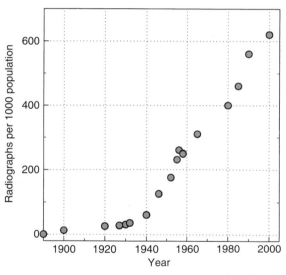

Figure 21.1 *The increasing use of X-rays as an imaging medium since their discovery in 1895 (UK data).*

ALPHA PARTICLES

These are helium nuclei so have a relatively large mass. They are easily stopped by tissue and can scarcely penetrate the dead outer layers of the skin. An alpha radionuclide is not hazardous externally but ingestion is of major concern either by swallowing, inhalation or as a result of wound contamination. Alpha particles with their much higher energy cause major radiation damage in tissue over a small range since all

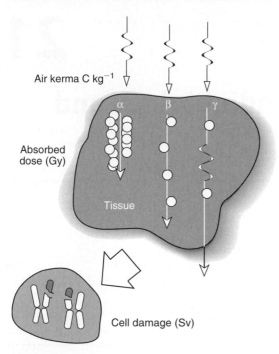

Air kerma C kg^{-1}

Absorbed dose (Gy)

Tissue

Cell damage (Sv)

Figure 21.2 *Ionizing events in tissue from electromagnetic radiation gamma, X-radiation and particulate radiation, alpha and beta.*

their energy is deposited in a very small tissue volume (α in Fig. 21.2).

BETA PARTICLES

These are high energy electrons from radioactive decay. They penetrate only about a centimeter or so of tissue; beta emitters are only hazardous to superficial tissues, unless ingested. The number of ionizing events depends on the β^- energy (β in Fig. 21.2). Low energy betas (^{3}H, ^{14}C) deposit all their energy in a small tissue volume. High energy β^- radiation has a more extensive pathway and produces Bremsstrahlung which can be an additional hazard (^{32}P). In general, particulate radiation only has a limited range in tissue so does not constitute an external hazard. It is a major hazard though when ingested, a feature utilized in therapy agents e.g. ^{32}P, ^{90}Y, and ^{131}I.

ELECTROMAGNETIC RADIATION

This is by far the most familiar ionizing radiation in radiology. Gamma photons are produced by radionuclides and can pass easily through soft tissues

only creating a small number of ionizing events (γ in Fig. 21.2). X-ray photons are similar but generally have lower energies so are attenuated more easily. In general, both gamma and X-photons leave behind a relatively small number of ionization events but cover a long tissue pathway. It is the density of ionization events that determines tissue damage.

21.1.2 Units of radiation dose

The interactions of radiation with matter and the concept of exposure have already been described in Chapter 5, Section 5.7.1.

EXPOSURE

Radiation exposure (X) is the ratio of the total electric charge (Q) which is the sum of all the electronic charges of either sign produced in air when all the electrons released by the ionizing events from a small volume of air of mass m are absorbed. So

$$X = \frac{Q}{m} \text{ coulombs kg}^{-1} \text{ (C kg}^{-1}) \quad (21.1)$$

Equal numbers of positive and negative charges are produced in any ionization event, since each electron ejected from one atom leaves a positively charged ion. Only the total charge of one sign is considered (e.g. electrons) in this definition.

An X-ray exposure is measured as the product of tube current (in mA) and duration (seconds) to give milliampere seconds (mAs). Since 1 mA is 1 milli-coulomb per second (1 mC s^{-1}) then mAs is equivalent to 1 mC s^{-1} × seconds = 1 mC. The exposure from an X-ray examination is described in Chapter 5, Box 5.10.

Exposure has SI units of coulomb per kilogram (C kg^{-1}) and only applies to air, and no other medium, and is measured with an air-filled ion chamber. It has an exact relationship to the **roentgen** and **gray** as: 1 R = 2.58 × 10^{-4} C kg^{-1} and 1 Gy = 2.9542 × 10^{-2} C kg^{-1} of air respectively. The roentgen is no longer used in radiation protection but there are still many dosimetry instruments calibrated in roentgen (R) or R h^{-1} or R min^{-1}. The conversion factor for roentgens can be derived by reference to the fundamental C kg^{-1} values, so that converting 1 R uses

$$\frac{2.58 \times 10^{-4}}{2.9542 \times 10^{-2}} = 8.733328 \text{ mGy}$$

Box 21.1 Exposure and photon number

Since 1 V exists if 1 J moves 1 C of charge, then, since the charge on an electron, e, is 1.6×10^{-19} C, so $1\,eV = 1.6 \times 10^{-19}$ J.

The ionization of air requires, on average, 34 eV. The radiation producing $1\,C\,kg^{-1} = 34\,J\,kg^{-1}$ in air. Since an exposure of $1\,Gy = 1\,J\,kg^{-1}$ then an exposure of $1\,C\,kg^{-1} = 34\,Gy$ in air. Using practical volumes, $1\,Gy = 1 \times 10^{-3}\,J\,g^{-1}$ and $10\,mGy$ (1 rad) $= 1 \times 10^{-5}\,J\,g^{-1}$. Hence, the number of photons N needed to produce 10 mGy exposure in 1 g air, where the exposure E in air is measured in grays and energy J is measured in joules, is then:

$$N = \frac{E}{J}$$

Assuming a photon energy of 60 keV, since $1\,eV = 1.6 \times 10^{-19}$ J then each X-ray photon of 60 keV represents 9.6×10^{-15} J. Using the basic equation, $E = hf$ (in Chapter 2), where $f = c/\lambda$, gives λ for 60 keV X-ray photons as $1.24/60 = 0.02$ nm, yielding a frequency of 1.5×10^{19} Hz. Using Planck's constant yields an energy value E of 9.6×10^{-15} J. Thus, for 60 keV the energy is 9.6×10^{-15} J. Hence,

$$N = \frac{1 \times 10^{-5}}{9.6 \times 10^{-15}} = 1 \times 10^{9} \text{ photons}$$

Similarly, for 140 keV and 1 MeV the number of photons is 4.5×10^{8} and 6.3×10^{7}, respectively.

Table 21.1 *Air kerma values for common diagnostic procedures.*

Procedure	Air kerma value
89 kV X-rays at 1 m	43 to 52 µGy mAs^{-1}
Fluoroscopy	0.5 µGy s^{-1}
	0.3 µGy frame^{-1}
Mammography at 28 kV	8.9 ×10^{-5}Gy mAs^{-1} or
	89 µGy mAs^{-1}
Nuclear medicine patient at 1 m (bone scintigraphy)	15.8 µGy h^{-1}

chamber where the wall of the chamber is an integral part of the device and produces secondary electrons that are important to the measurement.

Box 21.1 uses exposure values to calculate the number of photons of 60 keV, 140 keV and 1 MeV required to give a dose of 10 mGy (1 rad) to a tissue volume of 1 cm^3 (1 g). These photon quantities are useful when calculating detector absorption and conversion efficiency of various detector surfaces (image intensifier, intensifying screens etc.). The output from an X-ray tube is proportional to

$$\frac{\text{kilovoltage squared} \times (\text{mAs})}{d^2} \qquad (21.2)$$

where d is distance. This is measured in air kerma rate. Examples of air kerma values in practice are given in Table 21.1. Kerma is a measure of **energy released** and has previously been described in Chapter 5, Section 5.7.2 comparing its relationship to the **mass energy transfer coefficient** and **mass energy absorption coefficient**, which for diagnostic energies can be treated as equal.

For X- and gamma rays, kerma can be calculated from the mass energy transfer coefficient of the material and the energy fluence (MeV or J m^{-2}); the dose rate uses the energy flux (MeV or J m^{-2}s^{-1}). Both kerma and dose are measured in grays (Gy) or milligrays (mGy). The difference between kerma and dose for air is that the former is defined using the mass energy transfer coefficient whereas the latter uses the mass energy absorption coefficient.

for practical purposes therefore $1\,R = 8.7\,mGy$ and $1\,mR = 8.7\,\mu Gy$. Alternatively, $1\,Gy = 115\,R$ and $1\,mGy = 115\,mR$.

KERMA

The older term 'exposure' used above only applies to low energy X- or gamma photons which are stopped over a short distance in air. The term 'air kerma' does not have these restrictions and can be used for describing all ionizing events and all energies. The output of X-ray tubes is commonly quoted in terms of air kerma along with skin surface doses. The air kerma value is measured with a small ionization

ABSORBED DOSE

The basic quantities of radiation dosimetry are defined in the ICRP Report 60 of 1990. The dosimetric quantity for radiological protection is the absorbed dose, D, which is the energy absorbed per unit mass and its unit is the joule per kilogram, given the name gray (Gy) (L.H. Gray, 1905–65; British physicist). Absorbed dose is defined to mean the average dose over a tissue or organ. The use of the average dose as an indicator of the probability of subsequent stochastic effects depends on the linearity of the relationship between the probability of inducing an effect and the dose (the dose–response relationship) which is a reasonable approximation over a limited range of dose. The dose–response relationship is not linear for deterministic effects so the average absorbed dose is not directly relevant to deterministic effects unless the dose is distributed uniformly over the tissue or organ. The definition of exposure given in eqn 21.1 measures the quantity of electric charge ($C\ kg^{-1}$) produced by ionizing radiation and is not the same as the energy absorbed, although they are proportional. Absorbed dose is a measure of the energy absorbed by a volume of material (air or tissue).

The absorbed dose in $J\ kg^{-1}$ is the ratio of energy E absorbed by a mass M of tissue: E/M. The SI unit is the gray (Gy) as defined in Box 21.1 and photon flux can be calculated for any particular energy, which is useful when estimating dose or detector efficiency.

The amount of energy absorbed in the volume of mass M varies due to random photon and electron interactions taking place in the material. The SI unit of dose D is the $J\ kg^{-1}$ or gray (Gy). It replaces the obsolete unit the **rad** which is 100 $erg\ g^{-1}$ or $10^{-2}\ Gy$, so 100 rad = 1 Gy or 1 rad = 10 mGy. An unofficial unit, the centigray (cGy), is sometimes quoted which allows direct conversion between the rad and the gray (1 rad = 0.01 Gy or 1 cGy).

The total amount of energy deposited in the tissue (imparted energy) is: $J\ kg^{-1} \times kg$ (tissue). This measure is valuable when considering large volume exposure in computed tomography (CT). A single slice dose may be 50 mGy and this figure is used for representing the total volume (say 100 slices of 1 mm thickness). The imparted energy, however, which considers the total volume is much greater.

Kerma can be treated as identical to absorbed dose for energies <3 MeV which would, of course, apply to diagnostic energies. The average atomic number Z for air is 7.6, which is very close to water and soft tissue: 7.4. Therefore the mass attenuation and mass absorption coefficients for these materials are very similar and the dose in air can be treated the same as dose in tissue, along with other materials which are tissue equivalent (LiF in dosimeters).

LINEAR ENERGY TRANSFER

This is a measure of the density of ionization events along the ray's path. The linear energy transfer (LET) is correlated with the potential for tissue damage and depends on radiation type, e.g. alpha, beta, gamma or X-radiation, neutrons, protons and their radiation energy. LET is expressed as the quantity of energy (in keV) deposited per micron (μm) of tissue. Table 21.2 gives the LET for common ionizing radiation and shows approximate tissue penetration. Particulate radiations (alpha particles, neutrons, and protons) have higher LET values since they cause more ionization events over their path than either electromagnetic radiation (gamma and X-rays) or electrons (β^- radiation). Since high LET radiation is more damaging to tissues this radiation is used for radiation therapy. Internal conversion electrons and Auger electrons also have a high LET and this becomes important when considering *in vivo* radiation dose from various gamma-emitting radionuclides (e.g. ^{99m}Tc).

RADIATION WEIGHTING FACTORS

The damage imparted by radiation to living tissue and the probability of stochastic effects depend not only on the absorbed dose but also on the type and energy of the radiation. This is expressed by weighting the absorbed dose with a factor related to the quality of the radiation (alpha, beta, gamma or X-rays and neutrons). The value of the radiation weighting factor (w_R) for a specified type and energy of radiation represents the relative biological effectiveness (RBE) of that radiation in inducing stochastic effects at low doses.

The values of w_R are broadly related to the LET, a measure of the density of ionization along the track of an ionizing particle. A value w_R of unity is given for all radiations of low LET, including X- and gamma radiations of all energies; this would apply to diagnostic radiology. The choice for other radiations is based on observed values of the RBE, regardless of whether the reference radiation is X- or gamma radiation.

Auger electrons emitted from nuclei bound to DNA present a special problem. It is not realistic to average the absorbed dose over the whole mass of DNA as would be required by the present definition of equivalent dose, so the effects of Auger electrons are assessed by the techniques of microdosimetry.

Table 21.2 *Average linear energy transfer (LET) for alpha particles, beta radiation, gamma and X-rays, and tissue penetration.*

Radiation	Energy (keV)	Average LET (keV μm^{-1})	Tissue penetration (μm or HVL mm)	Example
Alpha particles	5000	95.0	35	^{241}Am, ^{239}Pu, ^{238}U
Beta radiation	1	12.3	0.01	Recoil electrons
	10	2.3	1	^{3}H (tritium)
	100	0.42	180	^{14}C
	1000	0.25	5000	^{198}Au, ^{131}I
	2000	0.23	10 000	$^{85-90}$Sr ^{90}Y ^{32}P
Gamma and X-rays	80	1.0	38 mm	Diagnostic X-rays
	120	1.4	43 mm	^{57}Co
	140	1.5	46 mm	^{99m}Tc
	364	2.8	65 mm	^{131}I
	511	3.5	70 mm	Positron emitters
	1000	5.2	100 mm	^{60}Co

Table 21.3 *Radiation weighting factors.*

Type of radiation and energy	Radiation weighting factor, w_R
Photons (all energies)	1
Electrons (including Auger)	1
Neutrons <10 keV	5
10 to 100 keV	10
100 keV to 2 MeV	20
2 MeV to 20 MeV	10
>20 MeV	5
Protons	5
Alpha particles	20

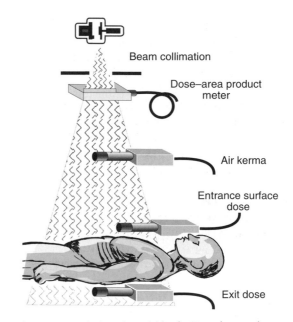

Figure 21.3 *The location within the X-ray beam where dose measurements are made. The dose–area product meter is fixed to the X-ray housing itself.*

Previously, the weighting factor was applied to the absorbed dose at a point and was called the **quality factor**, *Q*. The earlier version of the weighted absorbed dose was the **dose equivalent**; this term is now discontinued and replaced with the equivalent dose which represents an average dose and not a point dose. Table 21.3 lists some weighting factors for radiation.

DOSE MEASUREMENT

The quantity of energy deposited in a tissue by ionizing radiation can be estimated by using tissue equivalent monitoring devices, i.e. film dosimeters, thermoluminescent dosimeters, electronic detectors. Figure 21.3 indicates the position in the X-ray beam where relevant dose measurements are made. Both the dose rate and surface dose rate are expressed as air kerma; tissue dose is expressed in absorbed dose. While entrance surface dose (ESD) is a measure for the individual radiograph the dose–area product meter (DAP or Diamentor) gives a reading for the complete study (several radiographs).

When quantities cannot be measured directly, for instance when a radionuclide is deposited in an organ and irradiates that organ with alpha, beta or gamma radiation, the dose absorbed by that organ is calculated from the known activity of the radionuclide (Chapter 16).

EQUIVALENT DOSE

In radiological protection, it is the absorbed dose averaged over a tissue or organ (rather than at a point) and weighted for the radiation quality that is of interest. The weighting factor for this purpose is now called the radiation weighting factor, w_R, and is selected for the type and energy of the radiation incident on the body or, in the case of sources within the body, emitted by the radionuclide. The equivalent dose (H_T) in tissue T is given by

$$H_T = \sum_R w_R \cdot D_{T,R} \qquad (21.3)$$

where $D_{T,R}$ is the absorbed dose averaged over the tissue or organ T, due to radiation R.

The unit of equivalent dose is the joule per kilogram and called the sievert (Sv) (Rolf Sievert, 1896–1966; Swedish radiologist). The non-SI unit is the rem where 100 rem = 1 Sv. The basic units of radiation exposure are given in Table 21.4.

Table 21.4 *SI units of radiation exposure with their non-SI equivalents.*

Quantity	Name	Conversion
SI units of radiation and their conversion factors		
Exposure	C kg^{-1} air kerma (Gy)	1 C kg^{-1} = 34 Gy
Absorbed dose	gray (Gy)	1 Gy = J kg^{-1} 1 Gy = 2.9 × 10^{-2} C kg^{-1}
Equivalent dose	sievert (Sv)	Sv = Gy × w_R
Non-SI units of radiation and their conversion factors		
Exposure	roentgen (R)	1 C kg^{-1} = 3876 R 1 R = 2.58 × 10^{-4} C kg^{-1} 1 R = 8.7 mGy
Absorbed dose	rad	1 rad = 0.01 J kg^{-1} 10 mGy = 1 rad 1 μGy = 115 μR
Equivalent dose	rem	rem = rad × Q

21.2 BIOLOGICAL DAMAGE

Only a short time elapsed between the discovery of X-rays and reported cases of radiation damage from their use. The workers themselves (clinicians and technicians), who held the film cassettes in the X-ray beam, noticed damage to their hands that was slow to heal. Radiation workers were also suffering from general radiation exposure which sometimes led to cancers and early death. Relatively little radiation biology was done prior to 1940. Fundamental research in this area stemmed from the development of nuclear weapons, and the present strict guidelines and controls on the use of radiation originate from that time.

Of the various forms of radiation damage the most important is that to the DNA structure. Damage to DNA can prevent survival or reproduction of the cell but there is a repair mechanism (see later). If sufficient cells are killed or damaged there will be loss of organ function; an event that the ICRP calls **deterministic**. Somatic or hereditary effects which may start from a single modified or transformed cell are called **stochastic** effects.

21.2.1 Direct and indirect damage

Alpha and beta particles, being charged, lose energy by electrical interactions with the outer electrons of atoms in tissue. Electromagnetic radiation (gamma and X-rays), being uncharged, can behave differently but both produce ionizing events. The overall damage may be represented by:

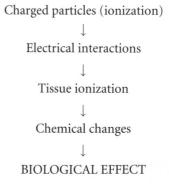

Charged particles (ionization)

↓

Electrical interactions

↓

Tissue ionization

↓

Chemical changes

↓

BIOLOGICAL EFFECT

DNA is responsible for cell growth and cell division and is the most important radiosensitive material in the cell. Other radiosensitive biological molecules are RNA, enzymes and the molecular structure of the cell wall.

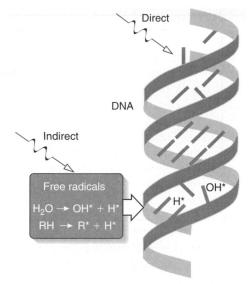

Figure 21.4 *Direct damage to the chromosome nuclear material (DNA) from ionizing radiation and indirect damage from free radical production (Box 21.2).*

DIRECT DAMAGE

DNA may be directly damaged by radiation, causing a break in a chain as shown in Fig. 21.4. It can also damage the nuclear cell membrane. Indirect damage is caused by free radicals produced by irradiation of water molecules some distance from the target. Free radicals attack the structure of DNA and other important biological complexes by forming unstable and very reactive compounds; these are listed in Box 21.2. Direct damage (stages 1, 2, and 3 in the box) leads to a chain of destruction involving a peroxy radical ($RO_2^\bullet$ in stages 2 and 3).

INDIRECT DAMAGE

This occurs when a charged particle passes through atoms in the tissue transferring some of its energy to atomic electrons in the medium (mostly water) without causing direct effects on radiosensitive targets.

Water molecules, the most common constituent of tissue, enter a state of excitation, forming free radicals ($H^\bullet$ and $OH^\bullet$). These are highly reactive and are responsible for indirect protein damage (stages 8 and 9). Simple ionization of the water can also occur ($H_2O \rightarrow H^+ + OH^-$). The main reactions with water are shown in stages 4 to 7. Both indirect and direct reactions can lead to self-perpetuating chain reactions.

Box 21.2 Direct and indirect radiation damage

Assume R represents the target molecule (e.g. DNA, RNA or enzyme system) and that * represents a radiation event.

Direct damage

In this example, R is a protein molecule and $RO_2^\bullet$ is the peroxy radical.

1 $RH^\bullet \rightarrow R + H$
2 $R^\bullet + O_2 \rightarrow RO_2^\bullet$
3 $RO_2^\bullet + RH \rightarrow RO_2H + R^\bullet$

(Return to start of 2.)

Indirect damage: the radiolysis of water

4 $H_2O^* \rightarrow H_2O^+ + e^-$
5 $H_2O + e^- \rightarrow H_2O^-$
6 $H_2O + \rightarrow H^+ + OH^\bullet$
7 $H_2O^- \rightarrow H^\bullet + OH^-$

The ions OH^- and H^+ are removed since they recombine to form water:

$H^+ + OH^- \rightarrow H_2O$

$H^\bullet$ and $OH^\bullet$ have unpaired electrons and therefore are free radicals. These extract hydrogen from organic molecules:

8 $RH + OH^\bullet \rightarrow R^\bullet + H_2O$
9 $RH + H^\bullet \rightarrow R^\bullet + H_2$

(This then joins the chain reaction in 1 above.)

REACTION TIME SPAN

Ionizing reactions in tissue can occur almost instantaneously or take place over a longer time. The extreme ranges listed in Table 21.5 show that the initial physical reactions are extremely fast, measured in femtoseconds (10^{-15}), these are followed by chemical reactions whose periods are measured in picoseconds (10^{-12}).

The biomolecular and biological cell damage appear at much slower rates, up to years afterwards, in some cases, which are considered in calculations of population risk.

Table 21.5 *Time span of radiation damage.*

Damage	Time span	Effect
Initial	10^{-17} to 10^{-15} s	Ionization Excitation
Chemical	10^{-14} to 10^{-3} s	Free radicals Excited molecules
Biomolecular	Seconds to hours	Protein damage Nucleic acid split
Biological	Hours to decades	Cell death Malignancy Animal death

Table 21.6 *Effects on biological materials.*

Level of complexity	Radiation effects and damage
Molecular	Macromolecules (enzymes, RNA, DNA)
Sub-cellular	Cell membrane, nucleus, chromosomes, mitochondria, lysosomes
Cellular	Inhibits cell division; leads to cell death, transformation, mutation
Tissue and organ	Nervous system, bone marrow, intestinal tract, cancer induction
Whole individual	Death, life shortening
Populations	Genetic change, mutations

LEVEL OF DAMAGE

The radiation harm to a living cell depends on the level of differentiation (complexity); whether a single cell, a group of cells or the whole organism. Frequency of cell division is also important. Radiation damage at the molecular and cellular levels can eventually become evident within the population. This progression is shown in Table 21.6.

21.2.2 Cellular response to radiation

The radiation sensitivity of a cell depends on whether it is haploid (unpaired chromosomes, e.g. bacteria) or diploid (paired chromosomes, e.g. mammalian cells).

BACTERIA

The response of simple bacterial cells to radiation damage shows a single exponential relationship

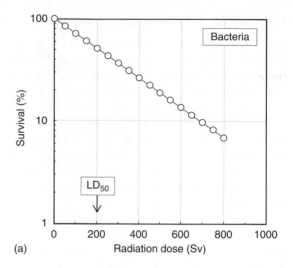

(a)

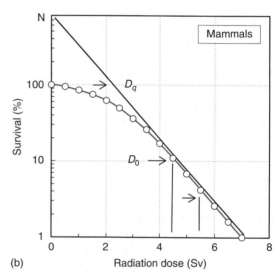

(b)

Figure 21.5 *(a) A simple exponential dose survival curve for haploid cells (bacteria). (b) Dose survival curves for diploid cells (mammalian) showing a repair 'shoulder'.* D_q *at point 100% and* D_0, *the dose reducing survival by 37%.*

(Fig. 21.5a). This is the **dose–response or survival curve**, the survival axis is plotted on a logarithmic scale and the radiation dose on a linear scale.

The overall effect of cellular damage is measured at the point where radiation dose causes a 50% cell loss. This is the **lethal dose** for 50% death or the LD_{50} point. Bacterial cells can survive high radiation doses (hundreds of sieverts). The LD_{50} for bacteria is typically 200 Sv; for viruses it is much more.

MAMMALIAN CELLS

These show a more complex dose–survival response to radiation than the simple single event exponential curve shown by bacteria. It is a multi-event response (Fig. 21.5b), where cellular repair at low radiation doses gives a shoulder to the start of the curve; this is characteristic of mammalian cells. The LD_{50} for mammalian cells shows they are more radiosensitive than bacteria (less resistant to radiation damage); the LD_{50} is between 3 and 5 Sv depending on the animal and cell type. From the curve certain important parameters can be identified: N, D_q and D_0.

The shape of the graph is described by reference to the two parameters N and D_0. The dimension D_0 is the slope of the exponential function (a straight line on this log–linear plot) and represents the dose necessary to reduce the surviving cell fraction by $1/e$ or 0.37 (37%); D_0 represents the mean lethal dose. If the exponential part of the curve is extrapolated toward the y-axis it will cross this axis at some point which is called N. This is a measure of the shoulder size of the curve. Where this line crosses the 100% survival point (arrow in Fig. 21.5b) is the threshold dose D_q, which approximates to the sub-lethal radiation dose.

TARGET THEORY

The mammalian cell survival–dose curve(s) suggest a multi-target model and the shoulder represents a repair process which becomes ineffective at higher doses. A simple multi-target model can be represented by incorporating the parameters N and D_0 into an equation describing the surviving fraction s after a dose D:

$$s = 1 - \left(1 - \exp\frac{D}{D_0}\right)^N \qquad (21.4)$$

The radiosensitivity of a cell or tissue affects the shoulder dimension and is proportional to its mitotic activity and inversely proportional to its state of differentiation. Rapidly dividing cell populations within an organ are most radiosensitive (e.g. bone marrow, gastrointestinal mucosa); tissues with little mitotic activity (e.g. brain, muscle) are more resistant. Following a radiation exposure the radiosensitive tissues will contain more target points and so suffer more damage than radioresistant tissues. Table 21.7

Table 21.7 *Damage to human tissues.*

Exposure	C kg^{-1}	Human exposure
0 to 200 mGy	0 to 0.0065	No effect detected
200 to 400 mGy	0.0065 to 0.013	Some blood changes
400 to 800 mGy	0.013 to 0.026	Blood changes and nausea
800 mGy to 2 Gy	0.026 to 0.05	Nausea, diarrhea, life shortening
3.5 Gy	0.1	Death in 50% of the population in 30 days
5 Gy	0.15	100% death in 30 days
10 Gy	0.25	Death in 2 weeks
25 Gy	0.8	Death in 2 days

gives radiation exposure levels and their observed effects on humans.

21.2.3 Organ response to radiation

A cell modified by radiation damage may transmit flawed genetic information via its DNA to other cell generations. This can cause both somatic and hereditary effects which may start from a single modified cell; this is the **stochastic** effect where radiation causes potential harm even at low doses. If enough cells in an organ or tissue are killed or prevented from functioning normally there will be a loss of organ function; this is the **deterministic** effect where there is a threshold dose (Th in Fig. 21.6a) below which these effects are not seen (e.g. cataracts and erythemas); a linear response region may still exist. These two radiation effects are illustrated in Fig. 21.6a where stochastic describes a linear relationship showing no lower limit or threshold to radiation damage: breast cancer and leukemia are examples.

These effects are a valuable guide to personnel radiation protection recommendations indicating maximum permissible radiation doses. Radiation protection measures aim to prevent deterministic (nonstochastic) effects and reduce the probability of stochastic effects to acceptable levels. Deterministic effects are shown where a loss of tissue function is seen at doses of a few hundred mSv (100 mSv = 10 rem). These are characterized by a dose–frequency relationship for which a dose threshold exists.

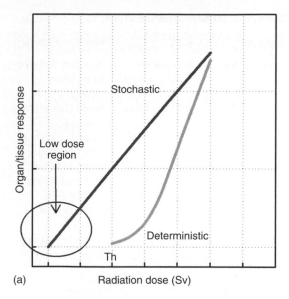

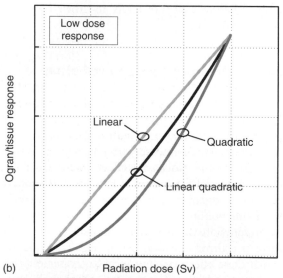

(a)

(b)

Figure 21.6 *(a) A stochastic effect with organ or tissue response at all dose levels. A deterministic response is seen when the dose reaches a certain threshold **Th**. (b) Three probable types of low dose stochastic response. Linear and two nonlinear models: quadratic and linear–quadratic.*

In order to produce a scheme for radiation protection it is necessary to know the probability of stochastic effects for a certain radiation dose (**risk estimates**). For healthy workers the probability for deterministic effects will be zero for doses up to hundreds of millisieverts but will increase steeply above this threshold. Table 21.8 lists some estimated dose levels for deterministic effects taken from ICRP 60.

Table 21.8 *Deterministic threshold dose equivalent (in Sv) for acute tissue (H_T) and chronic whole-body exposure (E).*

Tissue and effect	Brief exposure, H_T (Sv)	Long exposure, E (Sv y^{-1})
Gonads		
Testes		
Temporary	0.15	0.4
Permanent sterility	3.5 to 6.0	2.0
Ovaries		
Sterility	>2.5	>0.2
Lens		
Opacities	2 to 10	>0.1
Cataract	>2.0	>0.15
Bone marrow		
Hematopoesis	>0.5	>0.4

21.2.4 Population response to radiation

The response by human beings to low doses of radiation has been the subject of much study. Most hard evidence about radiation damage to human populations comes from high exposure rates (e.g. Japanese atomic-bomb survivors, therapy data) and estimated damage from low exposure rates is obtained by extrapolation from these high-dose data points. This provides much controversy and several theories exist which attempt to predict radiation damage to populations exposed to lower dose levels. The three possible curve shapes that can represent population dose responses are shown in Fig. 21.6b.

LINEAR

This is the simplest response. Radiation induced breast cancer is an example of a disease showing a linear dose relationship. Radiation protection standards take a linear response as their reference so that low dose responses can be simply calculated from high dose data, i.e.:

- 1000 people exposed to 1 Sv (100 rem) would show an increased cancer incidence of 20 cases.
- 10 000 people exposed to 100 mSv or 100 000 exposed to 10 mSv would show the same incidence.

QUADRATIC

This is proposed for describing the reduced damage shown by certain tissues (skin) to low radiation levels.

LINEAR QUADRATIC

This is an combined linear and quadratic model which takes into consideration the repair mechanism shown by diploid cells (Fig. 21.6b). It would not be included in a purely linear model. Leukemia induction is an example of a disease showing a linear–quadratic dose response.

21.2.5 Somatic and genetic effects

Radiation can damage body tissues causing somatic effects, seen mainly as carcinogenesis in individuals or populations, or affect their offspring causing genetic effects which are hereditary defects seen in populations.

SOMATIC CELL DAMAGE

This is the damage that is apparent during the lifetime of the organism, exclusive of effects on the reproductive system. Somatic cells include all cells except gametes. A great variety of changes can be seen, some temporary and others permanent, the latter often leading to cell death.

Somatic cells most commonly survive low radiation dose rates since the damage at molecular and sub-cellular levels is mostly repaired. Somatic damage could result in leukemia, breast cancer and other adult carcinomas in individuals and populations. Noncarcinoma damage, for instance cataract or pulmonary fibrosis, is seen in people exposed to local high radiation levels. Somatic effects occur mainly as a result of acute (short time-span) doses from atomic weapons or therapy. Chronic radiation exposure data from large populations in the USA and China have failed to show any unequivocal evidence that high natural background radiation levels increase the incidence of somatic or genetic effects.

Prior to 1921 radiologists exposed continuously to quite high levels of soft (low energy) radiation had an increased cancer mortality. This is not seen in present-day radiologists owing to safer equipment and decreased radiation exposures; indeed they may illustrate a 'healthy worker syndrome' as they have a lower incidence of cancer than the general population.

Somatic changes are seen in radiation sensitive adult tissues having high proliferation rates, for instance bone marrow, breast and gastrointestinal mucosa. Less damage is done to slowly proliferating

cells as in the adult central nervous system. Somatic damage is most dangerous at the embryo and fetus stages where cells have multiple descendants.

Inhibition of cell division by radiation mostly leads to cell death but some radiation damage causes cell transformation where normal cell functions are altered and carcinogenesis initiated. Soft radiation (UV, electrons), or soft (low energy) X-rays give a high surface dose and these would promote skin cancer.

The small incidence of **radiogenic** cancer that may be present in a population is indistinguishable from naturally occurring cancers (leukemia, breast, sarcoma, lung) and since the natural cancer rate is about 16% per 100 000 (16 000 deaths) the effect of low level radiation on the population (cancer incidence) is almost impossible to detect with statistical confidence.

GERM CELL DAMAGE

The influence of radiation on the gonads (testes or ovaries) can lead to inherited malfunction. Damage to reproductive cells (gametes) may be heritable, and could cause an abnormally functioning genotype, i.e. genetic effects. Most concern was initially focused on genetic damage to populations from radiation. Careful observation over a long period of time, however, has not established any trend in populations exposed to high levels of radiation (atomic bomb survivors and areas of high natural radiation) so inherited damage has been down-rated as a serious threat.

GENETICALLY SIGNIFICANT DOSE

This is a measure of genetic hazard to the population from radiation exposure, particularly medical radiation, and assumes a linear dose–effect relationship.

If the mean gonad dose to patients undergoing radiological examinations (between 0.5 mGy and 20 mGy) was received by every member of the population it would be expected to produce the same total genetic effect on the general population. So if 10% of the population received ×10 the mean gonad dose, the effect would be the same as the total population receiving just the mean dose.

Table 21.9 lists the estimated genetically significant doses for the USA, Japan, and some European countries. If the average gonad radiation dose to a relatively small exposed patient population is about 10 mGy then the genetically significant dose (GSD) adjusts

Table 21.9 *Genetically significant doses for some selected countries.*

Country	Dose (mGy)
Sweden	0.46
Germany	0.41
USA	0.20
Japan	0.17
UK	0.12

this to give the same relative hazard to the entire population. The GSD also takes into consideration the child bearing potential of the patient population. It is derived as:

$$SD = \frac{\sum (N_{xy}P_{xy}D_{xy})_m + \sum (N_{xy}P_{xy}D_{xy})_f}{\sum N_x P_x}$$

(21.5)

where:

N_{xy} = the number of patients in age groups x undergoing patient examination y

P_{xy} = the child expectancy for persons in age group x undergoing examination y

D_{xy} = the average gonad dose for patients in age group x undergoing examination y

N_x = the number of persons of age group x in the population

P_x = the child expectancy for age group x

21.3 NATURAL AND MAN-MADE RADIATION

Background radiation both natural and man-made is a consistent source of low exposure to all members of the population. Some areas of very high natural background levels (up to 100 mSv per year in Kerala, India, and some regions of Brazil) have served as benchmarks for studying population low dose exposure. The general population is exposed to a variety of natural and man-made radiation sources. These are listed in Table 21.10 for a typical location and represented as a pie chart in Fig. 21.7. The US values tend to be higher for radon (up to 55%) with proportionally less internal, external, and cosmic; the medical percentage is about the same but is seen to be increasing generally in the Western world.

Table 21.10 *Typical proportions of natural and man-made radiation in Europe (whole-body dose).*

Source	Dose (μSv)	Percent
Natural radiation		
Cosmic radiation (solar activity)	310	13
Terrestrial gamma radiation (soils, rock, water)	380	16
Radon decay products (houses and work area)	800	33
Internal radiation (e.g. ^{40}K, ^{14}C)	370	15
Total natural exposure	1860	78%
Man-made radiation		
Medical procedures	500	21
Weapons fall-out	10	0.4
Nuclear power	3	0.15
Occupational	9	0.36
Air travel	8	0.34
Total man-made	530	22
Natural and man-made	2390	100

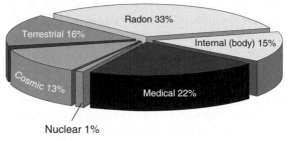

Figure 21.7 *Components of natural and man-made population exposure in the UK. The total dose range is between 3 and 10 mSv. The small sector represents exposure from nuclear products which is <1%.*

21.3.1 Natural radiation

The largest contributing factor to population exposure from natural radiation comes from radon gas (^{222}Rn), a decay product of uranium, a natural component of most soils and rocks. The exposure to other natural radiation sources normally cannot be altered but radon exposure is influenced by building design. A radon concentration of 200 Bq m^{-3} is currently considered a suitable limit.

A large variation in population dose arises from radon exposure and in some instances (hard rock areas, i.e. granite) this can be responsible for an individual annual dose of up to 100 mSv. Data on population exposure from all sources of radiation in most countries give an overall whole-body dose of 2.5 to 4 mSv. About 85% comes from natural sources, half of this from radon exposure in the home.

21.3.2 Man-made radiation

Background radiation acts as a reasonable benchmark for judging staff and patient radiation doses from medical exposures. Medical exposure accounts for a population dose of typically 20% of the total man-made radiation, nuclear discharges (in spite of popular misconception) add only a further 1%. Doses from individual medical exposures can range from 0.2 mSv for a chest radiograph to 10 or 20 mSv for extensive fluoroscopy.

21.4 RISK ESTIMATES

The slight increase in the incidence of cancer following irradiation can only be detected by studying large populations. It is from these studies that risk estimates are made. The largest set of data comes from the health records of atomic-bomb survivors who lived in Hiroshima and Nagasaki and radiation risks for medical workers are estimated from this comprehensive information. Box 21.3 gives a worked example of risk estimation showing that cancer induced from low radiation levels is almost impossible to detect within the high natural cancer incidence.

The two reports from the International Commission on Radiological Protection (**ICRP**) which have

Table 21.11 *A comparison of fatal risks.*

Event	Risk	Risk ratio
Anesthetic death	40×10^{-6}	1:25 000
Car driver (10 000 miles)	200×10^{-6}	1:5000
Age 55 years	$10\,000 \times 10^{-6}$	1:100
1 mSv exposure	10×10^{-6}	1:100 000
50 mSv exposure	1.5×10^{-6}	1:700

most influenced radiation dosimetry are ICRP 26 (1977) and ICRP 60 (1990). ICRP 26 is based on the early risk estimates from the original atomic-bomb survivor data (T65DR 'old' dosimetry). These data were reassessed during the 1980s, in the light of fresh information concerning the type and mixture of radiation given by the two nuclear explosions (DS86 'new' dosimetry). Based on the findings of DS86 the cancer risk associated with radiation was increased by about ×2 and recommendations to this effect were published in ICRP 60. The new calculations were necessary because the contribution from neutron radiation to the total population exposure was far less than originally thought. This increased the emphasis on gamma exposure and consequently the risks associated with gamma radiation were scaled upwards. There is still controversy over the neutron:gamma mix so ideas and recommendations may undergo more change. Although the new evidence has increased somatic risk the radiation risk associated with gonad exposure and hereditary defects has been derated.

21.4.1 Risk comparisons

The population is exposed to many risks. Some carry a beneficial component (car or air travel), others do not (e.g. aging). Table 21.11 compares a variety of radiation and nonradiation risks to the population. The risks are expressed as a 'risk ratio': 1.0×10^{-2} or 1 in 100 (1:100).

Radiation risks are usually standardized for a 1 Sv exposure. Risks for exposure levels less than this are derated linearly, demonstrated and calculated in Box 21.3.

21.4.1 Calculation of risks

If an irradiated group of people are studied (radiotherapy patients, atomic-bomb survivors etc.) and

---

Box 21.3 Radiation induced cancer risk

The risk for radiation induced cancer in 100 000 people exposed to 1 Sv would be 1250:

$$1.25 \times 10^{-2}\,Sv^{-1}, \text{ or } 1:80$$

For a lower dose of 1 mSv this would be 1.25 for 100,000 people exposed:

$$\approx 1 \times 10^{-5}\,mSv^{-1}, \text{ or } 1:100\,000$$

This has been revised by ICRP 60 and the risk for a 1 mSv exposure is now:

$$3.0 \times 10^{-5}\,mSv^{-1}, \text{ or } 1:33\,000$$

the radiation doses that they have received are known with a fair precision then if the number of cancers exceeds the number that would be expected (calculated from an identical unexposed population) then the excess number of cancers may be attributable to radiation effects and the risk of cancer per unit dose can be estimated. This is the risk factor and these form the basis of all radiation protection directives. There is a great deal of uncertainty in these calculations since the radiation dose to the population is not known accurately and the unexposed control is hardly ever identical to the exposed group. Box 21.3 calculates cancer induction from low dose levels and illustrates how difficult it would be to detect this cancer increase in a population.

ESTIMATION OF ACCEPTABLE RISK

For the purpose of dosimetry a risk can be:

- Unacceptable, which would unreasonably increase harm to a population
- Not unacceptable, where the small level of increased harm is balanced by a great deal of benefit

An increase in perceived somatic risks has placed more restrictive limits on worker and public exposure levels; these recent risk estimates are listed in Table 21.12. The re-evaluation of the Japanese data suggests a fatal risk of ≈ 3 in $100\,000\,\text{mSv}^{-1}$ or $\approx 1{:}33\,000\,\text{mSv}^{-1}$ (previously 1 in 100 000). The new data suggested that members of the public exposed to 1 mSv had a new risk estimate of 1 in 33,000 which was thought to be unacceptable, so the recommended maximum public exposure was lowered to 0.5 mSv, decreasing the perceived risk to 1 in 70 000.

Table 21.12 *Risk estimates (from ICRP 60).*

Risk	Risk estimate
Exposure at 50 mSv	1.5×10^{-3} (1 in 700)
Annual risk to workers	
Unacceptable	10^{-2} (1 in 100)
Not unacceptable	10^{-3} (1 in 1000)
Exposure at 15 mSv	5.0×10^{-4} (1 in 2000)
Risk to the public	
Unacceptable	10^{-4} (1 in 10 000)
Probably acceptable	10^{-5} (1 in 100 000)
Exposure 1 mSv	3.0×10^{-5} (1 in 33 000)
Exposure 0.5 mSv	1.4×10^{-5} (1 in 70 000)

NOMINAL RISK COEFFICIENTS

Since there is still uncertainty in the risk estimates given in ICRP 60 the probability of a fatal cancer was renamed the nominal risk coefficient (nominal: not real or actual). The nominal lifetime cancer risk coefficient for an adult is:

$$4 \times 10^{-2}\,\text{Sv}^{-1}\ (1{:}25)\ (1{:}25\,000\,\text{mSv}^{-1})$$

and for the whole population:

$$5 \times 10^{-2}\,\text{Sv}^{-1}\ (1{:}20)\ (1{:}20\,000\,\text{mSv}^{-1})$$

The nominal hereditary coefficient is much smaller:

$$\times 10^{-2}\,\text{Sv}^{-1}\ (1{:}100)\ (1{:}100\,000\,\text{mSv}^{-1})$$

RISK LIMIT

This is now analogous to the dose limit. The recommended long term dose limit for occupational exposure is:

$$\approx 8 \times 10^{-4}\ (1{:}1300 = 25\,\text{mSv per year})$$

and for the public:

$$\approx 3 \times 10^{-5}\ (1{:}33\,000 = 1\,\text{mSv per year})$$

These are maximum values. By practicing the ALARA principle, a typical diagnostic department can achieve 1.5×10^{-4} ($1{:}7000 = 5\,\text{mSv}$) for workers (technicians and radiologists) and 1.5×10^{-5} ($1{:}70{,}000 = 0.5\,\text{mSv}$) for the public (nonradiation workers). Table 21.13 summarizes the risk estimates

Table 21.13 *Summary of risks for various doses.*

Acceptable risk	Annual exposure (mSv)	Risk
Worker, 1:1000		
	50	1.5×10^{-3} (1:700)
	25	7.5×10^{-4} (1:1333)
	20	6.0×10^{-4} (1:1666)
	15	5.0×10^{-4} (1:2000)
Public, 1:100 000		
	5	1.6×10^{-4} (1:6000)
	1	3.0×10^{-5} (1:33 333)
	0.5	1.4×10^{-5} (1:70 000)

associated with radiation dose limits. Box 21.4 illustrates the calculation of risk assessment.

RISKS TO THE FETUS

Current information indicates that radiation risks to the developing fetus are small from diagnostic radiology. The probabilities, given in Table 21.14, are for developing cancer or an organ malfunction in later childhood. The natural incidence of these abnormalities in the Western world is 4.07% or approximately 1 in 25 live births. This incidence is hardly influenced

---

Box 21.4 Risk assessment

Assume that when 500 000 people are irradiated and receive 15 mSv whole-body irradiation they show four more cancers than normal. The risk factor is

$$\frac{\text{increased cancer incidence}}{\text{population} \times \text{dose}}$$

which is

$$\frac{4}{500\,000 \times 0.015}$$

or 5.3×10^{-4}, i.e. ≈ 1 in 2000

Since there is a spontaneous cancer incidence of about 1600 per 10 000 of the population there would be an expected cancer rate of 80 000 in 500 000 people. A population dose of 15 mSv would add 250 to this total and would be well hidden by the statistical fluctuation.

Table 21.14 *Added risks to fetus from radiation.*

Dose equivalent (mSv)	No abnormality (%)	Increased risk
0.0	95.930	0.0
0.5	95.928	0.002
1.0	95.922	0.008
2.5	95.910	0.02
5.0	95.880	0.05
10.0	95.830	0.10

even with an exposure of 10 mSv which would represent a fairly extensive abdominal X-ray investigation.

The risk of cancer induction in children from high level exposure *in utero* is $\approx 6 \times 10^{-2}\,\text{Sv}^{-1}$ (1:17), half these cases are expected to be fatal. There is also a risk of adult cancers originating from fetal exposure. There is a deterministic (nonstochastic) threshold of between 200 and 400 mGy for severe mental retardation resulting from fetal exposure.

CUMULATIVE RISK

The risks of damage to the gonads or fetus during diagnostic investigations are cumulative and patients who are undergoing successive investigations during diagnosis and follow-up will increase their risk of radiation damage to $\approx 1 \times 10^{-2}$ (1:100). This is obviously more serious in young patients undergoing repeat investigations and the level of risk must be justified by clinical benefit. The reduction of patient radiation exposure in diagnostic radiology is the prime responsibility of radiology staff since there are real risks to young patients and the population as a whole.

DOSE RATE EFFECTIVENESS FACTOR

This has been introduced so that high dose tissue responses, obtained from measurements, can be used to estimate low dose effects which cannot be easily measured. The dose rate effectiveness factor (DREF) allows for the enhanced effect seen at high dose rates (Japanese bomb survivors) so that risks for lower dose exposure can be derived.

A DREF value between 2 and 4 is commonly used as a divisor. A cancer mortality of $2.5 \times 10^{-2}\,\text{Sv}^{-1}$ (1:40), seen in bomb survivors, is reduced to $1.25 \times 10^{-2}\,\text{Sv}^{-1}$ (1:80) (DREF value of 2). There is considerable debate concerning the proper choice of DREF for human risk calculations.

THE LATENT PERIOD

The **reaction time span** (see Table 21.5) already describes the delay between radiation exposure and its effect (cancer or tissue damage). The time delay is the latent period. The latent period for leukemia is shorter than for other cancers; a minimum time of 2 years and a peak incidence at 8 years following high radiation doses. For other cancers 10 years and 15 years are typical minimal latent periods. Cancer risk can persist for a further 40 or more years.

KEYWORDS

absorbed dose: the ratio of energy absorbed by a volume of tissue. The unit is the gray (Gy)

air kerma: the energy released from all ionizing events in a volume of air. The unit is $C\,kg^{-1}$ or Gy

air kerma rate: measured as $\mu Gy\,mAs^{-1}$

ALI: annual limits on intake for internal exposure based on committed effective dose of 20 mSv

deterministic: loss of organ function due to multiple cell damage. Deterministic effects have a threshold below which no effect is seen

diploid: relates to cells having a double set of chromosomes. Usually relates to all mammalian cells except gametes

D_0: the dose that gives (on average) one lethal event per cell reducing survival to 37% of its previous value

dose equivalent (H_T): the product of the absorbed dose in tissue and quality factor. Measured in rem (non-SI) and sievert (SI)

DREF: dose rate effectiveness factor. Corrects for extrapolation from high to low dose effects

exposure: measured in roentgen (R) or air kerma

free radicals: molecules or ions with unpaired electrons and hence generally exceedingly reactive

germ cell: pertaining to the gametes: sperm, ovum or a cell from which they originate

gray (Gy): a measure of absorbed dose $1\,J\,kg^{-1}$

haploid: relates to single-stranded DNA cells: bacteria and gametes

hereditary: affecting future generations

LD_{50}: the lethal dose for 50% cell or population death

linear energy transfer (LET): a measure of the density of ionizing events along a radiation path as keV μm^{-1}

quality factor, Q or w_R: a dimensionless value used for weighting absorbed dose according to the radiation's biological effect. Now called the radiation weighting factor w_R

radiation weighting factor (w_R): as listed in Table 21.3 from ICRP 60. (See quality factor above)

röntgen (R): $2.58 \times 10^{-4}\,C\,kg^{-1}$ of air

sievert (Sv): a measure of dose equivalent: gray $\times$ Q or w_R

somatic: pertaining to all cells except reproductive cells

stochastic: somatic or hereditary effects which may start from a single cell. There is no threshold

tissue weighting factor: (w_T) as listed in Table 22.2 from ICRP 60

22

Radiation protection: legislation and clinical practice

22.1 DOSIMETRIC QUANTITIES

Organs and tissues are made up from cells having various general or special functions; these cells and their contents are considered the key targets for radiation damage. Low dose ionizing radiation has a non-uniform discontinuous interaction with matter. The related probabilistic nature of energy depositions results in distributions of imparted energy on a cellular and molecular level that are very uneven, due to the low photon density. Absorbed dose is the statistical mean of the distribution of energy imparted in small volumes divided by the mass of the corresponding volume. However, the smaller the average radiation dose to an organ or tissue, the fewer the number of cells that will be hit by an ionizing track. The fluctuations of energy imparted in individual cells and subcellular structures are the subject of microdosimetry.

X-radiation, and to some extent gamma radiation, undergoes three interactions which are important to diagnostic radiology:

1 Transmission through tissue, where the fluence variations carry information that forms the image
2 Absorption by the tissue, which influences image contrast and also causes radiation damage to the patient
3 Scatter within the tissue, spoiling image contrast, increasing patient radiation exposure and contributing to staff radiation exposure

All three can be optimized by employing the most efficient imaging equipment (fast film-screens or digital imaging) and scatter minimized by careful preparation. The aim of radiation protection is to provide an adequate standard of safety without unduly limiting its beneficial use as a clinical tool, both diagnostic and therapeutic. The dose restrictions currently applied to the workplace are sufficient to avoid deterministic effects and ensure that ionizing radiation remains a minor risk in the hospital.

22.1.1 Organ and tissue dose

Radiological protection for low dose exposures is primarily concerned with prevention of radiation-induced cancer and hereditary disease. These are termed **stochastic effects**, as they are probabilistic and are believed to have their origins in damage to single cells. For protection purposes the assumption is made that these effects increase with an increase with radiation dose; there is no threshold. Any increment of exposure above the natural background produces a linear increment of risk. There are two dose quantities for describing energy deposited in a tissue and distinguishing the effects of different radiation on tissue:

• Absorbed dose, measured in grays
• Equivalent dose, measured in sieverts

Both describe radiation damage to individual organs or tissues. The absorbed dose has been described in Chapter 21, Section 21.1.2.

EQUIVALENT DOSE

The equivalent dose (H_T) has been described in Section 21.1.2. In radiological protection, it is the absorbed dose averaged over a tissue or organ (rather than at a point) and weighted for the radiation quality that is of interest. The weighting factor for this purpose is now called the radiation weighting factor, w_R, and is selected for the type and energy of the radiation incident on the body or, in the case of sources within the body, emitted by the radionuclide. The equivalent dose in tissue T is given by

$$H_T = \sum_R w_R \cdot D_{T,R} \qquad (22.1)$$

where $D_{T,R}$ is the absorbed dose averaged over the tissue or organ T, due to radiation R. The unit of equivalent dose is the joule per kilogram and called the sievert (Sv) (Rolf Sievert, 1896–1966; Swedish radiologist). The non-SI unit is the rem where 100 rem = 1 Sv. The basic units of radiation exposure are given in Table 21.4.

The equivalent dose is measured in sieverts (Sv) and forms the foundation unit for other parameters in radiation protection. Some variations on the basic equivalent dose term are defined in Table 22.1 taking account of **deep** and **shallow** doses. ICRP 60 considers these other quantities describing them as individual dose equivalent (penetrating or deep dose) and individual dose equivalent (superficial or shallow dose). A further quantity, expressed as an eye dose equivalent, is sometimes used.

The equivalent dose measurement does not consider the different radiosensitivities of each tissue or organ so a further tissue weighting factor w_T is used which allows for the different radiosensitivities of the

various organs and tissues. **Radiation weighting factors** w_R modify the mean absorbed dose in any tissue or organ according to the detriment caused by different types of radiation (alpha, beta, neutrons) relative to photon radiation (gamma and X-rays). Values of w_R are taken to be independent of a specific tissue. Numerical values are specified in terms of type and energy of radiations either incident on the human body or emitted by radionuclides residing within the body. The same value of w_R is applicable to all tissues and organs of a body independent of the fact that the actual radiation field in the body may vary between different tissues and organs due to attenuation and degradation of the primary radiation and the production of secondary radiations of different radiation quality in the body. The selection of w_R is based on the relative biological effectiveness (RBE) of the different radiations with respect to stochastic effects. An RBE value is given by the ratio of the absorbed doses of two types of radiation producing the same specified biological effect (dose value of a reference radiation divided by the corresponding dose value of the radiation considered). The reference radiation is normally gamma or X-radiation with an accepted RBE of 1. For radiation protection, the RBE values at low doses and low dose rates are of particular interest.

TISSUE WEIGHTING FACTORS AND THE EFFECTIVE DOSE

The concept of 'effective dose' associated with a given exposure involves weighting individual tissues of interest, in the body, to reflect the relative **detriments**. Detriments are expressed typically as estimated mortality, loss of expected lifetime or some combination of these caused by a unit radiation weighted dose to each of the various tissues. Using such a system of tissue-specific weights, the sum of the tissue-specific radiation weighted doses, called the **effective dose**, is taken to be proportional to the total estimated detriment from the exposure, whatever the distribution of radiation weighted dose within the body.

The detriments are essentially the same for cancer and hereditary disease and, in certain instances, can be combined. These detrimental quantities are averaged over both genders and all ages at exposure, but with certain age-specific factors taken into account. A certain number of human tissues and organs are insufficient to judge the magnitude of their radiation risk, so they are consigned to a **remainder** category.

Table 22.1 *Equivalent dose variants.*

Variant	Definition
Shallow dose equivalent, H_s	Skin or extremity; 0.07 mm tissue depth (7 mg cm^{-2})
Deep dose equivalent, H_d	Whole body; 10 mm tissue depth (1000 mg cm^{-2})
Eye dose equivalent	Dose equivalent to eye lens; 3 mm tissue depth (300 mg cm^{-2})

Table 22.2 *Tissue weighting factors w$_T$ (ICRP 60) and proposed modifications to w$_T$ (ICRP 2005 report).*

ICRP 60		ICRP (proposed)	
Tissue or organ	**w$_T$**	**Tissue or organ**	**w$_T$**
Gonads	0.20	Bone marrow	0.12
Bone marrow (red)	0.12	Breast	0.12
Colon	0.12	Colon	0.12
Lung	0.12	Lung	0.12
Stomach	0.12	Stomach	0.12
Bladder	0.05	Bladder	0.05
Breast	0.05	Esophagus	0.05
Liver	0.05	Gonads	0.05
Esophagus	0.05	Liver	0.05
Thyroid	0.05	Thyroid	0.05
Skin	0.01	Bone surface	0.01
Bone surface	0.01	Brain	0.01
Remainder	0.05	Kidneys	0.01
		Salivary glands	0.01
		Skin	0.01
		Remainder*	0.10

*Adipose tissue, adrenals, connective tissue, extrathoracic airways, gall bladder, heart wall, lymphatic nodes, muscle, pancreas, prostate, small intestine, spleen, thymus, uterus/cervix.

Table 22.2 lists the radiosensitivity of organs defined by tissue weighting factors w$_T$. The radiation referred to is that incident on the body or emitted by a source within the body. The values of w$_T$ are used for calculating the **effective dose, E, or effective dose equivalent (EDE).**

ESTIMATION OF TISSUE WEIGHTING FACTORS AND DETRIMENT

Tissue-weighting factors, as recommended, are based on detriment-adjusted **nominal risk coefficients**. The unadjusted nominal risk coefficients were computed by averaging estimates of the radiation-associated lifetime risk for cancer incidence for two composite populations. For each of these tissues, detriment is modeled as a function of life lost, lethality and loss of quality of life. Since there is still uncertainty in the risk estimates given in ICRP 60 the probability of a fatal radiation induced cancer is termed the nominal risk coefficient. The nominal risk for an adult is $4 \times 10^{-2} \text{Sv}^{-1}$ (1:25) or $1:25\,000\,\text{mSv}^{-1}$ and for the whole population of all ages the risk is greater at $5 \times 10^{-2} \text{Sv}^{-1}$ (1:20) or $1:20\,000\,\text{mSv}^{-1}$. These estimates are based on data obtained from the National Registry for Radiation

Workers (UK) which covers 95 000 occupationally exposed workers.

In the draft revised edition ICRP 60 (2005) the tissue weighting factors are a single set of w$_T$ values that are averaged over both genders and all ages. The detriments for heritable effects and cancer following gonadal irradiation were aggregated to give a w$_T$ of 0.05. Cancer risk in salivary glands, brain and kidney, whilst not specifically quantifiable, is judged to be greater than that of other tissues in the 'remainder' fraction and for this reason each is ascribed a w$_T$ of 0.01.

This reassignment gives a w$_T$ value for the remainder tissues of 0.1 and it is proposed that this is distributed equally amongst fourteen named tissues giving approximately 0.007 each, which is lower than the w$_T$ for the lowest of the named tissues (0.01).

CANCER RISK IN DIFFERENT TISSUES

Nominal cancer risks and tissue weights were developed for twelve individual tissues and organs (esophagus, stomach, colon, liver, lung, bone surface, skin, breast, ovary, bladder, thyroid, bone marrow) with the remaining tissues and organs grouped into one 'remainder' category. These individual tissues and organs were selected because it was deemed that there was sufficient epidemiological information on the tumorgenic effects of radiation to make the judgments necessary for estimating cancer risks. Leukemia, excluding chronic lymphocytic leukemia (CLL) and multiple myeloma were included in the bone marrow category. The remainder category also includes all other tissues not explicitly evaluated as individual cancer sites.

HEREDITARY RISKS

The estimate of genetic (hereditary) risk from radiation has been substantially revised since the ICRP 60 report as a result of new information that has become available. Several factors have led to this change:

- Most radiation-induced mutations are more likely to cause multi-system developmental abnormalities rather than single gene (i.e. Mendelian) diseases; only a fraction of these are likely to be compatible with live births.
- Nearly all chronic diseases have a genetic component so the mutation component (i.e. the responsiveness of these diseases to an alteration in

mutation rate) is small. Chronic diseases respond only minimally to a radiation-induced increase in mutation rate.

- The ICRP 60 report made the implicit assumption that all genetic diseases are lethal. This impression has been revised and a lethality fraction for genetic diseases has now been designated as 80%.
- New genetic risk coefficients recommended by ICRP consider exposure and genetic risk for two generations only – this equilibrium value is now judged to be of questionable scientific validity.

The recalculated risk associated with gonadal dose is now estimated to be ≈ 20 cases per $10\,000\,\mathrm{Sv}^{-1}$ rather than ≈ 100 cases per $10\,000\,\mathrm{Sv}^{-1}$ in ICRP 60, and the corresponding relative contribution of the gonadal dose to the total detriment is now estimated as 4, versus the former 18.3. This revision is reflected in the lower tissue weighting value.

UNCERTAINTY AND SENSITIVITY ANALYSES

The estimated risk of radiation-induced cancer is uncertain and the sources of statistical uncertainty are many. For a chronic or low-dose exposure, the estimate and its statistical uncertainty is further complicated by an uncertain dose and dose-rate effectiveness factor (DDREF), a process that both reduces the estimate and further increases its uncertainty.

When an estimate based on a particular exposed population is applied to other populations or to other radiation sources, further uncertainty is introduced. Differences between radiation sources can produce uncertainty due to random or systematic error in dose estimates in either the original or secondary population.

Risk-based radiation protection depends heavily on the assumption that estimates based on studies of informative exposed populations, such as the Life Span Study cohort of atomic-bomb survivors, can be applied to other exposed populations. Transfers of risk estimates between populations pose a particularly difficult problem for cancer sites for which baseline rates differ widely between the two populations.

22.1.2 Whole-body effective dose or effective dose equivalent

The equivalent dose H_T enables individual organ or tissue radiation exposure to be described independent

of radiation type using weighting factors w_R. However, each tissue has a different radiosensitivity and in order to recognize these different sensitivities (e.g. for breast, lung, bone) **tissue weighting factors** w_T are used. These represent the risk of stochastic damage from irradiation of that organ or tissue as a total risk figure as if the **whole body** had been irradiated uniformly.

The quantity **effective dose** is introduced in order to measure the risk of stochastic effects. The measure of risk at exposures corresponding to the dose limits should be dependent on the manner of irradiation – whether the body is irradiated uniformly or non-uniformly from either external radiation or from intakes of radionuclides. This has been attempted by weighting the **absorbed dose** depending on the biological effectiveness of the different radiation qualities; this is the **radiation weighting factor** w_R. The summation of these radiation weighted doses to the various tissues and organs of the body is then modified by **tissue weighting factors**, w_T, which yields the **effective dose**. Tissue weighting factors allow for the varying radiation sensitivity of tissues and the induction of stochastic effects.

TISSUE WEIGHTING FACTORS (W_T)

These have been obtained from a representative population (wide age range and both sexes). The values published in ICRP 60 range from 0.01 (skin) up to 0.2 (gonads). The weighting factors listed have been estimated for important tissues. For purposes of calculation the remainder consists of adrenals, brain, intestine, uterus and other separate organs.

The values have changed from their introduction in ICRP 26 (1977) to revised values in ICRP 60 (1990). A more recent revision is presently being considered (ICRP revised 2005) which has reassessed the radiosensitivity of breast tissue and the gonads. The list includes those organs that are likely to be selectively irradiated and some of these organs are known to be susceptible to cancer induction. As more investigations are made and other tissues more closely investigated, and their radiosensitivity identified, they may also be included in later lists for w_T.

At higher doses, above certain **threshold** doses, **tissue reactions** (formally called **deterministic effects**) are induced which can be acute effects, and late effects such as cataracts of the lens of the eye, necrotic and fibrotic reactions in many tissues and organs. This threshold varies with the dose rate, especially for exposures to low LET radiation. High LET radiation (neutrons and alpha particles) cause more damage per unit of absorbed energy than low LET radiation. Values of **relative biological effectiveness** (RBE) for tissue reactions for high-LET compared with low-LET radiations have been determined for different biological effects for different tissues and organs.

Both w_R and w_T may change from time to time as new evidence accrues, so derived quantities that rely on these parameters may also change. This is the case for previous values of w_T published in ICRP 26 (1977) which were reviewed giving the revised figures published in ICRP 60 (1990). These have been studied again and suggested revisions given in an ICRP consultative document made available in 2005 (see Table 22.2).

EFFECTIVE DOSE (*E*) OR EFFECTIVE DOSE EQUIVALENT (*EDE*)

This is a quantity which describes the dose to the whole body and is derived from the equivalent dose. This quantity expresses the overall measure of health detriment associated with each irradiated tissue or organ as a whole body dose and considers the radiosensitivity of each irradiated organ or tissue. Both equivalent dose (for a single tissue or organ) and effective dose (for the whole body) are quantities intended for radiological protection use, providing a method for estimating the probability of stochastic effects at low doses.

If the risk per equivalent dose for the various exposed tissues or organs of the body ($H_T \times w_T$) is summed, a value is obtained for the overall risk per sievert of irradiating the whole body. This sum is the effective dose, E, and represents the summed organ or tissue doses as an overall whole-body dose:

$$E = \sum H_T \cdot w_T \qquad (22.2)$$

where, as before, H_T is the equivalent dose in tissue or organ T and w_T is the tissue weighting factor given in Table 22.2. Using the figure obtained from effective dose a radiation burden to the individual can be compared between various patient investigations, for instance a whole body dose from a nuclear medicine bone scan and CT or projection radiography. In both cases the patient dose can be compared as the same effective whole-body dose E using eqn 22.2.

As a simple example, a chest radiograph having a measured organ dose of 0.2 mSv and a w_T of 0.12 for the lung (from Table 22.2) would represent a whole-body dose equivalent of 0.2 × 0.12 or 0.024 mSv. Box 22.1 calculates E from eqn 22.2 for a nuclear medicine study and a CT of the chest involving multiple organs. Both groups of weighted sensitivities listed in Table 22.2 are used and the influence of the revised figures can be seen for both gonad and breast contributions.

The evolution of dose quantities used in radiation protection for individuals and the population is given

---

Box 22.1 Effective dose equivalents, *E*

Nuclear medicine

Consider a nuclear medicine bone investigation where 600 MBq (20 mCi) ^{99m}Tc-MDP is estimated to give the following equivalent dose values:

Organ	Dose (mSv)	w_T (ICRP 60)	w_T (ICRP revised)
Bone marrow	10	0.12	0.12
Bone surface	15	0.01	0.01
Bladder	65	0.05	0.05
Gonads	4	0.2	0.05

Using ICRP 60 the effective dose, E, is $\Sigma H_T \times w_T$, or 5.4 mSv. Using ICRP (revised) the effective dose, E, is $\Sigma H_T \times w_T$ or 4.8 mSv. Thus there is an 11% reduction in the estimated risk using revised w_T values.

Radiology

A CT study of the chest (CTDI*w* of 30 mSv) gives the following doses (ICRP 87):

Organ	Dose (mSv)	w_T (ICRP 60)	w_T (ICRP revised)
Breast	21.0	0.05	0.12
Lung	23.5	0.12	0.12
Bone marrow	5.17	0.12	0.12
Thyroid	2.30	0.12	0.05

Using ICRP 60 the effective dose, E, is $\Sigma H_T \times w_T$, or 4.6 mSv. Using ICRP (revised) the effective dose, E, is $\Sigma H_T \times w_T$ or 6.0 mSv. Thus, using the revised w_T values indicates there is 32% increase in the estimated risk.

Table 22.3 *Individual dosimetric terms.*

Measure	Unit	Derivation	Application
Organ or tissue dose			
Absorbed dose, D	gray	Energy/mass, $J\ kg^{-1}$	Average dose to organ
Equivalent dose, H_T	sievert	$H_T = \Sigma\ D_T \times w_R$	Radiation dose independent of radiation type
Individual whole-body dose			
Effective dose, E (effective dose equivalent, EDE)	sievert	$E = \Sigma\ H_T \times w_T$	Whole-body dose (see Box 22.1)
Accumulated organ or tissue dose			
Committed equivalent dose, $H_{T(\tau)}$	sievert	$H_{T(\tau)} = H_T \times \tau$	Equivalent dose H_T to a single organ over a stated time, τ
Accumulated whole-body dose			
Committed effective dose, $E(\tau)$	sievert	$E_{(\tau)} = \Sigma\ w_T \times H_{T(\tau)}$	Effective dose to the whole body over a stated time, τ
Accumulated population dose (where the population number = N)			
Collective equivalent dose, S_T	man-sievert	$S_T = H_{T(\tau)} \times N$	Dose to an individual organ for a population (Box 22.2)
Collective effective dose, S	man-sievert	$S = E_{(\tau)} \times N$	Dose to the whole body for a population

in Table 22.3. The effective dose estimate is intended as a principal protection quantity for establishing radiation protection guidance. It should not be used to assess risks of stochastic effects in retrospective situations for exposures in identified individuals, nor should it be used in epidemiological evaluations of human exposure. Certain diagnostic radiology procedures have been compared using the effective dose, by various manufacturers and clinicians; this is not valid. Its main use is to enable external and internal irradiation to be added as a means to demonstrate compliance with restrictions on dose, which are expressed in effective dose. In this sense effective dose is used for regulatory purposes worldwide.

Effective dose is a dose **estimate**, defined by doses to the body and so in principle and practice, it is a non-measurable quantity. For estimating values of effective dose, conversion coefficients are generally applied which relate the effective dose of a person to other measurable quantities, e.g. air kerma or particle fluence in the case of external exposure or activity concentrations etc. in the case of internal exposure.

22.1.3 Accumulated dose (committed doses)

If a person is subjected to a radiation burden over a period of time then **committed** dose quantities are

used. The time integral for the equivalent dose is the **committed equivalent dose** $H_{T(\tau)}$. If τ is not specified then it is assumed the dose is received over a 50 year period (70 years for children). Similarly, the **committed effective dose** E_τ is accumulated over a defined time period τ. This would describe long-term X-ray exposures in a radiology department to a member of staff where the time period is defined.

COMMITTED EQUIVALENT DOSE ($H_{T(\tau)}$)

This is a subsidiary dosimetric quantity of equivalent single organ or tissue dose and is the time integral over time τ in years, taken as 50 for adults and 70 for children, following an intake of radioactive material. The committed equivalent dose is defined as

$$H_{T(\tau)} = H_T \times \tau \qquad (22.3)$$

An example is calculated in Box 22.2 for radon inhalation over a 50 year period. Radon exposure varies depending on the underlying geology of the particular environment but comprises more than 40% of most people's background radiation.

COMMITTED EFFECTIVE DOSE, $E_{(\tau)}$

If the committed organ or tissue equivalent dose is multiplied by the appropriate tissue weighting factors then the sum of these products will be the committed

Box 22.2 Committed equivalent dose

The mean equivalent dose to the lung for inhaled radon is estimated as 6.6 mSv, giving an $H_{T(\tau)}$ value for 50 years as 330 mSv.

Box 22.3 Committed effective dose, $E_{(\tau)}$

The mean effective dose for inhaled radon is estimated as

$$6.6\,\text{mSv} \times 0.12w_T = 0.8\,\text{mSv}$$

This gives an $E_{(\tau)}$ value for a 50 year period of 40 mSv. A radiation worker receiving, on average, $1.5\,\text{mSv}\,\text{y}^{-1}$ with a working lifetime of 40 years would received an $E_{(\tau)}$ of 60 mSv.

effective dose. The committed effective dose is defined as

$$E_{(\tau)} = \sum w_T \cdot H_{T(\tau)} \qquad (22.4)$$

A calculation for committed effective dose is given in Box 22.3, following on from the radon theme in the previous example.

22.1.4 Population dose (collective dose)

For the purposes of assessing the overall effect of radiation dose on a large group of people or entire populations the individual equivalent or effective doses described in the previous section are multiplied by the population number exposed. This gives a collective dose figure. Overall increases or reductions in dose to the population can then be assessed and, in some instances, a financial costing given to attempts at exposure reduction.

COLLECTIVE EQUIVALENT DOSE (S_T)

This quantity describes the total radiation exposure to a specific tissue or organ in a group of individuals

$$S_T = \sum H_{T(\tau)} \times N \qquad (22.5)$$

where N is the number of individuals of a specified population receiving a mean organ equivalent dose H_T over a specified time (τ).

COLLECTIVE EFFECTIVE DOSE (S)

This is the whole-body exposure to a **population group** exposed to radioactive materials in the environment and can cover successive generations of the population being studied. An example of collective effective dose using this measurement would be a community of 40 000 people receiving 2 mSv and another 20 000 who receive 4 mSv. The collective dose in each case is 80 man-Sv (population × dose) which, on present estimates, would result in one radiation-induced cancer. Incidentally, the expected natural cancer incidence in a normal population of 40 000 would be 6400, so the effects of this low radiation dose could not be distinguished.

$$S = E_{(\tau)} \times N \qquad (22.6)$$

The UK population of 60 million people who receive approximately 2 mSv background radiation have a collective dose of 120 000 man-Sv. On the above estimate this would result in 1500 radiation-induced cancers over a period of time (cf. there are 6000 deaths per year as a result of road traffic accidents). The United States population of 240 million people exposed to a similar background would have a collective dose of 480 000 man-Sv, giving 6000 radiation-induced cancers (cf. 44 500 deaths in 1990 as a result of road traffic accidents). The example given in Box 22.4 describes the expected organ dose (lung) for a total UK population from radon inhalation, expressed as a 'collective equivalent dose'. Box 22.5 uses data from a nuclear power facility to calculate collective effective dose for the working population.

22.1.5 ICRU alternative dosimetry

The ICRU quantities listed in ICRU Report 39 (ICRU, 1985) give reasonable approximations of the effective dose and the equivalent dose to the skin. It is convenient to consider the determination of quantities related to the effective dose equivalent and to the dose equivalent in the skin which has been done separately for **environmental** and **individual** monitoring. These quantities are based on the concept of the dose equivalent at a point in the ICRU sphere.

Box 22.4 Collective equivalent dose, S_T

If the committed equivalent dose ($H_{T(\tau)}$) to the lung from inhaled radon is estimated as just over 6.6 mSv per year. For a population of 60 million (as in the UK, for example) the collective equivalent dose (S_T) would be

$$\frac{(60 \times 10^6) \times H_{T(\tau)}}{1000}$$

or approximately 400 000 man-Sv.

For a population of approximately 250 million (as in the USA) S_T would be 1 650 000 man-Sv. Present estimates indicate one radiation induced cancer per 80 man-Sv so for the UK population one would expect 5000 radon induced cancers. For the US population there would be an expected lung cancer rate of just over 20 000. However, in many areas the population radon dose is less than the 6.6 mSv quoted here.

From the relevant cancer registries the approximate incidence of lung cancer due to smoking is about 20 times that due to radon.

Box 22.5 Collective effective dose

Modified data from a nuclear facility reveal the following data:

Dose range (mSv)	Number of workers	Percentage
< 5	4225	65
5 to 15	1625	25
15 to 50	650	10
Total	6500	

The average annual dose is 5 mSv so the collective effective for this population is 32.5 man-Sv.

ENVIRONMENTAL MONITORING

Linking the external radiation field to the effective dose, and to the equivalent dose in the skin, is introduced for purposes of environmental and area monitoring. The first of these, the **ambient dose equivalent**, $H^*(d)$, is appropriate for strongly penetrating radiation, the second, the **directional dose equivalent**, $H'(d)$, is suitable for weakly penetrating radiation. The ambient dose equivalent, $H^*(d)$, at a point in a radiation field, is the dose equivalent that would be produced by the corresponding aligned and expanded field. The directional dose equivalent, $H'(d)$, at a point in a radiation field, is the dose equivalent that would be produced by the corresponding expanded field in the ICRU sphere at depth d on a radius in a specified direction.

INDIVIDUAL MONITORING

Two concepts are introduced for purposes of individual monitoring. The first of these concepts, the **individual dose equivalent**, penetrating, $H_p(d)$, is appropriate for organs and tissues deeply situated in the body which will be irradiated by strongly penetrating radiation; and the second, the individual dose equivalent, superficial, $H_s(d)$, is suitable for superficial organs and tissues which will be irradiated by both weakly and strongly penetrating radiation.

The US Nuclear Regulatory Commission (NRC) defines very similar quantities to ICRP. The committed dose equivalent ($H_{T.50}$) is the dose equivalent to organs or tissues during a 50 year period. Similarly committed effective dose equivalent ($H_{E.50}$) is $\Sigma H_{T.50} \cdot W_T$. The NRC also defines the **total effective dose equivalent** (TEDE) as the sum of the **deep dose** H_d for external radiation (Table 22.1) and **committed effective dose equivalent** $H_{E.50}$ for internal radiation exposure (Table 22.3).

Dose limits imposed by some authorities (USA) still retain the recommendations given by ICRP 26 although modifications have been made and the two sets of worker dose limits are now very similar except for the whole-body dose figure. An **agreement state** in the US complies with or exceeds federal standards which are basically ICRP 26.

22.2 OCCUPATIONAL EXPOSURE

In general, recommendation number 60 made by the ICRP in 1990 has been recognized internationally. Its ideas have been incorporated into the safety regulations of various countries and affect both staff and patients. The concept of 'as low as reasonably achievable' (the ALARA principle), justification of exposure, optimization and dose constraint, dose limits and the variety of other concepts originating or developed in ICRP 60 have found their way into European legislation via Euratom Directives, and into North American radiation safety legislation via their National Council on Radiation Protection and Measurements. Other national bodies in Africa, Asia, Australia, for example, have also been influenced by ICRP recommendations.

This section therefore uses the ICRP 60 and, in particular, the Euratom Directives as the foundation material for radiation protection of staff and patients. Any variation from this basic theme will be mentioned.

The primary aim of radiological protection is to provide an appropriate standard of protection for three categories – patients, staff, and public – without unduly limiting the beneficial practices giving rise to radiation exposure. The basic components of protection for all three categories are justification, optimization, and constraint.

Justification of a practice implies that it does more good than harm. No practice involving exposures to radiation should be adopted unless it produces at least sufficient benefit to the exposed individuals or to society to offset the radiation detriment it causes.

Optimization of protection implies that the margin of good over harm is maximized. All reasonable steps should be taken to adjust the protection so maximizing the net benefit, economic and social factors being taken into account. Procedures and equipment are updated from time to time, where practical, to achieve this.

Constraint is an important part of optimization and places a responsibility on practitioners to review dose levels and reduce them to as low as reasonably achievable or practical (ALARA and ALARP principles) providing that economic and social conditions allow.

The application of individual **dose limits** gives a standard of protection for exposed individuals, staff and public but these do not apply to medical exposures. However, applying the principle of constraint will have the effect of reducing dose levels significantly below the imposed dose limits.

When applied to a radiological or clinical environment that uses radiation, these principles determine the safe levels of radiation for:

- **Occupational exposure**, which is the exposure incurred at work, and principally as a result of work. It is defined as all exposures occurring at

work but limits its use to those exposures that are the responsibility of the operating management (i.e. hospital or clinic). All exposure to workers is occupational exposure and dose limits apply.
- **Medical exposures**, which occur when persons are exposed to radiation as part of their diagnosis or treatment.
- **Public exposure**, which comprises all other exposures.

Each exposure type embraces the principles of justification and optimization. Although dose limits strictly apply to occupational and public exposure the introduction of dose reference levels enables medical exposures to be as low as reasonably achievable and still maintain diagnostic quality images.

22.2.1 Legislation

The European Council Directive 96/29/EURATOM of May 1996 lays down the basic safety standards (BSS) for the protection of the health of workers and the general public against the dangers arising from ionizing radiation. Occupational exposures are those incurred at work that can reasonably be regarded as the responsibility of the operating management. Particular attention is given to the principle of optimization of protection, which is considered as being of central importance in the control of occupational exposure.

Management should establish radiological protection programs that explicitly recognize the importance of commitment to the principle at all levels recognizing that cost–benefit analysis may assist in reaching decisions on **optimization**. **Dose constraints** would support the optimization process. The content of the Directive for Basic Safety Standards (BSS) is listed in Table 22.4.

TRAINING

As in the existing statutory instrument, there will be requirements for training. Practitioners and others involved in medical exposures will be required to have adequate and practical training in their fields as well as competence in radiation protection. A new requirement will be for continuing education and training after qualification. While the medical and dental councils will have continuing responsibility for recognizing qualifications, the onus has been placed on member states to ensure the provision of

Table 22.4 *Important points identified in European legislation.*

Application	Directive articles
Dose limits for exposed workers	Risk estimates Classification of exposed workers – Category A – Category B Information and training Monitoring the workplace Individual monitoring
Dose constraints	Classification and delineation of areas – Controlled areas – Supervised areas Risk estimates
Dose limits for the public Special protection (pregnancy and breastfeeding)	Risk estimates Early declaration of pregnancy

suitable training programs by, for example, including training in radiation protection in core curricula of medical and dental schools.

RISK ESTIMATE

The Council Directive (BSS) requires a formal evaluation for identifying the nature and magnitude of the radiation risks to workers and other persons and of the measures necessary for their protection arising from any new practice or existing practice where such an evaluation has not been previously undertaken. Table 22.4 indicates that estimating the risks of any procedure can be influenced by dose limits and constraints for workers (see later). This evaluation must include consideration of potential exposures and will provide the basis for the establishment of written radiation safety procedures appropriate to the radiological risk and the nature of the work being undertaken.

EQUIPMENT FOR MEDICAL X-RAY EXPOSURES

X-ray equipment must be provided with the means of informing the user of the quantity of radiation produced during that procedure. Every user must have a quality assurance program in place which will include acceptance testing of new equipment before first use, performance testing at appropriate intervals, and dose assessments where appropriate. Suspected incidents

or over-exposures will be required to be notified. The new directive pays particular attention to the use of appropriate equipment and techniques for the medical exposure of children, for health screening, and for exposures involving high doses to the patient. There is a need to adopt detailed **quality assurance programs** and to ensure that staff are adequately trained in these practices.

22.2.2 Classification of workers: dose limits

A radiation worker is normally defined as an individual engaged in work under license issued by a national agency. The occupational dose is the dose received in the course of employment and does not include doses received from background radiation.

THE WORKING YEAR

When calculating a radiation worker's dose the time over which the person is potentially exposed is taken to be based on a common working day of 8 h (09:00 to 17:00) and a 5 day week with 50 weeks per year (allowing for 2 weeks' holiday); this gives 250 working days per year for a typical hospital employee, or a working period of 2000 h per year.

CLASSIFICATION OF WORKERS: DOSE LIMITS

There is a legal requirement for classifying radiation workers in both Europe and America. Estimated risks for radiation-induced cancer increased by a factor of 3 to 4 since ICRP 26 making it necessary to reconsider the annual dose limits for workers which is now presented in ICRP 60 (Table 22.5). Alternative dose limits are given in Table 22.6. These are sometimes observed in countries not influenced by European Union legislation. The restrictions on effective dose for workers are sufficient to ensure that deterministic effects will be avoided in all tissues and organs except the lens of the eye (which makes no contribution to the effective dose) and skin which may be subjected to localized high exposures such as radionuclide dispensing and angiography; separate equivalent dose limits are imposed on these tissues. Previous reports (ICRP 26) divided workers into:

- Category A workers, who are likely to receive a major proportion of the dose limit

Table 22.5 *Recommended annual dose limits.*

Application	Occupational (mSv)	Public (mSv)
Effective dose	20 (averaged over a defined period of 5 years)	1
Annual equivalent dose		
Lens of the eye	150	15
Skin	500	50
Hands and feet	500	50
Fetal dose	5 (see text)	1
Recommended constraint level		0.3 mSv y^{-1}

Table 22.6 *Alternative dose limits.*

Category	Dose (mSv)
Effective dose equivalent (EDE)	50
Dose equivalent to eye	150
Dose equivalent to any organ except eye (deep dose)	500
Dose equivalent to skin (shallow dose)	500
Minor ($\approx$ 18 years) respectively	5
	15
	50
	50
Embryo or fetus	5, over 9 months
Public	1, per year

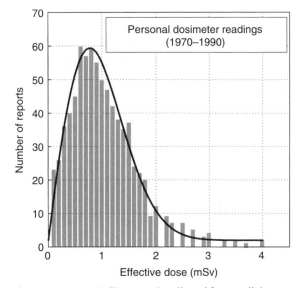

Figure 22.1 *Yearly film records collected from radiology sources for the 1970s, 1980s, and 1990s, showing a sharp decline in high dose rates over these decades.*

- Category B workers, who are likely to receive a minor proportion of the radiation dose

This clear division does not appear in ICRP 60 but it probably could continue in a modified form in order to distinguish those workers who are liable to receive higher radiation doses (fluoroscopy).

CATEGORY A

These workers would receive three tenths of any maximum. They are not normally seen in diagnostic radiology but high radiation levels can be approached in nuclear medicine (e.g. hands of a radiopharmacist) and in biplanar cine-angiography (e.g. cardiologists' eyes). They would receive up to a maximum of 15 mSv whole body according to ICRP 60. High exposure to the extremities can also place a worker in this category.

CATEGORY B

This is the general category commonly found in diagnostic radiology. Previous definitions (ICRP 26)

imposed dose limits for this category as above one tenth but below three tenths of any maximum. Most recent definitions redefine this category for a worker who does not exceed 5 mSv per year. The bar chart in Fig. 22.1 shows the greatest proportion of radiology workers return readings less than 1 mSv per year.

These dose limits do not apply to persons undergoing medical exposures or to carers, i.e. persons knowingly and willingly helping (other than as part of their work) in the support and comfort of patients undergoing medical diagnosis. This new flexibility is particularly needed for hospitals when radionuclides are administered to patients for therapeutic purposes.

CARERS

Members of the public and/or a patient's relatives are often required either to be present during a radiographic procedure or accompany a nuclear medicine patient. Once their exposure has been **justified**, it is proposed that a **dose constraint** of 5 mSv should be used at the planning stage. There is also a requirement to provide patients injected with radionuclides with a set of written instructions before leaving the hospital with a view to minimizing doses to persons who may come into in contact with them.

STAFF PREGNANCY

In the radiology workplace the ICRP recommends no particular restriction on women of child bearing age who are not pregnant. Radiology staff consistently show very low levels of radiation exposure therefore the previous controls for occupational exposure of women of child bearing age working in diagnostic radiology are no longer thought necessary at present. The consequence, however, of ICRP 60 and future legislation may affect future working practices for pregnant staff. The European current maximum for pregnant staff is 5 mSv (see Table 22.5) but since the fetus is to be treated as a member of the public its limit should be 1 mSv. ICRP 60 requires that once pregnancy has been declared the conceptus is protected by applying an equivalent dose limit to the surface of the abdomen of 2 mSv for the remainder of the pregnancy. The personal dosimeter record therefore should not exceed 0.14 mSv per month if the declared term exposure (7 months) is not to exceed 1 mSv (ICRP 84).

The principal criterion is that employment should be of a type that does not carry a significant probability of high accidental staff doses (e.g. fluoroscopy and perhaps nuclear medicine). Personal dosimeter records should be reported at 2 week intervals for this individual instead of each month.

Table 22.7 gives the expected natural incidence of abnormality for the fetus as 95.93% or 1:24.6. An exposure of 10 mSv increases this risk to only 1:23.9 although it has been estimated that a **risk of malignancy** before the 15th birthday from a 6 mSv exposure during the third trimester increases the nominal lifetime cancer risk to about 1:3000, of which half will be fatal (Doll and Wakeford, 1997).

Table 22.7 *Additional risk to the developing fetus from radiation. The probabilities have been calculated for developing cancer or an organ malfunction in later childhood.*

Dose (mSv)	Probability of a normal fetus (%)	Increased risk (%)
0.0	95.93	0.0
0.5	95.928	0.002
1.0	95.922	0.008
2.5	95.91	0.02
5.0	95.88	0.05
10.0	95.83	0.1

22.2.3 Dose optimization and constraint

If the procedures of justification of practices and of **optimization** of protection have been conducted effectively, there will be few cases where limits on individual (staff) dose will have to be applied. However, such limits provide a clearly defined boundary for these more subjective procedures and prevent excessive individual detriment, which might result from a combination of practices.

Accumulated evidence from film badge reports is now a more significant driving force for staff exposure reduction than recommendations from national and international radiation commissions. This evidence has encouraged **constraint levels** to be maintained in radiology departments.

With the widespread use of **dose constraints** and practical restrictions on the sources of public exposure (e.g. X-ray and nuclear medicine waiting rooms, toilets) generally applicable staff and public dose limits are rarely limiting in practice.

The recent European legislation encourages continuous review of dose levels in order to restrict exposures as far as reasonably achievable. This optimization process introduces a requirement for dose constraints in order to accomplish this. A dose constraint is a restriction on the predicted dose to persons from a defined source. Dose constraints must not be confused with dose limits. They are mainly used at the planning stage in radiation protection whenever optimization is involved and an investigation should be carried out by the user if a dose constraint is consistently exceeded.

DOSE OPTIMIZATION

This is specific to the radiation source, the work practice, and the workplace for which the protection is to be optimized. Optimization should anticipate radiation problems and so be used prospectively and not as a form of subsidiary dose limit to be applied retrospectively. Care in applying optimization for occupational exposure of medical and supporting staff is necessary when the protection arrangements would restrict the care given to patients.

DOSE CONSTRAINTS

The new recommendations introduce the term constraint which indicates a restriction to be applied to individual doses. A constraint on the upper limits of dose is seen as a regulatory requirement and should be set by regulatory agencies based on experience of the level of exposure likely to be met in the day to day operations. This is the ALARA principle in operation and can be viewed as a type of risk estimate.

The constraints used in the optimization of protection for those who work predominantly in X-ray diagnosis can be low. Specific consideration is given to the management of the exposure of women of reproductive age at work.

A constraint ensures that the sum of doses to an individual from different practices to which he/she may be exposed does not exceed the dose limit. This would include the design and shielding of rooms that are used for radiology and nuclear medicine. When the operation is up and running deployment of dose monitors (TLD wall badges) will measure whether the doses actually received are as low as reasonably achievable (ALARA). These TLDs would be placed outside shielded areas such as corridors and patient waiting areas.

There will therefore be a requirement to classify workers as **exposed workers** if a dose of 1 mSv per year might be received. This is a change from the current 5 mSv level. These exposed workers will be divided into Category B workers, those liable to receive a dose of 1 to 6 mSv in a year, and Category A workers, those liable to receive a dose of 6 mSv or greater in a year. This is a large reduction from the previous value of 5 mSv and 15 mSv in a year, respectively. It is emphasized that potential exposures must be taken into account in classifying workers. Medical surveillance and personnel monitoring will

Table 22.8 *Recommended dose limits for workers, when constraint principles are applied.*

Constraint limit	Occupational dose (mSv)
Effective dose (whole body)	5
Lens of the eye	50
Hands, feet, and skin	150
Fetus	1

Table 22.9 *Recommended constraint levels for various categories of staff.*

Staff category	Dose (mSv)
Radiotherapy staff	10
Diagnostic radiologists	5
Diagnostic radiographers	1
Nuclear medicine staff	5
Other hospital staff	1

continue to be required for exposed persons with more detailed requirements for Category A workers, as heretofore.

The trend shown by personnel dosimeter readings plotted in Fig. 22.1 indicates that low values can be implied and Table 22.8 suggests practical constraints that may be applied to clinical radiology. These are annual maximum dose limits that should not be exceeded routinely. Table 22.9 suggests practical constraint levels for various clinical staff members in radiology departments offering both diagnostic and therapy services.

The BSS Directive requires some form of radiation protection for all workplaces where there is a possibility of exposure to ionizing radiation in excess of 1 mSv. The previous practice of classifying working areas as **supervised** or **controlled** on the basis of potential dose is to be maintained, i.e. a controlled area being one in which a dose of 6 mSv might be received in a year and a supervised area one in which the dose is 1 mSv in a year.

22.2.4 Working environment

DESIGNATION OF WORKPLACES

Consideration has to be given to the definitions of **controlled** and **supervised areas**, to the monitoring of workers, and to the recording of doses. The control of occupational exposure in medicine can be simplified and made more effective by the designation of workplaces into two types:

- **Controlled areas** are those where special procedures apply and where radiation sources are likely to be present. Signs at the entrances to controlled areas should be used to convey this information to employees, especially maintenance staff. The use of mobile sources (e.g. mobile X-ray sets) or the existence of waiting rooms for nuclear medicine patients calls for some flexibility in the definition of designated areas.
- **Supervised areas** are those in which the working conditions are kept under review, but special procedures are not normally needed. The conditions in supervised areas should be such that any employee should be able to enter with a minimum of formality.

One difficult decision in all occupational exposure is the selection of workers who should be individually monitored. Two major factors should influence the decision:

- The expected level of dose or intake in relation to the relevant limits
- The likely variations in the doses and intakes

In medicine, it should be used for all those who work in controlled areas. It should be considered for those who work regularly in supervised areas unless it is clear that their doses will be consistently low. Alternative definitions commonly applied to radiation work areas are listed in Table 22.10.

ICRP 60 recommends these measures are kept under review but special procedures are not warranted. Controlled and supervised areas can be used as normal rooms when the X-ray units are switched off. This, of course, does not apply to nuclear medicine laboratories. Other radiation areas are distinguished in some US regulations: a **radiation area** would be where a dose rate is measured of $50\,\mu\mathrm{Sv}\,h^{-1}$ at 30 cm from the source (or barrier), a **high radiation area** where this is $1\,\mathrm{mSv}\,h^{-1}$ at 30 cm and a **very high radiation area** where $5\,\mathrm{Gy}\,h^{-1}$ at 1 m can occur.

MACHINE SHIELDING

Local shielding around equipment (under and overcouch fluoroscopy or cantilevered C-arm) can

Table 22.10 *Alternative classification of radiation areas.*

Area	Exposure
Radiation area	$50\,\mu\mathrm{Sv}\,h^{-1}$ at 30 cm
High radiation area	$1\,\mathrm{mSv}\,h^{-1}$ at 30 cm
Very high radiation area	$5\,\mathrm{Gy}\,h^{-1}$ at 1 m
Controlled area	Likely to exceed 0.3 of any limit
Supervised area	Likely to exceed 0.1 of any limit
Restricted area	Access limited by licensee
Unrestricted area	Uncontrolled access $< 20\,\mu\mathrm{Sv}$ year^{-1} (2 mrem year^{-1})

significantly reduce radiation dose to staff. The undercouch design usually comes equipped with a flexible lead screen surrounding the image intensifier. The overcouch unit can have a short flexible lead curtain fitted to the tube housing. Ceiling mounted lead glass shields, in the close vicinity of the X-ray housing can be used for cine-angiography.

22.2.5 Public exposure levels

The public are here defined as other hospital staff members (secretarial, portering, and nursing) who visit the radiology department from time to time and may become exposed. It also includes people who accompany the patients and who either wait in the department or assist with the investigation (e.g. mothers of pediatric patients). Radiation exposure limits for the public are needed since maximum worker limits will not necessarily protect against deterministic effects. An arbitrary reduction to 10% of the lens and extremity doses has been imposed; this would apply to nursing staff who assist from time to time in radiology procedures. The whole-body limit has been reduced from 5 to 1 mSv per year with a recommendation that this limit be reduced still further to $0.5\,\mathrm{mSv}\,y^{-1}$. Other variations include a short term dose rate of $20\,\mu\mathrm{Sv}\,h^{-1}$ which defines an unrestricted area.

Design constraint levels of $0.3\,\mathrm{mSv}\,y^{-1}$ for areas outside the immediate radiology zones (in offices and corridors) are now recommended (Table 22.5) and these areas would require special monitoring using low noise environmental dosimeters in order to confirm this low level; dose estimation may not be

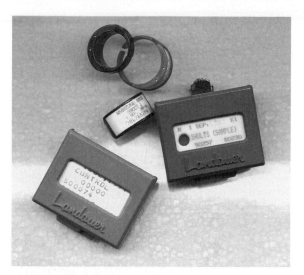

Figure 22.2 *A selection of film and thermoluminescence dosimeter radiation monitoring badges. (Courtesy of Landauer Inc.)*

acceptable. Examples of the dosimeters are given in Fig. 22.2.

22.2.6 Intervention

Intervention is the term applied to the remedial actions taken to reduce doses, or their consequences, resulting from an accident or from the misuse of a radiation source. Intervention is indicated only when the remedial actions are expected to do more good than harm. The decision to intervene should be influenced by the reduction achievable of the doses or consequences. Action to reduce the probability of subsequent accidents is important, but it is not part of intervention.

In medicine, such intervention is appropriate only for radioactive materials. Accidents and errors may occur with X-ray units but the termination of the exposures is easy and does not constitute intervention.

In diagnostic radiology the dose from a major spill of radioactive materials in nuclear medicine may be reduced by the early isolation of the contaminated area and by the controlled evacuation of staff and patients.

The decision to intervene following a major spill of radioactive materials should be specified in the emergency plans (local rules) and should be initiated immediately, without reference to formal intervention levels.

The basic principles of its System of Protection for interventions have been summarized by the ICRP as follows.

The system of radiological protection recommended by the Commission for intervention is based on the following general principles:

- The proposed intervention should do more good than harm, i.e. the reduction in detriment resulting from the reduction in dose should be sufficient to justify the harm and the costs, including social costs, of the intervention.
- Justification of interventions.
- Removal of unacceptable equipment.
- The form, scale, and duration of the intervention should be chosen so that the net benefit of the reduction of dose, i.e. the benefit of the reduction in dose less the costs of the intervention, should be as large as reasonably achievable.

INTERVENTION AND EMERGENCY PLANNING

The European Council Directive 96/29 on basic safety standards requires an assessment to be made by the user to identify all hazards with the potential to cause a radiation accident and to assess the magnitude of the risks to workers and other persons including members of the public from these hazards. Where this assessment identifies a situation where action would be required for the protection of workers or others, there will be requirements to prepare an emergency plan and to investigate the consequences of an accident. It will also be necessary to inform those concerned of the emergency plan and to carry out exercises of the arrangements in the plan at suitable intervals.

Individual dose limits have been set for occupational and public exposure. Dose limits apply to occupational and public exposures from medical procedures, but in most situations, the application of optimization of protection gives them limited relevance; personal dose levels received in practice are many times less than any dose limit. The dose limit for effective dose in occupational exposure is 20 mSv in a year, with the flexibility to go to 50 mSv in a single year provided that the total effective dose in 5 consecutive years does not exceed 100 mSv, an average annual dose of 20 mSv. Additional limits apply to the lens of the eye (150 mSv in a year), the skin (500 mSv in a year), and the hands and feet (500 mSv in a year), because these tissues may not be adequately protected by the limit on effective dose. The following points should be noted:

- The limits apply to the sum of the relevant doses from external exposure in the specified period and the 50 year committed dose (to age 70 years for children) from intakes in the same period.
- There is further provision that the effective dose should not exceed 50 mSv in any single year. Additional restrictions apply to the occupational exposure of pregnant women.
- In special circumstances, a higher value of effective dose could be allowed in a single year, provided that the average over 5 years does not exceed 1 mSv per year.
- The limitation on the effective dose provides sufficient protection for the skin against stochastic effects. An additional limit is needed for localized exposures in order to prevent deterministic effects.

STAFF DOSES IN NUCLEAR MEDICINE

These can be higher than conventional radiography staff doses if patients receiving high activity (e.g. 600 MBq ^{99m}Tc for bone or cardiac scans) are present in large numbers at any one time. Table 22.11 gives an indication of air kerma rates from such patients and if a radiographer/technologist/nurse is in close proximity, as a routine, then doses could exceed the annual radiation constraint value. For example, a department handling 25 such patients and the average proximity being 0.5 m, then over a working year this could contribute over 6 mSv to the staff member. The recommended limit for classified workers (as a result of ICRP 60) is likely to be 6 mSv.

Finger doses from syringes during dispensing and injection is reduced significantly by using syringe shields. Locating a 'butterfly needle' in the chosen vein prior to the injection also reduces the handling time of the loaded syringe and this practice can contribute

Table 22.11 *Staff exposure from a patient receiving 600 MBq of ^{99m}Tc.*

Distance (m)	C kg^{-1}h^{-1}	Air kerma (μGy h^{-1} (mR))
0.25	1.70×10^{-6}	58 (6.6)
0.5	0.92×10^{-6}	31 (3.6)
1.0	0.46×10^{-6}	15.8 (1.8)
2.0	0.13×10^{-6}	4.5 (0.5)

quite large dose savings. The annual dose limit for skin (the hand) is 500 mSv and this can be exceeded if an individual carries out most of the elution and dispensing. A finger dosimeter should be worn regularly in order to monitor these doses.

WAITING ROOMS

Radiation dose transfer from injected patient to adjacent patient is usually small provided the seating is separate and the waiting times short. Total doses range between <5 μSv to 35 μSv for the duration.

OUTPATIENTS

The major clinical advantage of nuclear medicine is its availability as an outpatient service. Non-hospitalized referrals are injected with a radionuclide preparation, undergo an imaging procedure and then leave. The short half-life of ^{99m}Tc ensures minimum radiation exposure to other members of the public but family members should be aware of contamination hazards from incontinent patients and proper precautions issued. Outpatients undergoing ^{131}I therapy are a very real hazard to the general public and clear instructions should be made available before they leave the hospital.

Exposure levels vary in radiology departments depending on equipment type and usage. There are also rooms within any department (offices and public waiting areas) that should not receive any radiation exposure.

Specified areas where radiation exposure will be experienced fall into categories of high and low exposure rates. These have been designated **controlled** and **supervised** areas, respectively. This has been abandoned in ICRP 60, however, and it is now recommended that design features or local (hospital) authorities should decide operational limits. These limits should be based on ambient exposure to radiation and intake of radionuclides. A controlled area could be defined as one where routine environmental monitoring is not sufficient to predict doses to individual workers. A supervised area could be one where doses can be predicted with confidence but may exceed the dose limit for members of the public.

Established definitions for a controlled area required workers to observe safety procedures in order to reduce their radiation exposure. These would be classified persons or patients undergoing investigation. Previous radiation thresholds required that these

Box 22.6 Exposure rates per working year (250 days)

General public (constraint)		Work area (1.0 μSv h^{-1})		Diagnostic staff (2.5 μSv h^{-1})		Category A worker (7.5 μSv h^{-1})	
Period	Total dose	Period	Total dose	Time	Total dose	Time	Total dose
1 day	1.2 μSv	1 day	8 μSv	1 day	20 μSv	1 day	60 μSv
1 week	5.0 μSv	1 week	40 μSv	1 week	0.1 mSv	1 week	0.3 mSv
1 month	24.0 μSv	1 month	160 μSv	1 month	0.4 mSv	1 month	1.2 mSv
1 year	0.3 mSv	1 year	2.0 mSv	1 year	5.0 mSv	1 year	15.0 mSv

areas would have an exposure rate exceeding one third of any maximum dose. Since the established maximum for ICRP 26 was 50 mSv one third is 15 mSv which gives an hourly exposure figure of 7.5 μSv h^{-1}. The following were commonly designated as controlled areas:

- ^{99m}Tc generator room
- Immediate vicinity of any X-ray machine (including mobiles)
- Nuclear medicine waste store

Lower radiation levels established definitions for a supervised area where the dose level is liable to exceed one tenth of the maximum dose, usually between 1 and 2.5 μSv h^{-1}. The area surrounding the control panel of X-ray equipment would be typically 1 μSv h^{-1}. Supervised areas would include:

- X-ray rooms
- Radiopharmacy
- Nuclear medicine waiting rooms

22.2.6 Radiation monitoring

ROOM MONITORING EQUIPMENT

Specification of radiation areas is given by the hospital radiation protection committee and decisions are made usually after long-term monitoring (typically a month). An easy method for deciding whether a room should have restricted access and be designated a controlled or supervised area is to position TLD badges on the walls. Immediate measurements can be obtained by a sensitive survey meter which has a large volume ionization chamber (350 cm^3 minimum). Large volume chambers have an almost flat

response with energy levels from 12 to 300 keV so are ideal for low level monitoring surveys. They have typical sensitivities from 3 μSv to 30 mSv min^{-1}. The exposure rates which define four important threshold levels are given in Box 22.6.

PERSONAL MONITORING

Radiation doses to designated workers are monitored on a regular basis by means of dosimeter badges which integrate the worker's radiation dose over a fixed period of time, usually 1 month but it could be over a shorter period (2 weeks for pregnant staff, as mentioned) or longer (2 months for occasional exposure, e.g. ancillary staff). There are three methods available for monitoring radiation:

- Film (film badge dosimeters)
- Thermoluminescence dosimeters (TLD badges)
- Direct readout electronic monitors

Film was the earliest form of radiation dosimeter. Commercially available film dosimeter badges have a sensitivity of 0.1 mSv over 1 month. Thermoluminescence dosimeters based on lithium fluoride are also commonly used and they have a similar sensitivity. Designs of these two dosimeters are itemized in Table 22.12 and a selection shown in Fig. 22.2.

TLDs are more versatile than film dosimeters since they can be manufactured in smaller dimensions, providing extremity readings (finger doses) as well as the usual whole-body dose. They are more expensive than film, however, and need an expensive reading device. Lithium fluoride (LiF), the fluorescent material used in badges, has a sensitivity slightly higher than film, at 0.08 mSv, and it also has a radiation absorption close to tissue. It is therefore regarded as **tissue equivalent** (see Chapter 6). A recent development has been the

Table 22.12 *Properties of film, thermoluminescence, and Landauer type dosimeters.*

Film dosimeter	Attenuation	Radiation measured
Window	None	All
Thin plastic	Low beta	High energy beta
Thick plastic	β, low gamma	Low energy X-rays
Dural	β, X-rays	High energy X-rays and low gamma
Cd–Pb	β, X-rays, some gamma	Slow neutrons
Sn–Pb	β, X-rays	Uniform response to gamma
Thermoluminescence dosimeter	**Filtration**	**Estimation**
Open window	None	Skin dose
Thick plastic	700 mg cm^{-2}	Whole-body dose
Optically stimulated luminescence	**Detection**	**Measured**
Luxel® Al$_2$O$_3$	Beta, X-rays, and gamma	Deep dose ($H_p(10)$) Shallow dose ($H_p(0.07)$)

use of **aluminum oxide** as a more sensitive radiation detector material.

ELECTRONIC MONITORS

Electronic pocket dosimeters are expensive but give immediate readout of radiation doses being received. Their accuracy is low, being typically ± 20% up to 500 mSv h^{-1}. The detector used in older models was a small, calibrated, Geiger tube but, more recently, PIN semiconductor diodes have been used complete with energy filters. They are able to measure deep and shallow dose ($H_p(10)$ and $H_p(0.7)$, respectively) and can store their readings in an on-board memory for subsequent readout. An example of a particular model is shown in Fig. 22.3. The dose range displayed is typically 1 μSv to 1000 mSv and their response is from 20 keV to 1.5 MeV. Overall accuracy ranges from ± 10% to ± 20%.

A staff-dose record from a personal dosimeter system should be kept for archive purposes (database) extending many years so a radiation exposure history is available. Staff who change jobs are required to carry a record of their radiation exposure with them so continuity of exposure record is maintained.

DOSE–AREA PRODUCT METERS (DAP/DIAMENTOR)

The dose–area product is measured with a special ionization chamber fixed to the X-ray tube housing shown in Chapter 4. It enables the total surface dose to

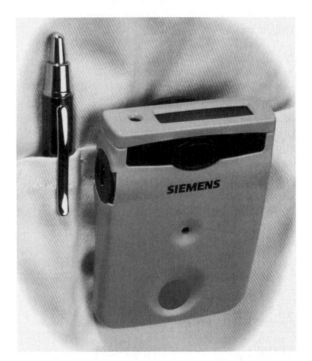

Figure 22.3 *An electronic dosimeter capable of storing dose information (courtesy of Siemens Inc.).*

be recorded for each examination; it can also display the total elapsed fluoroscopy time. With regular use the dose–area product meter can compare exposures for different patients and different techniques. It is particularly useful for training.

The detector consists of a large parallel-plate ionization chamber feeding a high input impedance

Table 22.13 *Advantages and disadvantages of film dosimeters.*

Advantages	Disadvantages
Cheap	Not tissue equivalent
Wide range of intensities	Long delay before result (≈1 month)
Mixed doses identifiable	Interpretation difficult
Robust detector	Can be used only once
Permanent record	Film varies in sensitivity

amplifier. The chamber is fixed close to the X-ray tube where the X-ray dose is high and backscattered radiation from the patient is minimal. The factors that alter the dose area product are:

- Tube kilovoltage (kV_p)
- Tube current (mA)
- Filtration (mm Al)
- Time (minutes)

The dose measurement is independent of distance from the X-ray source (see Chapter 4). Since the chamber is transparent it does not interfere with any light beam positioning device. Under-couch (under-table or UT) fluoroscopy units are not ideal for dose–area product meters since the table acts as an additional filter in front of the patient. A selection of common examinations with their typical dose–area values in Gy cm^2 are given in Section 22.5.1. Table 22.13 summarizes the advantages and disadvantages of film dosimeters.

MONITORING CLASSIFIED AREAS

The levels of ionizing radiation must be adequately monitored in classified areas, both supervised and controlled areas. There will be a requirement on the user to provide suitable and sufficient radiation monitoring equipment which must be properly maintained and adequately tested at appropriate intervals under the supervision of qualified persons. A qualified person must possess the necessary expertise in instrumentation theory and practice.

It is proposed that testing should be carried out once a year and that each instrument shall be individually calibrated before first use and as part of the annual testing. Proper calibrations should make use of radiation sources that ensure a known accuracy of calibration traceable to national standards. It will,

of course, be necessary to maintain records of all testing.

22.3 PERSONAL PROTECTION

22.3.1 Radiation exposure and distance

The simple reduction of intensity from an isotropic source obeys the inverse square law, derived in Chapter 1, which is

$$I_d \propto \frac{1}{d^2} \quad \text{or} \quad I_d = \frac{I_0}{d^2} \tag{22.7}$$

where I_0 is the intensity of the source and I_d the intensity at distance d. However, a more common problem in radiology is for an intensity to be given at a reference distance d and the intensity to be calculated for another new distance d_n. If the new intensity is I_{d_n} then eqn 22.7 can be restated as

$$I_{d_n} = \frac{I_0}{d_n^2} \tag{22.8}$$

Rearranging eqns 22.7 and 22.8 yields intensities $I_0 = I_d \times d^2$ and $I_0 = I_{d_n} \times d_n^2$ which together give

$$I_{d_n} = \frac{I_d \times d^2}{d_n^2} \tag{22.9}$$

Examples using this formula for problems commonly encountered in radiological protection are given in Box 22.7.

Staff working in controlled areas must wear protective clothing in the form of lead aprons. Several designs are available from complete wrap-around aprons to those that only cover the front of the body. The lead-equivalent thicknesses are normally 0.25, 0.33, and 0.5 mm lead equivalent. Lead as an attenuating medium has an inconvenient K-edge position as indicated in Fig. 22.4a. Energies above 88 kV are better attenuated than the lower energy scatter radiation. Composite aprons have been introduced which are manufactured from a lead/tin mixture. Tin has a lower K edge of 29 keV (Fig. 22.4a) which compensates for the higher K edge of lead. Over the range of 30 to 80 keV tin has a better attenuation than lead for a greatly reduced weight. Composite aprons therefore give improved protection over a fixed energy range than pure lead aprons but they are

Box 22.7 Radiation exposure and distance

Example 1

If the dose at 60 cm from an X-ray tube is 250 μGy then, by using eqn 22.9, the dose rate at 75 cm is

$$I_{d_n} = \frac{I_d \times d^2}{d_n^2} = \frac{250 \times 60^2}{75^2} = 160 \,\mu\text{Gy}$$

Example 2

The measured dose at 60 cm for a mammogram tube is 250 μGy. What is the dose during a magnification view at 50 cm?

$$I_{d_n} = 360 \,\mu\text{Gy}$$

Example 3

(Rearranging eqn 22.9). The distance limit can be found which reduces a dose rate of 1000 μSv h^{-1} at 30 cm from a radioactive source to 7.5 μSv h^{-1}. This is

$$d_n^2 = \frac{I_d \times d^2}{I_{d_n}} = \frac{1000 \times 30^2}{7.5} = 346 \,\text{cm}$$

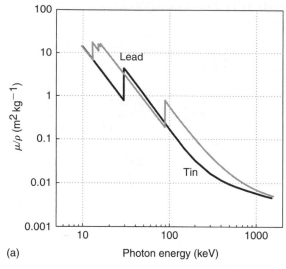

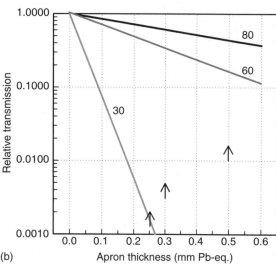

Figure 22.4 (**a**) The mass attenuation curve for lead and tin showing the position of the K edges. (**b**) The reduction in transmission for 0.25, 0.3, and 0.5 mm Pb equivalent protective aprons (arrows) at 30, 60, and 80 keV$_{eff}$.

inferior to 0.5 mm lead-equivalent aprons which should always be used for high dose procedures (e.g. fluoroscopy). The approximate weights for the different aprons are:

- 0.5 mm lead equivalent, 5.4 kg m^{-2}
- Composite (0.4 mm lead equivalent), 3.6 to 4.5 kg m^{-2}
- 0.3 mm lead, 3.24 kg m^{-2}

22.3.2 Personal dosimeter position

When measuring staff exposure radiation dose the position of the dosimeter on the clothing is important. Figure 22.4b shows the relative transmission for 30, 60, and 80 kV$_{eff}$ X-rays. The arrows indicate the common apron equivalent lead thickness of 0.25, 0.3, and 0.5 mm. An apron having a lead equivalent of 0.3 mm reduces transmission at these energies to

0.0002, 0.3, and 0.58 so a dosimeter badge placed under the apron would underestimate radiation exposure to the extremities.

ICRP Report 35 (1982) recommended that more than one dosimeter may be required when wearing protective lead aprons. A single dosimeter should be worn outside high on the trunk (collar level) to give an eye and skin unshielded dose. This dosimeter, placed outside the lead apron at collar level, will also give a better idea of ambient exposure

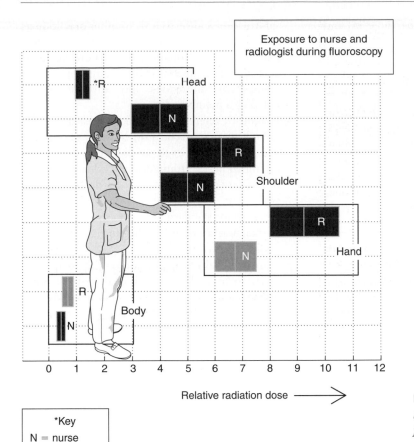

Figure 22.5 *Relative doses to a radiologist and a nurse during a fluoroscopy/angiography examination. The extremities show considerably greater exposure levels.*

because most of the scattered radiation is low energy and will be stopped by the apron itself. However, this dosimeter will overestimate the effective dose by about $\times 5$ so a second 'under apron badge' will be required to give the true whole-body dose for record keeping.

An 'above apron' badge is a very good indicator of efficient use of fluoroscopy equipment when used in parallel with a dose–area product area meter for the patient dose record. In some cases it is good practice to use an electronic dosimeter for recording individual doses since these can give an immediate idea of radiation exposure. The histogram in Fig. 22.5 shows relative radiation exposure for the body, shoulder, hand, and head for a radiologist and nurse during a fluoroscopy study. A reading from the body region would give a false idea of radiation exposure to the extremities; a shoulder badge position gives a better idea of radiation doses to the upper third of the body.

A summary of staff dose reduction for fluoroscopy examinations would be:

- Wear a protective lead apron (0.5 mm lead equivalent).
- Make use of image storage systems for review monitoring.
- Exposure timing devices should have an audible warning.
- Display elapsed fluoroscopic time on a monitor screen.

22.4 MEDICAL EXPOSURES

Individual countries at first introduced their own legislation for radiation protection but within the last two to three decades published measurements and risk assessments have influenced ICRP to offer recommendations which have been used as a basis for international directives in Europe, the USA, and Asia.

22.4.1 Framework legislation

The patient protection legislation for Europe is contained in the **European Council Directive 97/43/ EURATOM** on health protection of individuals against the dangers of ionizing radiation in relation to medical exposure. Table 22.14 summarizes the main Articles contained in this Directive. Some major definitions (from **Article 2**) introduce the important areas covered by this document:

1 **Clinical audit**: a systematic examination or review of medical radiological procedures with modification of practices where indicated and the application of new standards if necessary.
2 **Clinical responsibility**: responsibility regarding individual medical exposures attributed to a practitioner. Notably, justification, optimization, clinical evaluation of the outcome, and cooperation with other specialists and the staff, as appropriate, regarding practical aspects. Also includes obtaining appropriate clinical information of previous examinations, providing existing radiological

Table 22.14 *European Directive main headings.*

Application	Directive Articles
Patient exposure	Justification (Article 3)
	Optimization (Article 4)
	– Dose constraint (ALARA)
	– Diagnostic reference levels
	Responsibilities (Article 5)
	Written procedures (Article 6)
	– Medical physics expert
	– Clinical audit
Staff education	Training (Article 7)
	Recognized qualifications
Equipment (Article 8)	Commissioning
	Quality assurance
	Defective equipment
Special practices (Article 9)	Health screening
	Special protection during pregnancy and breast feeding (Article 10)
	Potential exposure (Article 11)
Population dose (Article 12)	Special practices
	Health screening programs

information and/or records to other practitioners and/or prescribers, as required, and giving information on the risk of ionizing radiation to patients and other individuals involved, as appropriate.
3 **Competent authorities**: any authority designated by a member state.
4 **Diagnostic reference levels**: dose levels in medical radiodiagnostic practices or, in the case of radiopharmaceuticals, levels of activity, for typical examinations for groups of standard-sized patients or standard phantoms for broadly defined types of equipment. These levels are expected not to be exceeded for standard procedures when good and normal practice regarding diagnostic and technical performance is applied.
5 **Dose constraint**: a restriction on the prospective doses to individuals which may result from a defined source (radiology or nuclear medicine). Used at the planning stage in radiation protection whenever optimization is applied.
6 **Health screening**: a procedure using radiological installations for early diagnosis in population groups at risk.
7 **Holder**: any organization or legal person who has the legal responsibility under national law for a given radiological installation.
8 **Individual detriment**: clinically observable deleterious effects that are expressed in individuals or their descendants, the appearance of which is either immediate or delayed.
9 **Medical physics expert**: an expert in radiation physics or radiation technology applied to exposure, within the scope of this Directive, whose training and competence to act is recognized by the competent authorities; and who, as appropriate, acts or gives advice on patient dosimetry (radiation protection adviser), on the development and use of complex techniques and equipment, on optimization, on quality assurance, including quality control, and on other matters relating to radiation protection, concerning exposure within the scope of the Directive.
10 **Medical radiological procedure**: any procedure concerning medical exposure.
11 **Medico-legal procedures**: procedures performed for insurance or legal purposes without a medical indication.
12 **Occupational health surveillance**: the medical surveillance for workers as specified by member states or competent authorities.

13 **Patient dose**: the dose concerning patients or other individuals undergoing medical exposure.

14 **Patient dosimetry**: the dosimetry concerning patients or other individuals undergoing medical exposure.

15 **Practitioner**: a medical doctor, dentist or other health professional who is entitled to take clinical responsibility for an individual medical exposure in accordance with national requirements.

16 **Prescriber**: a medical doctor, dentist or other health professional, who is entitled to refer individuals for medical exposure to a practitioner, in accordance with national requirements.

17 **Quality assurance**: all those planned and systematic actions necessary to provide adequate confidence that a structure, system, component or procedure will perform satisfactorily complying with agreed standards.

18 **Quality control**: is a part of quality assurance. The set of operations (programming, coordinating, implementing) intended to maintain or to improve quality. It covers monitoring, evaluation, and maintenance at required levels of all characteristics of performance of equipment that can be defined, measured, and controlled.

22.4.2 The justification of a medical exposure

A feature of the new Directive is that all individual medical exposures shall be in advance taking into account specific objectives of the exposure and the characteristics of the individual involved. It will be necessary to take into account alternative techniques having the same objective but involving no or less exposure to ionising radiation. In addition, the prescriber as well as the practitioner is required to be involved in this justification process at a level to be specified by the competent authority. Strong emphasis is placed on both the prescriber and practitioner seeking, wherever possible, to obtain previous diagnostic information or medical records relevant to the planned exposure and to consider these data with a view to avoiding unnecessary exposure.

The ICRP has provided recommendations on justification of practices, balancing benefits against costs and their disadvantages, concluding that a particular course of action or practice either is or is not worthwhile. In radiological protection, as in other areas, it is becoming possible to formalize and quantify procedures. Decisions concerning the adoption and continuation of a **practice** involve a choice between possible options including non-ionizing radiation examinations.

Choosing between the use of ionizing or non-ionizing clinical imaging is a complex decision. The harm (detriment) to be considered is not only confined to the use of radiation: economic and social costs of the practice are also considered. For this reason the term justification requires only that the net benefit be positive. This will be a new requirement that no practice resulting in exposure to ionizing radiation can be carried out unless it is of a type or class of practice carried out before the coming into force of the new statutory instrument or it has been accepted by the institute in advance as being justified by its economic, social or other benefits in relation to the health detriment it may cause. A list of existing practices will be provided in the statutory instrument for guidance.

It will be necessary, however, for the justification of existing classes or types of practices to be reviewed when new and important evidence about their efficacy or consequences becomes available. In the circumstances, the institute will be empowered to withdraw a licence for a particular practice.

There are three levels of justification of a practice in medicine:

1 **General justification** The use of radiation in medicine is accepted as doing more good than harm. This would include all the routine radiological investigations including chest radiographs, the common barium and iodine contrast studies, general nuclear medicine studies, and established computed tomography procedures.

2 **Generic justification** defines a specified radiology imaging procedure with a specified objective supplying additional diagnostic information. The aim of this is to judge whether this additional procedure will improve the diagnosis or treatment. The exposures to staff (occupational exposure) and to members of the public who are not connected with the procedures (public exposure) should be taken into account. Examples would include non-routine nuclear medicine studies involving radionuclides other than ^{99m}Tc. Other high dose procedures using CT or fluoroscopy would come under this heading.

3 Individual justification is applied to a procedure which justifies a radiology procedure for a single instance as a non-routine diagnostic procedure for a named patient. This includes clinical decisions to use a relatively high dose radiological procedure for investigating a young child or pregnant patient.

POTENTIAL EXPOSURES

All steps should be taken in order to reduce the likelihood of accidental exposure (machine switched on and controlled by authorized personnel; machine held in switch standby condition). The main emphasis is give to radiotherapy exposure levels but due consideration should also be given to diagnostic machines with high output (CT and fluoroscopy). Nuclear medicine is also included here where badly calibrated instrumentation allows higher activity levels to be injected.

RESPONSIBILITIES

It will be necessary to ensure that any medical exposure is effected under the clinical responsibility of a practitioner. Definitions of the prescriber and practitioner will be required. However, the practical aspects of the procedure may be delegated to competent individuals including those undergoing relevant training programs. The Directive places a requirement on practitioners and prescribers to take certain precautions in the cases of women of child-bearing age and during pregnancy or breastfeeding. If pregnancy cannot be excluded, special attention must be given to the justification and optimization of the medical exposure, taking into account the expectant mother and the unborn child. A physician must have adequate training to justify a request and therefore in the **Patient Directive** he/she is unlikely to be classified as a 'practitioner' under present European legislation but radiologists, who have had such training, can only justify an exposure if sufficient relevant clinical information is provided on the request form.

It has been reported (WHO Report 689) that up to 20% of radiographic examinations can be clinically unhelpful, and studies have shown a decrease in referral rates following the introduction of guidelines to physicians which, in turn, reduces the number of unhelpful radiographs.

22.4.3 Patient dose reduction and optimization

Diagnostic radiology is the largest artificial source of radiation exposure to the population. It contributes approximately 20% to overall human exposure worldwide. In Western countries this can be nearer 50%. A serious attempt should always be made to reduce patient radiation exposure whenever possible providing it does not compromise image quality.

UNNECESSARY INVESTIGATIONS

It has been estimated that at least 20% of X-ray examinations currently carried out in some Western countries are clinically unnecessary. Further unnecessary exposure results from repeat films due to film loss or poor image quality. Box 22.8 uses the man-sievert to

---

Box 22.8 The man-sievert

The annual collective dose for radiological examinations in the UK is 16 000 man-Sv of which 70% is film radiography, 30% is fluoroscopy, and smaller contributions are made by nuclear medicine (1000 man-Sv) and dental studies 200 man-Sv. Dose reduction and dose saving could be made in the following areas:

Dose reduction	Collective dose saving (man-Sv)
Unnecessary investigations	3200
Maintain number of films to national mean value (NMV)	2500
Reduce fluoroscopy time to NMV	1500
Reduce dose per examination to NMV	1300
Reduce repeat rate from 10% to 5%	600

Conclusion

For no financial outlay the collective dose to the patient population could be reduced by between 7000 and 8000 man-Sv, ≈40% with a concurrent reduction in staff dose. For the US population (230 million):

- Radiology 92 000 man-Sv
- Nuclear medicine 32 000 man-Sv

estimate dose savings in radiology and Table 22.15 lists procedures for reducing patient dose. Costs in this area are minimal. Other methods for reducing patient dose that require financial outlay are **rare-earth screens** when film screen recording is being made or to change entirely to **digital imaging (CR and DR)** which, when sensibly applied, can return substantial patient dose reduction. Most modern **table top materials** used for patient support in radiography equipment are now either carbon fiber (preferred) or strong plastic; mattresses are normally not necessary unless the procedure is itself high dose and of long duration.

Figure 22.6 shows the changes in radiology practice between 1991 and 2003 (UK data). There has been a general reduction in patient dose for all investigations due to more efficient imaging equipment and management. The exception to this is computed tomography (CT); the dramatic increase here has canceled all previous dose saving resulting in an overall increase in medical radiation exposure.

PATIENT DOSE REDUCTION TECHNIQUES

Fluoroscopy is a particularly high dose rate procedure. Dose reduction could be obtained by:

- Short periods of screening exposure
- Digital image store
- Temporary removal of antiscatter grid (less radiation needed for film exposure but poorer image quality)
- Automatic brightness control influencing X-ray exposure for different anatomy (varying absorption)
- 90 kV at 0.5 mA should be the exposure level delivering 10 mGy min^{-1} surface dose

Table 22.15 *Procedures for reducing patient dose.*

Method	Possible dose reduction (%)
1 Eliminate unjustified examinations	100
2 Minimize films per examination	20
3 Minimize fluoroscopy time	30
4 Reduce repeat rates	5
5 Availability of previous films	100
6 Collimate beam effectively	20
7 Shield sensitive organs	25
8 Patient compression	50
9 QC program	Influences No. 2 and 3 above

Collimating the beam to the smallest field with the current (in mA) and the voltage (in kV) as low as possible is also a very effective dose reduction technique using automatic collimation where possible.

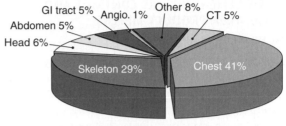

Frequency contribution 1991

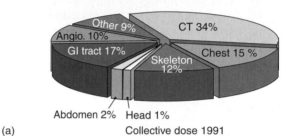

(a) Collective dose 1991

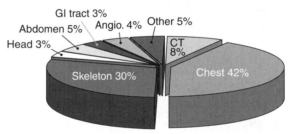

Frequency contribution 2003

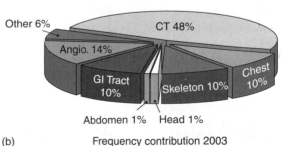

(b) Frequency contribution 2003

Figure 22.6 *Data from 1991 and 2003 showing the changes in frequency and collective dose for common radiological examinations. The dramatic increase in collective dose for computed tomography reflects the proliferation of these machines and the increased dose that multislice models deliver.*

Image storage devices added to fluoroscopy equipment can give major dose reduction for patient and staff (Chapter 9). If a non-storage system needs a 5 s screening exposure, a 'last image hold' would only require a 2 s exposure. This reduces the dose to 40%.

AUTOMATIC EXPOSURE CONTROLS AND DOSE–AREA PRODUCT METERS

The equipment section of the European Regulations (Article 8) requires that radiodiagnostic equipment is fitted with a device for informing the operator of the patient dose. This could be supplied by the automatic exposure control (as mGy surface dose and/or estimated mean glandular dose). A dose–area product (DAP) meter gives a more accurate measurement of overall dose during a patient procedure and registers this as a dose × area product (mGy or Gy cm^2). This latter figure is more easily used in any clinical audit.

22.4.4 Optimization of medical exposure

Once a practice has been justified and adopted it is necessary to consider how best to use resources in reducing the radiation risks to both patients and hospital staff. The broad aim should be to ensure that the magnitude of the individual doses and the number of people exposed are all kept as low as reasonably achievable (ALARA), economic and social factors being taken into account.

If reducing the **detriment** can only be achieved by expenditure that is seriously out of line with the consequent reduction (cost and convenience), it is not reasonable to take that step, provided that individuals have been adequately protected. The protection can then be said to be optimized and ALARA principles observed. Optimization should be applied to all stages of diagnostic imaging, from the design of premises, equipment, and procedures through to day-to-day applications. The primary question should be: 'Are there any reasonable steps that can be taken to improve protection?'; much depends on the interpretation of 'reasonable'.

CONSTRAINT OF MEDICAL EXPOSURES

The optimization of protection often involves the balancing of **collective detriment** and **collective benefits**. The exposure of families and friends who assist with patients undergoing radiology as carers is included as a

medical exposure, and in the exposure of volunteers in biomedical research programmes. These provide no direct benefit so dose constraints are needed to limit dose. Carers should be informed about any hazard and given appropriate guidance to reduce their exposure. Protection of carers from radiation exposure in the radiology department would include the sensible use of protective aprons and gloves. The procedure of optimization of protection for these groups is no different from that for public exposure, except that exposure need not be restricted by dose limits.

GENERAL MEDICAL IMAGING TASK

General medical imaging task refers to a task for a general clinical purpose, with minimum specification of other factors in order to reduce the frequency of unjustified high values. Table 22.16 lists these factors. An example would be a PA chest radiograph with the clinical purpose and technique factors unspecified. The following quantities and their applications are noted.

SPECIFIC MEDICAL IMAGING TASK

Specific medical imaging task refers to a task for a clearly defined clinical purpose promoting the attainment of a narrower range of values but allows for differences among medical facilities in other technical and clinical details. The clinical purpose is defined, but the X-ray equipment, technique factors, and image quality criteria may vary among facilities. An example would be a PA chest radiograph with the clinical purpose and the general technique (e.g. high kV$_p$) specified, but the detailed technique factors unspecified.

SPECIFIC MEDICAL IMAGING PROTOCOL

Specific medical imaging protocol refers to a clinical protocol with a fully defined set of specifications that is followed, or serves as a nominal baseline, at a single facility (or several allied facilities) promoting attainment of the optimum use of radiation exposure. An example would be a protocol for a PA chest radiograph that specifies the clinical purpose, the technical conduct of the procedure, the image quality criteria, any unique patient characteristics, and other appropriate factors.

DESIGN AND CONSTRUCTION OF EQUIPMENT AND INSTALLATIONS

These would include digital storage in the case of fluoroscopy and the use of fast film-screens, also the use

Table 22.16 *The radiation dose measurements used for clinical audit.*

Task	Measurement	Units
General medical imaging task	Entrance air kerma (no backscatter)	mGy
	Entrance surface dose (with backscatter)	mGy
	Dose–area product (DAP)	mGy cm^2
	Administered activity (*A*)	MBq
Specific medical imaging task	Entrance air kerma (no backscatter)	mGy
	Entrance surface dose (with backscatter)	mGy
	Dose–length product (DLP)	mGy cm^{-1}
	Dose–area product (DAP)	mGy cm^2
	Mean or average glandular dose (MGD or AGD)	mGy
Specific medical imaging protocol	Milliampere second	mAs
	Absorbed dose	Gy
	Administered activity	MBq

of a carbon fiber film cassette or table top and the appropriate thickness of radiation shielding in the room plan. The use of gonad shields and specific protocols for pediatric patients would play a significant role. Optimization of working procedures have a direct influence on patient care. The choice of the optimization pathway directly alters the level of exposure of the patient, the staff, and often the public. Since most procedures involving medical exposures using ionizing radiation are clearly justified and because the procedures are usually for the direct benefit of the exposed individual, less attention is given to the optimization of protection in medical exposure. However, there is considerable scope for dose reduction in diagnostic radiology. Simple, low-cost measures are available for reducing doses without loss of diagnostic information, but the extent to which these measures are used varies widely.

The use of antiscatter grids improves the contrast and resolution of the image, although removing the grid would allow a reduction in dose by a factor of 2 to 4. In many instances the benefit would be reduced by removing the grid due to the loss of image quality; optimization would not call for the removal of the grid in adult radiography. However, for radiography of small children, the amount of scattered radiation is less and the benefit of the dose reduction by removing the antiscatter grid is fully offset by the small deterioration of the image. The optimization of protection then calls for the reduction in dose allowed by the removal of the grid.

The exposure (other than occupational) of individuals helping to support and comfort patients is also medical exposure. This definition includes the exposures of families and friends of patients discharged from hospital after diagnostic or therapeutic nuclear medicine procedures.

Written protocols should be a part of every radiology department's optimization plan. The best technique and optimal settings can therefore be agreed. Box 22.9 gives an example of a written protocol for a specific diagnostic imaging procedure which can be used as a model for all imaging procedures including CT.

22.5 DIAGNOSTIC REFERENCE LEVELS

It is well recognized that, apart from natural background, medical exposures are at present by far the largest source of exposure to ionizing radiation of the population and radiation protection measures should be taken to prevent unnecessary medical radiation exposure. The main instrument is **justification** of clinical exposure, **optimization** of protection, and the use of **dose limits**. However, dose limits do not apply to medical exposures so individual justification from careful clinical assessment and optimization are even more important than in other practices using ionizing radiation. Doses to patients have been justified so applying any dose limits to medical exposures would restrict diagnostic quality and do more harm than good. Diagnostic reference levels (DRLs) apply to medical exposure, not to occupational and public exposure; they have no link to dose limits or constraints.

Patient radiation dose is determined principally by medical need, therefore dose constraints for

Box 22.9 Example of procedure documentation

Imaging requirements for lumbar spine AP projection

1 Linear reproduction of the upper and lower-plate surfaces in the centered beam area and visualization of the intervertebral spaces
2 Extensive coverage of the posterior linear vertebral edges
3 Definition of the oval arch roots
4 Intervertebral foramena and visually sharp reproduction of the pedicles
5 Small vertebral joints visible and distinguishable, depending on the region
6 Definition of the spinous processes
7 Reproduction of the transverse processes and costo-transverse joints
8 Visually sharp reproduction of the cortex and trabecular structures typical of the region
9 Visually sharp reproduction of the immediately adjacent soft tissues

Important image details are trabecular structures typical for the examined region: 0.3 to 0.5 mm.

Typical expected dose levels (lumbar spine AP)

Maximum acceptable entrance surface dose: 6 mGy.

View	Entrance surface dose	Dose–area product
Adult		
AP	6 mGy	1.6 Gy cm^2
Child		
neonate	70 μGy	6 mGy cm^2
1 year	190 μGy	10 mGy cm^2
5 year	370 μGy	48 mGy cm^2
10 year	980 μGy	230 mGy cm^2

Standard radiographic technique

Parameter	Specification
Radiographic device	Bucky table or vertical bucky or vertical stand with stationary grid
Radiographic voltage	75 to 90 kV
Total filtration	>2.5 mm Al equivalent
Focal spot size	0.6 mm (>1.2 mm)
Focus to film distance	115 (90 to 150) cm
Automatic exposure selection	Central measurement field
Exposure time	<100 ms
Antiscatter grid	r = 12; 40/cm Cr = 8; 40/cm
Film-screen	Rare earth, 400 speed (800 for children)
CR image plate	Standard (SR)
Radioprotection device	Gonad shields

patients are inappropriate but some limitation of diagnostic medical exposures is achieved by using **diagnostic reference levels** as first recommended in ICRP 73. Diagnostic medical exposures should be optimum, consistent with obtaining the best diagnostic information. Optimization in diagnostic radiology is best obtained using DRLs. They are reviewed from time to time in order to recognize equipment advances and dose saving capabilities. A DRL is set for standard procedures and for groups of standard-sized patients or a standard phantom measuring:

- Entrance surface dose per radiograph, for diagnostic radiography
- Entrance surface dose rate, for fluoroscopy
- Average glandular dose per cranio-caudal projection, for mammography
- Multiple scan average dose, for computed tomography

DRLs in practice should assist in the optimization of patient protection in the radiology department by helping to avoid unnecessarily high doses to the patient. The system requires:

- Estimation of patient doses, as part of a regular quality assurance program
- Comparison of obtained doses with the internationally recommended DRLs
- Corrective actions if guidance levels are consistently exceeded

Reference levels apply to both diagnostic radiology and diagnostic nuclear medicine, where radionuclide activity levels are controlled. In both cases, the DRL will be intended for use as a simple test for identifying situations where the levels of patient dose or administered activity are unusually high. If it is found that procedures are consistently high causing the relevant dose levels to be exceeded, then a local review of procedures and equipment is put in place.

Each department will need to know the typical doses delivered by its own equipment and techniques, in order to assess which examinations fall into the high dose category. Dose guidelines for a core set of examinations might include, for example:

- Lumbar spine
- Abdomen
- Barium enema
- Computed tomography of the head
- Dental panoramic radiography

- Mammography
- Skull, pelvis, chest radiography in children

Achievable doses based on department operational and technological factors should be gradually introduced to replace national reference doses.

DOSE INCREASES

The results of a recent survey (Hart and Wall, 2002) outlined the frequency of medical and dental X-ray examinations in the UK and contemporary data on the radiation doses typically received by patients. A total of about 41.5 million medical and dental X-ray examinations are conducted each year in the UK (0.70 examination per head of population) resulting in an annual per caput effective dose of 330 µSv; not significantly different from the previous rough estimate of 350 µSv for 1991. Over the last 10 years computed tomography (CT) has more than doubled its contribution and is now responsible for 40% of the total dose to the population from medical X-rays. In contrast, the contribution from conventional radiographic and fluoroscopic examinations has nearly halved to about 44%. Interventional and angiographic procedures together contribute the remaining 16%. The much increased contributions of CT, angiography, and interventional procedures to population dose indicate an urgent need to develop radiation protection and optimization activities for these high dose procedures to the same level as has been achieved for conventional radiology.

22.5.1 Range of doses from diagnostic examinations

Examples of radiological investigations and their typical doses, reported in the literature, are shown graphically in the following sections. The highest doses are for fluoroscopy and CT investigations; the lowest for chest radiography (CXR). Lowest patient dose levels are given by high voltage CXR techniques and successive increases in kV_p give substantial saving in radiation dose; high voltage chest radiographs should always be the method of choice.

Nuclear medicine studies give much lower whole-body doses than investigations involving X-rays; equivalent doses to target organs may be higher, however. The percentage collective dose of various radiological examinations given in Fig. 22.6 indicates the relative contributions made by various diagnostic X-ray investigations to the total patient collective dose and identifies those investigations that need careful planning in order to give a significant reduction in patient radiation exposure. Radiological investigations

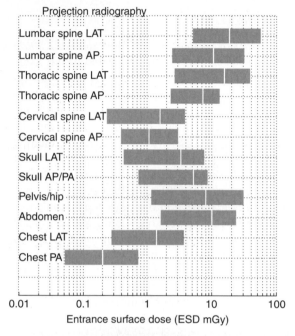

Figure 22.7 *Bar plots showing the published ranges of dose values for projection radiography. The white line gives the mean values. (Data obtained from Ng et al. (1998) and UNSCEAR (2000).)*

involving CT have become major additions to this collective dose figure.

22.5.2 The range of doses from conventional radiography

Achievable doses should be used as a supplement to the existing reference dose values of entrance surface dose per radiograph when departments are assessing the results of local dose surveys conducted for the purposes of reviewing patient protection. Figure 22.7 shows the ranges of expected exposure levels, measured by clinical audit, for common X-ray diagnostic investigations. Table 22.17 gives an idea of dose reference levels for common X-ray examinations derived from the third quartile values of clinical audits carried out by a large number of hospitals.

National reference dose values should be reset periodically in consultation with appropriate bodies. Further national reviews of radiographic practice should be conducted in order to extend both reference and achievable doses so as to continue to promote the optimization of patient protection.

FLUOROSCOPIC EXAMINATIONS

The present national reference dose values of dose–area product for common fluoroscopic procedures are unlikely to promote further improvements in current dosimetric performance. Methods should be developed for assessing the dose rate at the entrance

Table 22.17 *Rounded third quartile values from the current and previous reviews of national patient dose data. The year 2000 results form the basis of recommended national reference doses for individual radiographs on adult patients (UNSCEAR, 2000).*

Examination	Entrance surface dose per image (mGy)			Dose–area product per image (Gy cm²)
	Mid-1980s	1995	2000	
Skull AP/PA	5	4	3	
Skull LAT	3	2	1.6	
Chest PA	0.3	0.2	0.2	0.12
Chest LAT	1.5	0.7	1	
Thoracic spine AP	7	5	3.5	
Thoracic spine LAT	20	16	10	
Lumbar spine AP	10	7	6	1.6
Lumbar spine LAT	30	20	14	3
Lumbar spine LSJ	40	35	26	3
Abdomen AP	10	7	6	3
Pelvis AP	10	5	4	3

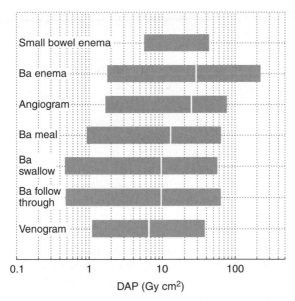

Figure 22.8 *Bar plots showing the published ranges of dose values for fluoroscopy. The white line gives the mean values. (Data obtained from Warren-Forward (1998) and UNSCEAR (2000).)*

surface of the patient and for the collection of such data during the more common procedures that involve prolonged fluoroscopy (Barium enema). Figure 22.8 shows the ranges for common fluoroscopic investigations and Table 22.18 gives suggestions for dose reference levels obtained from third quartile values and recommended timing.

ANGIOGRAPHIC AND COMPLEX INTERVENTIONAL EXAMINATIONS

All departments conducting angiographic and complex interventional examinations should undertake dose–area product monitoring. In view of the significant potential for damage to skin, methods should be developed to allow the reliable estimation of absorbed dose to skin from complex radiological procedures. There should be central collation of dose–area product data from local patient dose surveys of angiography and interventional procedures in order to allow the establishment of national reference dose values. Table 22.18 includes recommended DAP and timing for coronary angiography,

Table 22.18 *The third quartile figures are recommended national reference doses for complete examinations on adult patients using fluoroscopy (UNSCEAR, 2000).*

Procedure (mean weight range 75 to 85 kg)	Dose–area product distribution (Gy cm^2)			
	Mean	Third quartile	DRL (Gy cm^2)	Time (min)
Barium follow through	10.7	13.7	14	2.2
Barium enema	23.5	31.3	31	2.7
Barium meal	10.3	13.0	13	2.3
Barium swallow	8.0	10.2	11	2.3
ERCP	15.5	19.0		5.3
Femoral angiogram	25.9	32.5	33	5.0
Hysterosalpingogram	3.5	4.3	4	1.0
IVU	14.5	16.2	16	–
Venogram (leg)	4.5	5.0	5	2.3
Biliary drainage	34.1	53.9	54	17.0
MCU	16.7	17.3	17	2.7
Nephrostogram	10.4	12.9	13	4.6
Nephrostomy	15.5	18.9	19	8.8
Sialogram	1.1	1.6	1.6	1.6
Small bowel enema	39.3	50.5	50.0	10.7
T-tube cholangiogram	8.0	9.9	10	2.0
Coronary angiogram	30.4	36.3	36	5.6
Hickman line	2.9	4.1	4	2.2
Oesophageal dilation	18.5	15.6	16	5.5
Pacemaker	17.0	26.5	27	10.7
Retrograde pyelogram	10.0	13.0	13	3.0

ERCP, endoscopic retrograde cholangio-pancreatography; IVU, intravenous urogram; MCU, micturating cystourethrography.

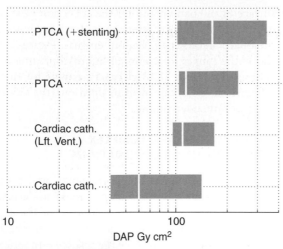

Figure 22.9 *Bar plots showing the published ranges of dose values for cardiac procedures. The white line gives the mean values. (Data obtained from van de Putte et al. (2000) and UNSCEAR (2000).)*

and Fig. 22.9 shows the ranges, with the mean values, expected from four cardiac investigations.

22.5.3 Range of doses from pediatric examinations

A further wide-scale review of dosimetric practice in pediatric radiology is required in order to assess the suitability of the initial reference dose values proposed by the European Union for promoting patient protection in the UK. Figure 22.10 shows the published ranges for conventional entrance surface doses and fluoroscopic DAP values.

Consideration should be given to the feasibility of establishing achievable doses on the basis of general recommendations for pediatric procedures. Table 22.19 shows the dose reduction that is possible if good techniques are applied to pediatric radiography.

22.5.4 Range of doses from dental radiography

It has been recommended that all dental X-ray sets should be assessed annually. All dentists should employ a system of quality assurance to ensure that radiographic images are consistently of a high standard. Reference doses should be established in collaboration with appropriate professional bodies on

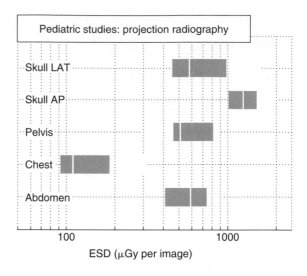

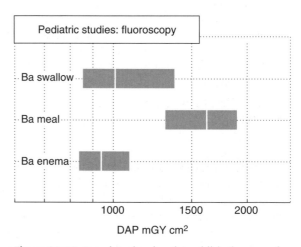

Figure 22.10 *Bar plots showing the published ranges of dose values for pediatric radiography. (Data obtained from UNSCEAR (2000).)*

the basis of published dose data from wide-scale surveys of dental practice.

The concept of dose–width product should be further developed so as to provide a practical means for monitoring patient exposure during panoramic radiography. Achievable doses should be developed on the basis of the lowest exposure factors that produce acceptable diagnostic images, following recommendations on simple, cost-effective changes in radiographic technique. The UNSCEAR 2000 report gives effective dose levels for two film intra-oral studies (0.005 mSv) and panoramic studies (0.01 mSv).

Table 22.19 *Examples of reduced doses in pediatric radiography with attention to good technique (UNSCEAR, 2000).*

Examination	Reduction of entrance surface dose (mGy)					
	Infant (10 months)		5-year-old child		10-year-old child	
	ESD	DAP (Gy cm²)	ESD	DAP (Gy cm²)	ESD	DAP (Gy cm²)
Chest AP (1 kg newborn)	0.02					
Chest AP/PA	0.02	0.003	0.03	0.005	0.04	0.016
Chest lateral						
Skull PA/AP	0.15	0.022	0.48	0.08	0.73	0.11
Skull lateral	0.09	0.014	0.30	0.053	0.36	0.06
Pelvis AP	0.07	0.005	0.08	0.011	0.42	0.15
Full spine PA/AP			0.21	0.069	0.22	0.07
Thoracic spine AP						
Thoracic spine lateral						
Lumbar spine AP	0.19	0.01	0.37	0.048	0.98	0.23
Lumbar spine lateral	0.14	0.012	0.21	0.10	1.52	0.30
Abdomen AP/PA	0.05	0.009	0.09	0.017	0.25	0.074
Barium meal/swallow		0.34		0.60		
MCU		0.26		0.25		0.45

MCU, micturating cystourethrography.

22.5.5 Range of doses from mammography

Mammography systems should have regular measurements of mean glandular dose for a standard breast model (MGDS) on a 6 monthly basis; population screening should have daily monitoring of the radiographic exposure (mAs) setting required for a standard phantom (such as 40 mm thickness of polymethyl methacrylate (PMMA)). Figure 22.11 gives the range of mean glandular dose for a 5 cm compressed breast when an optical density of 1.5 is used as a reference image density. All mammography systems with values of MGDS above 3 mGy should be subject to an immediate review of practice in order to justify their continued operation.

22.5.6 Range of doses from computed tomography

The doses to tissues from CT can often approach or exceed the levels known with certainty to increase the probability of cancer. CT examinations are increasing in frequency and newer spiral, multislice CT techniques have increased radiation dose levels when compared to older, single slice systems. Figure 22.12 gives the ranges from CTDI$_w$ and DLP for adults and

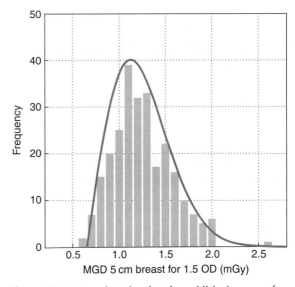

Figure 22.11 *Bar plots showing the published ranges of dose values for mammography. (Data adapted from Young et al. (1995).)*

children. The head is subject to the highest dose levels. Physicians and radiologists should make sure that the examination is indicated. Many practical possibilities currently exist to manage dose. The most important one is reduction in mA. Pediatric patients should have specific protocols with lower exposure factors.

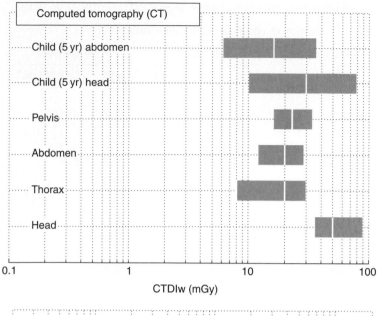

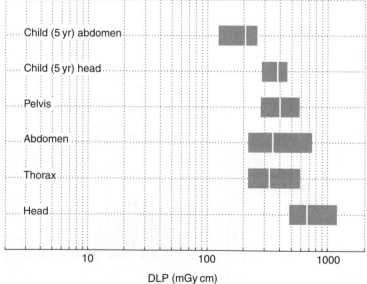

Figure 22.12 *Bar plots showing the published ranges of dose values for adults and 5-year-old children for computed tomography slice and dose–length product. (Data adapted from Shrimpton et al. (2003).)*

22.5.7 Range of doses from a nuclear medicine/PET department

A more formal system of audit is required in order to monitor effectively national practice in diagnostic nuclear medicine. Figure 22.13 gives the calculated effective dose levels for a selection of common nuclear medicine investigations.

The Administration of Radioactive Substances Advisory Committee (ARSAC) should continue to review and update on a regular basis the appropriateness of the recommended DRLs as an essential element of the optimization of protection for patients undergoing diagnostic nuclear medicine procedures.

22.6 THE PREGNANT PATIENT

Thousands of pregnant patients and radiation workers are exposed to ionizing radiation each year. Lack of knowledge is responsible for great anxiety and probably unnecessary termination of many pregnancies. For

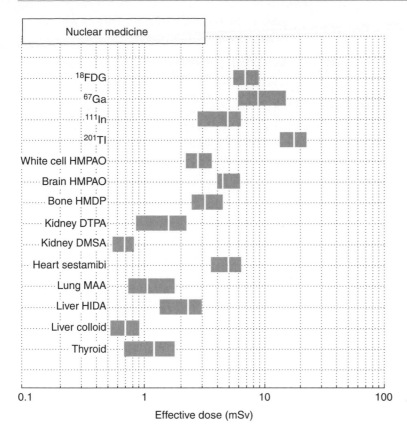

Figure 22.13 *Bar plots showing the published mean and range of dose values for nuclear medicine (^{99m}Tc agents unless otherwise stated).*

many patients the exposure is appropriate, while for others the exposure may be inappropriate, placing the unborn child at an unjustified increased risk.

In 1990 the International Commission on Radiological Protection (ICRP) modified its recommendations on the justification of medical exposures (ICRP Publication 60). The requirements for justification were based on two levels: those for diagnosis or therapy, i.e. broad principles, and those with respect to the case-by-case justification of medical exposures for individual patients. In the context of pregnant women the latter applied to the fetus as well.

The management of pregnant patients as well as pregnant workers in medical establishments where ionizing radiation is used demands special care (ICRP Publication 84). Many thousands of pregnant patients and medical radiation workers are exposed to radiation each year. It is the responsibility of the radiology staff to minimize the likelihood of inadvertent exposure of the conceptus before pregnancy is declared, and to prevent unnecessary exposure of the fetus when medical diagnostic procedures involving ionizing radiation are indicated during pregnancy.

22.6.1 Biological basics

The objectives on exposure of pregnant women to ionizing radiation are to:

- Minimize the likelihood of inadvertent exposure of the conceptus before pregnancy is declared
- Prevent unnecessary dose to the developing fetus

The stages of pregnancy for the first trimester are given in Fig. 22.14. The periods of organogenesis are identified between days 13 and 50.

Earlier NRPB advice was that no risks to the conceptus would follow irradiation during the first 10 days of the menstrual cycle and that subsequent risks in the remainder of the first 4 week period were likely to be so small that no special limitation on exposure was required.

Subsequently, NRPB revised its advice, with the objectives of minimizing the likelihood of inadvertent exposure of the conceptus before pregnancy is declared and of preventing an unnecessary dose to the fetus. Table 22.20 estimates the risk to the developing fetus from dose levels commonly seen in

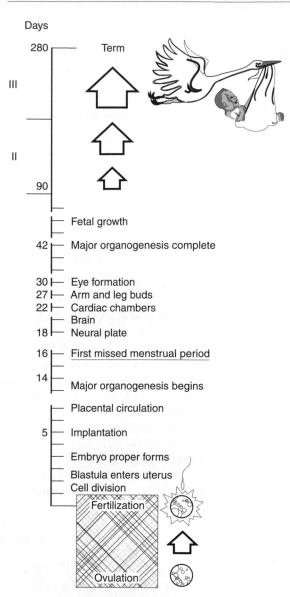

Figure 22.14 *The timing for ovulation and embryo/fetus development in days after fertilization and stages important to radiation protection protocols. Trimester divisions I, II and III are not to scale.*

Table 22.20 *The associated risk to the fetus for low radiation levels.*

Dose (mSv)	Probability of a normal fetus (%)	Increased risk (%)
0.0	95.93	0.0
0.5	95.928	0.002
1.0	95.922	0.008
2.5	95.91	0.02
5.0	95.88	0.05
10.0	95.83	0.1

diagnostic radiology. The unexposed fetus (0.0 mSv) has a natural occurrence of about 1 in 24 for abnormality.

It is necessary to assess the stochastic effects (cancer and hereditary disease) and the effects of irradiation *in utero* that are likely to arise following exposure to external radiation, or as a result of intakes of radionuclides. At diagnostic dose levels, the only adverse effect of radiation on the embryo/ fetus which is likely to pose a significant risk is that of cancer production. None of the other potential hazards (death, malformation, growth retardation, severe mental retardation, and heritable effects) presents a significant risk at these low diagnostic exposures.

The effects of high levels of radiation exposure to the developing fetus, obtained mostly from A-bomb data, are listed in Table 22.21. At diagnostic dose levels, the only adverse effect of radiation on the conceptus which is likely to pose a significant risk is that of cancer induction. None of the other potential hazards (death, malformation, growth retardation, severe mental retardation, and heritable effects) presents a significant problem at the low exposures used in diagnostic procedures. Table 22.22 lists the estimated doses to the uterus from some radiographic examinations.

22.6.2 Risk assessment

The risks to the developing embryo and fetus of death, malformation, mental impairment, cancer (solid tumors and leukemia) or heritable damage from irradiation are considered in cases before the mother can be aware of any pregnancy (see Fig. 22.14). Risks are also assessed in two other issues of particular relevance:

- Possible risks from irradiation of the early conceptus (3 to 4 weeks gestational age)
- Cases of preconception gonadal irradiation

Risk is assessed on the basis of dose. The induction of genetic disease and cancer by ionizing radiation is believed to show no dose threshold. The risks of these effects are judged relative to their natural incidences.

Risk can be expressed in several ways, including as relative risk or absolute risk. Relative risk indicates

Table 22.21 *Possible effects to the developing fetus from high levels of radiation.*

Days after fertilization	Period of development	Effects
1 to 9	Pre-implantation	Most probable effects: Death with little chance of malformation
10 to 12	Implantation	Reduced lethal effects
		Malformation unlikely
		Intra-uterine growth retardation predominant effect
13 to 50	Organogenesis	Production of congenital malformation
		Retarded growth
51 to 280	Fetal	Effects on central nervous system
		Growth retardation at high doses
All	Fetal/neonate	Increased incidence of cancer and leukemia

Table 22.22 *Estimated doses to the uterus from diagnostic procedures.*

Examination	Dose (mGy)
Upper gastrointestinal series	1
Cholecystography	1
Lumbar spine radiography	1
Pelvic radiography	1
Hip and femur radiography	1
Retrograde pyelography	1
Barium enema study	10
Abdominal (KUB) radiography	2.5
Hysterosalpingography	10
CT head	0.0
CT chest	0.16
CT abdomen	30

KUB, kidney/ureter/bladder.

the risk as a function of the 'background' cancer risk. A relative risk of 1.0 indicates that there is no effect of irradiation, whereas a relative risk of 1.5 for a given dose indicates that the radiation is associated with a 50% increase in cancer above background rates. Absolute risk estimates simply indicate the excess number of cancer cases expected in a population due to a certain radiation dose.

Almost always, if a diagnostic radiology examination is medically indicated, the risk to the mother of not doing the procedure is greater than the risk of potential harm to the fetus. Radiation doses resulting from most diagnostic procedures present no substantial risk of causing fetal death, malformation or impairment of mental development. If the fetus is in the direct beam, the procedure often can, and should, be tailored to reduce fetal dose.

EVALUATION OF RISK WITH RADIATION DOSE

Excess cancers as a result of *in-utero* exposure have not clearly been demonstrated among Japanese atomic-bomb survivor studies even though the population has been followed for about 50 years but the number exposed is not large.

As a result of radiation exposure after conception and until delivery there is felt to be an increased risk of childhood cancer and leukemia. The spontaneous incidence of childhood cancer and leukemia from ages 0 to 15, without radiation exposure above natural background, is about 2 to 3 per 1000. The magnitude of risk following low dose radiation exposure and whether the risk changes throughout pregnancy have been the subject of many publications and interpretation of these data remains open to debate.

There is accumulating evidence that the incidence of childhood cancer may be increased following *in-utero* irradiation before a period has been missed. A recent analysis of many of the epidemiological studies conducted on prenatal X-ray and childhood cancer is consistent with a relative risk of 1.4 (a 40% increase over the background risk) following a fetal dose of about 10 mGy. The best methodological studies, however, suggest that the risk is probably lower than this. The individual probability of childhood cancer after *in-utero* irradiation is known to be very low (about 0.3 to 0.4%) since the background incidence of childhood cancer is so low (about 0.2 to 0.3%). Recent absolute risk estimates for cancer risk from ages 0 to15 after *in-utero* irradiation have been estimated to be in the range of 600 per 10 000 persons each exposed to 1000 mGy (or 0.06% per 10 mGy). This is essentially equivalent to a risk of 1 cancer death per 1700 children exposed *in utero* to 10 mGy.

DIAGNOSTIC DOSE LEVELS

Although present knowledge of the effects of low radiation dose on the developing human embryo is very limited, it is possible, by making various assumptions, to arrive at an upper level of risk of fetal damage or childhood cancer. This is found to be about 1 in 1000 pregnant women irradiated at a dose level of 10 mGy to the embryo. This may be compared with the natural risk of malfunction or malignancies of 1 in 30. The excess absolute risk coefficient is approximately 6% per Gy (Doll and Wakeford, 1997).

The relationship between the level of risk of fetal damage or childhood cancer and the level of radiation dose to the embryo is not known with precision, but a proportional reduction in risk as the dose becomes smaller is widely accepted to be a conservative assumption. The dose level below which the estimated risk is considered to be so small as not to justify the administrative cost and inconvenience of operating a scheduling regime has been widely discussed. A working party of the UK Medical Research Council recommended a gonad dose limit (equivalent to early fetus) of 0.5 mGy. This is also recommended by the World Health Organization as a limit for volunteers involved in radiation research studies.

These MRC recommendations have been criticized for being too low and a proposal of 5 mGy is suggested as a more realistic dose level and considered acceptable by ICRP for the embryo of an occupational exposed woman in the first 2 months of pregnancy. If this limit of 5 mGy is observed then the maximum risk of fetal damage or childhood cancer is 1 in 100 000 women of reproductive capacity.

If a typical radiation dose for staff in a diagnostic radiology department is 0.2 mGy per month then over a 2 month period the exposure would be 0.4 mGy. This is 0.08 of the above limit or 1 in 1 250 000. European radiation protection organizations commonly require maximum limits of:

- 1 mSv for weeks 8 to 15 inclusive.
- 5 mSv for the entire pregnancy.
- Currently, the radiation dose to someone who is pregnant is allowed to be up to 10 mSv. In ICRP 60 the radiation dose limit for the fetus is 1 mSv.
- It is important to recognize that this large reduction in dose limit is not a direct consequence of any equivalent increased risk. It is mainly that the ICRP have taken the view that the fetus should be treated as a member of the public.

- It is important to note that the proposed 1 mSv dose limit to the abdomen of a pregnant worker applies only after pregnancy has been declared.
- Assuming that the declared term lasts for 7 months, then the proposed 1 mSv to the surface of the abdomen would average to a value of 0.14 mSv per month.
- A final point to note is that the value of 0.14 mSv is on the borderline of sensitivity for standard film badge dosimeters. Other more sensitive dosimeters are available. It must be re-emphasized that these issues are for future consideration and depend on the precise implementation of the ICRP 60 recommendations.

GENETIC DAMAGE

This would be seen as radiation-induced **genetic disease** demonstrated in the descendants of the unborn child. The risk for any individual pregnancy following fetal irradiation from medical diagnostic procedures is judged to be small relative to the natural risk of genetic disease (see Table 22.20); thus, there is no indication for termination of pregnancy or for the use of invasive fetal diagnostic techniques (such as amniocentesis).

CANCER INDUCTION

For most diagnostic procedures giving doses up to a few milligrays, the associated risks for the expression of childhood cancer are acceptable when compared with the natural risk. Radiation has been shown to cause leukemia and many types of cancer in both adults and children. Throughout most of pregnancy, the embryo/fetus is assumed to be at about the same risk for potential carcinogenic effects of radiation as are children.

MENTAL IMPAIRMENT

Doses resulting from most conventional diagnostic procedures have no substantial effect on the risk for the individual pregnancy regarding the incidence of fetal death, malformation or the impairment of mental development.

PRECONCEPTION RISKS

For gonadal exposure of the patient, dose minimization through correct alignment, collimation, and the use of gonadal shields whenever practical will minimize possible genetic effects. This applies to both female and male patients. With gonadal shielding then the risk of new mutations resulting from medical diagnostic exposures expressing as genetic disease in the descendants of patients is small, when compared with the risk of those arising naturally. Possible cancer risk to offspring following parental gonadal irradiation as a result of undergoing medical diagnostic procedures is so low that it does not provide any reason for termination of resulting pregnancies or employing invasive fetal diagnostic procedures.

22.6.3 Justification

When it is decided that a particular medical X-ray procedure is justified for a woman who may be pregnant, the procedure should be optimized, achieving the image quality with the appropriate dose. Too low a radiation dose will give poor diagnostic information. Too high a dose in diagnosis imaging increases the risk of tissue damage; this is possible in digital imaging where good quality images can be retrieved from abnormally high dose protocols. This latter point is of some concern in CR/DR techniques so very careful imaging protocols must be established.

THE PREGNANT PATIENT

In the case where patients are definitely or probably pregnant, the justification of the proposed examination should be reviewed very carefully. In some cases the direct clinical benefit for the mother, and therefore indirectly for the fetus, may justify the procedure being undertaken, but the dose to the fetus should be kept to the minimum consistent with the diagnostic purpose. Imaging procedures involving non-ionizing radiation (e.g. ultrasound, MRI) should always be considered as a valid alternative.

When a woman of reproductive age requires diagnostic radiology in which the primary beam irradiates the pelvic area, or for procedures involving radioactive isotopes, then appropriate steps should be taken to determine whether she is or may be pregnant, principally by requesting the date of the last menstrual period. If pregnancy is established or likely, individual justification for the proposed examination needs to be reviewed including whether the examination can be deferred, bearing in mind that a procedure of clinical benefit to the mother may also be of indirect benefit to her unborn child. In any resulting diagnostic examination it is important to keep the dose to the minimum consistent with diagnostic requirements.

For most diagnostic radiation exposures of the early conceptus the risks of cancer will be small, but those few procedures yielding doses above 10 mGy should be avoided, if possible, in early pregnancy. When the possibility of early pregnancy cannot be reasonably excluded, one way of avoiding such risks would be to restrict the use of high dose diagnostic procedures, such as barium enema, pelvic computed tomography (CT) or abdominal CT to the **early part** of the menstrual cycle (see **10-day rule** below) when pregnancy is unlikely.

At diagnostic dose levels, the only adverse effect of radiation on the conceptus which is likely to pose a significant risk is that of cancer induction. None of the other potential hazards (death, malformation, growth retardation, severe mental retardation, and heritable effects) presents a significant problem at the low exposures used in diagnostic procedures.

22.6.4 Implementation of guidelines

As part of the clinical routine patients should be asked if there is any chance that they might be pregnant. If the answer is 'No' the radiological examination can proceed. If there is uncertainty the radiographer/technologist/radiologist is asked to check the date of the last menstrual period. If this is overdue consideration should be given to delaying the examination and make a future appointment (if the clinical conditions allow). This is the so-called '28-day rule' and a suggested questionnaire is given in Fig. 22.15.

THE 28-DAY RULE

When a female patient of reproductive age presents for an examination in which the primary beam irradiates the pelvic area, or for a procedure involving radioactive isotopes, she should be asked whether she is or might be pregnant. If the patient cannot exclude the possibility of pregnancy, she should be asked whether her menstrual period is overdue. In line with accepted convention, this action should be recorded as required by the radiology department local rules. Depending on the answers, patients can then be assigned to one of the following groups:

- No possibility of pregnancy
- Proceed with the examination
- Patient definitely, or probably, pregnant

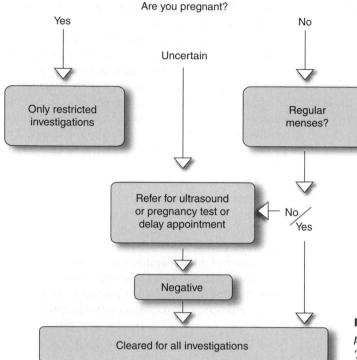

Figure 22.15 *A series of questions for the female patient who may be pregnant; the so-called '28-day rule' identifying the first missed period.*

If pregnancy is established, or a likely possibility then review the **justification** for the examination. Decide whether the investigation can be deferred until after delivery, bearing in mind that a procedure of clinical benefit to the mother may also be of indirect benefit to her unborn child and that delaying an essential procedure until later in pregnancy may present a greater risk to the fetus. If a procedure is undertaken, the fetal dose should be kept to the minimum consistent with the required diagnostic details. Particular problems may be experienced in obtaining this information from female patients under the age of 16 years; in such cases staff should refer to the guidance given by appropriate colleges and societies (e.g. UK College of Radiographers).

WHERE PREGNANCY IS ESTABLISHED (OR LIKELY)

Review the justification for the proposed examination, and decide whether to defer the investigation until after delivery, bearing in mind that a procedure of clinical benefit to the mother may also be of indirect benefit to her unborn child and that delaying an essential procedure until later in pregnancy may present a greater risk to the fetus. If a procedure is undertaken, the fetal dose should be kept to the minimum consistent with the diagnostic purpose(s). The number of such patients is likely to be small.

If it becomes obvious that a fetus has been inadvertently exposed, despite the above guidelines, the small risk to the fetus of the exposure does not justify the greater risks of invasive fetal diagnostic procedures to the fetus and mother (particularly as they are unlikely to pick up any induced effect), nor does the risk justify termination.

WHERE PREGNANCY CANNOT BE EXCLUDED

For **low dose diagnostic procedures** proceed with the examination, provided that the period is not overdue. If the period is overdue, follow the advice in the previous paragraph. **High dose procedures** (defined as examinations resulting in fetal doses of some tens of milligray such as fluoroscopy or CT) may carry significant risks: this reinforces the importance of knowing the magnitude of doses in individual departments. New evidence suggests that these may carry a small

risk of cancer induction for the unknown fetus. One of two courses could be adopted:

- Apply the rule that in women of childbearing age these examinations are booked for the first 10 days of the menstrual cycle, when conception is unlikely to have occurred (formerly known as the '10-day rule').
- Re-book patients who attend for such examinations and are identified as being in the second half of their cycle, of childbearing age and in whom pregnancy cannot be excluded. The number of such patients is likely to be small.

Although there may be a small risk to the developing fetus, this risk will increase in the months following the first missed period, and high dose examinations should only be re-booked if they can safely be postponed until after delivery, should the patient prove to be pregnant.

Doses resulting from most conventional diagnostic procedures have no substantial effect on the risk for the individual pregnancy regarding the incidence of fetal death, malformation or the impairment of mental development. The only examinations that would carry a risk would be those involving the abdomen or pelvis. Other routine examinations involving chest and extremities impose negligible radiation exposure to the uterus; this includes head CT.

If it becomes obvious that a fetus has been inadvertently exposed, despite the above guidance, the small risk to the fetus, caused by the exposure, does not justify the greater risks of invasive fetal diagnostic procedures to the fetus and mother (particularly as they are unlikely to pick up any induced effect), nor does the risk justify the termination of pregnancy.

Skeletal surveys can be achieved by employing the 'scout-view' or 'Toposcan' longitudinal scan given by a CT machine. This is a very low dose technique giving typical dose levels of 40 µGy (4 mrad). Other investigations in the abdominal region should use the fastest screen/film combinations or digital radiography that give a diagnostic image. Chest and extremity investigations are not restricted since the dose to the conceptus or fetus is negligible.

THE '10-DAY RULE'

An early recommendation from the ICRP for examinations involving the lower abdomen of women was '… *is least likely to pose any hazard to a developing*

embryo if carried out during the 10-day interval following the onset of menstruation …'. This recommendation was adopted by certain national regulatory organizations but was subsequently questioned since it was found that the developing ovum prior to fertilization was equally radiosensitive. The shaded portion in Fig. 22.14 represents the stage of follicle production and ovulation prior to fertilization which can be threatened by radiation exposure. The 10-day rule serves a very useful purpose when considering high dose diagnostic procedures (e.g. fluoroscopy or CT).

LOW DOSE PROCEDURES

When pregnancy cannot be excluded, but the menstrual period is **not** overdue, low dose procedures (resulting in doses of a few milligrays to the fetus) may proceed, as the additional risk of problems in childhood, from exposure to any very early fetus, is judged to be acceptable when compared with the natural risk in childhood. If the period is overdue assume pregnancy and follow the advice in the following paragraph.

HIGH DOSE PROCEDURES

Procedures that result in doses of some tens of milligray to the fetus do carry an additional risk, as stated previously. In most departments, the only routine examinations in this category will probably be abdominal and pelvic computed tomography. However, any procedure that delivers doses to the fetus of some tens of milligray (e.g. some barium studies) may carry significant risks. This reinforces the importance of knowing the magnitude of doses in individual departments. The new evidence suggests that these may carry a small risk of cancer induction for the unknown fetus. One of two courses could be adopted:

- Apply the rule that in female patients of childbearing age these examinations are booked for the first 10 days of the menstrual cycle, when conception is unlikely to have occurred (formerly known as the '10-day rule').
- Re-book patients who attend for such examinations and are identified as being in the second half of their cycle, are of childbearing age, and in whom pregnancy cannot be excluded. **The number of such patients is likely to be small.**

It should be emphasized that although there may be a small risk to the unknown fetus, this risk will increase in the months following the first missed period, and high dose examinations should only be re-booked if they can safely be postponed until after delivery, should the patient prove to be pregnant.

COMPUTED TOMOGRAPHY

There is a strong case for restricting high dose examinations such as CT, which can give *in-utero* radiation doses between 20 and 50 mGy. A '10-day rule' could be employed in such cases which restricts high dose investigations to the first part of the menstrual cycle. If the patient is comatose (trauma patient) or clinical conditions demand a radiological investigation then the lowest possible radiation doses should be employed.

For exposure of pregnant women to the higher doses (some tens of milligray) associated with, for example, pelvic CT, there may be more than a doubling of the natural cancer risk in the unborn child. This level of excess risk is about 1 in 1000 for the individual fetus and is unlikely to be a reason for termination of the pregnancy or for the use of invasive fetal diagnostic procedures.

Monitoring of national practice in CT would be facilitated by the introduction of a national dosimetry protocol for CT in parallel with the system in successful operation for conventional X-ray examinations. Consideration should be given to the feasibility of establishing achievable doses on the basis of general recommendations for CT procedures.

22.7 SHIELDING MATERIALS

22.7.1 Lead sheet

Lead sheet is the standard shielding material and is readily available in a standard thicknesses for building and plumbing requirements. These thicknesses have traditional code numbers which correspond to their mass measured in units of lb ft^2. Table 22.23 lists the coding and lead thicknesses. In the UK lead sheet is manufactured to BS EN 12588 (BSI, 1999), which controls composition and thickness tolerance. Lead (Pb) is the usual shielding material being high density and easily worked. Sheet lead is

fixed inside a plywood sandwich (plymax) forming an ideal material for partitions. Thicknesses range from 1 to 4 mm for diagnostic radiology. This ease of installation may offset its expense but although other materials are cheaper they are more labor intensive. Other materials used as effective shielding are concrete and brick. Their shielding efficiency is expressed as '**lead equivalent**' in mm Pb ranging from 1 mm to 4 mm.

22.7.2 Concrete and concrete blocks

This is a complex hydrated calcium silicate of varying density. For load bearing floors and ceilings 150 and 300 mm of concrete will be needed and this usually provides sufficient radiation protection provided the density is at least 2350 kg m^{-3}. Any irregularity in construction (embedded ducting or pipework) is unacceptable if uniform shielding has to be achieved. Sufficient radiation shielding for walls in diagnostic X-ray facilities can often be achieved using high density (2350 kg m^{-3}) solid concrete blocks. Figure 22.16 gives the equivalent thickness of concrete for a stated thickness of lead sheet. Concrete block walls may need additional shielding (lead sheet) if a required thickness cannot be accepted.

Clay bricks have a typical density of about 1600 kg m^{-3}. Denser bricks are available of 2100 kg m^{-3}. Since brick is less dense than concrete a greater thickness is required to achieve the necessary lead equivalence. A wall can be built of one or two rows of bricks in order to provide greater shielding.

Table 22.23 *Standard lead thicknesses and weights (kg) per square meter.*

Thickness (mm)	Code number*	Weight per square meter
0.50		5.70
1.00		11.40
1.32	3	15.00
1.80	4	20.40
2.00		22.70
2.24	5	25.40
2.65	6	30.10
3.15	7	35.70
3.55	8	40.30

*The code number is an old rating that corresponds to the weight per unit area in lb ft^{-2}.

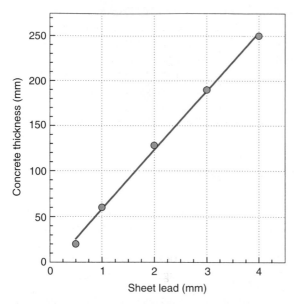

Figure 22.16 *The equivalent thicknesses of lead and concrete compared.*

22.7.4 Gypsum wallboard

Gypsum wallboard (plasterboard) is the name for a family of panel products manufactured mainly from hydrated calcium sulfate ($CaSO_4 \cdot 2H_2O$) sandwiched in a paper covering. Like concrete it owes its shielding properties to the calcium content. The wallboard is typically a noncombustible core made primarily of gypsum with a paper surfacing on the face, back, and long edges. Standard board thicknesses are 9.5, 12.5, and 15 mm. It is common practice to fix two or three layers of wallboard to one side of a partition wall, and this is a convenient method of room shielding for low energy X-ray applications such as in mammography or dental radiology.

22.7.5 Barium plaster

This is usually a mixture of conventional gypsum plaster incorporating barytes aggregate ($BaSO_4$); the mixture is treated the same as plaster and requires only the addition of water for its preparation. A total plaster thickness of up to 25 mm can be achieved. The plaster application requires particular skills which may not be readily available and is labor intensive. It is worth noting that with adequate room sizes and modern machines, concrete block or brick construction offers a very effective barrier against scattered radiation. The added expense of barium plaster (materials and fixing time) seldom warrants the added protection and should be specified cautiously. Mobile lead screens or strategically placed lead sheet plywood (plymax) can usefully be installed in sensitive areas or as room partitions for temporary room designs. Sensible and informed planning can save a great deal of unnecessary cost.

22.7.6 Lead glass

This is similar in appearance to plate glass but it is specially formulated with a high lead and barium content to give the glass its shielding properties; density and lead content can vary as shown in Table 22.24. The glass is particularly brittle and great care is needed in handling and supporting it with rubber seals in its frame. It is also softer than normal glass, so that it can be scratched and chipped easily. The relation between the thickness of lead glass and its lead equivalence is given in Table 22.25. Common applications of lead glass are observer windows in control rooms and mobile screens.

22.7.7 Transparent lead acrylic

Transparent lead acrylic is an acrylic co-polymer resin with lead salts added to the plastic mix. It is

Table 22.24 *Physical properties of lead glass.*

Property	
Density	4800 to 5050 kg m^{-3}
Lead content (PbO)	48 to 65%

Table 22.25 *Dimensions and lead equivalence of lead glass.*

Glass thickness (mm)	Lead equivalent (mm) 80 to 150 kV
3.5 to 5.0	1.5
5.0 to 6.5	1.6
7.0 to 8.5	2.2
8.5 to 10	2.7
10.0 to 11.5	3.2
11.5 to 13.0	3.6
16.0 to 18.0	5.1
20.0 to 22.0	6.3
26.0 to 29.0	8.2
33.0 to 36.0	10.5

Table 22.26 *Dimensions and lead equivalence of transparent lead acrylic.*

Lead equivalence (mm)	Acrylic lead thickness (mm)
0.3	7
0.5	12
0.8	18
1.0	22
1.5	35
2.0	46

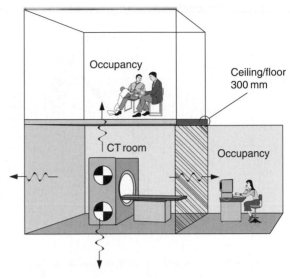

Figure 22.17 *Room position within the building. Radiation from the X-ray machine will penetrate walls, floors, and ceilings into adjacent areas (e.g. offices).*

commonly manufactured in six sheet thicknesses and the key characteristics of each type are presented in Table 22.26. The sheets are more robust and easier to machine and bond than lead glass; it is also lighter, easier, and cheaper to install. It is a softer material and easier to scratch. For low kV radiation shielding (mammography, bone densitometry, and dentistry) lead acrylic sheet is generally less expensive than lead glass. For conventional rooms, in which 1.5 mm or 2 mm of lead protection is commonly specified, lead glass is cheaper. Lead glass also offers a much wider lead equivalence.

Shielded observation windows as secondary barriers can be provided by both lead glass and lead plastic. Glass impregnated with lead and barium oxides or acrylic plastic impregnated with an organo-lead compound can be used. Plastic has the advantage of less cost, so larger areas are possible allowing large open-plan room designs. It is shatterproof, unlike glass, and can be machined.

22.8 RADIATION SHIELDING SPECIFICATION

Several methods have been recommended for calculating the required shielding for an X-ray room. The safe design principles include a proper understanding of the workload (intended and projected for increasing patient numbers) together with the position of the X-ray room with respect to other users (consulting rooms and offices) (see Fig. 22.17). Modern construction methods commonly specify significant thicknesses of concrete in the ceilings and floors that offer sufficient lead equivalence on their own (see Fig. 22.16).

22.8.1 Scattered radiation

Scattered radiation is always present in diagnostic radiology when an absorber is placed in the primary beam and is a direct result of Compton scattering. In clinical applications the fluence of scattered radiation depends on three major factors:

- The volume of the patient irradiated
- The spectrum (quality) of the primary beam
- The field size

Both the fluence and the quality of the scattered radiation are dependent on the angle at which they are measured; the half-value layer (beam quality) also varies with scatter angle.

22.8.2 Leakage radiation

Leakage radiation arises if the X-ray tube housing is badly designed or misplaced. The X-ray tube housing is generally constructed of aluminum or steel lined with lead. Any radiation transmitted through this protective shield is termed leakage radiation. Manufacturers generally provide more protection than is needed to meet the regulatory requirements, with the possible exception of mobile radiographic equipment where weight is

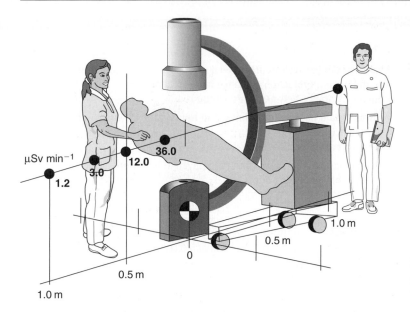

μSv min⁻¹

1.2
3.0
12.0
36.0

1.0 m
0.5 m
0
0.5 m
1.0 m

Figure 22.18 *Mobile C-arm radiation contours, showing the low dose rates at 1.0 m from the machine.*

especially important. Dental X-ray units are prone to losing collimation, leading to leaked radiation. Leakage is usually given for a maximum operating kV$_p$. Typically measurable leakage will be much lower than the regulatory maximum of 1 mGy at 1 m in 1 h. The presence of leakage radiation can be established by holding a film cassette or image plate next to the housing during an X-ray exposure made with collimators closed; any leakage seen by the cassette will be revealed by black streak marks.

22.8.3 Mobile X-ray machines

The use of small mobile X-ray machines outside the radiology department need pose no radiation exposure problems since these machines are deliberately designed to have a decreased primary beam intensity. Portable machines can be found in intensive care units (ICUs) which use mobile X-ray units operating at 60 to 80 kV$_p$ with a low tube current. Rare-earth screens should always be used with these units. Unprotected members of staff should be 2 m from the tube housing; at this distance scatter radiation is negligible. An example of local rules for the use of portable equipment in wards would be:

- The primary beam should only be directed at the patient.
- Ward staff should stand at least 2 m from the machine unless contrary to the patient's wellbeing.

Aprons and gloves should be available in this case.
- The radiographer or technician must wear a protective apron (0.25 mm Pb).
- Small mobile screens should be available if adjacent patients need to be protected.

Mobile C-arm fluoroscopy units are used for orthopedic and cardiac pacemaker work. The exposure from these machines shows that at 2 m the scattered radiation is negligible (Fig. 22.18).

22.8.4 Room design

The position of the X-ray room within the building identifies adjacent areas which may need particular attention (e.g. offices, kitchens); radiation will penetrate walls, ceilings, and floors into these locations (Fig. 22.17). The principles associated with room design and equipment layout generally cover the following points:

- Construction of barriers to attenuate both primary (direct beam) and secondary (scatter) radiation
- Restriction of X-ray beam dimensions (collimation)
- Observing the inverse square law during planning stages and equipment positioning
- Using the minimum radiation for the diagnostic information required
- Warning signs and indicator lights in operation

Table 22.27 *Fluoroscopy workload.*

Usage	Remarks
Low 30 mA min week^{-1}	Theaters and intensive care units need no special construction requirements Staff and patient protection guidance from local rules Adequate clearance between beds is required
Medium 30 to 300 mA min week^{-1}	Theaters should have walls, ceilings, and floors 1 mm Pb eqivalent Restricted access Screen protection for adjacent patients
High >300 mA min week^{-1}	Walls, ceilings, and floors of 2 mm Pb equivalent and more Warning lights on outside doors

Table 22.28 *Parameters for calculating primary shielding using eqn 22.10 in Box 22.11.*

Parameter and value	Area
P: yearly constraint dose (mSv)	
1.0	Control areas in X-ray room
0.3	Public areas in radiology department
T: Occupancy	
1.0	Control areas and offices
0.25	Corridors and wards
0.06	Toilets and outside areas
U: Use factor	
1	Surfaces exposed to the primary beam
0.25	Areas not exposed to the primary beam
0.06	Occasional exposure (ceilings)

When designing radiation protection for a room the following points should also be known:

- The workload expected in the room in mA min per week (see Table 22.27)
- The direction of the primary beam
- The occupancy factor of the X-ray room and any adjoining non-X-ray rooms (Table 22.28)

An occupancy or use factor is given to the exposed surfaces (floors, walls, ceilings) so that the amount of shielding can be calculated. The expected workload in mA min per week can be estimated from the X-ray examination and the number of patients examined. It is categorized in terms of usage: low, moderate, and high. The limits are given in Table 22.27.

The general design of an X-ray room should consider easy access for the staff behind the shielded area of the control console. The primary beam of the X-ray unit should be restricted so that occupants in adjoining rooms are not exposed. Ideally the room should be of adequate size, typically 36 m^2 (350 ft^2) with a ceiling height of 3.6 m (12 ft) and any external windows 2 m (6.5 ft) above ground level. The walls should be concrete block or brick; particular attention should be made to any corridor walls. There should be a shielded cubicle surrounding the control panel with a clear, lead glass observation window of adequate lead equivalent thickness (typically 1.5 to 2 mm Pb equivalent for conventional units). The primary beam should be directed away from doors and the control cubicle. Wall areas that may be exposed to the primary beam should be shielded depending on the activity in the adjacent room. The doors leading into the room should be lead-lined but this is not necessary for the staff access door since this should already be protected by the shielding of the control area.

The design and construction of an X-ray room decides not only the safe working conditions for the radiology personnel working in that room but also for non-radiological staff (secretaries, porters, and nurses) outside the immediate vicinity. Visitors and the general public are also afforded optimum protection.

The skill involved in shielding design maintains optimum protection without over-specification, since lead sheet and barium plaster are very heavy and require substantial and very expensive foundation support. Lead-lined doors should only be specified if essential since these too are very expensive and because of their inertia when closing can constitute a hazard in themselves.

Uniformity of room shielding should be an important consideration. Although each wall may receive different exposure levels from the existing X-ray unit and calculations suggest varying thicknesses of lead sheet or concrete/brick for each wall, the highest figure should be used for all the walls since during the lifetime of the room different X-ray systems may be installed in different orientations.

22.8.5 Clinical workload

The workload value is a measure of expected exposure levels obtained from the expected number of patients and the total mAs per patient. Table 22.27 indicates the **mA min per week** (mA min w^{-1}) expected for low, medium, and high usage facilities and Box 22.10 uses some clinical workloads in order to express these as mA min w^{-1}.

Since most X-ray units now have dose–area product meters fitted this has become the method of choice for estimating clinical workload. Table 22.29 lists some values for guidance. The workload for CT is given by the number of slices performed in any one year for a single slice machine; a multislice machine would need a modified calculation (see later).

22.8.6 Occupancy

The dose constraint principle should be applied regarding the occupancy of areas adjacent to the radiation source (control area, next door rooms etc.). Radiation sources can also be nuclear medicine patients or patients undergoing PET studies. The occupancy factor for an area is taken as a worst case for the fraction of time spent by the single person who is in the area the longest. The critical groups for shielding purposes will not be patients or patients' visitors but radiology department workers, both clinical and non-clinical (secretaries, porters etc.). It is estimated from the fraction of an 8-h day or 2000-h year for which a particular area may be occupied by a single individual.

When considering occupancy it is important to remember the constraint level of $3/10$ of the maximum limit areas where exposure can be greater than 6 mSv per year should be controlled. Any design factors and assumptions on occupancy should reflect this limit. A lower limit of 0.5 mSv per annum or an occupancy factor of 0.05 (5%) is sometimes recommended and Table 22.28 suggests some working values for yearly constraint dose levels, occupancy and use factors. These values do not represent fixed rules but are suggestions. Any assessment should remember the

---

Box 22.10 Workload estimation

Low use

For 100 patients X-rayed in ICU per week the average exposure is

$$15 \, \text{mAs} = 1500 \, \text{mAs}$$
$$\text{or} \quad 25 \, \text{mA min week}^{-1}$$

Moderate use

For 15 patients undergoing fluoroscopy per week, each patient is exposed for 3 to 5 min screening at 3 mA, giving 15 mA min per patient. This gives a maximum of

$$225 \, \text{mA min week}^{-1}$$

High use

For 10 patients per week undergoing cine-angiography assume there are five cine runs per patient, giving 5 s at 1200 mA, or

$$5000 \, \text{mA min week}^{-1}$$

Table 22.29 *Values for the dose–area product (DAP) for some representative examinations.*

Examination	DAP (Gy cm²)	
	Average	Upper limit
Lumbar spine AP	3.2	5
Lumber spine Lat	3.4	7
Lumbar spine LSJ	3.6	5
Chest PA	0.15	0.25
Chest Lat	0.5	1
Abdomen AP	3.8	7
Pelvis AP	3.3	7
Skull AP/PA	0.8	1.5
Skull Lat	0.5	1
Thoracic spine AP	1.8	3
Thoracic spine Lat	3.3	6
IVU	16.0	40.0

0.3 mSv constraint value for public places and careful appraisal of the architectural drawings should be made including the surrounding area/rooms in order to identify areas that need added protection.

Although corridors may have a low occupancy value, a waiting area may be allocated in a corridor serving an X-ray installation (CT or chest unit). This must be taken into account when specifying the construction of the corridor wall.

LARGE C-ARM FLUOROSCOPY UNITS

Large cantilevered C-arm machines which are tending to replace fixed under or over-table units present their own problems for staff radiation protection. Figure 22.19 shows a typical unit being used with the X-ray tube both under-table (a) and over-table (b). The contour A in both cases shows significant radiation dose rates to the operator without local machine shielding. Figure 22.19b shows the marked reduction in dose rate when a 1.5 to 2 mm Pb equivalent acrylic shield is used.

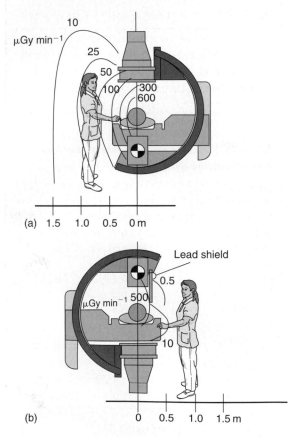

Figure 22.19 *Two C-arm positions. (a) The X-ray tube under the table and (b) the X-ray tube over the table where contours show the change in radiation exposure to the operator with shielding.*

22.8.7 Primary barrier

Protection from the primary beam must be incorporated into any part of the ceiling, floor, and walls that the primary beam can be directed toward. The equipment itself will be supplied with shielding for the tube housing, image intensifier and table covers. In order to limit the radiation dose to an acceptable level shielding must be provided to walls, floors, ceilings, and room doors:

- **Walls**: Shielding should take into account the distance between the X-ray tube and the type of adjoining room.
- **Floors and ceilings**: These are commonly concrete and usually need no additional material. The level of extra shielding depends on the occupancy in areas below and above the X-ray room. If concrete construction is not used then local lead shielding may be necessary above and below the X-ray unit.
- **Doors**: Both single and double width patient access doors should be lead lined; this can be 1 mm in most cases since distance from the equipment would have reduced scattered radiation reaching doors.

Lead-lined doors are very expensive and should be planned with care. Warning lights outside doors are essential. The doors should be lockable on the inside. The upright cassette holder/chest stand should have a primary shield (2 mm lead) on the wall behind.

PRIMARY BARRIER CALCULATION

The information that is necessary in order to calculate the primary barrier requirements is:

- Yearly dose limit under constraint (P)
- Workload in mA min per week (W)
- Maximum kilovoltage likely to be experienced
- Occupancy factors for adjoining rooms (T)
- Use factor (U)

The recommended constraint values (P) can be modified to suit local requirements. The workload is measured in mA min. A 5-min screening at 5 mA is 25 mA min per patient. For 20 patients a week this would be 500 mA min per week. The maximum kilovoltage is usually taken as 100 kV for routine diagnostic work but 90 and 70 keV are considered; computed tomography uses the 150 kV$_p$ curve. The allowable transmission B for maintaining radiation levels, corrected for weekly dose levels, is calculated within the set limits from factors listed in Table 22.28:

$$B = \frac{P \times d^2}{W \times U \times T \times 52} \qquad (22.10)$$

where d is the distance from the X-ray tube housing. The other factors are identified in the bulleted list above. The B factor is translated into lead thickness by reference to Fig. 22.20. The shielding for a primary barrier specification is calculated in Box 22.11 using these graphs for the room shown in Fig. 22.21.

The maximum lead thickness for the left wall in this room is 2 mm. A prudent physicist or radiation adviser would specify shielding to comply with Code 5 (see Table 22.23) for walls, doors, ceiling, and floor. This higher specification and its uniformity would allow future increase in workload and any repositioning of the X-ray system.

22.8.8 Secondary barrier

This protects personnel from scattered radiation and applies to any part of the room receiving scattered radiation. Barrier requirements are far less than for primary barrier since scattered radiation 1 m from the X-ray source has an intensity about 0.1% of the primary beam. Secondary shielding is typically half

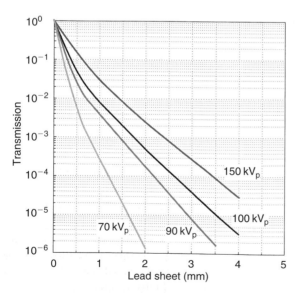

Figure 22.20 *Factor 'B' calculated in Box 22.11 related to shielding thickness (mm Pb) for energies 70, 90, 100, and 150 kV$_p$. A constant current supply is assumed.*

the shielding thickness of primary barriers and is normally satisfied if the walls are brick or concrete.

Scatter levels have steadily become lower due to the introduction of faster film-screens, digital radiography, modern machine design and more effective collimation of the beam. Although calculated barrier requirements have decreased, the patient safety levels have become more stringent requiring greater safety levels for staff and public areas. Safety measures that influence patient dose reduction have a direct effect on radiation exposure to staff.

22.8.9 Computed tomography shielding

The introduction of multislice machines has widened the scatter contours within the CT room (see Fig. 22.22). The 'bow-tie' shaped contour

---

Box 22.11 Primary barrier thickness

Calculate the radiation shielding necessary for the X-ray room depicted in Fig. 22.21. It has a workload of 400 mA min per week. Values are taken from Table 22.28.

Top wall

P is 0.3 mSv since there is a public area on the other side of this wall; the U value is 0.25 (exposed to scatter) and T is 0.25. The X-ray housing has a minimum distance of 2 m. From eqn 22.10 this gives a transmission value of 0.001 which translates as 1.75 mm Pb for 100 kV$_p$.

Left wall

Since this contains the vertical chest bucky it is exposed to the primary beam, so $U = 1$. Other factors are the same yielding a B value of 0.0002 which requires 2.4 mm or approximately 2.0 mm if the shielding offered by the cassette and patient is taken into account.

Control console window

At 4 m distance from the housing the lead glass would be about 1.25 mm Pb equivalent.

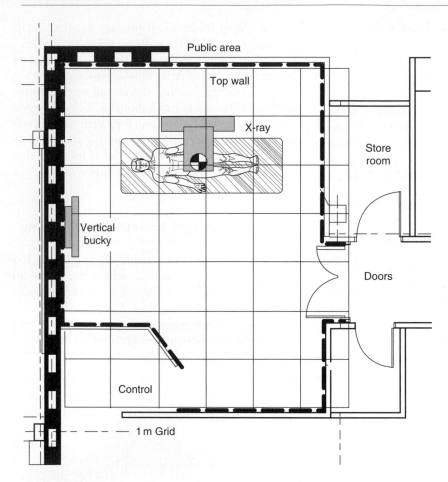

Public area

Top wall

X-ray

Store room

Vertical bucky

Doors

Control

1 m Grid

Figure 22.21 *A general X-ray room with an X-ray housing situated 2 m from the top wall. A control window is positioned 4 m from the housing. This is the example used in Box 22.11.*

surrounding the gantry center is usually shown as microgray per rotation. Both increased acquisition speed and efficiency of spiral CT scanners demand high output X-ray tubes. These higher rated tubes place additional radiation burden on the radiology and immediate hospital environment. The constraint dose limits for workers and public require great care when deciding specification for radiation shielding around spiral CT installations. Current hospital building regulations in Europe typically require solid floor and ceiling construction with a concrete thickness of 300 mm (equivalent to about 3 mm lead: see Fig. 22.16) and a floor to ceiling height of 3.6 m.

In order to calculate the weekly dose rate at this contour the following parameters are used (using data for a 64-slice machine):

1 Exposure per rotation typically 210 mAs
2 Number of rotations per patient: five rotations for this example

3 Number of body studies per week: 150 for this example

From (2) and (3) above, the number of gantry rotations per week is $150 \times 5 = 750$. The dose at ceiling level (using the 1.3 μGy contour in Fig. 22.22) is $750 \times 1.3 = 975$ μGy (or approximately 1 mSv per week). A transmission figure of $0.3/(1 \times 52)$ or 0.006 suggests shielding of 1.6 mm Pb or 120 mm concrete would be sufficient (see Fig. 22.16). Since modern construction thicknesses are typically 300 mm concrete no extra shielding is required. This applies also to the floor where the 10.4 μGy plays a part; shielding of 2.5 mm Pb is reasonable which is more than satisfied with 300 mm concrete. If Code 6 specification is adopted then the 2.65 mm Pb or equivalent would maintain radiation levels well within any constraint limits.

The hospital radiation protection physicist (adviser) will determine whether the specified shielding will provide adequate protection in adjacent

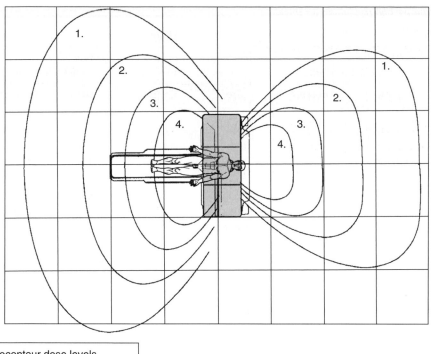

isocontour dose levels
microGy per rotation
1.   1.3
2.   2.6
3.   5.2
4.   10.4

1 m grid

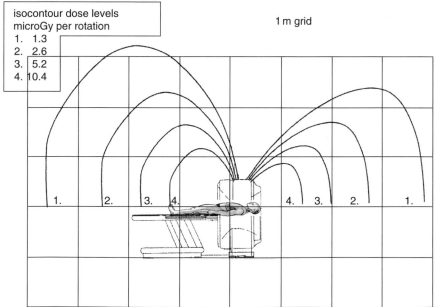

Figure 22.22 *The radiation air kerma contours for a 64-slice computed tomography machine.*

areas, particularly in high occupancy areas such as the control room and reporting areas. Whilst this form of shielding may provide adequate protection from radiation directly scattered from the patient the CT machine is a rotating X-ray source and effective protection from conic-pattern scattered beam is necessary by specifying adequate floor and ceiling thicknesses.

Standard guidance figures for radiation shielding are offered particularly in the USA (Table 28.30). This simplifies design specification although it does not take into consideration the size of the room. Setting down the dimensions of the room and placement of the X-ray unit within the room will have significant effects on the shielding requirement. So computation of the shielding for a practical workload could save

Table 28.30 *Some alternative USA regulations for shielding.*

Location	Anticipated workload					
	High (250 to 1000 mA min week^{-1})		Moderate (15 to 250 mA min week^{-1})		Low (0 to 15 mA min week^{-1})	
	Lead	Concrete	Lead	Concrete	Lead	Concrete
Primary beam						
Walls	1.5 to 3.2	130 to 230	1.5	130	1.5	130
Doors	1.5 to 3.2	130 to 230	1.5	130	1.5	130
Floors	2.5 to 3.2	165 to 230	1.5 to 2.5	130 to 165	1.5	130
Secondary radiation						
Walls	1.5	130	1.0 to 1.5	60 to 130	0 to 1	0 to 6
Doors	1.5	130	1.0 to 1.5	60 to 130	0 to 1	0 to 6
Floors	1.5	130	1.0 to 1.5	60 to 130	0 to 1	0 to 6
Ceilings	1.5	60	1.0	60	0 to 1	0 to 6

retro-fitting additional shielding when the workload increases or a higher output machine installed.

22.9 THE ORGANIZATION OF HOSPITAL RADIATION SAFETY

22.9.1 The radiation safety committee

The proper implementation of safety measures throughout a hospital, including radiology, nuclear medicine, and laboratories using radiation equipment is the responsibility of a committee or informed group appointed by the hospital board.

Every hospital that uses radiation equipment or substances must establish a **hospital radiation protection committee** comprising radiologist, hospital administrator, physicist, and radiation safety officers from each department using radiation. There should be definite pathways to this committee for any member of the hospital staff who wishes to clarify problems or events concerning radiation exposure to either staff or patients.

Radiation safety officers are sometimes termed 'authorized' users, either a licensed physician certified in radiology, radiation oncology or who has been trained and certified in the use of radiation or radioactive materials and listed in the hospital's license. Hospital doctors, other than radiologists, who are responsible for using or directing medical exposures (e.g. orthopedic surgeons) should undergo a recognized training course.

28.9.2 Hospital and local regulations

A set of simple instructions to staff members must be published in-house for reference. Controlled and supervised areas can be defined in this document along with procedures for the safe use of radiation. Brief 'local rules' for each laboratory or section of radiology should be displayed along with the name(s) of the safety officers. Suggested outlines for radiographic local rules would be:

- Close the room door before making an exposure.
- Staff not taking part in a procedure should be behind control panel shielding.
- Gonad shields should be used on patients whenever appropriate.
- Beam field size to be collimated consistent with investigation. Fluoroscopy procedures should operate under limited tube current (1 mA at 100 kV).
- Staff who are needed to support patients during an exposure must wear a lead-fabric apron (0.3 mm Pb equivalent). Lead-fabric gloves may also be necessary.
- A record should be kept of the dose given.

A larger version of the department local rules should also include a list of diagnostic reference levels (DRLs) as well as a collection of procedure protocols.

A continuous program for the training of hospital staff in the details of radiation safety should be available in all large hospitals, organized by the radiation physicist in conjunction with radiology clinical staff. The European Commission radiation protection document 116 offers guidelines on education and training in radiation protection for medical exposures which could form the basis of any teaching program, either basic or advanced, for radiology staff, hospital doctors using X-ray equipment and technologists.

KEYWORDS

accidental exposure*: an exposure of individuals as a result of an accident. It does not include emergency exposure

action level: an intervention level applied to exposure to radiation; when a public exposure action level is consistently exceeded, remedial action to reduce exposure should be considered; when an occupational exposure action level is consistently exceeded within a practice, a program of radiation protection should apply to that practice

ALARA: as low as reasonably achievable. Making every reasonable effort to reduce radiation levels below the stated dose limits within economic and social limits

ALARP: as low as reasonably practical. The limiting factor being existing facilities due for update or replacement. (An unofficial term)

annual limit on intake (ALI): that quantity of a radionuclide which, taken into the body during 1 year, would lead to a committed effective dose equal to the occupational annual limit on effective dose

approved dosimetric service*: a body responsible for the calibration, reading or interpretation of individual monitoring devices, or for the measurement of radioactivity in the human body or in biological samples, or for assessment of doses, whose capacity to act in this respect is recognized by the competent authorities

approved medical practitioner*: a medical practitioner responsible for the medical surveillance of category A workers, as defined in Article 21, whose capacity to act in that respect is recognized by the competent authorities

authorization*: a permission granted in a document by the competent authority, on application, or granted by national legislation, to carry out a practice or any other action within the scope of this Directive

becquerel (Bq): a measure of radioactivity: one disintegration per second, 1 dps

BEIR: biological effects of ionizing radiation

clearance levels*: values established by national competent authorities and expressed in terms of activity concentrations and/or total activity, at or below which radioactive substances or materials containing radioactive substances arising from any practice subject to the requirement of reporting or authorization may be released from the requirements of this Directive

clinical audit†: a systematic examination or review of medical radiological procedures which seeks to improve the quality and the outcome of patient care through structured review whereby radiological practices, procedures and results are examined against agreed standards for good medical radiological procedures, with modification of practices where indicated and the application of new standards if necessary

clinical responsibility†: responsibility regarding individual medical exposures attributed to a practitioner, notably: justification; optimization; clinical evaluation of the outcome; cooperation with other specialists and the staff, as appropriate, regarding practical aspects; obtaining information, if appropriate, of previous examinations; providing existing radiological information and/or records to other practitioners and/or prescribers, as required, giving information on the risk, of ionizing radiation to patients and other individuals involved, as appropriate

code of practice: for radiation protection a document prescribing specific requirements for radiation protection in a particular application

collective effective dose (collective dose): sum of individual doses received by a population in a given time from a specified radioactive source. A measure of the total radiation exposure of a group of people which is obtained by summing their individual effective doses. The collective dose, S, is measured in man-sieverts (manSv) and is given by the equation

$$S = E_{(\tau)} \times N$$

collective equivalent dose: a measure of the total radiation exposure of a specific organ type or tissue type in a group of people which is obtained by summing the equivalent doses received by those individual organs or tissues of the people exposed. The collective equivalent dose, S_T, is measured in man-sieverts (manSv) and is given by the equation

$$S_T = \sum H_{T(\tau)} \times N$$

committed equivalent dose: the equivalent dose which an organ or tissue is committed to receive from an intake of radioactive material. The committed equivalent dose, $H_{T(\tau)}$, is defined as

$$H_{T(\tau)} = H_T \times \tau$$

where H_T is the equivalent dose, and τ is the time period, which is taken to be 50 years or, for children, 70 years

committed effective dose: the effective dose which a person is committed to receive from an intake of radioactive material. The committed effective dose, $E_{(\tau)}$ is defined as:

$$E_{(\tau)} = \sum w_T \times H_{T(\tau)}$$

where τ is the period over which the integral of the equivalent dose rate for organ or tissue T is made to obtain the committed equivalent dose $H_{T(\tau)}$. For adults, an integration period of 50 years is assumed; for children, the integration period is taken to age 70 years

competent authority*: any authority designated by a member state

controlled area: an area with limited access within a department; an area subject to special rules for the purpose of protecting against ionizing radiation or of preventing the spread of radioactive contamination and to which access is controlled

constraint: either dose constraint in the case of exposures anticipated to be received, or risk constraint in the case of potential exposures (see dose constraint and risk constraint)

controlled area: an area to which access is subject to control and in which employees are required to follow specific procedures aimed at controlling exposure to radiation

critical group: a group of members of the public comprising individuals who are relatively homogeneous with regard to age, diet and those behavioral characteristics that affect the doses received and who receive the highest radiation doses from a particular practice

curie (Ci): a non-SI unit which is a measure of radioactivity. 1 Ci = 3.7 H 10^{10} Bq

deep dose equivalent: external whole-body dose-equivalent at 1 cm depth. The symbol used is H_d

detriment: a measure, or measures, of harm caused by exposure to radiation and usually taken to mean health detriment. It has no single definition, but can be taken to be an attribute or a collection of attributes which measure harm, such as attributable probability of death and reduction of life expectancy

diagnostic reference levels[†]: dose levels in medical radiodiagnostic practices or, in the case of radiopharmaceuticals, levels of activity, for typical examinations for groups of standard-sized patients or standard phantoms for broadly defined types of equipment. These levels are expected not to be exceeded for standard procedures when good and normal practice regarding diagnostic and technical performance is applied

diploid: relates to cells having a double set of chromosomes, usually applies to all mammalian cells except gametes

disposal*: the emplacement of waste in a repository, or a given location, without the intention of retrieval. Disposal also covers the approved direct discharge of wastes into the environment, with subsequent dispersion

D_o: the dose that gives (on average) one lethal event per cell reducing survival to 37% of its previous value

dose: a generic term which may mean absorbed dose, equivalent dose or effective dose depending on context

dose constraint: a prospective restriction on anticipated dose, primarily intended to be used to discard undesirable options in an optimization calculation. In occupational exposure, a dose constraint may be used to restrict the options considered in the design of the working environment for a particular category of employee in medical exposure, a dose constraint for volunteers in medical research may be used to restrict the options considered in the design of an experimental protocol in public exposure, a dose constraint maybe used to restrict the exposure of the critical group from a particular source of radiation

dose equivalent: an old term that refers to the product of the absorbed dose in tissue (at a point) and the radiation quality factor. Measured in rem (a non-SI unit) and sievert (SI unit). It has been replaced by the **equivalent dose** which uses the absorbed dose averaged over the tissue of interest

dose limits*: maximum references laid down in Title IV for the doses resulting from the exposure of workers, apprentices and students and members of the public to ionizing radiation covered by this Directive that apply to the sum of the relevant doses from external exposures in the specified period and the 50-year committed doses (up to age 70 for children) from intakes in the same period

DREF: dose rate effectiveness factor corrects for extrapolation from high to low dose effects

effective dose or effective dose equivalent: the sum of the products of the equivalent doses and the tissue weighting factors (w_T) for each organ or tissue. This sum is the effective dose, E, and represents the summed organ or tissue doses as an overall whole-body dose:

$$E = \sum H_T \times w_T$$

where, as before, H_T is the equivalent dose in tissue or organ T and w_T is the tissue weighting factor

equivalent dose: in radiological protection, it is the absorbed dose averaged over a tissue or organ and weighted for the radiation quality that is of interest. The equivalent dose, (H_T), in tissue T is given by

$$H_T = \sum_R w_R \times D_{T,R}$$

where $D_{T,R}$ is the absorbed dose averaged over the tissue or organ T, due to radiation R. The unit of equivalent dose is the joule per kilogram and called the sievert (Sv)

eye dose equivalent: external exposure of the lens of the eye. The dose equivalent at 0.3 cm depth

excluded exposure: in the context of occupational exposure, the component of exposure which arises from natural background radiation, provided that any relevant action level, or levels, for the workplace are not exceeded and that the appropriate authority does not prohibit its exclusion

exclusion: in the context of assessing radiation exposure, the deliberate omission of a specified component, or components, of total exposure to radiation

exemption: the deliberate omission of a practice from regulatory control, or from some aspects of regulatory control, by the appropriate authority

exposed workers*: persons, either self-employed or working for an employer, subject to an exposure incurred at work from practices covered by this Directive and liable to result in doses exceeding one or other of the dose levels equal to the dose limits for members of the public

exposure†: the process of being exposed to ionizing radiation

free radical: a chemical compound containing an unpaired electron

gray (Gy): a measure of absorbed dose 1 J kg^{-1}

guidance level for medical exposure: a reference level of dose or of administered activity likely to be appropriate for average-sized patients undergoing medical diagnosis or treatment

haploid: relates to single stranded DNA cells: bacteria and gametes

health detriment*: an estimate of the risk of reduction in length and quality of life occurring in a population following exposure to ionizing radiations. This includes loss arising from somatic effects, cancer, and severe genetic disorders

health screening†: a procedure using radiological installations for early diagnosis in population groups at risk

ICRP: International Commission on Radiological Protection

incident: an event which causes, or has the potential to cause, abnormal exposure of employees or of members of the public and which requires investigation of its causes and consequences and may require corrective action within the program for control of radiation, but which is not of such scale as to be classified as an accident

individual detriment†: clinically observable deleterious effects that are expressed in individuals or their descendants, the appearance of which is either immediate or delayed and, in the latter case, implies a probability rather than a certainty of appearance

intervention: action taken to decrease exposures to radiation which arise from existing situations

intervention level: a reference level of an environmental or dosimetric quantity, such as absorbed dose rate; if measured values of that quantity are found to consistently exceed the intervention level, remedial action should be considered

investigation level: a reference level of an environmental or dosimetric quantity, such as absorbed dose rate; if measured values of that quantity are found to consistently exceed the investigation level, the cause or implications of the situation should be investigated

justification: the notion that human activities which lead to exposure to radiation should be justified, before they are permitted to take place, by showing that they are likely to do more good than harm

license: a written authorization issued to an operator which allows the operator to carry out an operation legally

limitation: the requirement that radiation doses and risks should not exceed a value regarded as unacceptable

medical exposure: exposure of a person to radiation received as a patient undergoing medical diagnosis or therapy, or as a volunteer in medical research, or non-occupational exposure received as a consequence of assisting an exposed patient

medical physics expert[†]: an expert in radiation physics or radiation technology applied to exposure, within the scope of this Directive, whose training and competence to act is recognized by the competent authorities; and who, as appropriate, acts or gives advice on patient dosimetry, on the development and use of complex techniques and equipment, on optimization, on quality assurance, including quality control, and on other matters relating to radiation protection, concerning exposure within the scope of this Directive

NCRP: National Council on Radiological Protection and Measurements (in the USA)

nominal risk coefficients: the unadjusted nominal risk coefficients are computed by averaging estimates of the radiation-associated lifetime risk for cancer incidence for two composite populations

NRPB: National Radiological Protection Board (in the UK)

occupational exposure: exposure of a person to radiation which occurs in the course of that person's work and which is not excluded exposure. They can reasonably be regarded as the responsibility of the operating management. Particular attention is given to the principle of optimization of protection which is considered as being of central importance in the control of occupational exposure

operation: an instance of a practice; a particular human activity which may result in exposure to ionizing radiation and to which a program of radiation protection applies

operator: any person or entity responsible for an operation which may lead to exposure to ionizing radiation

optimization: the process of maximizing the net benefit arising from human activities which lead to exposure to radiation

population dose: to obtain the overall effect of radiation dose on a large group of people or entire populations the individual equivalent or effective doses are multiplied by the population number exposed. Population doses are measured in man-sieverts (manSv). See: collective equivalent dose and collective effective dose

potential exposure*: exposure that is not expected to be delivered with certainty, with a probability of occurrence that can be estimated in advance

practice: a type of human activity; in a radiological context, a human activity which may result in exposure

to ionizing radiation and to which a system of radiation protection applies

practitioner[†]: a medical doctor, dentist or other health professional, who is entitled to take clinical responsibility for an individual medical exposure in accordance with national requirements

prescriber[†]: a medical doctor, dentist or other health professional, who is entitled to refer individuals for medical exposure to a practitioner, in accordance with national requirements

program of radiation protection: a system of radiation protection, designed for a particular operation

public exposure: exposure of a person, or persons, to radiation which is neither occupational nor medical exposure

quality assurance[†]: all those planned and systematic actions necessary to provide adequate confidence that a structure, system, component or procedure will perform satisfactorily complying with agreed standards

quality control[†]: is a part of quality assurance. The set of operations (programming, coordinating, implementing) intended to maintain or to improve quality. It covers monitoring, evaluation and maintenance at required levels of all characteristics of performance of equipment that can be defined, measured, and controlled

radiation area: an area within the department where individuals could receive $0.05\,\text{mSv}\,\text{h}^{-1}$ at 30 cm ($50\,\mu\text{Sv}$ or 5 mrem) from the radiation source

radiation weighting factor: values of radiation weighting factors (w_R) are given in ICRP 60

restricted area: a limited access area where exposure to individuals may occur

radionuclide: a species of atomic nucleus which undergoes radioactive decay

radon: used generically, all isotopes of the element radon, having atomic number 86, but typically used to refer to the radioactive gas ^{222}Rn

radon progeny: the short-lived products of the radioactive decay of radon, namely ^{218}Po, ^{214}Pb, ^{214}Bi, and ^{214}Po

risk constraint: a restriction applied to potential exposure (see dose constraint)

röntgen/roentgen: a non-SI unit of ionizing electromagnetic radiation. Symbol, R. It is the quantity of X-rays or gamma rays that, through ionization, produces $2.58 \times 10^{-4}\,\text{C}\,\text{kg}^{-1}$ of air

shallow dose equivalent: the external exposure to the skin is the dose equivalent at a tissue depth of 0.007 cm averaged over an area of 1 cm². Symbol: H_S

specific activity: the activity of a radionuclide per unit mass of the element, or the activity of a radioactive material per unit mass of that material

supervised area: an area in which working conditions are kept under review but in which special procedures to control exposure to radiation are not normally necessary

system of radiation protection: a generic process of radiation risk management designed to limit the health risks arising from exposure to radiation to acceptable levels in a manner which takes economic and social considerations into account

sievert (Sv): an SI unit that is a measure of dose equivalent. It is given by absorbed dose (in Gy) $\times$ the RBE of the radiation. $1\,\mathrm{Sv} = 1\,\mathrm{J\,kg^{-1}}$

total effective dose equivalent (TEDE): the sum of the deep dose equivalent (external exposures) and committed effective dose equivalent (internal exposures)

tissue weighting factor: a factor which modifies equivalent dose in an organ or tissue to yield effective dose and which is the partial contribution from the organ or tissue to the total detriment resulting from uniform irradiation of the whole body. Values for tissue weighting factors (w_T) are given in Table 22.2

thoron: the radioactive gas $^{220}\mathrm{Rn}$

thoron progeny: the short-lived products of the radioactive decay of thoron, namely $^{216}\mathrm{Po}$, $^{212}\mathrm{Pb}$, $^{212}\mathrm{Bi}$, $^{212}\mathrm{Po}$, and $^{208}\mathrm{Tl}$

*Terms that occur in Council Directive 96/29 of the European Commission.

†Terms that occur in Council Directive 97/43 of the European Commission.

REFERENCES

European Commission (1996) Council Directive 96/29 EURATOM of 13 May 1996 laying down basic safety standards for the protection of the health of workers and the general public against the dangers arising from ionizing radiation. *Official Journal of the European Communities* L 159, vol. **39** (29 June 1996).

European Commission (1997) Council Directive 97/43 EURATOM of 30 June 1997 on health protection of individuals against the dangers of ionizing radiation in relation to medical exposure, and repealing Directive 84/466 Euratom. *Official Journal of the European Communities* L 189 (July 1997).

Doll R and Wakeford R (1997) Risk of childhood cancer from fetal irradiation. *Br J Radiol* **70**: 130–139.

Hart D and Wall BF (2002) *Radiation Exposure of the UK Population from Medical and Dental Examinations.* NRPB-W4 Report. Chilton, UK: National Radiological Protection Board.

ICRP Publication 26 (1977) *Recommendations of the International Commission on Radiological Protection.* (Reprinted, with additions, in 1987.)

ICRP Publication 35 (1982) *General Principles for Monitoring for Radiation Protection of Workers.*

ICRP Publication 60 (1990) *1990 Recommendations of the International Commission on Radiological Protection.*

ICRP Publication 84 (2000) *Pregnancy and Medical Radiation.*

ICRP Publication 87 (2002) *Managing Patient Dose in Computed Tomography.*

ICRU Report 39 (1985) *Determination of Dose Equivalents Resulting from External Radiation Sources.* Bethesda, MA: International Commission on Radiation Units and Measurements.

Ng K-H *et al.* (1998) *Br J Radiol* **71**: 654–660.

Shrimpton PC *et al.* (2003) *Dose from Computed Radiography (CT).* NRPB-W67 report. Chilton, UK: National Radiological Protection Board.

UNSCEAR (2000) *Report, Annex D: Medical Radiation Exposures.* New York: United Nations.

van de Putte *et al.* (2000) *Br J Radiol* **73**: 504–513.

Warren-Forward HM (1998) *Br J Radiol* **71**: 961–967.

World Health Organization (1983) *A Rational Approach to Diagnostic Investigations.* Report number 689. Geneva: WHO.

Young KC *et al.* (1995) *Mammographic Dose and Image Quality in the UK Breast Screening Programme.* NHSBSP Publication 35.

FURTHER READING

Administration of Radioactive Substances Advisory Committee (1993) *Notes for Guidance on the Administration of Radioactive Substances to Persons for Purposes of Diagnosis, Treatment or Research.* London: ARSAC.

British Institute of Radiology (2000) *Radiation Shielding for Diagnostic X-rays.* Joint report by the BIR and IPEM. London: BIR.

ICRP Publication 73 (1996) *Radiological Protection and Safety in Medicine.*

ICRP Publication 76 (1998) *Protection from Potential Exposures: Application to Selected Radiation Sources.*

ICRP Publication 77 (1998) *Radiological Protection Policy for the Disposal of Radioactive Waste.*

ICRP Publication 78 (1999) *Individual Monitoring for Internal Exposure of Workers.*

ICRP Publication 79 (1999) *Genetic Susceptibility to Cancer.*

ICRP Publication 80 (2000) *Radiation Dose to Patients from Radiopharmaceuticals.*

ICRP Publication 81 (2000) *Radiation Protection Recommendations as Applied to the Disposal of Long-lived Solid Radioactive Waste.*

ICRP Publication 82 (2000) *Protection of the Public in Situations of Prolonged Radiation Exposure.*

ICRP Publication 83 (2001) *Risk Estimation for Multifactorial Diseases.*

ICRP Publication 85 (2001) *Avoidance of Radiation Injuries from Medical Interventional Procedures.*

ICRP Publication 86 (2002) *Prevention of Accidents to Patients Undergoing Radiation Therapy.*

ICRP Publication 88 (2002) *Doses to the Embryo and Fetus from Intakes of Radionuclides by the Mother.*

ICRP Supporting Guidance 2 (2003) *Radiation and Your Patient: A Guide for Medical Practitioners.*

ICRP Supporting Guidance 3 (2003) *Guide for the Practical Application of the ICRP Human Respiratory Tract Model.*

ICRP Publication 89 (2003) *Basic Anatomical and Physiological Data for Use in Radiological Protection: Reference Values.*

ICRP Publication 90 (2004) *Biological Effects after Prenatal Irradiation (Embryo and Fetus).*

ICRP Publication 91 (2004) *A Framework for Assessing the Impact of Ionizing Radiation on Non-Human Species.*

ICRP Publication 92 (2004) *Relative Biological Effectiveness (RBE), Quality Factor (Q), and Radiation Weighting Factor* (w_R).

ICRP Publication 93 (2004) *Managing Patient Dose in Digital Radiology.*

Institute of Physics and Engineering in Medicine (1991) *Radiation Protection in Nuclear Medicine and Pathology.* IPEM Report no. 63. York, UK: IPEM.

National Council on Radiological Protection and Measurements (1995) *Principles and Application of Collective Dose in Radiation Protection.* NCRP Report no. 121. Bethesda, MD: NCRP.

National Council on Radiological Protection and Measurements (1996) *Sources and Magnitude of Occupational and Public Exposures from Nuclear Medicine Procedures.* NCRP Report no. 124. Bethesda, MD: NCRP.

National Council on Radiological Protection and Measurements (1998) *Operational Radiation Safety Program.* NCRP Report no. 127. Bethesda, MD: NCRP.

National Radiological Protection Board (1990) Patient dose reduction in diagnostic radiology. *Doc. NRPB* **1(3)**: 1–46.

National Radiological Protection Board (1993) Diagnostic medical exposures: exposure to ionising radiation of pregnant women. *Doc. NRPB* **4(4)**: 5–14.

Nias AHW (1990) *An Introduction to Radiobiology.* Chichester: John Wiley.

Note. All reports from the International Commission on Radiological Protection (ICRP) are available from Elsevier Health, on http://www.elsevierhealth.com

INDEX

Note: Page numbers followed by 'f' indicate figures: followed by 't' indicate tables: followed by 'b' indicate boxed material. *vs.* indicates a comparison.

(CR – computed radiography; CT – computed tomography; MRI – magnetic resonance imaging; MSCT – multislice computed tomography; NMR – nuclear magnetic resonance; PACS – picture archiving and communication systems; PET – positron emission tomography; SPECT – single photon emission computed tomography)